From the publisher of *Nursing* journal

# Nursing™

### THE SERIES FOR CLINICAL EXCELLENCE

# Deciphering
# Diagnostic
# Tests

From the publisher of *Nursing* journal

# Nursing™

## THE SERIES FOR CLINICAL EXCELLENCE

# Deciphering Diagnostic Tests

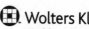 Wolters Kluwer | Lippincott Williams & Wilkins
Health

Philadelphia • Baltimore • New York • London
Buenos Aires • Hong Kong • Sydney • Tokyo

# Staff

**Executive Publisher**
Judith A. Schilling McCann, RN, MSN

**Editorial Director**
H. Nancy Holmes

**Clinical Director**
Joan M. Robinson, RN, MSN

**Art Director**
Elaine Kasmer

**Editorial Project Manager**
Ann E. Houska

**Clinical Project Manager**
Jennifer Meyering, RN, BSN, MS, CCRN

**Editors**
Julia M. Catagnus, Linda Hager

**Copy Editors**
Kimberly Bilotta (supervisor), Jane Bradford,
Heather Ditch, Elizabeth Mooney,
Carolyn Petersen, Pamela Wingrod

**Designers**
Matie Anne Patterson (project manager),
Lynn Foulk (book design),
Joseph John Clark (cover design)

**Digital Composition Services**
Diane Paluba (manager), Joyce Rossi Biletz,
Donna S. Morris

**Manufacturing**
Beth J. Welsh

**Editorial Assistants**
Megan L. Aldinger, Karen J. Kirk,
Linda K. Ruhf

**Design Assistant**
Georg W. Purvis IV

**Indexer**
Barbara Hodgson

NSDXT010407

**Library of Congress
Cataloging-in-Publication Data**

Nursing. Deciphering diagnostic tests.
      p. ; cm.
   Includes bibliographical references and index.
   1. Diagnosis, Laboratory—Handbooks, manuals, etc. 2. Nursing—Handbooks, manuals, etc. I. Lippincott Williams & Wilkins.
   [DNLM: 1. Diagnostic Tests, Routine—nursing—Handbooks. WY 49 N9744 2007]
   RT48.5.N89 2007
   616.07'56—dc22
ISBN-13: 978-1-58255-662-8 (alk. paper)
ISBN-10: 1-58255-662-8 (alk. paper)
                                    2006101877

# Contents

# Contributors and consultants

**Elizabeth (Libby) A. Archer,** RN, EdD
Associate Professor
Baptist College of Health Sciences
Memphis

**Debra F. Chastang,** APRN, MSN, CNS, CS-C
Clinical Nurse Specialist
Providence Hospital
Mobile, Ala.

**Lillian Craig,** RN, MSN, FNP-C
Nursing Instructor
Oklahoma Panhandle State University
Goodwill

**Peggy S. Denning,** RN, MSN
Assistant Director of Nursing
Tri-State School of Practical Nursing
Erie, Pa.

**April N. Hart,** RN, MSN, FNP, BC
Assistant Professor
Bethel College
Mishawaka, Ind.

**Rebecca E. Heyne,** RN, MSN
Clinical Instructor, Nursing
Walsh University
North Canton, Ohio

**Julia Anne Isen,** RN, MS, FNP, CNS
Assistant Clinical Professor
University of California—San Francisco
    School of Nursing

**Jaclynn A. Johnson,** RNC, MSN
Lead Instructor Freshman Nursing
Otero Junior College
La Junta, Colo.

**Christine Kennedy,** RN, MSN
LPN Instructor
Eli Whitney Vocational School—State of
    Connecticut
Hamden

**Carol T. Lemay,** RN
Consultant
Brattleboro, Vt.

**Kendra S. Seiler,** RN, MSN
Nursing Instructor
Rio Hondo Community College
Whittier, Calif.

**Georgia Simmons,** RN, BSN
Practical Nursing Instructor
Ivy Tech State College
Madison, Ind.

**Allison J. Terry,** RN, MSN, PhD
Director of Center for Nursing Workforce
    Research
Alabama Board of Nursing
Montgomery

**Janet E. Williams,** RN, BSN
Assistant Master Technical Instructor
University of Texas at Brownsville and Texas
    Southmost College
Brownsville

# I

# Blood tests

# 1

# Hematology and coagulation tests

## Red blood cell tests

### Erythrocyte sedimentation rate

The erythrocyte sedimentation rate (ESR) measures the degree of erythrocyte settling in a blood sample during a specified period. The ESR is a sensitive but nonspecific test that's commonly the earliest indicator of disease when other chemical or physical signs are normal. The ESR usually increases significantly in widespread inflammatory disorders; elevations may be prolonged in localized inflammation and malignant disease.

#### Reference values
- In men, the normal ESR is 0 to 15 mm/hour (SI, 0 to 15 mm/hour).
- In women, it's 0 to 20 mm/hour (SI, 0 to 20 mm/hour).
- The ESR gradually increases with age.

#### Abnormal results
- The ESR rises in pregnancy, anemia, acute or chronic inflammation, tuberculosis, paraproteinemias (especially multiple myeloma and Waldenström's macroglobulinemia), rheumatic fever, rheumatoid arthritis, and some cancers.
- Polycythemia, sickle cell anemia, hyperviscosity, and low plasma fibrinogen or globulin levels tend to depress the ESR.

#### Purpose
- To monitor inflammatory or malignant disease
- To aid in the detection and diagnosis of occult disease, such as tuberculosis, tissue necrosis, or connective tissue disease

#### Patient preparation
- Explain that the ESR test is used to evaluate the condition of red blood cells.
- Tell the patient that a blood sample will be taken. Explain who will perform the venipuncture and when it will be done.
- Explain to the patient that he may feel slight discomfort from the tourniquet and needle puncture.
- Tell him that he doesn't need to restrict food or fluids.

#### Procedure and posttest care
- Confirm the patient's identity using two patient identifiers according to facility policy.
- Perform a venipuncture and collect the sample in a 4.5-ml tube with EDTA added or a tube with sodium citrate added. (Check with the laboratory to determine its preference.)

- Make sure subdermal bleeding has stopped before removing pressure.
- If a hematoma develops at the venipuncture site, apply warm soaks. If the hematoma is large, monitor pulses distal to the venipuncture site.

### Precautions

- Because hemostasis of the sample decreases the ESR, examine the sample for clots or clumps and send it to the laboratory immediately. It must be tested within 2 to 4 hours.
- Use of a small-gauge needle may alter test results.

# Hematocrit

The hematocrit (HCT) test measures percentage by volume of packed red blood cells (RBCs) in a whole blood sample (for example, an HCT of 40% indicates that a 100-ml sample of blood contains 40 ml of packed RBCs). The test may be done alone or as part of a complete blood count. RBCs are tightly packed without causing hemolysis by centrifuging anticoagulated whole blood in a capillary tube. Test results may be used to calculate two RBC indices: mean corpuscular volume and mean corpuscular hemoglobin concentration.

### Reference values

- HCT is usually measured electronically. Such results are 3% lower than manual measurements, which trap plasma in the column of packed RBCs.
- In adult men, HCT is 42% to 52% (SI, 0.42 to 0.52).
- In adult women, HCT is 36% to 48% (SI, 0.36 to 0.48).
- Neonates
  - In neonates ages 0 to 2 weeks, HCT is 44% to 64% (SI, 0.44 to 0.64).
  - In neonates ages 2 to 8 weeks, HCT is 39% to 59% (SI, 0.39 to 0.59).
- In infants ages 2 to 6 months, HCT is 35% to 49% (SI, 0.35 to 0.49).
- In infants ages 6 months to 1 year, HCT is 30% to 40% (SI, 0.30 to 0.40).
- In children ages 1 to 6 years, HCT is 30% to 40% (SI, 0.30 to 0.40).
- In children ages 6 to 16 years, HCT is 32% to 42% (SI, 0.32 to 0.42).
- In adolescents ages 16 to 18 years, HCT is 34% to 44% (SI, 0.34 to 0.44).

### Abnormal results

- Low HCT suggests anemia, hemodilution, or massive blood loss.
- High HCT indicates polycythemia or hemoconcentration from blood loss and dehydration.

### Purpose

- To help diagnose polycythemia, anemia, or abnormal states of hydration
- To help calculate RBC indices

### Patient preparation

- Explain that HCT is tested to detect anemia and other abnormal blood conditions.
- Tell the patient that the test requires a blood sample. Explain who will perform the venipuncture and when it will be done.
- Tell him he doesn't need to restrict food or fluids.
- If the patient is an infant or child, explain to his parents that a small amount of blood will be taken from his finger or earlobe.
- If the patient is an older child or adult, tell him that he may feel slight discomfort from the tourniquet and needle puncture.

### Procedure and posttest care

- Confirm the patient's identity using two patient identifiers according to facility policy.

- Perform a fingerstick using a heparinized capillary tube with a red band on the anticoagulant end.
- Fill the capillary tube from the red-banded end to about two-thirds capacity; seal this end with clay.
- Alternatively, perform a venipuncture and fill a 3- or 4.5-ml EDTA tube.

### Do's & don'ts

 Don't draw the blood from above an I.V. infusion site to avoid hemodilution.

- Make sure that subdermal bleeding has stopped before removing pressure.
- If a hematoma develops at the venipuncture site, apply warm soaks. If the hematoma is large, monitor pulses distal to the venipuncture site.

## Osmotic fragility

Osmotic fragility measures red blood cell (RBC) resistance to hemolysis when exposed to a series of increasingly dilute saline solutions. The sooner hemolysis occurs, the greater the osmotic fragility of the cells. Osmotic fragility is based on osmosis—the movement of water across a membrane from a more concentrated one in a natural tendency to correct the imbalance.

RBCs suspended in an isotonic saline solution—one with the same salt concentration (osmotic pressure) as normal plasma (0.85 g/dl)—keep their shape. If RBCs are added to a hypotonic (less concentrated) solution, they take up water until they burst; if placed in a hypertonic solution, they shrink. (See *Understanding concentration and fluid flow*.)

The degree of hypotonicity needed to produce hemolysis varies inversely with the RBCs' osmotic fragility; the closer the saline tonicity is to normal physiologic values when hemolysis occurs, the more fragile the cells. In some cases,

RBCs don't hemolyze immediately and their incubation in solution for 24 hours improves test sensitivity.

Osmotic fragility testing offers quantitative confirmation of RBC morphology and should be used to supplement the stained cell examination.

### Reference values

- Osmotic fragility values (percentage of RBCs hemolyzed) that have been obtained photometrically are plotted against decreasing saline tonicity to produce an S-shaped curve with a slope characteristic of the disorder. Reference values differ with tonicities.

### Abnormal results

- Low osmotic fragility (increased resistance to hemolysis) occurs after splenectomy and in thalassemia, iron deficiency anemia, sickle cell anemia, and other RBC disorders in which target cells are found.
- High osmotic fragility (increased tendency toward hemolysis) occurs in hereditary spherocytosis, hemolytic disease of the newborn (erythroblastosis fetalis), and spherocytosis associated with autoimmune hemolytic anemia, severe burns, or chemical poisoning.

### Purpose

- To help diagnose hereditary spherocytosis
- To confirm morphologic RBC abnormalities

### Patient preparation

- Explain that osmotic fragility testing is used to identify the cause of anemia.
- Tell the patient that a blood sample will be taken. Explain who will perform the venipuncture and when it will be done.
- Explain to the patient that he may feel slight discomfort from the tourniquet and needle puncture.

## Understanding concentration and fluid flow

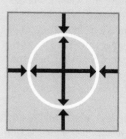

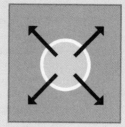

### Isotonic
An isotonic fluid has a concentration of dissolved particles, or tonicity, equal to that of intracellular fluid. When isotonic fluids, such as 5% dextrose in water and normal saline solution, enter the circulation, they cause no net movement of water across the semipermeable cell membrane. Because the osmotic pressure is the same inside and outside the cells, they neither swell nor shrink.

### Hypertonic
A hypertonic fluid has a concentration greater than that of intracellular fluid. When a hypertonic solution, such as 50% dextrose or 3% sodium chloride, is rapidly infused into the body, water rushes out of the cells to the area of greater concentration, and the cells shrivel. Dehydration can also make extracellular fluid hypertonic, leading to the same kind of cellular shrinkage.

### Hypotonic
A hypotonic fluid has a concentration less than that of intracellular fluid. When a hypotonic solution, such as 2.5% dextrose or half-normal saline solution, surrounds a cell, water diffuses into the intracellular fluid, causing the cell to swell. Inappropriate use of I.V. fluids or severe electrolyte loss makes body fluids hypotonic.

■ Tell the patient he doesn't need to restrict food or fluids.

### Procedure and posttest care
■ Confirm the patient's identity using two patient identifiers according to facility policy.
■ Perform a venipuncture, collecting the sample in a 4.5-ml heparinized tube.
■ If a hematoma develops at the venipuncture site, apply warm soaks. If the hematoma is large, monitor pulses distal to the venipuncture site.

### Precautions
■ Because this test isn't routinely performed, notify the laboratory before

drawing the sample. Reference laboratories have certain guidelines and testing dates that you'll need to follow.
■ If the patient has severe anemia, there may not be enough RBCs for accurate testing results.

## Red blood cell count

The red blood cell (RBC) count is part of a complete blood count. It's used to detect the number of RBCs in a microliter ($\mu$l) or cubic millimeter ($mm^3$) of whole blood. The RBC count itself provides no qualitative information regarding the size, shape, or concentration of hemoglobin (Hb) within the corpuscles, but it may be used to calculate two RBC indices: mean corpuscular volume (MCV) and mean corpuscular hemoglobin (MCH).

## Reference values

- For men, normal values are 4.2 to 5.4 million RBCs/µl (SI, 4.2 to 5.4 × $10^{12}$/L) of venous blood.
- For women, normal values are 3.6 to 5 million RBCs/µl (SI, 3.6 to 5 × $10^{12}$/L) of venous blood.
- For full-term neonates, normal values are 4.1 to 6.1 million RBCs/µl (SI, 4.1 to 6.1 × $10^{12}$/L) of capillary blood at birth, decreasing to 3.8 to 5.6 million/µl (SI, 3.8 to 5.6 × $10^{12}$/L) at age 2 months, and increasing slowly thereafter.
- For children, normal values are 4 to 5.2 million/µl (SI, 4 to 5.2 × $10^{12}$/L) of venous blood.
- For patients who live at high altitudes or are very active, normal values may exceed these levels.

## Abnormal results

- An elevated RBC count may indicate absolute or relative polycythemia.
- A reduced RBC count may indicate anemia, fluid overload, or hemorrhage lasting longer than 24 hours.
- Further tests, such as stained cell examination, hematocrit, Hb, RBC indices, and white blood cell studies, are needed to confirm the diagnosis.

## Purpose

- To provide data for calculating MCV and MCH, which reveal RBC size and Hb content
- To support other hematologic tests for diagnosing anemia or polycythemia

## Patient preparation

- Explain that the RBC count is used to evaluate the number of RBCs and to detect possible blood disorders.

- Tell the patient that a blood sample will be taken. Explain who will perform the venipuncture and when it will be done.
- If the patient is a child, explain to him (if he's old enough) and his parents that a small amount of blood will be taken from his finger or earlobe. Have the parents stay with the child to decrease his level of anxiety.
- If the patient is an older child or adult, tell him that he may feel slight discomfort from the tourniquet and needle puncture.
- Tell the patient that he doesn't need to restrict food or fluids.

## Procedure and posttest care

- Confirm the patient's identity using two patient identifiers according to facility policy.
- For adults and older children, draw venous blood into a 3- or 4.5-ml EDTA sodium metabisulfite solution tube.
- For younger children, collect capillary blood in a microcollection device.

### DO'S & DON'TS

 Don't draw the blood from above an I.V. infusion site to avoid hemodilution.

- Make sure that subdermal bleeding has stopped before removing pressure.
- If a hematoma develops at the venipuncture site, apply warm soaks. If the hematoma is large, monitor pulses distal to the venipuncture site.

# Red blood cell indices

Using the results of the red blood cell (RBC) count, hematocrit (HCT), and total hemoglobin (Hb) tests, RBC indices (erythrocyte indices) provide important information about the size, Hb concentration, and Hb weight of an average RBC.

## Comparative red blood cell indices in anemias

|       | Normal values (Normocytic, normochromic) | Iron deficiency anemia (Microcytic, hypochromic) | Pernicious anemia (Macrocytic, normochromic) |
|-------|------------------------------------------|--------------------------------------------------|----------------------------------------------|
| **MCV**  | 84 to 99 $\mu m^3$ | 60 to 80 $\mu m^3$ | 96 to 150 $\mu m^3$ |
| **MCH**  | 26 to 32 pg/cell | 5 to 25 pg/cell | 33 to 53 pg/cell |
| **MCHC** | 30 to 36 g/dl | 20 to 30 g/dl | 33 to 38 g/dl |

Key:
MCV = mean corpuscular volume
MCH = mean corpuscular hemoglobin
MCHC = mean corpuscular hemoglobin concentration

### Reference values

- Mean corpuscular volume (MCV)—the ratio of HCT (packed cell volume) to the RBC count—expresses the average size of the erythrocytes and indicates whether they're undersized (microcytic), oversized (macrocytic), or normal (normocytic).
- Mean corpuscular hemoglobin (MCH)—the ratio of Hb to RBC—gives the weight of Hb in an average RBC.
- Mean corpuscular hemoglobin concentration (MCHC)—the ratio of Hb weight to HCT—defines the concentration of Hb in 100 ml of packed RBCs. It helps to distinguish normally colored (normochromic) RBCs from paler (hypochromic) RBCs.
- Normal MCV values are 84 to 99 $\mu m^3$ (SI, 84 to 99 fl).
- Normal MCH values are 26 to 32 pg/cell (SI, 0.40 to 0.49 fmol/cell).
- Normal MCHC values are 30 to 36 g/dl (SI, 300 to 360 g/L).

### Abnormal results

- Low MCV and MCHC indicate microcytic, hypochromic anemias caused by iron deficiency, pyridoxine-responsive anemia, or thalassemia.
- High MCV suggests macrocytic anemias caused by megaloblastic disorders, folic acid or vitamin $B_{12}$ deficiency, inherited disorders of deoxyribonucleic acid synthesis, or reticulocytosis.
- Because the MCV reflects the average volume of many cells, a value within the normal range can encompass RBCs of varying size, from microcytic to macrocytic. (See *Comparative red blood cell indices in anemias*.)

### Purpose

- To help diagnose and classify anemias

### Patient preparation

- Explain that RBC indices help determine if the patient has anemia.
- Tell him that a blood sample will be taken. Explain who will perform the venipuncture and when it will be done.
- Explain to the patient that he may feel slight discomfort from the tourniquet and needle puncture.

### Procedure and posttest care

- Confirm the patient's identity using two patient identifiers according to facility policy.

- Perform a venipuncture and collect the sample in a 3- or 4.5-ml EDTA tube.
- Make sure that subdermal bleeding has stopped before removing pressure.
- If a hematoma develops at the venipuncture site, apply warm soaks. If the hematoma is large, monitor pulses distal to the venipuncture site.

### Precautions
- A falsely elevated Hb value will invalidate the MCH and MCHC results.

## Reticulocyte count

Reticulocytes are nonnucleated, immature red blood cells (RBCs) that remain in the peripheral blood for 24 to 48 hours while maturing. They're usually larger than mature RBCs. In the reticulocyte count test, reticulocytes in a whole blood sample are counted and expressed as a percentage of the total RBC count. Because this manual method of reticulocyte counting uses only a small sample, values may be imprecise and should be compared with the RBC count or hematocrit. The reticulocyte count is useful for evaluating anemia and is an index of effective erythropoiesis and bone marrow response to anemia.

### Reference values
- Normal reticulocyte count is 0.5% to 2.5% (SI, 0.005 to 0.025) of the total RBC count.
- In infants, the normal reticulocyte count is 2% to 6% (SI, 0.02 to 0.06) at birth, decreasing to adult levels in 1 to 2 weeks.

### Abnormal results
- A low reticulocyte count indicates hypoproliferative bone marrow (hypoplastic anemia) or ineffective erythropoiesis (pernicious anemia).

- A high reticulocyte count indicates a bone marrow response to anemia caused by hemolysis or blood loss.
- The reticulocyte count may also increase after therapy for iron deficiency anemia or pernicious anemia.

**DRUG CHALLENGE**

Azathioprine, chloramphenicol, dactinomycin, sulfonamides, and methotrexate (possible false-low); corticotropin, antimalarials, antipyretics, levodopa, and sulfonamides (possible false-high)

### Purpose
- To help distinguish between hypoproliferative and hyperproliferative anemias
- To help assess blood loss, bone marrow response to anemia, and therapy for anemia

### Patient preparation
- Explain that the reticulocyte count is used to detect anemia or to monitor its treatment.
- Tell the patient that a blood sample will be taken. Explain who will perform the venipuncture and when it will be done.
- If the patient is an infant or child, explain to his parents that a small amount of blood will be taken from his finger or earlobe.
- If the patient is an adult, tell him that he may feel slight discomfort from the tourniquet and needle puncture.
- Notify the laboratory and practitioner of medications the patient is taking that may affect test results; these medications may need to be restricted.
- Tell the patient he doesn't need to restrict food or fluids.

## Procedure and posttest care

■ Confirm the patient's identity using two patient identifiers according to facility policy.
■ Perform a venipuncture and collect the sample in a 3- or 4.5-ml EDTA tube.
■ Make sure that subdermal bleeding has stopped before removing pressure.
■ If a hematoma develops at the venipuncture site, apply warm soaks. If the hematoma is large, monitor pulses distal to the venipuncture site.
■ Instruct the patient that he may resume medications discontinued before the test as ordered.
■ Monitor the patient with an abnormal reticulocyte count for trends or significant changes in repeated tests.

# Hemoglobin tests

Ferritin

Ferritin, a major iron-storage protein, normally appears in small quantities in serum. In healthy adults, serum ferritin levels are directly related to the amount of available iron stored in the body and can be measured accurately by radioimmunoassay.

### Reference values

■ For men, normal ferritin values are 20 to 300 ng/ml (SI, 20 to 300 µg/L).
■ For women, values are 20 to 120 ng/ml (SI, 20 to 120 µg/L).
■ For neonates, values are 25 to 200 ng/ml (SI, 25 to 200 µg/L).
■ For infants age 1 month, values are 200 to 600 ng/ml (SI, 200 to 600 µg/L).
■ For infants ages 2 to 5 months, values are 50 to 200 ng/ml (SI, 50 to 200 µg/L).
■ For children ages 6 months to 15 years, values are 7 to 140 ng/ml (SI, 7 to 140 µg/L).

## Abnormal results

■ High serum ferritin levels may indicate acute or chronic hepatic disease, iron overload, leukemia, acute or chronic infection or inflammation, Hodgkin's disease, or chronic hemolytic anemias.
■ Low serum ferritin levels indicate chronic iron deficiency.

### Purpose

■ To screen for iron deficiency and iron overload
■ To measure iron storage
■ To distinguish between iron deficiency (a condition of low iron storage) and chronic inflammation (a condition of normal storage)

### Patient preparation

■ Explain to the patient that the serum ferritin test is used to assess the available iron stored in the body.
■ Tell the patient that a blood sample will be taken. Explain who will perform the venipuncture and when it will be done.
■ Explain to the patient that he may feel slight discomfort from the tourniquet and needle puncture.
■ Review the patient's history for transfusion within the past 4 months.
■ Tell the patient he doesn't need to restrict food or fluids.

### Procedure and posttest care

■ Confirm the patient's identity using two patient identifiers according to facility policy.
■ Perform a venipuncture, collecting the sample in a 10-ml tube without additives.
■ Make sure that subdermal bleeding has stopped before removing pressure.
■ If a hematoma develops at the venipuncture site, apply warm soaks. If the hematoma is large, monitor pulses distal to the venipuncture site.

# Fetal hemoglobin
## [Kleihauer-Betke test]

Fetal hemoglobin (Hb), or Hb F, is a normal Hb produced in the red blood cells of a fetus and in smaller amounts in infants. It constitutes 50% to 90% of the Hb in a neonate; the remaining Hb consists of Hb $A_1$ and Hb $A_2$—the Hb in adults.

Under normal conditions, the body ceases to manufacture Hb F during the first years of life and begins to manufacture adult Hb. If this changeover doesn't occur and Hb F continues to constitute more than 5% of the Hb after age 6 months, an abnormality should be suspected, particularly thalassemia.

## Reference values

- For infants ages 0 to 30 days, normal Hb F value is 60% to 90% (SI, 0.60 to 0.90).
- For infants ages 1 to 23 months, the normal Hb F value is 2% (SI, 0.02).
- For those ages 24 months to adult, normal Hb F value is 0% to 2% (SI, 0 to 0.02).
- Hb F commonly increases to as much as 5% during a normal pregnancy.

## Abnormal results

- In beta-thalassemia major, Hb F may constitute 30% or more of the total Hb.
- Slight increases in Hb F concentration appear in many unrelated hematologic disorders, such as aplastic anemia, homozygous sickle cell disease, and myeloproliferative disorders.

## Purpose

- To diagnose thalassemia

## Patient preparation

- Explain that the Hb test is used to detect thalassemia disease.
- Tell the patient that a blood sample will be taken.

- Explain who will perform the venipuncture and when it will be done.
- If the patient is a child, explain to his parents that a small amount of blood will be taken from his finger or earlobe.
- If the patient is an older child or adult, tell him that he may feel slight discomfort from the tourniquet and needle puncture.
- Inform the patient or his parents that he need not restrict food or fluid intake.

## Procedure and posttest care

- Confirm the patient's identity using two patient identifiers according to facility policy.
- Perform a venipuncture and collect the sample of blood in a 4.5-ml EDTA tube.
- For a young child, collect capillary blood in a microcollection device.
- If a hematoma develops at the venipuncture site, apply warm soaks. If the hematoma is large, monitor pulses distal to the venipuncture site.
- Make sure that subdermal bleeding has stopped before removing pressure.

# Heinz bodies

Heinz bodies are particles of decomposed hemoglobin (Hb) that precipitate from the cytoplasm of red blood cells (RBCs) and accumulate on RBC membranes. They form as a result of drug injury to RBCs, the presence of unstable Hb, unbalanced globin chain synthesis due to thalassemia, or a RBC enzyme deficiency (such as glucose-6-phosphate dehydrogenase deficiency). Although Heinz bodies are removed from RBCs by the spleen, they're a major cause of hemolytic anemias. (See *Identifying Heinz bodies.*)

Heinz bodies can be detected in a whole blood sample using phase microscopy or supravital stains; when they don't form spontaneously, various oxidant drugs may be added to the sample to induce their formation.

## Reference values

- A negative test result indicates an absence of Heinz bodies.

## Abnormal results

- Heinz bodies may be present after splenectomy or may indicate an inherited RBC enzyme deficiency, unstable Hb, thalassemia, or drug-induced RBC injury.

### DRUG CHALLENGE

 Antimalarials, nitrofurantoin, phenacetin, procarbazine, and sulfonamides (possible false-positive)

## Purpose

- To help detect causes of hemolytic anemia

## Patient preparation

- Explain that this test is used to determine the cause of anemia.
- Tell the patient that a blood sample will be taken. Explain who will perform the venipuncture and when it will be done.
- Tell him that he may feel slight discomfort from the tourniquet and needle puncture.
- Notify the laboratory and practitioner of medications the patient is taking that may affect test results; these medications may need to be restricted.
- Tell the patient that he doesn't need to restrict food or fluids.

## Procedure and posttest care

- Confirm the patient's identity using two patient identifiers according to facility policy.
- Perform a venipuncture and collect the sample in a 3- or 4.5-ml EDTA tube.

## Identifying Heinz bodies

After special supravital staining, Heinz bodies (particles of denatured hemoglobin that are usually attached to the cell membrane) appear as small, purple inclusions at cell margins. Heinz bodies are present in certain hemolytic anemias.

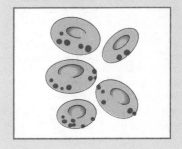

- If a hematoma develops at the venipuncture site, apply warm soaks. If the hematoma is large, monitor pulses distal to the venipuncture site.
- Make sure that subdermal bleeding has stopped before removing pressure.
- Instruct the patient to resume medications discontinued before the test as ordered.

# Hemoglobin electrophoresis

Hemoglobin (Hb) electrophoresis is probably the most useful laboratory method for separating and measuring normal and abnormal Hb. Through electrophoresis, different types of Hb are separated to form a series of distinctly pigmented bands in a medium. Results are then compared with those of a normal sample.

Hb A, Hb A$_2$, Hb S, and Hb C are routinely checked, but the laboratory may change the medium or its pH to expand the range of this test.

## Variations of hemoglobin type and distribution

| Hemoglobin | Percentage of total hemoglobin | Clinical implications |
| --- | --- | --- |
| Hb A | 95% to 100% (SI, 0.95 to 1.00) | Normal |
| Hb A₂ | 4% to 5.8% (SI, 0.04 to 0.058) | Beta-thalassemia minor |
| | 1.5% to 3% (SI, 0.015 to 0.03) | Normal |
| | Less than 1.5% (SI, < 0.015) | Hb H disease |
| Hb F | Less than 1% (SI, < 0.01) | Normal |
| | 2% to 5% (SI, 0.02 to 0.05) | Beta-thalassemia minor |
| | 10% to 90% (SI, 0.10 to 0.90) | Beta-thalassemia major |
| | 5% to 15% (SI, 0.05 to 0.15) | Beta-δ-thalassemia minor |
| | 5% to 35% (SI, 0.05 to 0.35) | Heterozygous hereditary persistence of fetal Hb (HPFH) |
| | 100% (SI, 1.0) | Homozygous HPFH |
| | 15% (SI, 0.15) | Homozygous Hb S |
| Homozygous Hb S | 70% to 98% (SI, 0.70 to 0.98) | Sickle cell disease |
| Homozygous Hb C | 90% to 98% (SI, 0.90 to 0.98) | Hb C disease |
| Heterozygous Hb C | 24% to 44% (SI, 0.24 to 0.44) | Hb C trait |

### Reference values

■ In adults, Hb A accounts for 95% (SI, 0.95) of all Hb; Hb A₂, 1.5% to 3% (SI, 0.015 to 0.030); and Hb F, < 2% (SI, < 0.02).
■ In neonates, Hb F normally accounts for one-half of the total Hb. Hb S and Hb C are normally absent.

### Abnormal results

■ Hb electrophoresis allows identification of various types of Hb. Certain types may indicate a hemolytic disease. (See *Variations of hemoglobin type and distribution*.)

### Purpose

■ To measure the amount of Hb A and to detect abnormal Hb
■ To aid in the diagnosis of thalassemia

### Patient preparation

■ Explain to the patient that Hb electrophoresis is used to evaluate Hb.
■ Tell the patient that a blood sample will be taken. Explain who will perform the venipuncture and when it will be done.
■ If the patient is a child, explain to his parents that a small amount of blood will be taken from his finger or earlobe.
■ If the patient is an older child or adult, tell him that he may feel slight discomfort from the tourniquet and needle puncture.
■ Explain that the patient doesn't need to restrict food or fluids.

### Procedure and posttest care

■ Confirm the patient's identity using two patient identifiers according to facility policy.

- Ask him if he has received a blood transfusion within the past 4 months.
- Perform a venipuncture and collect the sample in a 3- or 4.5-ml EDTA tube.
- For young children, collect capillary blood in a microcollection device.
- If a hematoma develops at the venipuncture site, apply warm soaks. If the hematoma is large, monitor pulses distal to the venipuncture site.
- Make sure that subdermal bleeding has stopped before removing pressure.

# Iron and total iron-binding capacity

Iron is essential to the formation and function of hemoglobin as well as many other heme and nonheme compounds. After iron is absorbed by the intestines, it's distributed to various body compartments for synthesis, storage, and transport. (See *Normal iron metabolism,* page 14.)

Because serum iron level is usually highest in the morning and declines gradually during the day, the sample should be drawn in the morning. An iron assay is used to measure the amount of iron bound to transferrin in blood plasma. The total iron-binding capacity (TIBC) test measures the amount of iron that would appear in plasma if all the transferrin were saturated with iron.

Serum iron level and TIBC tests are of greater diagnostic usefulness when performed with the serum ferritin assay, but together these tests may not accurately reflect the state of other iron compartments, such as myoglobin iron and the labile iron pool. Bone marrow or liver biopsy and iron absorption or excretion studies may yield more information.

## Reference values

- Serum iron
  - In men, normal values are 60 to 170 mcg/dl (SI, 10.7 to 30.4 µmol/L).
  - In women, normal values are 50 to 130 mcg/dl (SI, 9.0 to 23.3 µmol/L).
- TIBC: In men and women, normal values are 300 to 360 mcg/dl (SI, 54 to 64 µmol/L).
- Saturation: In men and women, normal values are 20% to 50% (SI, 0.2 to 0.5).

## Abnormal results

- In iron deficiency, serum iron levels decrease and TIBC levels increase, decreasing saturation.
- In cases of chronic inflammation (such as in rheumatoid arthritis), serum iron levels may be low in the presence of adequate body stores, but TIBC levels may remain unchanged or may decrease to preserve normal saturation.
- Iron overload may not alter serum levels until relatively late but, in general, serum iron levels increase and TIBC levels remain the same, which increases the saturation.

### DRUG CHALLENGE

 Iron supplements (possible false-positive serum iron values but false-negative TIBC values)

## Purpose

- To estimate total iron storage
- To help diagnose hemochromatosis
- To help distinguish iron deficiency anemia from anemia of chronic disease (For information on another test used to differentiate anemias, see *Siderocyte stain,* page 15.)
- To help evaluate nutritional status

## Patient preparation

- Explain that this test evaluates the body's capacity to store iron.

## Normal iron metabolism

Ingested iron, absorbed and oxidated in the bowel, bonds with the protein transferrin for circulation to the bone marrow, where hemoglobin (Hb) synthesis occurs, and to all iron-hungry body cells. In the spleen, Hb breakdown recycles iron back to the bone marrow or into storage. The body conserves iron, losing small amounts through skin, stool, urine, and menses. Storage areas in the liver, spleen, bone marrow, and reticuloendothelial system hold iron as ferritin until the body needs it; the liver alone stores about 60% of the body's iron.

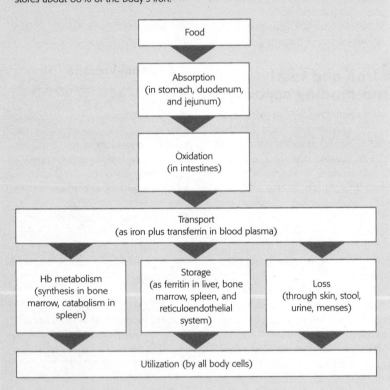

- Tell the patient that a blood sample will be taken. Explain who will perform the venipuncture and when it will be done.
- Explain to the patient that he may feel slight discomfort from the tourniquet and needle puncture.
- Notify the laboratory and practitioner of medications the patient is taking that may affect test results; these medications may need to be restricted.
- Tell the patient that he doesn't need to restrict food or fluids.

### Procedure and posttest care
- Confirm the patient's identity using two patient identifiers according to facility policy.
- Perform a venipuncture and collect the sample in a 4.5-ml clot-activator tube.
- If a hematoma develops at the venipuncture site, apply warm soaks. If the

## Siderocyte stain

Siderocytes are red blood cells (RBCs) containing particles of nonhemoglobin iron known as siderocytic granules. In neonates, siderocytic granules are normally present in normoblasts and reticulocytes during hemoglobin synthesis; however, the spleen removes most of these granules from normal RBCs, and they disappear rapidly with age.

In adults, an elevated siderocyte level usually indicates abnormal erythropoiesis, which may occur in congenital spherocytic anemia, chronic hemolytic anemias (such as the thalassemias), pernicious anemia, hemochromatosis, toxicities (such as lead poisoning), infection, and severe burns. Elevated levels may also follow splenectomy because the spleen normally removes siderocytic granules.

### Performing the test

The siderocyte stain test measures the number of circulating siderocytes. Venous blood is drawn into a 3- or 4.5-ml EDTA tube or, for infants and children, collected in a microtainer or pipette and smeared directly on a $3'' \times 5''$ glass slide. When the blood smear is stained, siderocytic granules appear as purple-blue specks clustered around the periphery of mature erythrocytes. Cells containing these granules are counted as a percentage of total RBCs. The results aid in the differential diagnosis of the anemias and hemochromatosis and help in detecting toxicities.

### Interpreting results

Normally, neonates have a slightly elevated siderocyte level that reaches the normal adult value of 0.5% (SI, 0.005) of total RBCs in 7 to 10 days. In patients with pernicious anemia, the siderocyte level ranges from 8% to 14% (SI, 0.08 to 0.14); in chronic hemolytic anemia, 20% to 100% (SI, 0.20 to 1.00); in lead poisoning, 10% to 30% (SI, 0.10 to 0.30); and in hemochromatosis, 3% to 7% (SI, 0.03 to 0.07). A high siderocyte level calls for additional testing (including bone marrow examination) to determine the cause of abnormal erythropoiesis.

---

hematoma is large, monitor pulses distal to the venipuncture site.
▪ Make sure that subdermal bleeding has stopped before removing pressure.
▪ Instruct the patient to resume medications stopped before the test, as ordered.

## ▌Methemoglobin

Methemoglobin is a structural hemoglobin (Hb) variant that's formed when the heme portion of deoxygenated Hb is oxidized to a ferric state. When this occurs, the heme can't combine with oxygen and carry it to the tissues, and the patient becomes cyanotic.

### Reference values

▪ Normal methemoglobin levels range from 0% to 1.5% (SI, 0 to 0.015) of total Hb.

### Abnormal results

▪ Increased methemoglobin levels may indicate acquired or hereditary methemoglobinemia or carbon monoxide poisoning. Taking certain drugs or being exposed to certain substances can also cause these levels.

### ACTION STAT!

 Levels greater than 40% (SI, 0.40) are critical values that require immediate intervention.

- Decreased methemoglobin levels may occur in pancreatitis.

### DRUG CHALLENGE

Nitroglycerin, benzocaine, chlorates, lidocaine, nitrates, nitrites, phenacetin, sulfonamides, primaquine, and resorcinol (possible increase)

### Purpose
- To detect methemoglobinemia acquired from excessive radiation or the toxic effects of chemicals or drugs
- To detect congenital methemoglobinemia

### Patient preparation
- If possible, obtain a history of the patient's hematologic status and Hb disorder, conditions that produce nitrite, and exposure to sources of nitrites in drugs.
- Explain that this test is used to detect abnormal Hb in the blood.
- Tell the patient that a blood sample will be taken. Explain who will perform the venipuncture and when it will be done.
- Explain to the patient that he may feel slight discomfort from the tourniquet and needle puncture.
- Notify the laboratory and practitioner of medications the patient is taking that may affect test results; these medications may need to be restricted.

### Procedure and posttest care
- Confirm the patient's identity using two patient identifiers according to facility policy.
- Perform a venipuncture and collect the sample in a 4.5-ml heparinized tube.
- If a hematoma develops at the venipuncture site, apply warm soaks. If the hematoma is large, monitor pulses distal to the venipuncture site.

- Make sure that subdermal bleeding has stopped before removing pressure.

### Precautions
DO'S & DON'TS

Place the collection tube on ice and send it to the laboratory immediately.

## Sickle cells

The sickle cell test (also known as *hemoglobin [Hb] S test*) is used to detect sickle cells, which are severely deformed, rigid erythrocytes that may slow blood flow. Sickle cell trait (characterized by heterozygous Hb S) is found almost exclusively in blacks; 0.2% of blacks born in the United States have sickle cell disease. (See *Inheritance patterns in sickle cell anemia.*)

Although the Hb S test is useful as a rapid screening procedure, it may produce erroneous results. Hb electrophoresis should be performed to confirm the diagnosis if sickle cell disease is strongly suspected.

### Reference values
- Results of the Hb S test are reported as positive or negative. A negative result suggests the absence of Hb S.

### Abnormal results
- A positive test result may indicate the presence of sickle cells, but Hb electrophoresis is needed to further diagnose the sickling tendency of cells.
- Rarely, in the absence of Hb S, other abnormal Hb may cause sickling.

### Purpose
- To identify sickle cell disease and sickle cell trait (see *Identifying sickle cell trait*)

# Inheritance patterns in sickle cell anemia

When both parents have sickle cell anemia (left), childbearing—if possible at all—is dangerous for the mother, and all offspring will have sickle cell anemia. When one parent has sickle cell anemia and one is normal (right), all offspring will be carriers of sickle cell anemia.

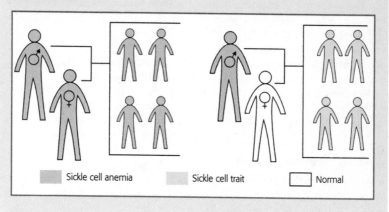

■ Sickle cell anemia        ■ Sickle cell trait        □ Normal

## Patient preparation

■ Explain to the patient that the Hb S test is used to detect sickle cell disease.
■ Tell the patient that a blood sample will be taken. Explain who will perform the venipuncture and when it will be done.
■ If the patient is an infant or child, explain to his parents that a small amount of blood will be taken from his finger or earlobe.
■ If the patient is an older child or adult, tell him that he may feel slight discomfort from the tourniquet and needle puncture.
■ Check the patient's history for a blood transfusion within the past 3 months.
■ Tell him he doesn't need to restrict food or fluids.

## Procedure and posttest care

■ Confirm the patient's identity using two patient identifiers according to facility policy.
■ Perform a venipuncture and collect the sample in a 3- or 4.5-ml EDTA tube.

## Identifying sickle cell trait

This relatively benign condition results from heterozygous inheritance of the abnormal hemoglobin (Hb) S-producing gene. Like sickle cell anemia, it's most common in blacks.

In people with sickle cell trait, 20% to 40% of the total Hb is Hb S; the rest is normal. These people, called carriers, usually have no symptoms. They have normal Hb and hematocrit values and can expect a normal life span. Nevertheless, they must avoid situations that provoke hypoxia, which occasionally causes a sickling crisis similar to that in sickle cell anemia.

Genetic counseling is essential for sickle cell carriers. Every child of two sickle cell carriers has a 25% chance of inheriting sickle cell anemia and a 50% chance of being a carrier.

For young children, collect capillary blood in a microcollection device.

■ If a hematoma develops at the venipuncture site, apply warm soaks. If the hematoma is large, monitor pulses distal to the venipuncture site.
■ Make sure that subdermal bleeding has stopped before removing pressure.

### Precautions
■ A blood transfusion within 3 months may cause a false-negative test result.

## Total hemoglobin

Total hemoglobin (Hb) is used to measure the amount of Hb found in a deciliter (dl, or 100 ml) of whole blood. It's usually part of a complete blood count. Hb concentration correlates closely with the red blood cell (RBC) count and affects the Hb-RBC ratio (mean corpuscular hemoglobin [MCH] and mean corpuscular hemoglobin concentration [MCHC]).

### Reference values
■ In adult men, normal total Hb values range from 14 to 17.4 g/dl (SI, 140 to 174 g/L).
■ In men after middle age, normal total Hb values range from 12.4 to 14.9 g/dl (SI, 124 to 149 g/L).
■ In adult women, normal total Hb values range from 12 to 16 g/dl: (SI, 120 to 160 g/L).
■ In women after middle age, normal total Hb values range from 11.7 to 13.8 g/dl (SI, 117 to 138 g/L).
■ In neonates, normal total Hb values range from 17 to 22 g/dl (SI, 170 to 220 g/L).
■ In infants age 1 week, normal total Hb values range from 15 to 20 g/dl (SI, 150 to 200 g/L).
■ In infants age 1 month, normal total Hb values range from 11 to 15 g/dl (SI, 110 to 150 g/L).
■ In children, normal total Hb values range from 11 to 13 g/dl (SI, 110 to 130 g/L).
■ Those who are more active or who live in high altitudes may have higher values.

### Abnormal results
■ Low Hb concentration may indicate anemia, recent hemorrhage, or fluid retention, causing hemodilution.
■ Elevated Hb suggests hemoconcentration from polycythemia or dehydration.

### Purpose
■ To measure the severity of anemia or polycythemia and to monitor response to therapy
■ To obtain data for calculating the MCH and MCHC

### Patient preparation
■ Explain to the patient that the total Hb test is used to detect anemia or polycythemia or to assess his response to treatment.
■ Tell the patient that a blood sample will be taken. Explain who will perform the venipuncture and when it will be done.
■ If the patient is an infant or child, explain to his parents that a small amount of blood will be taken from his finger or earlobe.
■ If the patient is an older child or adult, tell him that he may feel slight discomfort from the tourniquet and needle puncture.
■ Explain that the patient doesn't need to restrict food or fluids.

### Procedure and posttest care
■ Confirm the patient's identity using two patient identifiers according to facility policy.

- For adults and older children, perform a venipuncture, and collect the sample in a 3- or 4.5-ml EDTA tube.

**DO'S & DON'TS**

 For younger children and infants, collect the sample by fingerstick or heelstick in a microcollection device with EDTA.

- If a hematoma develops at the venipuncture site, apply warm soaks. If the hematoma is large, monitor pulses distal to the venipuncture site.
- Make sure that subdermal bleeding has stopped before removing pressure.

# Unstable hemoglobin

Unstable hemoglobin (Hb) is a rare, congenital defect caused by amino acid substitutions in the structure of Hb. It's called "unstable" because of the ease with which the Hb decomposes. The presence of unstable Hb may lead to the formation of small masses called Heinz bodies, which accumulate on red blood cell membranes. Although Heinz bodies are usually removed by the spleen or liver, they may cause mild to severe hemolysis. (See *Signs and symptoms of unstable hemoglobin.*) Unstable Hb is best detected by precipitation tests (heat stability or isopropanol solubility).

## Reference values

- The heat stability test result is negative; the isopropanol solubility test result is reported as stable.

## Abnormal results

- A positive heat stability test result or unstable solubility test result, especially with hemolysis, strongly suggests the presence of unstable Hb.

## Signs and symptoms of unstable hemoglobin

More than 60 varieties of unstable hemoglobin (Hb) exist, each named after the city in which it was discovered. Their effects vary according to their number, the degree of instability, the condition of the spleen, and the oxygen-binding abilities of the unstable Hb.

Patients with unstable Hb typically exhibit pallor, jaundice, splenomegaly, and (with severely unstable Hb) cyanosis, pigmenturia, and hemoglobinuria. Thalassemia commonly causes similar signs and symptoms, but the molecular bases of the two diseases differ greatly.

**DRUG CHALLENGE**

 Antimalarials, furazolidone (in infants), nitrofurantoin, phenacetin, procarbazine, and sulfonamides (possible false-positive or unstable results)

## Purpose

- To detect unstable Hb

## Patient preparation

- Explain that the unstable Hb test is used to detect abnormal Hb in the blood.
- Tell the patient that a blood sample will be taken. Explain who will perform the venipuncture and when it will be done.
- Explain to the patient that he may feel slight discomfort from the tourniquet and needle puncture.
- Notify the laboratory and practitioner of medications the patient is taking that may affect test results; these medications may need to be restricted.
- Tell the patient that he doesn't need to restrict food or fluids.

### Procedure and posttest care

- Confirm the patient's identity using two patient identifiers according to facility policy.
- Perform a venipuncture and collect the sample in a 3- or 4.5-ml EDTA tube.
- If a hematoma develops at the venipuncture site, apply warm soaks. If the hematoma is large, monitor pulses distal to the venipuncture site.
- Make sure that subdermal bleeding has stopped before removing pressure.
- Instruct the patient to resume medications stopped before the test, as ordered.

# White blood cell tests

## White blood cell count

A white blood cell (WBC) count, also called a leukocyte count, is part of a complete blood count. It indicates the number of white cells in a microliter (µl) or cubic millimeter (mm³) of whole blood.

WBC counts may vary by as much as 2,000 cells/µl (SI, 2 × 10⁹/L) on any given day due to strenuous exercise, stress, or digestion. The WBC count may increase or decrease significantly in certain diseases but is diagnostically useful only when the patient's white cell differential and clinical status are considered.

### Reference values

- WBC count values are 4,000 to 10,000/µl (SI, 4 to 10 × 10⁹/L).

### Abnormal results

- An elevated WBC count (leukocytosis) commonly signals infection, such as an abscess, meningitis, appendicitis, or tonsillitis. It may also result from leukemia

and tissue necrosis from burns, myocardial infarction, or gangrene.

- A low WBC count (leukopenia) indicates bone marrow depression that may result from viral infections or from toxic reactions, such as those following treatment with antineoplastics, ingestion of mercury or other heavy metals, and exposure to benzene or arsenicals. Leukopenia characteristically accompanies influenza, typhoid fever, measles, infectious hepatitis, mononucleosis, and rubella.

#### DRUG CHALLENGE

 Most antineoplastics; anti-infectives, such as metronidazole and flucytosine; anticonvulsants, such as phenytoin derivatives; thyroid hormone antagonists; and nonsteroidal anti-inflammatory drugs such as indomethacin (decrease)

### Purpose

- To detect infection or inflammation
- To determine the need for further tests, such as the WBC differential or bone marrow biopsy
- To monitor response to chemotherapy or radiation therapy

### Patient preparation

- Explain that the WBC count test is used to detect an infection or inflammation.
- Tell the patient that a blood sample will be taken. Explain who will perform the venipuncture and when it will be done.
- Explain to the patient that he may feel slight discomfort from the tourniquet and needle puncture.
- Tell him to avoid strenuous exercise for 24 hours before the test and to avoid eating a heavy meal before the test.

- If the patient is being treated for an infection, advise him that this test will be repeated to monitor his progress.
- Notify the laboratory and practitioner of medications the patient is taking that may affect test results; these medications may need to be restricted.

### Procedure and posttest care
- Confirm the patient's identity using two patient identifiers according to facility policy.
- Perform a venipuncture and collect the sample in a 3- or 4.5-ml EDTA tube.
- If a hematoma develops at the venipuncture site, apply warm soaks. If the hematoma is large, monitor pulses distal to the venipuncture site.
- Make sure that subdermal bleeding has stopped before removing pressure.
- Instruct the patient that he may resume his usual diet, activity, and medications discontinued before the test as ordered.

DO'S & DON'TS

 A patient with severe leukopenia may have little or no resistance to infection and therefore requires protective isolation.

# White blood cell differential

The white blood cell (WBC) differential is used to evaluate the distribution and morphology of WBCs, providing more specific information about a patient's immune system than the WBC count alone.

WBCs are classified as one of five major types of leukocytes—neutrophils, eosinophils, basophils, lymphocytes, and monocytes—and the percentage of each type is determined. The differential count is the percentage of each type of WBC in the blood. The total number of

each type of WBC is obtained by multiplying the percentage of each type by the total WBC count.

High levels of these leukocytes are associated with various allergic diseases and reactions to parasites. An eosinophil count is sometimes ordered as a follow-up test when an elevated or depressed eosinophil level is reported.

### Reference values
- For normal values for the five types of WBCs classified in the differential for adults and children, see *Interpreting WBC differential values,* page 22.
- For an accurate diagnosis, differential test results must always be interpreted in relation to the total WBC count.

### Abnormal results
- Abnormal differential patterns provide evidence for many disease states and other conditions. (See *Influence of disease on blood cell count,* pages 23 and 24.)

DRUG CHALLENGE

 Methysergide and desipramine (increase or decrease eosinophil count); indomethacin and procainamide (decrease eosinophil count); anticonvulsants, capreomycin, cephalosporins, D-penicillamine, gold compounds, isoniazid, nalidixic acid, novobiocin, para-aminosalicylic acid, paromomycin, penicillins, phenothiazines, rifampin, streptomycin, sulfonamides, and tetracyclines (increase count by provoking an allergic reaction)

### Purpose
- To evaluate the body's capacity to resist and overcome infection
- To detect and identify various types of leukemia (see *Performing a LAP stain,* page 24)
- To determine the stage and severity of an infection

## Interpreting WBC differential values

The differential count measures the types of white blood cells (WBCs) as a percentage of the total WBC count (the relative value). The absolute value is obtained by multiplying the relative value of each cell type by the total WBC count. The relative and absolute values must be considered to obtain an accurate diagnosis.

For example, consider a patient whose WBC count is 6,000/µl (SI, $6 \times 10^9$/L) and whose WBC differential shows 30% (SI, 0.30) neutrophils and 70% (SI, 0.70) lymphocytes. His relative lymphocyte count seems to be quite high (lymphocytosis), but when this figure is multiplied by his WBC count (6,000 × 70% = 4,200 lymphocytes/µl) (SI, [$6 \times 10^9$/L] × 9.79 = $4.2 \times 10^9$/L lymphocytes), it's well within the normal range.

However, this patient's neutrophil count (30%; SI, 0.30) is low. When this figure is multiplied by the WBC count (6,000 × 30% = 1,800 neutrophils/ml) (SI, [$6 \times 10^9$/L] × 0.30 = $1.8 \times 10^9$/L neutrophils), the result is a low absolute number, which may mean depressed bone marrow.

The normal percentages of WBC types in adults are the following:

Neutrophils: 54% to 75% (SI, 0.54 to 0.75)

Eosinophils: 1% to 4% (SI, 0.01 to 0.04)

Basophils: 0% to 1% (SI, 0 to 0.01)

Monocytes: 2% to 8% (SI, 0.02 to 0.08)

Lymphocytes: 25% to 40% (SI, 0.25 to 0.40)

---

■ To detect allergic reactions and parasitic infections and assess their severity (eosinophil count)
■ To distinguish viral from bacterial infections

### Patient preparation

■ Explain to the patient that the WBC differential test is used to evaluate the immune system.
■ Tell the patient that a blood sample will be taken. Explain who will perform the venipuncture and when it will be done.
■ Explain to the patient that he may feel slight discomfort from the tourniquet and needle puncture.
■ Notify the laboratory and practitioner of medications the patient is taking that may affect test results; these medications may need to be restricted.
■ Inform the patient that he need not restrict food or fluid intake but that he should refrain from strenuous exercise for 24 hours before the test.

### Procedure and posttest care

■ Confirm the patient's identity using two patient identifiers according to facility policy.
■ Perform a venipuncture and collect the sample in a 3- or 4.5-ml EDTA tube.
■ If a hematoma develops at the venipuncture site, apply warm soaks. If the hematoma is large, monitor pulses distal to the venipuncture site.
■ Make sure that subdermal bleeding has stopped before removing pressure.

# Influence of disease on blood cell count

The white blood cell (WBC) differential test aids diagnosis because some disorders affect only one WBC type. Each WBC type, as well as the corresponding effect and its cause, is listed below.

| Cell type | How affected |
| --- | --- |
| **Basophils**<br /> | **IIncreased by:**<br />■ CML, Hodgkin's disease, ulcerative colitis, chronic hypersensitivity states<br />**Decreased by:**<br />■ Hyperthyroidism<br />■ Ovulation, pregnancy<br />■ Stress |
| **Eosinophils**<br /> | **Increased by:**<br />■ Allergic disorders: asthma, hay fever, food or drug sensitivity, serum sickness, angioneurotic edema<br />■ Parasitic infections: trichinosis, hookworm, roundworm, amebiasis<br />■ Skin diseases: eczema, pemphigus, psoriasis, dermatitis, herpes<br />■ Neoplastic diseases: chronic myelocytic leukemia (CML), Hodgkin's disease, metastases and necrosis of solid tumors<br />**Decreased by:**<br />■ Stress response<br />■ Cushing's syndrome |
| **Lymphocytes**<br /> | **Increased by:**<br />■ Infections: tuberculosis (TB), hepatitis, infectious mononucleosis, mumps, rubella, cytomegalovirus<br />■ Thyrotoxicosis, hypoadrenalism, ulcerative colitis, immune diseases, lymphocytic leukemia<br />**Decreased by:**<br />■ Severe debilitating illnesses: heart failure, renal failure, advanced TB<br />■ Defective lymphatic circulation, high levels of adrenal corticosteroids, immunodeficiency due to immunosuppressives |
| **Monocytes**<br /> | **Increased by:**<br />■ Infections: subacute bacterial endocarditis, TB, hepatitis, malaria<br />■ Collagen vascular disease: SLE, rheumatoid arthritis<br />■ Carcinomas<br />■ Monocytic leukemia<br />■ Lymphomas<br />**Decreased by:**<br />■ Infections<br />■ Acute lymphocytic leukemia, chronic lymphocytic leukemia, leukemic reticuloendotheliosis<br />■ Aplastic anemia<br />■ Anorexia nervosa |

*(continued)*

## Influence of disease on blood cell count *(continued)*

| Cell type | How affected |
| --- | --- |

**Neutrophils**

**Increased by:**
- Infections: osteomyelitis, otitis media, salpingitis, septicemia, gonorrhea, endocarditis, smallpox, chickenpox, herpes, Rocky Mountain spotted fever
- Ischemic necrosis due to myocardial infarction, burns, carcinoma
- Metabolic disorders: diabetic acidosis, eclampsia, uremia, thyrotoxicosis
- Stress response due to acute hemorrhage, surgery, excessive exercise, emotional distress, third trimester of pregnancy, childbirth
- Inflammatory diseases: rheumatic fever, rheumatoid arthritis, acute gout, vasculitis, myositis

**Decreased by:**
- Bone marrow depression due to radiation or cytotoxic drugs
- Infections: typhoid, tularemia, brucellosis, hepatitis, influenza, measles, mumps, rubella, infectious mononucleosis
- Hypersplenism: hepatic disease, storage diseases
- Collagen vascular disease: systemic lupus erythematosus (SLE)
- Folic acid or vitamin $B_{12}$ deficiency

# Performing a LAP stain

Levels of leukocyte alkaline phosphatase (LAP), an enzyme found in neutrophils, may be altered by infection, stress, chronic inflammatory diseases, Hodgkin's disease, and hematologic disorders. Most of these conditions elevate LAP levels; only a few—notably chronic myelogenous leukemia (CML)—depress them. Thus, this test is usually used to differentiate CML from other disorders that produce an elevated white blood cell count.

## Procedure

To perform the LAP stain, a blood sample is obtained by venipuncture or fingerstick. The venous blood sample is collected in a 7-ml green-top tube and transported immediately to the laboratory, where a blood smear is prepared; the peripheral blood sample is smeared on a 3″ glass slide and fixed in cold formalin-methanol. The blood smear is then stained to show the amount of LAP present in the cytoplasm of the neutrophils; 100 neutrophils are counted and assessed, and each is assigned a score of 0 to 4, according to the degree of LAP staining. Normally, values for LAP range from 40 to 100, depending on the laboratory's standards.

## Implications of results

Depressed LAP values typically indicate CML; however, values may also be low in paroxysmal nocturnal hemoglobinuria, aplastic anemia, and infectious mononucleosis. Elevated levels may indicate Hodgkin's disease, polycythemia vera, or a neutrophilic leukemoid reaction—a response to such conditions as infection, chronic inflammation, or pregnancy.

After a diagnosis of CML, the LAP stain may also be used to help detect onset of the blastic phase of the disease, when LAP levels typically rise. LAP levels also increase toward normal in response to therapy; because of this, test results must be correlated with the patient's condition.

# Hemostasis

## Platelet activity tests

### Bleeding time

The bleeding time test measures the duration of bleeding after a measured skin incision. One of three methods—template, Ivy, or Duke—may be used. The template method is the most commonly used and the most accurate because the incision size is standardized. Bleeding time depends on the elasticity of the blood vessel wall and on the number and functional capacity of platelets.

Although the bleeding time test is usually performed on a patient with a personal or family history of bleeding disorders, it's also useful—along with a platelet count—for preoperative screening. The test isn't usually recommended for a patient with a platelet count of less than 75,000/µl (SI, 75 × 10⁹/L).

#### Reference values

- Normal bleeding time ranges from 3 to 6 minutes (SI, 3 to 6 minutes) using the template method, from 3 to 6 minutes using the Ivy method, and from 1 to 3 minutes (SI, 1 to 3 minutes) using the Duke method.

#### Abnormal results

- Prolonged bleeding time may indicate the presence of disorders associated with thrombocytopenia, such as Hodgkin's disease, acute leukemia, disseminated intravascular coagulation, hemolytic disease of the newborn, Schönlein-Henoch purpura, severe hepatic disease (for example, cirrhosis), or severe deficiency of factors I, II, V, VII, VIII, IX, and XI.
- Prolonged bleeding time in a patient with a normal platelet count suggests a platelet function disorder (thrombasthenia, thrombocytopathia) and requires further investigation with clot retraction, prothrombin consumption, and platelet aggregation tests.

#### DRUG CHALLENGE

 Sulfonamides, thiazide diuretics, antineoplastics, anticoagulants, nonsteroidal anti-inflammatory drugs, vitamin E supplementation, aspirin and aspirin compounds, and some non-narcotic analgesics (prolonged bleeding time)

#### Purpose

- To assess overall hemostatic function (platelet response to injury and functional capacity of vasoconstriction)
- To detect congenital and acquired platelet function disorders

#### Patient preparation

- Explain that the bleeding time test measures the time required to form a clot and stop bleeding.

- Tell the patient who will be performing the test and when it will be done.
- Tell him that he doesn't need to restrict food or fluids.
- Explain that he may feel some discomfort from the incisions, the antiseptic, and the tightness of the blood pressure cuff. Also inform the patient that, depending on the method used, incisions or punctures may leave tiny scars that should be barely visible when healed.
- Notify the laboratory and practitioner of medications the patient is taking that may affect test results; these medications may need to be restricted.

### Procedure and posttest care

- Confirm the patient's identity using two patient identifiers according to facility policy.
- *Template method*
  - Wrap the pressure cuff around the upper arm and inflate the cuff to 40 mm Hg.
  - Select an area on the forearm with no superficial veins and clean it with antiseptic. Allow the skin to dry completely before making the incision.
  - Apply the appropriate template lengthwise to the forearm. Use the lancet to make two incisions 1 mm deep and 9 mm long.
  - Start the stopwatch. Without touching the cuts, gently blot the drops of blood with filter paper every 30 seconds until the bleeding stops in both cuts.
  - Average the bleeding time for the two cuts and record the result.
- *Ivy method*
  - After applying the pressure cuff and preparing the test site, make three small punctures with a disposable lancet.
  - Start the stopwatch immediately.
  - Taking care not to touch the punctures, blot each site with filter paper every 30 seconds until the bleeding stops.
  - Average the bleeding time of the three punctures and record the result.
- *Duke method:*
  - Drape the patient's shoulder with a towel.
  - Clean the earlobe and let the skin air-dry.
  - Make a puncture wound 2 to 4 mm deep on the earlobe with a disposable lancet.
  - Start the stopwatch.
  - Being careful not to touch the ear, blot the site with filter paper every 30 seconds until the bleeding stops.
  - Record the result.
- In a patient with a bleeding tendency (hemophilia), maintain a pressure bandage over the incision for 24 to 48 hours to prevent further bleeding. Check the test area frequently; keep the edges of the cuts aligned to minimize scarring.
- In other patients, a piece of gauze held in place by an adhesive bandage is sufficient.
- Instruct the patient that he may resume any medications stopped before the test as ordered.

### Precautions

- Be sure to maintain a cuff pressure of 40 mm Hg throughout the test.
- If the bleeding doesn't diminish after 15 minutes, stop the test.
- After the test, apply direct pressure to the test site until bleeding ceases.

### Complications

- Bleeding that doesn't slow after 15 minutes

# Capillary fragility

The capillary fragility test is a nonspecific method for evaluating bleeding tendencies. This test measures the capillaries' ability to remain intact under increased intracapillary pressure. The pressure is controlled by a blood pressure cuff placed around the patient's upper arm and inflated to 70 to 90 mm Hg, or midway between the diastolic and systolic pressure. The pressure is maintained for 5 minutes. This temporary increase in pressure may cause rhexis bleeding of the capillaries and formation of petechiae on the arm, wrist, or hand. The number of petechiae within a given circular space is recorded as the test result.

### Reference values

▪ A few petechiae may normally be present before the test. Fewer than 10 petechiae on the forearm 5 minutes (SI, 5 minutes) after the test is considered normal, or negative; more than 10 petechiae is considered a positive result. The following scale may also be used to report test results.

### Abnormal results

▪ A positive finding (more than 10 petechiae, or a score of 2+ to 4+) indicates weakness of the capillary walls (vascular purpura) or a platelet defect. It may occur in such conditions as thrombocytopenia, thrombasthenia, purpura senilis, scurvy, disseminated intravascular coagulation (DIC), von Willebrand's disease, vitamin K deficiency, dysproteinemia, and polycythemia vera and in severe deficiencies of factor VII, fibrinogen, or prothrombin. Conditions unrelated to bleeding defects, such as scarlet fever, measles, influenza, chronic renal disease, hypertension, and diabetes with coexisting vascular disease, may also increase capillary fragility.
▪ An abnormal number of petechiae sometimes appear before menstruation and at other times in some healthy persons, especially in women older than age 40.

**DRUG CHALLENGE**

 Decreasing estrogen levels in postmenopausal women (possible increase)

### Purpose

▪ To assess the fragility of capillary walls
▪ To identify a platelet deficiency (thrombocytopenia)

### Patient preparation

▪ Explain that the capillary fragility test identifies abnormal bleeding tendencies.
▪ Tell the patient who will be performing the procedure and when it will be done.
▪ Inform the patient that he doesn't need to restrict food or fluids.
▪ Explain to the patient that he may feel discomfort from the pressure of the blood pressure cuff.

### Procedure and posttest care

▪ Confirm the patient's identity using two patient identifiers according to facility policy.
▪ The patient's skin temperature and the room temperature should be normal to ensure accurate results.
▪ Select and mark a 2″ (5-cm) space on the patient's forearm. Ideally, the site should be free from petechiae; otherwise, record the number of petechiae before starting the test.
▪ Fasten the cuff around the arm and raise the pressure to a point midway between the systolic and diastolic blood pressures. Maintain this pressure for 5 minutes, then release the cuff.
▪ Count the number of petechiae that appear in the 2″ space.
▪ Record the test results.
▪ Encourage the patient to open and close his hand a few times to hasten return of blood to the forearm.

## Precautions

- Don't repeat this test on the same arm within 1 week.
- This test is contraindicated in patients with DIC or other bleeding disorders and in those with significant petechiae already present.

# Platelet aggregation

After vascular injury, platelets gather at the injury site and clump together to form an aggregate or plug that helps maintain hemostasis and promotes healing. The platelet aggregation test, an in vitro procedure, measures the rate at which the platelets in a plasma sample form a clump after the addition of an aggregating reagent.

## Reference values

- Normal platelet aggregation occurs in 3 to 5 minutes (SI, 3 to 5 minutes), but findings are temperature dependent and vary with the laboratory.
- Aggregation curves obtained by using different reagents help to distinguish various qualitative platelet defects.

## Abnormal results

- Abnormal findings may indicate congenital disorders, such as Glanzmann's thrombasthenia, von Willebrand's disease, Bernard-Soulier syndrome, and storage pool disease, or acquired conditions, such as polycythemia vera, severe liver disease, uremia, autoimmune disorders, myeloproliferative disorders, and vasculitis.

### DRUG CHALLENGE

 Aspirin and aspirin compounds, phenylbutazone, sulfinpyrazone, phenothiazines, anti-inflammatories, antihistamines, and tricyclic antidepressants (decrease)

## Purpose

- To assess platelet aggregation
- To detect congenital and acquired platelet bleeding disorders
- To distinguish between congenital and acquired bleeding disorders

## Patient preparation

- Explain that the platelet aggregation test determines if blood clots properly.
- Tell the patient that the test requires a blood sample. Explain who will perform the venipuncture and when it will be done. (See *Aspirin and platelet aggregation*.)
- Explain to the patient that he may feel slight discomfort from the tourniquet and needle puncture.
- Instruct the patient to fast or to maintain a nonfat diet for 8 hours before the test because lipemia can affect the test results.
- Notify the laboratory and practitioner of medications the patient is taking that may affect test results; these medications may need to be restricted.

## Procedure and posttest care

- Confirm the patient's identity using two patient identifiers according to facility policy.
- Perform a venipuncture and collect the sample in a 4.5-ml siliconized tube.
- Completely fill the collection tube and invert it gently several times to mix the sample and the anticoagulant thoroughly.
- Apply pressure to the venipuncture site for 5 minutes or until bleeding stops.
- If a hematoma develops at the venipuncture site, apply warm soaks. If the hematoma is large, monitor pulses distal to the venipuncture site.
- Instruct the patient that he may resume his usual diet and medications stopped before the test as ordered.

# Aspirin and platelet aggregation

Unlike other salicylates, aspirin inhibits platelet aggregation. The inhibition occurs in the second phase of platelet aggregation, when it prevents the release of adenosine diphosphate from platelets. Mean bleeding time may double in healthy individuals after ingestion of aspirin. In children or in patients with bleeding disorders, such as hemophilia, bleeding time may be even more prolonged.

## Effect on platelets

The effect of aspirin on platelets seems to result from the inhibition of prostaglandin synthesis. A single 325-mg oral dose of aspirin results in about a 90% inhibition of the enzyme cyclooxygenase in circulating platelets, preventing the synthesis of compounds that induce platelet aggregation. The inhibition of cyclooxygenase is irreversible; thus, its effect lasts for 4 to 6 days—the life span of platelets. Bleeding time peaks within 12 hours. Altered hemostasis persists about 36 hours after the last dose of aspirin, sometimes longer for the patient receiving long-term therapy.

## Effect on blood vessels

Aspirin's action on blood vessels may oppose that seen in platelets because cyclooxygenase plays a different role in the vascular endothelium. Here, the enzyme produces prostacyclin, a compound that inhibits platelet aggregation and causes vasodilation. Inhibition of cyclooxygenase in the vascular endothelium, in effect, reverses aspirin's antithrombotic effect on platelets. Studies suggest that cyclooxygenase in the platelets is more sensitive than that in the vascular endothelium and that, therefore, a low aspirin dosage (for example, 80 mg daily or 325 mg every other day) may prove more effective in preventing thrombosis than higher dosages.

## Precautions

▪ Because the list of medications known to alter the results of this test is long and continually growing, the patient should be as drug-free as possible before the test.

▪ If the patient has taken aspirin within the past 14 days and the test can't be postponed, ask the laboratory to verify the presence of aspirin in the plasma. If test results are abnormal for such a sample, the use of aspirin must be stopped and the test repeated in 2 weeks.

▪ Avoid excessive probing at the venipuncture site.

▪ Remove the tourniquet promptly to avoid bruising.

▪ Handle the sample gently to prevent hemolysis and keep it between 71.6° F and 98.6° F (22° C and 37° C) to prevent aggregation.

# ▌Platelet count
[thrombocyte count]

Platelets are the smallest formed elements in the blood. They promote coagulation and the formation of a hemostatic plug in vascular injury.

Platelet count is one of the most important screening tests of platelet function. Accurate counts are vital.

## Reference values

▪ In adults, normal platelet counts are 140,000 to 400,000/µl (SI, 140 to 400 × 10⁹/L).

▪ In children, normal platelet counts are 150,000 to 450,000/µl (SI, 150 to 450 × 10⁹/L).

## Abnormal results

▪ A platelet count below 50,000/µl can cause spontaneous bleeding; a count below 5,000/µl may cause fatal central nervous system bleeding or massive GI hemorrhage.

▪ A decreased platelet count (thrombocytopenia) can result from aplastic or hypoplastic bone marrow; infiltrative bone marrow disease, such as leukemia, or disseminated infection; megakaryocytic hypoplasia; ineffective thrombopoiesis due to folic acid or vitamin $B_{12}$ deficiency; pooling of platelets in an enlarged spleen; increased platelet destruction due to drugs or immune disorders; disseminated intravascular coagulation; Bernard-Soulier syndrome; or mechanical injury to platelets.

▪ A transient increased platelet count (thrombocytosis) may occur during hemorrhage, infectious disorders, iron deficiency anemia, recent surgery, pregnancy, splenectomy, or inflammatory disorders, but the count returns to normal after recovery.

▪ A constantly elevated platelet count occurs in primary thrombocythemia, myelofibrosis with myeloid metaplasia, polycythemia vera, and chronic myelogenous leukemia.

▪ When the platelet count is abnormal, further studies are needed for diagnosis (such as complete blood count, bone marrow biopsy, direct antiglobulin test [direct Coombs' test], and serum protein electrophoresis).

### DRUG CHALLENGE

Heparin (decrease); acetazolamide, acetohexamide, antineoplastics, brompheniramine maleate, carbamazepine, chloramphenicol, ethacrynic acid, furosemide, gold salts, hydroxychloroquine, indomethacin, isoniazid, mephenytoin, mefenamic acid, methazolamide, methimazole, methyldopa, oral diazoxide, penicillamine, penicillin, phenylbutazone, phenytoin, pyrimethamine, quinidine sulfate, quinine, salicylates, streptomycin, sulfonamides, thiazide and thiazide-like diuretics, and tricyclic antidepressants (possible decrease)

## Purpose

▪ To measure the number of platelets in the blood
▪ To evaluate platelet production
▪ To assess the effects of chemotherapy or radiation therapy on platelet production
▪ To diagnose and monitor severe thrombocytosis or thrombocytopenia
▪ To confirm a visual estimate of platelet number and morphology from a stained blood film

## Patient preparation

▪ Explain that the platelet count test determines if the patient's blood clots normally.
▪ Tell the patient that a blood sample will be taken. Explain who will perform the venipuncture and when it will be done.
▪ Inform the patient that he doesn't need to restrict food or fluids.
▪ Explain to the patient that he may feel slight discomfort from the tourniquet and needle puncture.
▪ Notify the laboratory and practitioner of medications the patient is taking that may affect test results; these medications may need to be restricted.

## Procedure and posttest care

▪ Confirm the patient's identity using two patient identifiers according to facility policy.
▪ Perform a venipuncture and collect the sample in a 3- or 4.5-ml EDTA tube.
▪ If a hematoma develops at the venipuncture site, apply warm soaks. If the

hematoma is large, monitor pulses distal to the venipuncture site.
- Make sure that subdermal bleeding has stopped before removing pressure.
- Instruct the patient that he may resume any medications stopped before the test as ordered.

### Precautions
- Use the proper anticoagulant and mix the sample and anticoagulant promptly and adequately.
- Rough handling of the sample or excessive probing at the venipuncture site may cause hemolysis.

# Coagulation tests

## ■ Activated clotting time
### [ACT, automated coagulation time]

The activated clotting time (ACT) test measures whole blood clotting time. It's commonly performed during procedures that require extracorporeal circulation, such as cardiopulmonary bypass, ultrafiltration, hemodialysis, and extracorporeal membrane oxygenation (ECMO), and during invasive procedures, such as cardiac catheterization and percutaneous transluminal coronary angioplasty.

### Reference values
- In a nonanticoagulated patient, normal ACT is 107 seconds plus or minus 13 seconds (SI, 107 ± 13 seconds).
- During cardiopulmonary bypass, heparin is titrated to maintain an ACT of between 400 and 600 seconds (SI, 400 to 600 seconds).
- During ECMO, heparin is titrated to maintain an ACT of between 220 and 260 seconds (SI, 220 to 260 seconds).

### Abnormal results
- An elevated ACT without the presence of heparin indicates severe clotting factor deficiencies and requires further testing.

### Purpose
- To monitor the effect of heparin
- To monitor the effect of protamine sulfate in heparin neutralization
- To detect severe deficiencies in clotting factors (except factor VII)

### Patient preparation
- Explain that the ACT test monitors the effect of heparin on the blood's ability to coagulate.
- Tell the patient that the test requires a blood sample but that it's usually drawn from an existing vascular access site, so no venipuncture is needed.
- Explain who will perform the test and that it's usually done at the bedside.
- Explain that two blood samples will be drawn and that the first one will be discarded so that any heparin in the tubing doesn't interfere with the results.

### Procedure and posttest care
- Confirm the patient's identity using two patient identifiers according to facility policy.
- If the sample is drawn from a line with a continuous infusion, stop the infusion before drawing the sample.
- Withdraw 5 to 10 ml of blood from the line and discard it.
- Withdraw a clean sample of blood into the special tube containing celite provided with the ACT unit.
- Start the ACT unit and wait for the signal to insert the tube.
- Flush the vascular access site according to your facility's policy.

## Precautions

 Guard against contamination with heparin if blood is drawn from an access site containing heparin.

# D-dimer

D-dimer is an asymmetrical carbon compound fragment formed after thrombin converts fibrinogen to fibrin, factor XIIIa stabilizes fibrin into a clot, and plasma acts on the cross-linked, or clotted, fibrin. The test is specific for fibrinolysis because it confirms the presence of fibrin split products.

## Reference values

• Normal D-dimer results are negative or less than 250 mcg/L (SI, less than 250 mcg/L).

## Abnormal results

• Increased D-dimer values may indicate disseminated intravascular coagulation (DIC), pulmonary embolism (PE), arterial or venous thrombosis, neoplastic disease, pregnancy (late and postpartum), surgery occurring up to 2 days before testing, subarachnoid hemorrhage (spinal fluid only), or secondary fibrinolysis.

## Purpose

• To diagnose DIC
• To distinguish subarachnoid hemorrhage from a traumatic lumbar puncture in spinal fluid analysis
• To diagnose and monitor diseases and conditions that cause a hypercoagulation state
• To rule out deep vein thrombosis, PE, and ventricular or atrial thrombi

## Patient preparation

• Obtain the patient's history of hematologic diseases, the records of recent surgery, and the results of other tests performed.
• Explain that the D-dimer test determines if the blood is clotting normally.
• Tell the patient that the test requires a blood sample. Explain who will perform the venipuncture and when it will be done.
• Explain to the patient that he may feel slight discomfort from the tourniquet and needle puncture.

## Procedure and posttest care

• Confirm the patient's identity using two patient identifiers according to facility policy.
• Perform a venipuncture and collect the sample in a 4.5-ml tube with sodium citrate added.
• For a spinal fluid analysis, the sample is collected during a lumbar puncture and placed in a plastic vial. See "Cerebrospinal fluid analysis," page 476, for details of the procedure.
• Apply pressure to the venipuncture site for 5 minutes or until bleeding stops.
• If a hematoma develops at the venipuncture site, apply warm soaks. If the hematoma is large, monitor pulses distal to the venipuncture site.

## Precautions

• For a patient with coagulation problems, you may need to apply additional pressure at the venipuncture site to control bleeding.
• If a patient has a high rheumatoid factor titre or an increased CA-125 level, a positive result may be a false-positive.

# Fibrinogen
## [factor I]

Fibrinogen originates in the liver and is converted to fibrin by thrombin during clotting. Because fibrin is necessary for clot formation, fibrinogen deficiency can produce mild to severe bleeding disorders.

## Reference values
- Fibrinogen levels are 200 to 400 mg/dl (SI, 2 to 4 g/L).
- Postoperative patients or women in the third trimester of pregnancy may have increased fibrinogen levels.

### Abnormal results
- Depressed fibrinogen levels may indicate congenital afibrinogenemia; hypofibrinogenemia or dysfibrinogenemia; disseminated intravascular coagulation; fibrinolysis; severe hepatic disease; cancer of the prostate, pancreas, or lung; or bone marrow lesions.
- Obstetric complications or trauma may cause low fibrinogen levels.
- Markedly decreased fibrinogen levels impede the accurate interpretation of coagulation tests that have a fibrin clot as an end point.
- Elevated fibrinogen levels may indicate cancer of the stomach, breast, or kidney or inflammatory disorders, such as pneumonia or membranoproliferative glomerulonephritis.
- Prolonged partial thromboplastin time, prothrombin time, and thrombin time may also indicate a fibrinogen deficiency.

### Purpose
- To aid in the diagnosis of suspected clotting or bleeding disorders caused by fibrinogen abnormalities

### Patient preparation
- Explain that the plasma fibrinogen test determines if blood clots normally.
- Tell the patient that a blood sample will be taken. Explain who will perform the venipuncture and when it will be done.
- Explain to the patient that he may feel slight discomfort from the tourniquet and needle puncture.
- Notify the laboratory and practitioner of medications the patient is taking that may affect test results; these medications may need to be restricted.
- Inform the patient that he doesn't need to restrict food or fluids.

### Procedure and posttest care
- Confirm the patient's identity using two patient identifiers according to facility policy.
- Perform a venipuncture and collect the sample in a 3- or 4.5-ml tube with sodium citrate added.
- If a hematoma develops at the venipuncture site, apply warm soaks. If the hematoma is large, monitor pulses distal to the venipuncture site.
- Make sure that subdermal bleeding has stopped before removing pressure.
- Instruct the patient that he may resume medications stopped before the test as ordered.

### Precautions
- This test is contraindicated in the patient with active bleeding or acute infection or illness and in a patient who has had a blood transfusion within 4 weeks.
- Avoid excessive probing during venipuncture and handle the sample gently.

## ▌Fibrin split products
### [FSPs]

After vascular injury causes a fibrin clot to form, the clot is eventually degraded by the enzyme plasmin. The resulting fragments are known as fibrin split products (FSPs). Their measurement helps analyze fibrinolytic (clot-dissolving) system activity. In this test, FSPs are detected in the diluted serum that's left in a blood sample after clotting occurs.

# Causes of disseminated intravascular coagulation

| | |
|---|---|
| Cardiovascular | Fat embolism, acute venous thrombosis, cardiopulmonary bypass surgery, hypovolemic shock, cardiac arrest, and hypotension |
| Infectious | Acute bacteremia, septicemia, and rickettsemia; viral, fungal, and protozoal infection |
| Necrotic | Trauma, destruction of brain tissue, extensive burns, heatstroke, rejection of transplant, and hepatic necrosis |
| Neoplastic | Sarcoma, metastatic carcinoma, acute leukemia, prostate cancer, and giant hemangioma |
| Obstetric | Amniotic fluid embolism, eclampsia, retained dead fetus, retained placenta, abruptio placentae, and gestational hypertension |
| Other | Snakebite, cirrhosis, transfusion of incompatible blood, purpura, and glomerulonephritis |

## Reference values
- Serum contains FSP levels of less than 10 mcg/ml (SI, < 10 mg/L). A quantitative assay shows levels of less than 3 mcg/ml (SI, < 3 mg/L).

## Abnormal results
- FSP levels increase in primary fibrinolytic states caused by increased levels of circulating profibrinolysin; in secondary states caused by disseminated intravascular coagulation (DIC) and subsequent fibrinolysis; and in alcoholic cirrhosis, preeclampsia, abruptio placentae, congenital heart disease, sunstroke, burns, intrauterine death, pulmonary embolus, deep vein thrombosis (transient increase), and myocardial infarction (after 1 or 2 days).
- FSP levels usually exceed 100 mcg/ml (SI, greater than 100 mg/L) in active renal disease or renal transplant rejection.

**DRUG CHALLENGE**

 Pretest administration of heparin (false-high); fibrinolytic drugs, such as urokinase, streptokinase, and tissue plasminogen activator (increase); and large doses of barbiturates (increase)

## Purpose
- To detect FSP in the circulation
- To help determine the presence and the approximate severity of a hyperfibrinolytic state (such as DIC) that may result in primary fibrinogenolysis or hypercoagulability (see *Causes of disseminated intravascular coagulation*)

## Patient preparation
- Explain that the FSP test determines if the blood is clotting normally.
- Tell the patient that a blood sample will be taken. Explain who will perform the venipuncture and when it will be done.
- Explain that the patient may feel slight discomfort from the tourniquet and needle puncture.
- Notify the laboratory and practitioner of medications the patient is taking that may affect test results; these medications may need to be restricted.

- Tell him that he doesn't need to restrict food or fluids.

## Procedure and posttest care

- Confirm the patient's identity using two patient identifiers according to facility policy.
- Perform a venipuncture and draw 2 ml of blood into a plastic syringe.
- Transfer the sample to the laboratory-provided tube, which contains a soybean trypsin inhibitor and bovine thrombin.
- If a hematoma develops at the venipuncture site, apply warm soaks. If the hematoma is large, monitor pulses distal to the venipuncture site.
- Make sure that subdermal bleeding has stopped before removing pressure.
- Instruct the patient that he may resume any medications stopped before the test as ordered.

## Precautions

- Draw the sample before administering heparin to avoid false-positive test results.
- The blood clots within 2 seconds; after clotting, the sample must be sent immediately to the laboratory to be incubated at 98.6° F (37° C) for 30 minutes before testing proceeds.

# International Normalized Ratio
## [INR]

The International Normalized Ratio (INR) system is viewed as the best means of standardizing measurement of prothrombin time to monitor oral anticoagulant therapy. It isn't used as a screening test for coagulopathies.

## Reference values

- For those receiving warfarin therapy, nomal INR values are 2.0 to 3.0 (SI, 2.0 to 3.0).

- For those with mechanical prosthetic heart valves, normal INR values are 2.5 to 3.5 (SI, 2.5 to 3.5).

## Abnormal results

- Increased INR values may indicate disseminated intravascular coagulation, cirrhosis, hepatitis, vitamin K deficiency, salicylate intoxication, uncontrolled oral anticoagulation, or massive blood transfusion.

## Purpose

- To evaluate the effectiveness of oral anticoagulant therapy

## Patient preparation

- Explain that the INR test determines the effectiveness of the patient's oral anticoagulant therapy.
- Tell the patient that a blood sample will be taken. Explain who will perform the venipuncture and when it will be done.
- Tell him that he may feel slight discomfort from the tourniquet and needle puncture.
- Explain that this test will be performed regularly while he's receiving anticoagulant therapy.

## Procedure and posttest care

- Confirm the patient's identity using two patient identifiers according to facility policy.
- Perform a venipuncture and collect the sample in a 4.5-ml tube with sodium citrate added.
- If a hematoma develops at the venipuncture site, apply warm soaks. If the hematoma is large, monitor pulses distal to the venipuncture site.
- Make sure that subdermal bleeding has stopped before removing pressure.

# One-stage factor assay: Extrinsic coagulation system

When prothrombin time (PT) and partial thromboplastin time (PTT) are prolonged, a one-stage assay is used to detect a deficiency of factor II, V, or X. If PT is abnormal but PTT is normal, a deficiency of factor VII may exist.

## Reference values

- The reference range for most factors is 50% to 150% of normal (SI, 0.5 to 1.5).

## Abnormal results

- Deficiency of factor X may also indicate disseminated intravascular coagulation (DIC).
- Factor V deficiency suggests severe hepatic disease, DIC, or fibrinogenolysis.
- Deficiencies of any of the four factors may be congenital.

Alert

Absence of factor II is lethal.

Drug challenge

Oral anticoagulants (possible increase due to inhibition of vitamin K–dependent synthesis and activation of clotting factors II, VII, and X, which form in the liver)

## Purpose

- To identify a specific factor deficiency in a person with prolonged PT or PTT
- To study the patient with congenital or acquired coagulation defects
- To monitor the effects of blood component therapy in the factor-deficient patient

## Patient preparation

- Explain that the one-stage assay test assesses the function of the blood coagulation mechanism.
- Tell the patient that a blood sample will be taken. Explain who will perform the venipuncture and when it will be done.
- Explain to the patient that he may feel slight discomfort from the tourniquet and needle puncture.
- Explain to the factor-deficient patient who is receiving blood component therapy that he may need a series of tests. (See *Factor XIII assay: The missing link.*)
- Notify the laboratory and practitioner of medications the patient is taking that may affect test results; these medications may need to be restricted.
- Inform the patient that he doesn't need to restrict food or fluids.

## Procedure and posttest care

- Confirm the patient's identity using two patient identifiers according to facility policy.
- Perform a venipuncture and collect the sample in a 3- or 4.5-ml siliconized tube.
- Apply direct pressure to the venipuncture site until bleeding stops.
- If a hematoma develops at the venipuncture site, apply warm soaks. If the hematoma is large, monitor pulses distal to the venipuncture site. A patient with a bleeding disorder may require a pressure bandage to stop bleeding at the venipuncture site.
- Instruct the patient that he may resume his usual diet and medications stopped before the test as ordered.

## Factor XIII assay: The missing link

When a patient shows poor wound healing and other symptoms of a bleeding disorder despite normal coagulation test results, a factor XIII assay is recommended. In this test, a plasma sample is incubated with either chloroacetic acid or a urea solution after normal clotting takes place. The clot is observed for 24 hours; if it dissolves, a severe factor XIII deficiency exists.

Factor XIII is responsible for stabilizing the fibrin clot—the final step in the clotting process. If the clot is unstable, it breaks loose, resulting in scarring and poor wound healing. Deficiency of this factor is usually transmitted as an autosomal recessive trait but may result from hepatic disease or tumors.

### Effects of deficiency

The clinical effects of factor XIII deficiency include umbilical bleeding in the neonate; prolonged bleeding after trauma; hemarthrosis; spontaneous abortion (rarely); intraovarial bleeding (more common in factor XIII deficiency than in other bleeding disorders); and recurrent ecchymoses, hematomas, and poor wound healing. Bleeding after trauma may begin immediately or may be delayed for as long as 12 to 36 hours.

### Improving prognosis

Treatment with infusions of plasma or cryoprecipitate has improved the prognosis of the patient with factor XIII deficiency; in some cases, the patient may even live a normal life. However, before appropriate treatment can begin, diagnostic evaluation must rule out other bleeding disorders. Dysfibrinogenemia, hyperfibrinogenemia, and disseminated intravascular coagulation also cause rapid clot dissolution in this assay but, unlike factor XIII deficiency, they also cause an abnormal fibrinogen level and thrombin time.

### Precautions

▪ If the patient has a suspected coagulation defect, avoid excessive probing during venipuncture, don't leave the tourniquet on too long (it will cause bruising), and apply pressure to the puncture site for 5 minutes or until the bleeding stops.

## One-stage factor assay: Intrinsic coagulation system

When prothrombin time is normal but partial thromboplastin time is abnormal, a one-stage assay is used to identify a deficiency in the intrinsic coagulation system (factor VIII, IX, XI, or XII).

### Reference values

▪ The reference range for most factors is 50% to 150% of normal activity (SI, 0.5 to 1.5).
▪ Factor VIII may be increased in pregnant patients.

### Abnormal results

▪ Factor VIII deficiency may indicate hemophilia A, von Willebrand's disease, or a factor VIII inhibitor. An acquired deficiency of factor VIII may result from disseminated intravascular coagulation or fibrinolysis. Factor VIII antigen and ristocetin cofactor tests distinguish between hemophilia A (and its carrier state) and von Willebrand's disease.
▪ A factor IX deficiency may suggest hemophilia B, or it may be acquired as a result of hepatic disease, a factor IX in-

hibitor, a vitamin K deficiency, or coumadin therapy.
■ Factor VIII and IX inhibitors, which occur after blood transfusions in patients deficient in either factor, are antibodies specific to each factor.
■ A factor XI deficiency may appear after the stress of trauma or surgery or transiently in a neonate.
■ A factor XII deficiency may be inherited or acquired (such as nephrosis) and may also appear transiently in a neonate.

### Purpose
■ To identify a specific factor deficiency
■ To study a patient with a congenital or an acquired coagulation defect
■ To monitor the effects of blood component therapy in the factor-deficient patient

### Patient preparation
■ Explain that the one-stage assay test assesses the function of the blood coagulation mechanism.
■ Tell the patient that a blood sample will be taken. Explain who will perform the venipuncture and when it will be done.
■ Explain that the patient may feel slight discomfort from the tourniquet and needle puncture.
■ Notify the laboratory and practitioner of medications the patient is taking that may affect test results; these medications may need to be restricted.
■ Explain to the factor-deficient patient who is receiving blood component therapy that a series of tests may be needed to monitor therapeutic progress.
■ Inform the patient that he doesn't need to restrict food or fluids.

### Procedure and posttest care
■ Confirm the patient's identity using two patient identifiers according to facility policy.

■ Perform a venipuncture and collect the sample in a 3- or 4.5-ml siliconized tube.
■ Apply direct pressure to the venipuncture site until bleeding subsides.
■ If a hematoma develops at the venipuncture site, apply warm soaks. If the hematoma is large, monitor pulses distal to the venipuncture site. A patient with a bleeding disorder may require a pressure bandage to stop bleeding at the venipuncture site.
■ Instruct the patient that he may resume any medications stopped before the test as ordered.

### Precautions
■ If a coagulation defect is suspected, avoid excessive probing during venipuncture, don't leave the tourniquet on too long (it will cause bruising), and apply pressure to the puncture site for 5 minutes or until the bleeding stops.

# ■ Partial thromboplastin time
### [PTT]

The partial thromboplastin time (PTT) evaluates all the clotting factors of the intrinsic pathway (except platelets) by measuring how long it takes for a fibrin clot to form after calcium and a phospholipid emulsion are added to a plasma sample. An activator such as kaolin is used to shorten clotting time.

### Reference values
■ A fibrin clot forms 21 to 35 seconds (SI, 21 to 35 seconds) after reagents are added.
■ For a patient receiving anticoagulant therapy, ask the practitioner to specify the reference values.

### Abnormal results
■ A prolonged PTT may indicate a deficiency of certain plasma clotting factors,

the presence of heparin or fibrin split products, fibrinolysins, or circulating anticoagulants that are antibodies to specific clotting factors.

## Purpose
- To screen for deficiencies of the clotting factors in the intrinsic pathways
- To evaluate excessive clotting and excessive bleeding disorders
- To monitor response to heparin therapy

## Patient preparation
- Explain that the PTT test determines if the blood is clotting normally.
- Tell the patient that a blood sample will be taken. Explain who will perform the venipuncture and when it will be done.
- Explain to the patient that he may feel slight discomfort from the tourniquet and needle puncture.
- Tell him that he doesn't need to restrict food or fluids.
- Tell the patient receiving heparin therapy that this test may be repeated at regular intervals to assess his response to treatment.

## Procedure and posttest care
- Confirm the patient's identity using two patient identifiers according to facility policy.
- Perform a venipuncture and collect the sample in a 7-ml tube with sodium citrate added.
- If a hematoma develops at the venipuncture site, apply warm soaks. If the hematoma is large, monitor pulses distal to the venipuncture site.
- Make sure that subdermal bleeding has stopped before removing pressure.

## Precautions
- Completely fill the collection tube, invert it gently several times, and send it to the laboratory on ice.

- For a patient receiving anticoagulant therapy, additional pressure may be needed at the venipuncture site to control bleeding.

# Plasminogen
[profibrinolysis]

Plasma plasminogen testing assesses plasminogen levels in a plasma sample. During fibrinolysis, plasmin dissolves fibrin clots to prevent excessive coagulation and impaired blood flow. Because plasmin doesn't circulate in active form, it can't be directly measured. Its circulating precursor, plasminogen, can be measured and used to evaluate the fibrinolytic system.

## Reference values
- Plasminogen levels are 10 to 20 mg/dl (SI, 0.1 to 0.2 g/L).

## Abnormal results
- Diminished plasminogen levels can result from disseminated intravascular coagulation, tumors, preeclampsia, and eclampsia, all of which accelerate plasminogen conversion to plasmin and increase fibrinolysis. Some liver diseases prevent formation of sufficient plasminogen, decreasing fibrinolysis.

### DRUG CHALLENGE

 Thrombolytic drugs, such as streptokinase and urokinase (possible decrease)

## Purpose
- To assess fibrinolysis
- To detect congenital and acquired fibrinolytic disorders

## Patient preparation
- Explain that the plasminogen test evaluates blood clotting.

- Tell the patient that a blood sample will be taken. Explain who will perform the venipuncture and when it will be done.
- Explain to the patient that he may feel slight discomfort from the tourniquet and needle puncture.
- Notify the laboratory and practitioner of medications the patient is taking that may affect test results; these medications may need to be restricted.
- Tell the patient that he doesn't need to restrict food or fluids.

### Procedure and posttest care

- Confirm the patient's identity using two patient identifiers according to facility policy.
- Perform a venipuncture and collect the sample in a 4.5-ml siliconized tube.
- If a hematoma develops at the venipuncture site, apply warm soaks. If the hematoma is large, monitor pulses distal to the venipuncture site.
- Make sure that subdermal bleeding has stopped before removing pressure.
- Instruct the patient that he may any resume medications stopped before the test as ordered.

### Precautions

- Collect the sample as quickly as possible to prevent stasis, which can slow blood flow, causing coagulation and plasminogen activation.
- To prevent hemolysis, avoid excessive probing during venipuncture and rough handling of the sample.
- Invert the tube gently several times and send the sample to the laboratory immediately. If testing must be delayed, plasma must be separated and frozen at $-94°$ F ($-67.8°$ C).

## Protein C
### [protein C antigen]

Vitamin K–dependent, protein C is produced in the liver and circulates in the plasma. It acts as a potent anticoagulant by suppressing activated factors V and VIII. Deficiencies of protein C may be acquired or congenital.

If a deficiency of protein C is identified, further immunologic tests may be needed to determine the type of deficiency. Identifying the role of protein C deficiency in idiopathic venous thrombosis may help prevent thromboembolism.

### Reference values

- Normal values of protein C are 70% to 140% (SI, 0.70 to 1.40).

### Abnormal results

- Rare, homozygous protein C deficiency causes rapidly fatal thrombosis in the perinatal period, a condition known as purpura fulminans.
- More common heterozygous deficiency is associated with genetic susceptibility to venous thromboembolism before age 30 and continuing throughout life.
- Protein C deficiency is also seen in cirrhosis, in vitamin K deficiency, and in those receiving warfarin.

### Purpose

- To investigate the mechanism of idiopathic venous thrombosis

### Patient preparation

- Explain that the protein C test evaluates blood clotting.
- Tell the patient that a blood sample will be taken. Explain who will perform the venipuncture and when it will be done.
- Tell him that he may feel slight discomfort from the tourniquet and needle puncture.

- Tell him that he doesn't need to restrict food or fluids.
- Notify the laboratory and practitioner of medications the patient is taking that may affect test results; these medications may need to be restricted.

### Procedure and posttest care
- Confirm the patient's identity using two patient identifiers according to facility policy.
- Perform a venipuncture. Collect a 3-ml sample in a siliconized vacuum specimen tube or in a special syringe with anticoagulant provided by the laboratory.
- Apply direct pressure to the venipuncture site until bleeding stops. If a hematoma develops at the venipuncture site, apply warm soaks. If the hematoma is large, monitor pulses distal to the venipuncture site.
- Instruct the patient to resume any medications stopped before the test as ordered.

## ▌Prothrombin time
### [PT]

Prothrombin time (PT) measures the time required for a fibrin clot to form in a citrated plasma sample after addition of calcium ions and tissue thromboplastin (factor III).

### Reference values
- PT values are 10 to 14 seconds (SI, 10 to 14 seconds), depending on the source of tissue thromboplastin and the type of sensing devices used to measure clot formation.
- In a patient receiving oral anticoagulants, PT is usually maintained between 1 and 2.5 times the normal control value.

### Abnormal results
- Prolonged PT may indicate deficiencies in fibrinogen; prothrombin; factors V, VII, or X (specific assays can pinpoint such deficiencies); or vitamin K. It may also result from ongoing oral anticoagulant therapy.
- A prolonged PT that exceeds 2.5 times the normal control value is commonly associated with abnormal bleeding.

**DRUG CHALLENGE**

 Salicylates, more than 1 g/day (increase); antihistamines, chloral hydrate, corticosteroids, digoxin, diuretics, glutethimide, griseofulvin, progestin-estrogen combinations, pyrazinamide, vitamin K, and xanthines, such as caffeine and theophylline (possible decrease); corticotropin, anabolic steroids, cholestyramine resin, heparin I.V. (within 5 hours of sample collection), indomethacin, mefenamic acid, para-aminosalicylic acid, methimazole, oxyphenbutazone, phenylbutazone, phenytoin, propylthiouracil, quinidine, quinine, thyroid hormones, vitamin A, or alcohol in excess (prolonged PT); antibiotics, barbiturates, hydroxyzine, sulfonamides, mineral oil, or clofibrate (possible increase or decrease)

### Purpose
- To evaluate the extrinsic coagulation system (factors II, V, VII, and X and prothrombin and fibrinogen)
- To monitor response to oral anticoagulant therapy

### Patient preparation
- Explain that the PT test determines if the blood is clotting normally.
- Notify the laboratory and practitioner of medications the patient is taking that may affect test results; these medications may need to be restricted.

- Tell the patient that a blood sample will be taken. Explain who will perform the venipuncture and when it will be done.
- Explain to him that he may feel slight discomfort from the tourniquet and needle puncture.
- Explain that this test monitors the effects of oral anticoagulants; the test will be performed daily when therapy begins and repeated at longer intervals as medication levels stabilize.
- Tell the patient that he doesn't need to restrict food or fluids.

### Procedure and posttest care

- Confirm the patient's identity using two patient identifiers according to facility policy.
- Perform a venipuncture and collect the sample in a 3- or 4.5-ml siliconized tube.
- If a hematoma develops at the venipuncture site, apply warm soaks. If the hematoma is large, monitor pulses distal to the venipuncture site.
- Make sure that subdermal bleeding has stopped before removing pressure.
- Instruct the patient that he may resume his usual diet and medications stopped before the test as ordered.

### Precautions

- Completely fill the collection tube and invert it gently several times to mix the sample and the anticoagulant thoroughly. If the tube isn't filled to the correct volume, an excess of citrate appears in the sample.
- To prevent hemolysis, avoid excessive probing during venipuncture and handle the sample gently.

# Thrombin time
## [thrombin clotting time]

Plasma thrombin time measures how quickly a clot forms when a standard amount of bovine thrombin is added to a platelet-poor plasma sample from the patient and to a normal plasma control sample. This measures the last step of the coagulation cascade, which is the conversion of fibrinogen to fibrin. After thrombin is added, the clotting times for each sample are recorded and compared. This test allows a quick but imprecise estimation of plasma fibrinogen levels, which are a function of clotting time. (For information about another test that helps determine the cause of coagulation disorders, see *Understanding the antithrombin III test.*)

### Reference values

- Normal thrombin time values are 10 to 15 seconds (SI, 10 to 15 seconds).

### Abnormal results

- A prolonged thrombin time may indicate heparin therapy, hepatic disease, disseminated intravascular coagulation (DIC), hypofibrinogenemia, or dysfibrinogenemia.
- The patient with a prolonged thrombin time may require measurement of fibrinogen levels; in suspected DIC, the test for fibrin split products is also necessary.

**DRUG CHALLENGE**

 Heparin, fibrinogen, or fibrin degradation products (possible increase)

### Purpose

- To detect a fibrinogen deficiency or defect

## Understanding the antithrombin III test

The antithrombin III (AT III) test helps detect the cause of impaired coagulation, especially hypercoagulation, by measuring levels of AT III, a protein that inactivates thrombin and inhibits coagulation. AT III may be evaluated by a functional clotting assay or synthetic substrates. Exogenous heparin is added to a fresh, citrated blood sample to accelerate activity, then excess thrombin (factor Xa) is added to the plasma. The amount of factor Xa not activated by AT III is quantitated and compared with that of a normal control sample. Reference values, which may vary for each laboratory, should lie between 80% and 120% of normal.

Decreased AT III levels can indicate disseminated intravascular coagulation or thromboembolic disorders, hypercoagulation disorders, or hepatic disorders. Slightly decreased levels can result from hormonal contraceptives. Elevated levels can result from kidney transplantation and the use of oral anticoagulants or anabolic steroids.

■ To aid in the diagnosis of DIC and hepatic disease
■ To monitor the effectiveness of treatment with heparin or thrombolytic agents

### Patient preparation

■ Explain that the thrombin time test determines whether the blood is clotting normally.
■ Notify the laboratory and practitioner of medications the patient is taking that may affect test results; these medications may need to be restricted.
■ Tell the patient that a blood sample will be taken. Explain who will perform the venipuncture and when it will be done.
■ Explain to the patient that he may feel slight discomfort from the tourniquet and needle puncture.
■ Tell him that he doesn't need to restrict food or fluids.

### Procedure and posttest care

■ Confirm the patient's identity using two patient identifiers according to facility policy.
■ Perform a venipuncture and collect the sample in a 3- to 4.5-ml siliconized tube.

■ If a hematoma develops at the venipuncture site, apply warm soaks. If the hematoma is large, monitor pulses distal to the venipuncture site.
■ Make sure that subdermal bleeding has stopped before removing pressure.
■ Tell the patient to resume any medications stopped before the test as ordered.

### Precautions

■ If the tube isn't filled to the correct volume, an excess of citrate appears in the sample. Completely fill the collection tube and invert it gently several times to mix the sample and the anticoagulant thoroughly.
■ To prevent hemolysis, avoid excessive probing during venipuncture and rough handling of the sample.

# Blood gas analysis and electrolytes

## Blood gas analysis

### Alveolar-to-arterial oxygen gradient
[A-aDo$_2$]

The alveolar-to-arterial oxygen gradient (A-aDo$_2$) test can help identify the cause of hypoxemia and intrapulmonary shunting by approximating the partial pressure of oxygenation of the alveoli and arteries. It may help differentiate among the possible causes (ventilated alveoli but no perfusion, unventilated alveoli with perfusion, and collapse of the alveoli and capillaries).

#### Reference values
- A-aDo$_2$ at rest is normally less than 10 mm Hg and at maximum exercise ranges from 20 to 30 mm Hg.

#### Abnormal results
- Increased A-aDo$_2$ values may be caused by mucus plugs, bronchospasm, or airway collapse (asthma, bronchitis, emphysema).
- Hypoxemia results in increased A-aDo$_2$ values and may be caused by arterial septal defects, pneumothorax, atelectasis, emboli, or edema.

#### Purpose
- To evaluate the efficiency of gas exchange
- To assess the integrity of the ventilatory control system
- To monitor respiratory therapy

#### Patient preparation
- Explain that the A-aDo$_2$ test evaluates how well the lungs are delivering oxygen to and eliminating carbon dioxide from the blood.
- Tell the patient that the test requires a blood sample. Explain who will perform the arterial puncture and when it will be done.
- Tell the patient that he doesn't need to restrict food or fluids.
- Instruct him to breathe normally during the test and warn him that he may experience cramping or throbbing pain at the puncture site.

#### Procedure and posttest care
- Confirm the patient's identity using two patient identifiers according to facility policy.
- Perform an arterial puncture or draw blood from an arterial line using a heparinized blood gas syringe.

Eliminate all air from the sample and place it on ice immediately.

■ Apply pressure to the puncture for 3 to 5 minutes or until bleeding stops.
■ Place a gauze pad over the site and tape it in place but don't tape the entire circumference.
■ Monitor vital signs and observe for signs of circulatory impairment, such as swelling, discoloration, pain, numbness, and tingling distal to the puncture site.
■ Watch for bleeding from the puncture site.
■ The arterial sample is analyzed for partial pressure of arterial oxygen ($Pao_2$), partial pressure of arterial carbon dioxide ($Paco_2$), barometric pressure (PB), water vapor pressure ($PH_2O$), and fraction of inspired oxygen ($Fio_2$) (21% for room air). From these values, the alveolar oxygen tension ($PAo_2$), the arterial-to-alveolar oxygen ratio (a/A ratio), and the $A\text{-}aDo_2$ are derived by solving these mathematical formulas:

$$PAo_2 = Fio_2 (PB - PH_2O) - 1.25 (Paco_2)$$

$$\text{a/A ratio} = Pao_2 \div PAo_2$$

$$A\text{-}aDo_2 = PAo_2 - Pao_2$$

■ Based on the results of the formulas, appropriate interventions to correct patient problems are initiated.

### Precautions

■ Before sending the sample to the laboratory, note on the laboratory request whether the patient was breathing room air or receiving oxygen therapy when the sample was collected.
■ If the patient was receiving oxygen therapy, note the flow rate and method of delivery. If he was on a ventilator, note the $Fio_2$, tidal volume, mode, respiratory rate, and positive end-expiratory pressure.

■ Note the patient's core temperature.

# Arterial blood gas analysis
## [ABG analysis]

Arterial blood gas (ABG) analysis measures the partial pressure of arterial oxygen ($Pao_2$), the partial pressure of arterial carbon dioxide ($Paco_2$), the pH of an arterial sample, oxygen content ($O_2CT$), arterial oxygen saturation ($Sao_2$), and bicarbonate ($HCO_3^-$) values. A blood sample for ABG analysis may be drawn by percutaneous arterial puncture or from an arterial line.

The $Pao_2$ indicates how much oxygen the lungs are delivering to the blood. The $Paco_2$ indicates how efficiently the lungs eliminate carbon dioxide. The pH indicates the acid-base or hydrogen ion ($H^+$) level of the blood. Acidity indicates $H^+$ excess; alkalinity indicates $H^+$ deficit. (See *Balancing pH*, page 46.) $O_2CT$, $Sao_2$, and $HCO_3^-$ values also aid diagnosis.

### Reference values

■ $Pao_2$ values are 80 to 100 mm Hg (SI, 10.6 to 13.3 kPa).
■ $Paco_2$ values are 35 to 45 mm Hg (SI, 4.7 to 5.3 kPa).
■ pH values are 7.35 to 7.45 (SI, 7.35 to 7.45).
■ $O_2CT$ values are 15% to 23% (SI, 0.15 to 0.23).
■ $Sao_2$ values are 94% to 100% (SI, 0.94 to 1.00).
■ $HCO_3^-$ values are 22 to 25 mEq/L (SI, 22 to 25 mmol/L).

### Abnormal results

■ Low $Pao_2$, $O_2CT$, and $Sao_2$ levels and a high $Paco_2$ level may result from conditions that impair respiratory function, such as respiratory muscle weakness or paralysis, respiratory center inhibition (from head injury, brain tumor, or drug

# Balancing pH

To measure the acidity or alkalinity of a solution, chemists use a pH scale of 1 to 15 that measures hydrogen ion ($H^+$) level. As $H^+$ and acidity increase, pH falls below 7.0, which is neutral. Conversely, when $H^+$ decreases, pH and alkalinity increase. Acid-base balance, or homeostasis of $H^+$, is necessary if the body's enzyme systems are to work properly.

The slightest change in $H^+$ level changes the rate of cellular chemical reactions; a severe enough change can be fatal. To maintain a normal blood pH—generally between 7.35 and 7.45—the body relies on three mechanisms.

## Buffers

Chemically composed of two substances, buffers prevent radical pH changes by replacing strong acids added to a solution (such as blood) with weaker ones. For example, strong acids capable of yielding many hydrogen ions are replaced by weaker ones that yield fewer hydrogen ions. Because of the principal buffer coupling of bicarbonate ($HCO_3^-$) and carbonic acid ($H_2CO_3$)—normally in a ratio of 20:1—the plasma acid-base level rarely fluctuates. Increased $HCO_3^-$ indicates alkalosis, whereas decreased $HCO_3^-$ points to acidosis. Increased $H_2CO_3$ indicates acidosis, and decreased $H_2CO_3$ indicates alkalosis.

## Respiration

Respiration is important in maintaining blood pH. The lungs convert $H_2CO_3$ to carbon dioxide ($CO_2$) and water ($H_2O$). With every expiration, $CO_2$ and $H_2O$ leave the body, decreasing the $H_2CO_3$ content of the blood. Consequently, fewer hydrogen ions are formed, and blood pH increases. When the blood's $H^+$ or $H_2CO_3$ content increases, neurons in the respiratory center stimulate respiration.

Hyperventilation eliminates $CO_2$, and hence $H_2CO_3$, from the body; reduces $H^+$ formation; and increases pH. Conversely, increased blood pH from alkalosis—decreased $H^+$ concentration—causes hypoventilation, which restores blood pH to its normal level by retaining $CO_2$ and thus increasing $H^+$ formation.

## Urinary excretion

The third factor in acid-base balance is urine excretion. Because the kidneys excrete varying amounts of acids and bases, they control urine pH, which in turn affects blood pH. For example, when blood pH is decreased, the distal and collecting tubules remove excessive $H^+$ ions ($H_2CO_3$ forms in the tubular cells and dissociates into H and $HCO_3^-$) and displace them in urine, thereby eliminating H from the body. In exchange, basic ions in the urine—usually sodium—diffuse into the tubular cells, where they combine with $HCO_3^-$. This sodium bicarbonate is then reabsorbed in the blood, resulting in decreased urine pH and, more important, increased blood pH.

abuse), and airway obstruction (possibly from mucus plugs or a tumor).
■ Decreased values may result from bronchiole obstruction caused by asthma or emphysema, from an abnormal ventilation-perfusion ratio due to partially blocked alveoli or pulmonary capillaries, or from alveoli that are damaged or filled with fluid because of disease, hemorrhage, or near-drowning.
■ When inspired air contains insufficient oxygen, $Pao_2$, $O_2CT$, and $Sao_2$ decrease, but $Paco_2$ may be normal. Such findings are common in pneumothorax, impaired diffusion between alveoli and blood (due to interstitial fibrosis, for ex-

ample), or an arteriovenous shunt that permits blood to bypass the lungs.
- Low $O_2CT$—with normal $PaO_2$, $SaO_2$, and possibly $PaCO_2$ values—may result from severe anemia, decreased blood volume, and reduced hemoglobin oxygen-carrying capacity.
- ABGs can also give considerable information about acid-base disorders. (See *Acid-base disorders*, pages 48 and 49.)

### DRUG CHALLENGE

$HCO_3^-$, ethacrynic acid, hydrocortisone, metolazone, prednisone, and thiazides (may increase $PaCO_2$); acetazolamide, methicillin, nitrofurantoin, and tetracycline (may decrease $PaCO_2$)

### Purpose

- To evaluate the efficiency of pulmonary gas exchange
- To assess the integrity of the ventilatory control system
- To determine the acid-base level of the blood
- To monitor respiratory therapy

### Patient preparation

- Explain that ABG analysis evaluates how well the lungs are delivering oxygen to and eliminating carbon dioxide from the blood.
- Tell the patient that the test requires a blood sample. Explain who will perform the arterial puncture and when, and which site—radial, brachial, or femoral artery—has been selected for the puncture.
- Tell the patient that he doesn't need to restrict food or fluids.
- Instruct him to breathe normally during the test and warn him that he may experience a brief cramping or throbbing pain at the puncture site.

### Procedure and posttest care

- Confirm the patient's identity using two patient identifiers according to facility policy.
- Perform an arterial puncture, or draw blood from an arterial line. Use a heparinized blood gas syringe to draw the sample. Eliminate air from the sample, place it on ice immediately, and transport it for analysis.
- After applying pressure to the puncture site for 3 to 5 minutes or until bleeding has stopped; tape a gauze pad firmly over it. (If the puncture site is on the arm, don't tape the entire circumference; this may restrict circulation.)
- If the patient is receiving anticoagulants or has a coagulopathy, apply pressure to the puncture site longer than 5 minutes, if necessary.
- Monitor vital signs and observe for signs of circulatory impairment, such as swelling, discoloration, pain, numbness, and tingling distal to the puncture site.
- Watch for bleeding from the puncture site.

### Precautions

- Wait at least 20 minutes before drawing arterial blood when starting, changing, or stopping oxygen therapy; after starting or changing settings of mechanical ventilation; or after extubation.
- Before sending the sample to the laboratory, note on the laboratory request whether the patient was breathing room air or receiving oxygen therapy when the sample was collected.
- If the patient was receiving oxygen therapy, note the flow rate and method of delivery. If he was on a ventilator, note the fraction of inspired oxygen, tidal volume, mode, respiratory rate, and positive-end expiratory pressure.
- Note the patient's core temperature.

# Acid-base disorders

| Disorders and ABG findings | Possible causes |
|---|---|
| **Respiratory acidosis (excess $CO_2$ retention)**<br>pH < 7.35 (SI, < 7.35)<br>$HCO_3^-$ >26 mEq/L (SI, > 26 mmol/L)<br>(if compensating)<br>$Paco_2$ > 45 mm Hg (SI, > 5.3 kPa) | ■ Central nervous system depression from drugs, injury, or disease<br>■ Asphyxia<br>■ Hypoventilation due to pulmonary, cardiac, musculoskeletal, or neuromuscular disease<br>■ Obesity<br>■ Postoperative pain<br>■ Abdominal distention |
| **Respiratory alkalosis (excess $CO_2$ excretion)**<br>pH > 7.45 (SI, > 7.45)<br>$HCO_3^-$ < 22 mEq/L (SI, < 22 mmol/L)<br>(if compensating)<br>$Paco_2$ < 35 mm Hg (SI, < 4.7 kPa) | ■ Hyperventilation due to anxiety, pain, or improper ventilator settings<br>■ Respiratory stimulation caused by drugs, disease, hypoxia, fever, or high room temperature<br>■ Gram-negative bacteremia<br>■ Compensation for metabolic acidosis (chronic renal failure) |
| **Metabolic acidosis ($HCO_3^-$ loss, acid retention)**<br>pH < 7.35 (SI, < 7.35)<br>$HCO_3^-$ < 22 mEq/L (SI, < 22 mmol/L)<br>$Paco_2$ < 35 mm Hg (SI, < 4.7 kPa)<br>(if compensating) | ■ $HCO_3^-$ depletion due to renal disease, diarrhea, or small-bowel fistulas<br>■ Excessive production of organic acids due to hepatic disease; endocrine disorders, including diabetes mellitus, hypoxia, shock, and drug intoxication<br>■ Inadequate excretion of acids due to renal disease |
| **Metabolic alkalosis ($HCO_3^-$ retention, acid loss)**<br>pH > 7.45 (SI, > 7.45)<br>$HCO_3^-$ > 26 mEq/L (SI, > 26 mmol/L)<br>$Paco_2$ > 45 mm Hg (SI, > 5.3 kPa) | ■ Loss of hydrochloric acid from prolonged vomiting or gastric suctioning<br>■ Loss of potassium due to increased renal excretion (as in diuretic therapy) or steroid overdose<br>■ Excessive alkali ingestion<br>■ Compensation for chronic respiratory acidosis |

## Signs and symptoms

Diaphoresis, headache, tachycardia, confusion, restlessness, apprehension

Rapid, deep breathing; paresthesia; light-headedness; twitching; anxiety; fear

Rapid, deep breathing; fruity breath; fatigue; headache; lethargy; drowsiness; nausea; vomiting; coma (if severe)

Slow, shallow breathing; hypertonic muscles; restlessness; twitching; confusion; irritability; apathy; tetany; seizures; coma (if severe)

# ■ Arterial-to-alveolar oxygen ratio
## [a/A ratio]

Using calculations based on the patient's laboratory values, the arterial-to-alveolar oxygen ratio (a/A ratio) test can help identify the cause of hypoxemia and intrapulmonary shunting by providing an approximation of the partial pressure of oxygenation of the alveoli and arteries. It may help differentiate among the possible causes (ventilated alveoli but no perfusion, unventilated alveoli with perfusion, and collapse of the alveoli and capillaries).

### Reference values
■ The normal a/A ratio is 75%.

### Abnormal results
■ Increased values may be caused by mucus plugs, bronchospasm, or airway collapse (asthma, bronchitis, emphysema).
■ Increased $A-aDo_2$ from hypoxemia may be caused by arterial septal defects, pneumothorax, atelectasis, emboli, or edema.

### Purpose
■ To evaluate the efficiency of gas exchange
■ To assess the integrity of the ventilatory control system
■ To monitor respiratory therapy

### Patient preparation
■ Explain that the a/A ratio test evaluates how well the lungs are delivering oxygen to and eliminating carbon dioxide from the blood.
■ Tell the patient that the test requires a blood sample. Explain who will perform the arterial puncture and when it will be done.
■ Tell the patient that he doesn't need to restrict food or fluids.

■ Instruct him to breathe normally during the test and warn him that he may experience cramping or throbbing pain at the puncture site.

### Procedure and posttest care

■ Confirm the patient's identity using two patient identifiers according to facility policy.
■ Perform an arterial puncture or draw blood from an arterial line using a heparinized blood gas syringe.
■ Eliminate all air from the sample and place it on ice immediately.
■ Apply pressure to the puncture for 3 to 5 minutes or until bleeding has stopped.
■ Place a gauze pad over the site and tape it in place but don't tape the entire circumference.
■ Monitor vital signs and observe for signs of circulatory impairment, such as swelling, discoloration, pain, numbness, and tingling distal to the puncture site.
■ Watch for bleeding from the puncture site.
■ The arterial sample is analyzed for partial pressure of arterial oxygen ($Pa_{O_2}$), partial pressure of arterial carbon dioxide ($Pa_{CO_2}$), barometric pressure ($P_B$), water vapor pressure ($PH_2O$), and fractional concentration of inspired oxygen ($FI_{O_2}$) (21% for room air). From these values, the alveolar oxygen tension ($PA_{O_2}$), the a/A ratio, and the alveolar-to-arterial oxygen gradient ($A\text{-}aD_{O_2}$) are derived by solving these mathematical formulas:

$$PA_{O_2} = FI_{O_2} (P_B - PH_2O) - 1.25 (Pa_{CO_2})$$
$$\text{a/A ratio} = Pa_{O_2} \div PA_{O_2}$$
$$A\text{-}aD_{O_2} = PA_{O_2} - Pa_{O_2}$$

■ Based on the results of the formulas, appropriate interventions are started to correct patient problems.

### Precautions

■ Before sending the sample to the laboratory, note on the laboratory request whether the patient was breathing room air or receiving oxygen therapy when the sample was collected.
■ If the patient was receiving oxygen therapy, note the flow rate and method of delivery. If he was on a ventilator, note the $FI_{O_2}$, tidal volume, mode, respiratory rate, and positive end-expiratory pressure.
■ Note the patient's core temperature.

# ▌Total carbon dioxide content

When carbon dioxide ($CO_2$) pressure in red blood cells exceeds 40 mm Hg, $CO_2$ spills out of the cells and dissolves in plasma. There it may combine with water to form carbonic acid, which in turn may dissociate into hydrogen and bicarbonate ions.

The total $CO_2$ content test measures the total concentration of all forms of $CO_2$ in serum, plasma, or whole blood samples. It's commonly ordered for patients with respiratory insufficiency and is usually included in an assessment of electrolyte balance. Test results are most significant when considered with pH and arterial blood gas values.

Because about 90% of $CO_2$ in serum is in the form of bicarbonate ($HCO_3^-$), this test closely assesses $HCO_3^-$ levels. Total $CO_2$ content reflects the adequacy of gas exchange in the lungs and the efficiency of the carbonic acid–bicarbonate buffer system, which maintains acid-base balance and normal pH.

### Reference values

■ Total $CO_2$ levels are 22 to 26 mEq/L (SI, 22 to 26 mmol/L).
■ Levels may vary, depending on the patient's gender and age.

### Abnormal results

■ High total $CO_2$ levels may occur in metabolic alkalosis, respiratory acidosis, primary aldosteronism, and Cushing's syndrome.

- Total $CO_2$ levels may also increase after excessive loss of acids, as with severe vomiting and continuous gastric drainage.
- Decreased total $CO_2$ levels are common in metabolic acidosis. Decreased total $CO_2$ levels in metabolic acidosis also result from loss of $HCO_3^-$.
- Total $CO_2$ levels may decrease in respiratory alkalosis.

### DRUG CHALLENGE

 Excessive use of corticotropin, cortisone, or thiazide diuretics; excessive ingestion of alkali or licorice (increase); salicylates, paraldehyde, methicillin, dimercaprol, ammonium chloride, and acetazolamide; ingestion of ethylene glycol or methyl alcohol (decrease)

### Purpose
- To help evaluate acid-base balance

### Patient preparation
- Explain that the total $CO_2$ content test measures the amount of $CO_2$ in the blood.
- Tell the patient that the test requires a blood sample. Explain who will perform the venipuncture and when it will be done.
- Explain to the patient that he may experience discomfort from the tourniquet and needle puncture.
- Tell the patient that he doesn't need to restrict food or fluids.
- Notify the laboratory and practitioner of medications the patient is taking that may affect test results; these medications may need to be restricted.

### Procedure and posttest care
- Confirm the patient's identity using two patient identifiers according to facility policy.
- Perform a venipuncture.
- When $CO_2$ content is measured along with electrolytes, a 3- or 4-ml clot activator tube may be used.
- When this test is performed alone, a heparinized tube is appropriate.
- Apply direct pressure to the venipuncture site until the bleeding has stopped.
- If a hematoma develops at the venipuncture site, apply warm soaks. If the hematoma is large, monitor pulses distal to the venipuncture site.
- Instruct the patient to resume medications stopped before the test as ordered.

### Precautions
- Fill the tube completely to prevent diffusion of $CO_2$ into the vacuum.

---

## Electrolyte tests

### Anion gap

Total levels of cations and anions are usually equal, making serum electrically neutral. Measuring the gap between measured cation and anion levels provides information about the level of anions (including sulfate; phosphate; organic acids, such as ketone bodies and lactic acid; and proteins) that are not routinely measured in laboratory tests. In metabolic acidosis, measuring the anion gap helps to identify the type of acidosis and possible causes. Further tests are usually needed to determine the specific cause of metabolic acidosis.

### Reference values
- Normal anion gaps are 8 to 14 mEq/L (SI, 8 to 14 mmol/L). A normal anion gap doesn't rule out metabolic acidosis,

## Anion gap and metabolic acidosis

Metabolic acidosis with a *normal anion gap* (8 to 14 mEq/L) occurs in conditions characterized by loss of bicarbonate, such as:

■ Hypokalemic acidosis due to renal tubular acidosis, diarrhea, or ureteral diversions

■ Hyperkalemic acidosis due to acidifying agents (for example, ammonium chloride, hydrochloric acid), hydronephrosis, sickle cell nephropathy)

Metabolic acidosis with an *increased anion gap* (>14 mEq/L) occurs in conditions characterized by accumulation of organic acids, sulfates, or phosphates, such as:

■ Renal failure

■ Ketoacidosis due to starvation, diabetes mellitus, or alcohol abuse

■ Lactic acidosis

■ Ingestion of toxins, such as salicylates, methanol, ethylene glycol (antifreeze), and paraldehyde.

including hyperchloremic acidosis, renal tubular acidosis, and severe bicarbonate-wasting conditions, such as biliary or pancreatic fistulas and poorly functioning ileal loops. Normal anion gap acidosis results from loss of bicarbonate in the urine or other body fluids, which causes the anion gap to remain unchanged. (See *Anion gap and metabolic acidosis*.)

### Abnormal results

■ An increased anion gap indicates an increase in one or more of the unmeasured anions (sulfate; phosphates; organic acids, such as ketone bodies and lactic acid; and proteins). This may occur with acidoses that are characterized by excessive organic or inorganic acids, such as lactic acidosis or ketoacidosis.

■ When acidosis results from an accumulation of metabolic acids—as occurs in lactic acidosis, for example—the anion gap increases (> 14 mEq/L) with the increase in unmeasured anions. Metabolic acidosis caused by such an accumulation is known as high anion gap acidosis.

■ A decreased anion gap is rare but may occur with hypermagnesemia and paraproteinemic states, such as multiple myeloma and Waldenström's macroglobulinemia.

### Drug challenge

 Diuretics, lithium, chlorpropamide, and vasopressin (possible decrease due to decreased serum sodium levels); corticosteroids and antihypertensives (possible increase due to increased serum sodium levels); salicylates, paraldehyde, methicillin, dimercaprol, ammonium chloride, acetazolamide, ethylene glycol, and methyl alcohol (possible increase due to decreased serum bicarbonate levels); adrenocorticotropic hormone, cortisone, and mercurial or chlorothiazide diuretics (possible decrease due to increased serum bicarbonate levels); ammonium chloride, cholestyramine, boric acid, oxyphenbutazone, and phenylbutazone, and excessive I.V. infusion of sodium chloride (possible decrease due to increased serum chloride levels); thiazide diuretics, ethacrynic acid, furosemide, and bicarbonates, and prolonged I.V. infusion of dextrose 5% in water (possible increase due to decreased serum chloride levels)

### Purpose

■ To distinguish among types of metabolic acidosis

■ To monitor renal function and total parenteral nutrition

## Patient preparation

- Explain that the anion gap test determines the cause of metabolic acidosis.
- Tell the patient that the test requires a blood sample. Explain who will perform the venipuncture and when it will be done.
- Explain to the patient that he may experience slight discomfort from the tourniquet and needle puncture.
- Tell the patient that he doesn't need to restrict food or fluids.
- Notify the laboratory and practitioner of medications the patient is taking that may affect test results; these medications may need to be restricted.

## Procedure and posttest care

- Confirm the patient's identity using two patient identifiers according to facility policy.
- Perform a venipuncture and collect the sample in a 3- or 4-ml clot-activator tube.
- Apply direct pressure to the venipuncture site until bleeding stops.
- If a hematoma develops at the venipuncture site, apply warm soaks. If the hematoma is large, monitor pulses distal to the venipuncture site.
- Instruct the patient to resume medications stopped before the test as ordered.

# Calcium
[Ca+]

About 99% of the body's calcium is found in the teeth. About 1% of total calcium in the body circulates in the blood. About 50% of this serum calcium is bound to plasma proteins and 40% is ionized, or free. Evaluation of serum calcium levels measures the total amount of calcium in the blood, and evaluation of ionized calcium measures the fraction of serum calcium occurring in the ionized form.

## Reference values

- In adults, total serum calcium levels are 8.2 to 10.2 mg/dl (SI, 2.05 to 2.54 mmol/L).
- Ionized calcium levels are 4.65 to 5.28 mg/dl (SI, 1.10 to 1.25 mmol/L).
- In children, total serum calcium levels are 8.6 to 11.2 mg/dl (SI, 2.15 to 2.79 mmol/L).

## Abnormal results

- High serum calcium levels (hypercalcemia) may occur in hyperparathyroidism and parathyroid tumors, Paget's disease of the bone, sarcoidosis, vitamin D intoxication, multiple myeloma, metastatic carcinoma, multiple fractures, and prolonged immobilization.
- High levels may also result from inadequate excretion of calcium, as with adrenal insufficiency and renal disease; from excessive calcium ingestion; and from overuse of antacids such as calcium carbonate.

Alert

 Observe the patient with hypercalcemia for deep bone pain, flank pain due to renal calculi, and muscle hypotonicity. Hypercalcemic crisis begins with nausea, vomiting, and dehydration, leading to stupor and coma, and can end in cardiac arrest.

- Low serum calcium levels (hypocalcemia) may result from hypoparathyroidism, total parathyroidectomy, or malabsorption. Decreased serum calcium levels may also occur with Cushing's syndrome, renal failure, osteomalacia, renal failure, vitamin D deficiency, acute pancreatitis, peritonitis, malnutrition with hypoalbuminemia, and blood transfusions (due to citrate).

ALERT

In the patient with hypocalcemia, be alert for circumoral and peripheral numbness and tingling, muscle twitching, Chvostek's sign (facial muscle spasm), tetany, muscle cramping, Trousseau's sign (carpedal spasm), seizures, arrhythmias, laryngeal spasm, decreased cardiac output, prolonged bleeding time, fractures, and prolonged QT interval.

## Purpose
- To evaluate endocrine function, calcium metabolism, and acid-base balance
- To guide therapy in patients with renal failure, renal transplant, endocrine disorders, malignancies, cardiac disease, and skeletal disorders

## Patient preparation
- Explain that the calcium test determines blood calcium levels.
- Tell the patient that the test requires a blood sample. Explain who will perform the venipuncture and when it will be done.
- Explain to the patient that he may experience slight discomfort from the tourniquet and needle puncture.
- Tell him that he doesn't need to restrict food or fluids.

## Procedure and posttest care
- Confirm the patient's identity using two patient identifiers according to facility policy.
- Perform a venipuncture (without a tourniquet if possible) and collect the sample in a 3- or 4-ml clot-activator tube.
- Apply direct pressure to the venipuncture site until bleeding stops.
- If a hematoma develops at the venipuncture site, apply warm soaks. If the hematoma is large, monitor pulses distal to the venipuncture site.

# ▌Chloride
## [Cl⁻]

The chloride test measures serum levels of chloride, the major extracellular fluid anion. Chloride helps maintain osmotic pressure of blood and, therefore, helps regulate blood volume and arterial pressure. Chloride levels also affect acid-base balance. Chloride is absorbed from the intestines and excreted primarily by the kidneys.

## Reference values
- For adults, serum chloride levels are 100 to 108 mEq/L (SI, 100 to 108 mmol/L).

## Abnormal results
- Chloride levels are inversely related to bicarbonate levels, reflecting acid-base balance.
- Excessive loss of gastric juices or other secretions containing chloride may cause hypochloremic metabolic alkalosis; excessive chloride retention or ingestion may lead to hyperchloremic metabolic acidosis.
- An increase in chloride levels may be evident in severe dehydration, complete renal shutdown, respiratory alkalosis, metabolic acidosis, head injury (producing neurogenic hyperventilation), and primary aldosteronism.
- Decreased levels of chloride may result from low sodium and potassium levels due to prolonged vomiting, gastric suctioning, intestinal fistula, chronic renal failure, and Addison's disease. Heart failure or edema resulting in excess extracellular fluid can cause dilutional hypochloremia.

ALERT

Observe the patient with hypochloremia for hypertonicity of muscles, tetany, depressed respirations, and decreased blood pressure with dehydration. In the patient with hyperchloremia, be alert for signs of developing stupor, rapid deep breathing, and weakness, which may lead to coma.

## DRUG CHALLENGE

Ammonium chloride, cholestyramine, boric acid, oxyphenbutazone, and phenylbutazone, and excessive I.V. infusion of sodium chloride (possible increase); thiazide diuretics, ethacrynic acid, furosemide, and bicarbonates, and prolonged I.V.-infusion of dextrose 5% in water (decrease)

### Purpose
▪ To detect acid-base imbalance (acidosis or alkalosis) and to aid in evaluation of fluid status and extracellular cation-anion balance

### Patient preparation
▪ Explain that the serum chloride test evaluates the chloride content of blood.
▪ Tell the patient that the test requires a blood sample. Explain who will perform the venipuncture and when it will be done.
▪ Explain to the patient that he may experience slight discomfort from the tourniquet and needle puncture.
▪ Tell the patient that he doesn't need to restrict food or fluids.
▪ Notify the laboratory and practitioner of medications the patient is taking that may affect test results; these medications may need to be restricted.

### Procedure and posttest care
▪ Confirm the patient's identity using two patient identifiers according to facility policy.
▪ Perform a venipuncture and collect the sample in a 3- or 4-ml clot-activator tube.

▪ Apply direct pressure to the venipuncture site until bleeding stops.
▪ If a hematoma develops at the venipuncture site, apply warm soaks. If the hematoma is large, monitor pulses distal to the venipuncture site.
▪ Instruct the patient to resume medications stopped before the test as ordered.

# ▌Magnesium
[Mag, Mg++]

The magnesium test measures serum levels of magnesium, an electrolyte that's vital to neuromuscular function. It also helps in intracellular metabolism, activates many essential enzymes, and affects the metabolism of nucleic acids and proteins. Magnesium also helps transport sodium and potassium across cell membranes and influences intracellular calcium levels. Most magnesium is found in bone and intracellular fluid; a small amount is found in extracellular fluid. Magnesium is absorbed by the small intestine and excreted in urine and stool.

### Reference values
▪ Serum magnesium levels are 1.3 to 2.1 mg/dl (SI, 0.65 to 1.05 mmol/L).

### Abnormal results
▪ High magnesium levels (hypermagnesemia) most commonly occur in renal failure, when the kidneys excrete inadequate amounts of magnesium, and also occur with magnesium administration or ingestion. Adrenal insufficiency (Addison's disease), dehydration, and diabetic acidosis can also increase serum magnesium levels.

## ALERT

Observe the patient for lethargy; flushing; diaphoresis; decreased blood pressure; slow, weak pulse; muscle weakness;

diminished deep tendon reflexes; slow, shallow respiration; and electrocardiogram (ECG) changes (prolonged PR interval, wide QRS complex, elevated T waves, atrioventricular block, premature ventricular contractions [PVCs]).

■ Low magnesium levels (hypomagnesemia) most commonly result from chronic alcoholism. Other causes include malabsorption syndrome, diarrhea, delirium tremens, excessive insulin administration, cirrhosis, toxemia of pregnancy, ulcerative colitis, faulty absorption after bowel resection, prolonged bowel or gastric aspiration, acute pancreatitis, primary aldosteronism, severe burns, hypercalcemic conditions (including hyperparathyroidism), malnutrition, and certain diuretic therapy.

ALERT

 Watch for leg and foot cramps, hyperactive deep tendon reflexes, arrhythmias, muscle weakness, seizures, twitching, tetany, tremors, and ECG changes (PVCs and ventricular fibrillation).

### Purpose
■ To evaluate electrolyte status

### Patient preparation
■ Explain that the magnesium test determines the magnesium content of the blood.
■ Instruct the patient not to use magnesium salts (such as milk of magnesia or Epsom salt) for at least 3 days before the test, but tell him that he doesn't need to restrict food or fluids.
■ Tell the patient that the test requires a blood sample. Explain who will perform the venipuncture and when it will be done.

■ Explain to the patient that he may experience slight discomfort from the tourniquet and needle puncture.

### Procedure and posttest care
■ Confirm the patient's identity using two patient identifiers according to facility policy.
■ Perform a venipuncture without a tourniquet, if possible, and collect the sample in a 3- or 4-ml clot-activator tube.
■ Apply pressure to the venipuncture site until bleeding stops.
■ If a hematoma develops at the venipuncture site, apply warm soaks. If the hematoma is large, monitor pulses distal to the venipuncture site.

# Phosphate
## [PO₄, phosphorus]

The phosphate test measures serum levels of phosphates, the primary anions in intracellular fluid. Phosphates are essential in the storage and use of energy, calcium regulation, red blood cell function, acid-base balance, formation of bone, and the metabolism of carbohydrates, protein, and fat. The intestines absorb most phosphates from dietary sources; the kidneys excrete phosphates and provide a regulatory mechanism. Abnormal levels of serum phosphates usually result from improper excretion rather than faulty ingestion or absorption from dietary sources.

Normally, calcium and phosphate have an inverse relationship; if one is increased, the other is decreased.

### Reference values
■ For adults, phosphate levels are 2.7 to 4.5 mg/dl (SI, 0.87 to 1.45 mmol/L).
■ For children, phosphate levels are 4.5 to 6.7 mg/dl (SI, 1.45 to 1.78 mmol/L).

## Abnormal results

- Decreased phosphate levels (hypophosphatemia) may result from malnutrition, malabsorption syndromes, alcohol abuse, severe burns, hyperparathyroidism, renal tubular acidosis, and treatment of diabetic ketoacidosis (DKA).
- Increased phosphate levels (hyperphosphatemia) may result from skeletal disease, healing fractures, hypoparathyroidism, acromegaly, DKA, high intestinal obstruction, lactic acidosis (due to hepatic impairment), and renal failure.

### Drug challenge

 Acetazolamide, insulin, epinephrine, and phosphate-binding antacids; vitamin D deficiency; and extended I.V. infusion of dextrose 5% in water (possible decrease)

## Purpose

- To help diagnose renal disorders and acid-base imbalance
- To detect endocrine, skeletal, and calcium disorders

## Patient preparation

- Explain that the phosphate test measures phosphate levels in the blood.
- Tell the patient that the test requires a blood sample. Explain who will perform the venipuncture and when it will be done.
- Explain to the patient that he may experience slight discomfort from the needle puncture.
- Tell him that he doesn't need to restrict food or fluids.
- Notify the laboratory and practitioner of medications the patient is taking that may affect test results; these medications may need to be restricted.

## Procedure and posttest care

- Confirm the patient's identity using two patient identifiers according to facility policy.
- Perform a venipuncture without using a tourniquet, if possible, and collect the sample in 3- or 4-ml clot-activator tube.
- Apply pressure to the venipuncture site until bleeding stops.
- If a hematoma develops at the venipuncture site, apply warm soaks. If the hematoma is large, monitor pulses distal to the venipuncture site.
- Instruct the patient to resume medications stopped before the test as ordered.

# Potassium
## [K+]

The potassium test measures serum levels of potassium, the major intracellular cation. Potassium helps to maintain cellular osmotic equilibrium; regulates muscle activity, enzyme activity, and acid-base balance; and influences renal function.

The body can't conserve potassium, as it does sodium. The kidneys excrete nearly all ingested potassium, even when the body's supply is depleted, so potassium deficiency can arise quickly.

Potassium levels are affected by variations in the secretions of adrenal steroid hormones and by fluctuations in pH, glucose levels, and sodium levels. A reciprocal relationship exists between potassium and sodium; a substantial intake of one causes a decrease in the other.

Because the kidneys excrete nearly all ingested potassium daily, a dietary intake of at least 40 mEq/day is essential. A normal diet usually includes 60 to 100 mEq of daily potassium. (See *Dietary sources of potassium,* page 58. See also *Treating potassium imbalance,* page 59.)

# Dietary sources of potassium

A healthy person needs to consume at least 40 mEq of potassium daily. This table highlights foods and beverages, their serving size, and the amount of potassium each contains.

| Foods and beverages | Serving size | Amount of potassium (mEq) |
|---|---|---|
| **Beverages** | | |
| Apricot nectar | 1 cup (240 ml) | 9 |
| Grapefruit juice | 1 cup | 8.2 |
| Orange juice | 1 cup | 11.4 |
| Pineapple juice | 1 cup | 9 |
| Prune juice | 1 cup | 14.4 |
| Tomato juice | 1 cup | 11.6 |
| Milk (whole or skim) | 1 cup | 8.8 |
| **Fruits** | | |
| Apricots (dried) | 4 halves | 5 |
| Apricots (raw) | 3 small | 8 |
| Bananas | 1 medium | 12.8 |
| Cantaloupe | 6 oz | 13 |
| Figs (dried) | 7 small | 17.5 |
| Peaches (raw) | 1 medium | 6.2 |
| Pears (raw) | 1 medium | 6.2 |
| **Meats** | | |
| Beef | 4 oz (112 g) | 11.2 |
| Chicken | 4 oz | 12 |
| Scallops | 5 large | 30 |
| Veal | 4 oz | 15.2 |
| **Vegetables** | | |
| Artichokes | 1 large bud | 7.7 |
| Asparagus (frozen, cooked) | ½ cup | 5.5 |
| Asparagus (raw) | 6 spears | 7.7 |
| Beans (dried, cooked) | ½ cup | 10 |
| Beans (lima) | ½ cup | 9.5 |
| Broccoli (cooked) | ½ cup | 7 |
| Carrots (cooked) | ½ cup | 5.7 |
| Carrots (raw) | 1 large | 8.8 |
| Mushrooms (raw) | 4 large | 10.6 |
| Potatoes (baked) | 1 small | 15.4 |
| Spinach (raw or cooked) | ½ cup | 8.5 |
| Squash (winter and baked) | ½ cup | 12 |
| Tomatoes (raw) | 1 medium | 10.4 |

# Treating potassium imbalance

Hypokalemia and hyperkalemia can cause serious problems if not treated promptly.

## Hypokalemia

A patient with a potassium deficiency can be treated with oral potassium chloride replacement and increased dietary intake. In severe cases, potassium can be replaced by I.V. infusion at a rate not exceeding 20 mEq/hour and at a concentration of no more than 80 mEq/L of I.V. fluid. When hanging I.V. potassium, shake the I.V. solution because it can settle near the neck of the bottle or plastic bag. Failure to mix the solution adequately or to infuse it properly can cause a burning sensation at the I.V. site and possibly even fatal hyperkalemia.

Monitor the electrocardiogram, urine output, and serum potassium levels frequently during the infusion. Never give I.V. potassium replacement to a patient with inadequate urine flow because diminished excretion can rapidly lead to hyperkalemia.

## Hyperkalemia

Dangerously high potassium levels may be reduced with sodium polystyrene sulfonate—a potassium-removing resin—given orally, rectally, or through a nasogastric tube. Hyperkalemia may also be treated with an I.V. infusion of sodium bicarbonate or of glucose and insulin, which lowers blood potassium by causing it to move into cells.

A calcium I.V. infusion provides fast but transient relief from the cardiotoxic effects of hyperkalemia; however, it doesn't directly lower serum potassium levels. In renal failure, dialysis may help remove excess potassium, but this corrects the imbalance much more slowly.

## Reference values

- Serum potassium values are 3.5 to 5 mEq/L (SI, 3.5 to 5 mmol/L).

## Abnormal results

- High potassium levels (hyperkalemia) occur when excess cellular potassium enters the blood, as in burn injuries, crush injuries, diabetic ketoacidosis, transfusions of large amounts of blood, and myocardial infarction. Hyperkalemia may also indicate reduced sodium excretion, possibly due to renal failure (preventing normal exchange of sodium and potassium) or Addison's disease (due to potassium buildup and sodium depletion).

**ALERT**

 Observe the patient with hyperkalemia for weakness, malaise, nausea, diarrhea, colicky pain, muscle irritability progressing to flaccid paralysis, oliguria, and bradycardia. The electrocardiogram (ECG) reveals flattened P waves; a prolonged PR interval; a wide QRS complex; tall, tented T waves; and ST-segment depression. Cardiac arrest may occur without warning.

- Low potassium levels (hypokalemia) commonly result from aldosteronism or Cushing's syndrome, loss of body fluids (as with long-term diuretic therapy, vomiting, or diarrhea), and excessive licorice ingestion.

**ALERT**

 Observe the patient with hypokalemia for decreased reflexes; a rapid, weak, irregular pulse; mental confusion; hypotension; anorexia; muscle weakness; and paresthesia. The ECG shows a flattened T wave, ST-segment depression, and U-wave elevation. In severe cases, ventricular fibrillation, respiratory paralysis, and cardiac arrest can develop.

 Excessive or rapid potassium infusion, spironolactone or penicillin G potassium therapy, and renal toxicity from administration of amphotericin B, methicillin, or tetracycline (increase); insulin and glucose administration; diuretic therapy (especially with thiazides but not with triamterene, amiloride, or spironolactone); and I.V. infusions without potassium (decrease)

## Purpose

- To evaluate clinical signs of potassium excess (hyperkalemia) or potassium depletion (hypokalemia)
- To monitor renal function, acid-base balance, and glucose metabolism
- To evaluate neuromuscular and endocrine disorders
- To detect the origin of arrhythmias

## Patient preparation

- Explain that the serum potassium test determines the potassium content of blood.
- Tell the patient that the test requires a blood sample. Explain who will perform the venipuncture and when it will be done.
- Explain to the patient that he may experience slight discomfort from the tourniquet and needle puncture.
- Tell him that he doesn't need to restrict food or fluids.
- Notify the laboratory and practitioner of medications the patient is taking that may affect test results; these medications may need to be restricted.

## Procedure and posttest care

- Confirm the patient's identity using two patient identifiers according to facility policy.
- Perform a venipuncture and collect the sample in a 3- or 4-ml clot-activator tube.
- Apply direct pressure to the venipuncture site until the bleeding stops.
- If a hematoma develops at the venipuncture site, apply warm soaks. If the hematoma is large, monitor pulses distal to the venipuncture site.
- Instruct the patient to resume medications stopped before the test as ordered.

## Precautions

- Draw the sample immediately after applying the tourniquet because a delay may increase the potassium level by allowing intracellular potassium to leak into the serum.

 ## Sodium
### [Na+]

The sodium test measures serum sodium levels in relation to the amount of water in the body. Sodium, the major extracellular cation, affects body water distribution, maintains osmotic pressure of extracellular fluid, helps promote neuromuscular function, helps maintain acid-base balance, and influences chloride and potassium levels.

Because the extracellular sodium level helps the kidneys to regulate body water (decreased levels promote water excretion and increased levels promote retention), sodium levels are evaluated in relation to the amount of water in the body. For example, a sodium deficit (hyponatremia) refers to a decreased level of sodium in relation to the body's water level. (See *Fluid imbalances*.)

The body normally regulates this sodium-water balance through aldosterone, which inhibits sodium excretion

# Fluid imbalances

This chart lists the causes, signs and symptoms, and laboratory test findings associated with hypervolemia (increased fluid volume) and hypovolemia (decreased fluid volume).

| Causes | Signs and symptoms | Laboratory findings |
| --- | --- | --- |
| **Hypervolemia** | | |
| ▪ Increased water intake<br>▪ Decreased water output due to renal disease<br>▪ Heart failure<br>▪ Excessive ingestion or infusion of sodium chloride<br>▪ Long-term administration of adrenocortical hormones<br>▪ Excessive infusion of isotonic solutions | ▪ Increased blood pressure, pulse rate, body weight, and respiratory rate<br>▪ Bounding peripheral pulses<br>▪ Moist pulmonary crackles<br>▪ Moist mucous membranes<br>▪ Moist respiratory secretions<br>▪ Edema<br>▪ Weakness<br>▪ Seizures and coma due to swelling of brain cells | ▪ Decreased red blood cell (RBC) count, hemoglobin concentration, packed cell volume, serum sodium concentration (dilutional decrease), and urine specific gravity |
| **Hypovolemia** | | |
| ▪ Decreased water intake<br>▪ Fluid loss due to fever, diarrhea, or vomiting<br>▪ Systemic infection<br>▪ Impaired renal concentrating ability<br>▪ Fistulous drainage<br>▪ Severe burns<br>▪ Hidden fluid in body cavities | ▪ Increased pulse and respiratory rates<br>▪ Decreased blood pressure and body weight<br>▪ Weak and thready peripheral pulses<br>▪ Thick, slurred speech<br>▪ Thirst<br>▪ Oliguria<br>▪ Anuria<br>▪ Dry skin | ▪ Increased RBC count, hemoglobin concentration, packed cell volume, serum sodium concentration, and urine specific gravity |

and promotes its resorption (with water) by the renal tubules to maintain balance. Low sodium levels stimulate aldosterone secretion; high sodium levels suppress it.

## Reference values

▪ Serum sodium values are 135 to 145 mEq/L (SI, 135 to 145 mmol/L).

## Abnormal results

▪ Sodium imbalance can result from a loss or gain of sodium or from a change in the patient's state of hydration.

▪ High serum sodium levels (hypernatremia) may be due to inadequate water intake, excessive sodium intake, water loss in excess of sodium (as with diabetes insipidus, impaired renal function, prolonged hyperventilation, and occasionally, severe vomiting or diarrhea), and sodium retention (as with aldosteronism).

ALERT

 In a patient with hypernatremia and associated loss of water, observe for signs of thirst, restlessness, dry and sticky mucous membranes, flushed skin, oliguria, and diminished reflexes. If increased total body sodium causes water retention, observe for hypertension, dyspnea, edema, and heart failure.

■ Low serum sodium levels (hyponatremia) may result from inadequate sodium intake or excessive sodium loss due to profuse sweating, GI suctioning, diuretic therapy, diarrhea, vomiting, adrenal insufficiency, burns, or chronic renal insufficiency with acidosis. Urine sodium determinations are usually more sensitive to early changes in sodium balance and should be evaluated simultaneously with serum sodium findings.

ALERT

 In a patient with hyponatremia, watch for apprehension, lassitude, headache, decreased skin turgor, abdominal cramps, and tremors that may progress to seizures.

DRUG CHALLENGE

 Most diuretics (decrease, by promoting sodium excretion); lithium, chlorpropamide, and vasopressin (decrease, by inhibiting water excretion); corticosteroids (increase, by promoting sodium retention); antihypertensives, such as methyldopa, hydralazine, and reserpine (possible increase due to sodium and water retention)

## Purpose
■ To evaluate fluid-electrolyte and acid-base balance and related neuromuscular, renal, and adrenal functions

## Patient preparation
■ Explain that the sodium test determines the sodium content of the blood.
■ Tell the patient that the test requires a blood sample. Explain who will perform the venipuncture and when it will be done.
■ Explain to the patient that he may experience slight discomfort from the tourniquet and needle puncture.
■ Tell him that he doesn't need to restrict food or fluids.
■ Notify the laboratory and practitioner of medications the patient is taking that may affect test results; these medications may need to be restricted.

## Procedure and posttest care
■ Confirm the patient's identity using two patient identifiers according to facility policy.
■ Perform a venipuncture and collect the sample in a 3- or 4-ml clot-activator tube.
■ Apply direct pressure to the venipuncture site until bleeding stops.
■ If a hematoma develops at the venipuncture site, apply warm soaks. If the hematoma is large, monitor pulses distal to the venipuncture site.
■ Instruct the patient to resume medications stopped before the test as ordered.

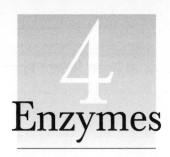

# Enzymes

## Cardiac enzyme tests

### B-type natriuretic peptide
[BNP]

B-type natriuretic peptide (BNP) is a neurohormone produced predominantly by the heart ventricle. BNP is released from the heart in response to blood volume expansion or pressure overload.

Plasma BNP increases with the severity of heart failure. Studies have demonstrated that the heart is the major source of circulating BNP. It's an excellent hormonal marker of ventricular systolic and diastolic dysfunction.

#### Reference values
- Normal serum BNP levels are less than 100 pg/ml.

#### Abnormal results
- Levels greater than 100 pg/ml are an accurate predictor of heart failure.
- The level of BNP in the blood is related to the severity of heart failure.
- The higher the BNP level, the worse the symptoms of heart failure. (See *Linking BNP levels to heart failure symptom severity*, page 64.)

DRUG CHALLENGE

 Natrecor (increased levels)

#### Purpose
- To help diagnose and determine the severity of heart failure

#### Patient preparation
- Explain that the BNP assay identifies the presence and severity of heart failure.
- Tell the patient that the test requires a blood sample. Explain who will perform the venipuncture and when it will be done.
- Explain to the patient that he may experience slight discomfort from the tourniquet and needle puncture.
- Tell him that he doesn't need to restrict food or fluids.

#### Procedure and posttest care
- Confirm the patient's identity using two patient identifiers according to facility policy.
- Perform a venipuncture and collect the sample in a 3.5-ml EDTA tube.
- Apply direct pressure to the venipuncture site until bleeding stops.
- If a hematoma develops at the venipuncture site, apply warm soaks. If the hematoma is large, monitor pulses distal to the venipuncture site.

### C-reactive protein
[CRP]

C-reactive protein (CRP) is an abnormal protein that appears in the blood during an inflammatory process. It's absent

# Linking BNP levels to heart failure symptom severity

The following chart shows the level of B-type natriuretic peptide (BNP) levels and the correlation with symptoms of heart failure. The higher the level of BNP, the more severe the symptoms.

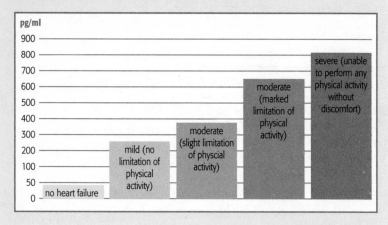

from the blood of healthy people. This nonspecific protein is synthesized mainly in the liver and is found in many body fluids (pleural, peritoneal, pericardial, and synovial). It appears in the blood 18 to 24 hours after the onset of tissue damage, with levels that increase up to 1,000-fold and then decline rapidly when the inflammatory process regresses. CRP has been found to rise before antibody titers and erythrocyte sedimentation rate (ESR) levels rise; it also decreases sooner than ESR levels.

## Reference values
- CRP isn't present in the blood.
- During the third trimester of pregnancy, the CRP level may increase.
- In adults, normal results may be reported as less than 0.8 mg/dl (SI, less than 8 mg/L).

## Abnormal results
- An elevated CRP level may be present in rheumatoid arthritis, rheumatic fever, myocardial infarction (MI), cancer (ac-

tive, widespread), acute bacterial and viral infections, inflammatory bowel disease, Hodgkin's disease, systemic lupus erythematosus, and postoperatively (declines after the fourth day).

### DRUG CHALLENGE

 Steroids and salicylates (false normal level); hormonal contraceptives (false increase)

## Purpose
- To evaluate the inflammatory disease course and severity (including tissue necrosis) in conditions (such as MI, malignancy, rheumatoid arthritis)
- To monitor acute inflammatory phases of rheumatoid arthritis and rheumatic fever, so early treatment can be initiated
- To monitor the patient's response to treatment or determine if the acute phase is declining
- To help interpret the ESR

■ To monitor the wound healing process of internal incisions, burns, and organ transplantation

### Patient preparation

■ Explain that the CRP test identifies the presence of infection or monitors treatment.

■ Inform the patient that he must restrict fluids, except for water, for 8 to 12 hours before the test.

■ Tell him that the test requires a blood sample. Explain who will perform the venipuncture and when it will be done.

■ Explain to the patient that he may experience slight discomfort from the tourniquet and needle puncture.

■ Notify the laboratory and practitioner of medications the patient is taking that may affect test results; these medications may need to be restricted.

### Procedure and posttest care

■ Confirm the patient's identity using two patient identifiers according to facility policy.

■ Perform a venipuncture and collect the sample in a 5-ml clot-activator tube.

■ Apply direct pressure to the venipuncture site until bleeding stops.

■ If a hematoma develops at the venipuncture site, apply warm soaks. If the hematoma is large, monitor pulses distal to the venipuncture site.

■ Instruct the patient to resume his usual diet and medications stopped before the test as ordered.

### Precautions

■ Keep the blood sample away from heat.

DO'S & DON'TS

Collect blood sample at least 2 weeks after the resolution of an inflammatory disease process.

# Creatine kinase and isoforms
## [CK]

Creatine kinase (CK) is an enzyme that catalyzes the creatine-creatinine metabolic pathway in muscle cells and brain tissue. Because of its intimate role in energy production, CK reflects normal tissue catabolism; increased serum levels indicate trauma to cells.

Fractionation and measurement of three distinct CK isoenzymes—CK-BB ($CK_1$), CK-MB ($CK_2$), and CK-MM ($CK_3$)—have replaced the use of total CK levels to accurately localize the site of increased tissue destruction. $CK_1$ is most commonly found in brain tissue; $CK_2$ and $CK_3$ are found primarily in heart and skeletal muscle. In addition, subunits of $CK_2$ and $CK_3$, called isoforms or isoenzymes, can be assayed to increase the test's sensitivity.

### Reference values

■ Total CK values determined by ultraviolet or kinetic measurement are 55 to 170 units/L (SI, 0.94 to 2.89 µkat/L) for men and from 30 to 135 units/L (SI, 0.51 to 2.30 µkat/L) for women.

■ Total CK levels may be significantly higher in muscular people.

■ Infants up to age 1 have levels two to four times higher than adult levels, possibly reflecting birth trauma and striated muscle development.

■ Normal ranges for isoenzyme levels are as follows: $CK_1$ undetectable; $CK_2$ less than 5% (SI, less than 0.05); $CK_3$ 90% to 100% (SI, 0.90 to 1.00).

### Abnormal results

■ Detectable $CK_1$ isoenzyme may indicate, but doesn't confirm, a diagnosis of brain tissue injury, widespread malignant tumors, severe shock, or renal failure.

# Release of cardiac enzymes and proteins

Because they're released by damaged tissue, serum proteins and isoenzymes (catalytic proteins that vary in concentration in specific organs) can help identify the compromised organ and assess the extent of damage. After an acute myocardial infarction, cardiac enzymes and proteins rise and fall in a characteristic pattern, as shown in the graph below.

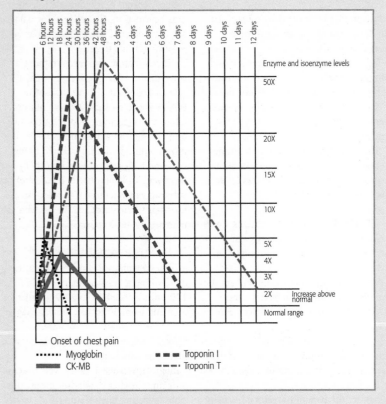

- $CK_2$ levels greater than 5% of the total CK level indicate a myocardial infarction (MI).
- In an acute MI and after cardiac surgery, $CK_2$ begins to increase within 2 to 4 hours, peaks within 12 to 24 hours, and usually returns to normal within 24 to 48 hours; persistent elevations and increasing levels indicate ongoing myocardial damage. Total CK follows roughly the same pattern but increases slightly

later. (See *Release of cardiac enzymes and proteins*.)
- Serious skeletal muscle injury that occurs in certain muscular dystrophies, polymyositis, and severe myoglobinuria may produce a mild $CK_2$ increase because a small amount of this isoenzyme is present in some skeletal muscles.
- Increasing $CK_3$ values follow skeletal muscle damage from trauma, such as surgery and I.M. injections, and from diseases, such as dermatomyositis and

muscular dystrophy (values may be 50 to 100 times normal).

■ A moderate increase in $CK_3$ levels develops in a patient with hypothyroidism; sharp increases occur with muscle activity caused by agitation, such as during an acute psychotic episode.

■ Total CK levels may be increased in patients with severe hypokalemia, carbon monoxide poisoning, malignant hyperthermia, rhabdomyolysis, and alcoholic cardiomyopathy. They may also be increased after seizures, and occasionally, in patients who have suffered pulmonary or cerebral infarctions.

### DRUG CHALLENGE

 Halothane and succinylcholine, alcohol, lithium, large doses of aminocaproic acid, and I.M. injections (increase in total CK)

### Purpose

■ To detect and diagnose acute MI and reinfarction ($CK_2$ primarily used)
■ To evaluate possible causes of chest pain and to monitor the severity of myocardial ischemia after cardiac surgery, cardiac catheterization, and cardioversion ($CK_2$ primarily used)
■ To detect early dermatomyositis and musculoskeletal disorders that aren't neurogenic in origin such as Duchenne's muscular dystrophy (total CK primarily used)

### Patient preparation

■ Explain that the CK test assesses myocardial and musculoskeletal function and that multiple blood samples are required to detect fluctuations in serum levels.
■ Tell the patient who will perform the venipunctures and when it will be done.
■ Explain to him that he may experience slight discomfort from the tourniquet and needle puncture.

■ If the patient is being evaluated for musculoskeletal disorders, advise him to avoid exercising for 24 hours before the test.
■ Notify the laboratory and practitioner of medications the patient is taking that may affect test results; these medications may need to be restricted.

### Procedure and posttest care

■ Confirm the patient's identity using two patient identifiers according to facility policy.
■ Perform a venipuncture and collect the sample in a 4-ml tube without additives.
■ Apply direct pressure to the venipuncture site until bleeding stops.
■ If a hematoma develops at the venipuncture site, apply warm soaks. If the hematoma is large, monitor pulses distal to the venipuncture site.
■ Instruct the patient to resume exercise and medications stopped before the test as ordered.

### Precautions

■ Draw the blood sample before or 1 hour after giving I.M. injections because muscle trauma increases the total CK level.

### DO'S & DON'TS

 Obtain the blood sample on schedule. Note on the laboratory request the time the sample was drawn and the hours elapsed since the onset of chest pain.

■ Send the sample to the laboratory immediately because CK activity diminishes significantly after 2 hours at room temperature.

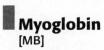 ## Myoglobin
### [MB]

Myoglobin is an oxygen-binding muscle protein usually found in skeletal and cardiac muscle. It's released into the bloodstream in ischemia, trauma, and inflammation of the muscle. Creatine kinase and its isoform $CK_2$ are released more slowly than myoglobin during myocardial infarction (MI). Myoglobin can be detected as soon as 2 hours after the onset of chest pain and peaks in 8 to 12 hours, so it's useful as an early indicator of MI.

### Reference values
- Myoglobin levels are 0 to 0.09 mcg/ml (SI, 5 to 70 µg/L).

### Abnormal results
- Increased myoglobin levels may result from acute alcohol intoxication, dermatomyositis, hypothermia (with prolonged shivering), MI, muscular dystrophy, polymyositis, rhabdomyelitis, severe burns, trauma, severe renal failure, and systemic lupus erythematosus.

### Purpose
- To determine if MI has occurred
- To estimate damage to skeletal or cardiac muscle tissue
- To predict flare-ups of polymyositis

### Patient preparation
- Explain that the myoglobin test estimates damage to muscle tissue.
- Obtain a patient history, including disorders that may be associated with increased myoglobin levels.
- Tell the patient that the test requires a blood sample. Explain who will perform the venipuncture and when it will be done.
- Explain that the patient may experience slight discomfort from the tourniquet and needle puncture.
- Inform him that the results need to be correlated with other tests for a definitive diagnosis.

### Procedure and posttest care
- Confirm the patient's identity using two patient identifiers according to facility policy.
- Perform a venipuncture and collect the sample in a 4-ml tube with no additives.
- Apply direct pressure to the venipuncture site until bleeding stops.
- If a hematoma develops at the venipuncture site, apply warm soaks. If the hematoma is large, monitor pulses distal to the venipuncture site.

## ▌Troponin
### [cTnI, cTnT]

Cardiac troponin I (cTnI) and cardiac troponin T (cTnT) are proteins in the striated cells that are extremely specific markers of cardiac damage. When injury occurs to the myocardial tissue, these proteins are released into the bloodstream. Elevations in troponin levels can be seen within 4 hours of myocardial infarction (MI) and will persist for a week or longer. Troponin measurements have a greater sensitivity than $CK_2$ measurements.

### Reference values
- cTnI levels are less than 0.35 mcg/L (SI, < 0.35 µg/L).
- cTnT levels are less than 0.1 mcg/L (SI, < 0.1 µg/L).

### Abnormal results
- Laboratory results may vary. Some laboratories may call a test positive if it shows any detectable levels, and others may give a range for abnormal results.
- Troponin levels rise rapidly, are detectable within 4 to 6 hours of myocardial cell injury, and peak within 12 to 24 hours.
- cTnI levels greater than 2 mcg/L (SI, > 2 µg/L) suggest cardiac injury.
- Qualitative cTnT rapid immunoassay results greater than 0.1 mcg/L (SI, > 0.1

μg/L) are considered positive for cardiac injury.

## Drug challenge

 Cardiotoxic drugs such as dox-orubicin (increase)

# Alanine aminotransferase
### [ALT, SGPT]

The alanine aminotransferase (ALT) test measures serum levels of ALT, one of two enzymes that catalyze a reversible amino group transfer reaction in the Krebs cycle. ALT is necessary for tissue energy production. It's found primarily in the liver, with lesser amounts in the kidneys, heart, and skeletal muscles, and is a sensitive indicator of acute hepatocellular disease.

When such hepatic damage occurs, ALT is released from the cytoplasm into the bloodstream, typically before jaundice appears, resulting in abnormally high serum levels that may not return to normal for days or weeks. This test measures serum ALT levels using the spectrophotometric method.

## Purpose
- To detect and diagnose acute MI and reinfarction
- To evaluate possible causes of chest pain

## Patient preparation
- Explain that the troponin test helps assess myocardial injury and that multiple samples may be drawn to detect fluctuations in serum levels.
- Tell the patient that he doesn't need to restrict food or fluids.
- Tell him that the test requires a blood sample. Explain who will perform the venipuncture and when it will be done.
- Explain to the patient that he may feel slight discomfort from the tourniquet and needle puncture.

## Procedure and posttest care
- Confirm the patient's identity using two patient identifiers according to facility policy.
- Perform a venipuncture and collect the specimen in a 7-ml clot-activator tube.
- If a hematoma develops at the venipuncture site, apply warm soaks. If the hematoma is large, monitor pulses distal to the venipuncture site.

## Precautions
- Obtain each specimen on schedule and note the date and collection time on each one.

## Reference values
- For adults, ALT levels are 10 to 35 units/L (SI, 0.17 to 0.60 µkat/L).
- For neonates, ALT levels are 13 to 45 units/L (SI, 0.22 to 0.77 µkat/L).

## Abnormal results
- Very high ALT levels (up to 50 times normal) suggest viral or severe drug-induced hepatitis or other hepatic disease with extensive necrosis.
- Moderate to high levels may indicate infectious mononucleosis, chronic hepatitis, intrahepatic cholestasis or cholecystitis, early or improving acute viral hepatitis, or severe hepatic congestion due to heart failure.
- Slight to moderate elevations of ALT may appear in any condition that produces acute hepatocellular injury, such as active cirrhosis and drug-induced or alcoholic hepatitis.

▪ Marginal elevations occasionally occur in acute myocardial infarction, reflecting secondary hepatic congestion or the release of small amounts of ALT from myocardial tissue.

**DRUG CHALLENGE**

 Barbiturates, griseofulvin, isoniazid, nitrofurantoin, methyldopa, phenothiazines, phenytoin, salicylates, tetracycline, chlorpromazine, para-aminosalicylic acid, and other drugs that cause hepatic injury by competitively interfering with cellular metabolism (false-high)

## Purpose
▪ To detect and evaluate treatment of acute hepatic disease, especially hepatitis and cirrhosis without jaundice
▪ To distinguish between myocardial and hepatic tissue damage (used with aspartate aminotransferase test)
▪ To assess the hepatotoxicity of some drugs

## Patient preparation
▪ Explain that the ALT test assesses liver function.
▪ Tell the patient that the test requires a blood sample. Explain who will perform the venipuncture and when it will be done.
▪ Explain that the patient may experience slight discomfort from the tourniquet and needle puncture.
▪ Tell him that he doesn't need to restrict food or fluids.
▪ Notify the laboratory and practitioner of medications the patient is taking that may affect test results; these medications may need to be restricted.

## Procedure and posttest care
▪ Confirm the patient's identity using two patient identifiers according to facility policy.

▪ Perform a venipuncture and collect the sample in a 4-ml tube without additives.
▪ Apply direct pressure to the venipuncture site until bleeding stops.
▪ If a hematoma develops at the venipuncture site, apply warm soaks. If the hematoma is large, monitor pulses distal to the venipuncture site.
▪ Instruct the patient to resume medications stopped before the test, as ordered.

# Alkaline phosphatase
[ALP, alk phos]

The alkaline phosphatase (ALP) test measures serum levels of ALP, an enzyme that influences bone calcification and lipid and metabolite transport. ALP measurements reflect the combined activity of several ALP isoenzymes found in the liver, bones, kidneys, intestinal lining, and placenta. Bone and liver ALP are always present in adult serum, with liver ALP most prominent, except during the third trimester of pregnancy (when the placenta originates about half of all ALP). Intestinal ALP can be normal (almost exclusively in blood groups B and O), but it's usually an abnormal finding linked to hepatic disease.

The ALP test is particularly sensitive to mild biliary obstruction and is a primary indicator of space-occupying hepatic lesions. Additional liver function studies are usually required to identify hepatobiliary disorders. Although skeletal and hepatic diseases can raise ALP levels, this test is most useful for diagnosing metabolic bone disease.

## Reference values
▪ ALP values are 45 to 115 International Units/ml (SI, 45 to 115 units/L).

## Abnormal results
▪ Although significant ALP elevations are possible with diseases that affect many organs, they usually indicate

skeletal disease or extrahepatic or intrahepatic biliary obstruction causing cholestasis.

■ Many acute hepatic diseases cause ALP elevations before they affect serum bilirubin levels.

■ Moderate increases in ALP levels may reflect acute biliary obstruction from hepatocellular inflammation in active cirrhosis, mononucleosis, or viral hepatitis.

■ Moderate increases also in osteomalacia and deficiency-induced rickets.

■ Sharp elevations in ALP levels may indicate complete biliary obstruction by malignant or infectious infiltrations or fibrosis, most common in Paget's disease, and occasionally in biliary obstruction, extensive bone metastases, and hyperparathyroidism.

■ Metastatic bone tumors resulting from pancreatic cancer raise ALP levels without a concomitant rise in serum alanine aminotransferase levels.

■ Isoenzyme fractionation and additional enzyme tests (gamma-glutamyl transferase, lactate dehydrogenase, 5′ nucleotidase, and leucine aminopeptidase) are sometimes performed when the cause of ALP elevations is in doubt.

■ Rarely, low levels of serum ALP are associated with hypophosphatasia and protein or magnesium deficiency.

**DRUG CHALLENGE**

 Drugs that influence liver function or cause cholestasis, such as barbiturates, chlorpropamide, hormonal contraceptives, isoniazid, methyldopa, phenothiazines, phenytoin, and rifampin (possible mild increase); halothane sensitivity (possible drastic increase); clofibrate (decrease)

## Purpose

■ To detect and identify skeletal diseases primarily characterized by marked osteoblastic activity

■ To detect focal hepatic lesions causing biliary obstruction, such as tumors or abscesses

■ To assess the patient's response to vitamin D in the treatment of rickets

■ To supplement information from other liver function studies and GI enzyme tests

## Patient preparation

■ Explain that the ALP test assesses liver and bone function.

■ Instruct the patient to fast for at least 8 hours before the test because fat intake stimulates intestinal ALP secretion.

■ Tell him that this test requires a blood sample. Explain who will perform the venipuncture and when it will be done.

■ Inform him that he may experience slight discomfort from the tourniquet and needle puncture.

## Procedure and posttest care

■ Confirm the patient's identity using two patient identifiers according to facility policy.

■ Perform a venipuncture and collect the sample in a 4-ml clot-activator tube.

■ Apply direct pressure to the venipuncture site until bleeding stops.

■ If a hematoma develops at the venipuncture site, apply warm soaks. If the hematoma is large, monitor pulses distal to the venipuncture site.

■ Instruct the patient to resume his usual diet.

## Precautions

■ Send the sample to the laboratory immediately; ALP activity increases at room temperature because of a rise in pH.

# ▌Alpha₁-antitrypsin
### [AAT, alpha₁-AT]

A protein produced by the liver, alpha₁-antitrypsin (AAT) is believed to inhibit the release of protease into body fluids by dying cells and is a major component of alpha$_1$-globulin. AAT is measured using radioimmunoassay or isoelectric focusing. Congenital absence or deficiency of AAT has been linked to high susceptibility to emphysema in adults and cirrhosis in children.

### Reference values
- AAT levels are 110 to 200 mg/dl (SI, 1.1 to 2 g/L).

### Abnormal results
- Decreased AAT levels may occur in early-onset emphysema and cirrhosis, nephrotic syndrome, malnutrition, congenital alpha$_1$-globulin deficiency, and transiently in the neonate.
- Increased AAT levels can occur in chronic inflammatory disorders, necrosis, pregnancy, acute pulmonary infections, hyaline membrane disease in infants, hepatitis, systemic lupus erythematosus, and rheumatoid arthritis.

D**RUG** **CHALLENGE**

 Hormonal contraceptives and corticosteroids (possible false-high)

### Purpose
- To screen the patient at high risk for emphysema
- To use as a nonspecific method of detecting inflammation, severe infection, and necrosis
- To test for congenital AAT deficiency

### Patient preparation
- Explain to the patient (or parents if the patient is a child) that the AAT test helps diagnose respiratory or liver disease, inflammation, infection, or necrosis.
- Tell the patient that the test requires a blood sample. Explain who will perform the venipuncture and when it will be done.
- Explain that the patient may experience slight discomfort from the tourniquet and needle puncture.
- Tell him to avoid smoking because irritants in tobacco stimulate leukocytes in the lungs to release protease.
- Tell the patient to avoid hormonal contraceptives and steroids for 24 hours before the test.
- Tell the patient to fast for at least 8 hours before the test.

### Procedure and posttest care
- Confirm the patient's identity using two patient identifiers according to facility policy.
- Perform a venipuncture and collect the sample in a 4-ml tube without additives.
- In a child, puncture the clean area with a sharp needle or lancet, then collect the blood sample in a pipette, in a small container, or onto a slide.
- Apply direct pressure to the venipuncture site until bleeding stops.
- If a hematoma develops at the venipuncture site, apply warm soaks. If the hematoma is large, monitor pulses distal to the venipuncture site.
- Instruct the patient to resume his usual diet and medications stopped before the test as ordered.

### Precautions
- If clinically indicated, the patient with AAT levels less than 125 mg/dl (SI, 1.25 g/L) should be phenotyped to confirm homozygous and heterozygous deficiencies. (The patient with heterozygous deficiencies doesn't appear to be at increased risk for early emphysema.)

# Aspartate aminotransferase
## [AST, SGOT]

Aspartate aminotransferase (AST) is one of two enzymes that catalyze the conversion of the nitrogenous portion of an amino acid to an amino acid residue. It's essential to energy production in the Krebs cycle. AST is found in the cytoplasm and mitochondria of many cells, primarily in the liver, heart, skeletal muscles, kidneys, pancreas, and red blood cells. It's released into serum in proportion to cellular damage.

Although a high correlation exists between myocardial infarction (MI) and elevated AST levels, this test is sometimes considered superfluous for diagnosing MI because of its relatively low organ specificity; it doesn't allow differentiation between acute MI and the effects of hepatic congestion due to heart failure.

### Reference values

- For men, AST levels are 14 to 20 units/L (SI, 0.23 to 0.33 µkat/L).
- For women, AST levels are 10 to 36 units/L (SI, 0.17 to 0.6 µkat/L).
- For children, AST levels are 9 to 80 units/L (SI, 0.15 to 1.3 µkat/L).
- For neonates, AST levels are 47 to 150 units/L (SI, 0.78 to 2.5 µkat/L).

### Abnormal results

- AST levels fluctuate in response to the extent of cellular necrosis, increasing gradually early in the disease process and becoming extremely high during the most acute phase. Depending on when the first blood sample is drawn, serial AST levels may increase, indicating increasing disease severity and tissue damage, or they may decrease, indicating disease resolution and tissue repair.
- Maximum elevations in AST levels (more than 20 times normal) may indicate acute viral hepatitis, severe skeletal muscle trauma, extensive surgery, drug-induced hepatic injury, or severe passive liver congestion.
- High AST levels (10 to 20 times normal) may indicate severe MI, severe infectious mononucleosis, or alcoholic cirrhosis.
- High AST levels also occur during the prodromal and resolving stages of conditions that cause maximum elevations.
- Moderate to high AST levels (5 to 10 times normal) may indicate dermatomyositis, Duchenne's muscular dystrophy, or chronic hepatitis.
- Moderate to high levels also occur during prodromal and resolving stages of conditions that cause high elevations.
- Low to moderate AST levels (2 to 5 times normal) occur at some time during the preceding conditions or diseases, or may indicate hemolytic anemia, metastatic hepatic tumors, acute pancreatitis, pulmonary emboli, alcohol withdrawal syndrome, or fatty liver. AST levels rise slightly after the first few days of biliary duct obstruction.

### DRUG CHALLENGE

 Chlorpropamide, hormonal contraceptives, opioids, methyldopa, erythromycin, sulfonamides, pyridoxine, dicumarol, and antitubercular agents; large doses of acetaminophen, salicylates, or vitamin A; and many other drugs known to affect the liver (increase)

### Purpose

- To aid in the detection and differential diagnosis of acute hepatic disease
- To monitor patient progress and prognosis in cardiac and hepatic diseases

### Patient preparation

- Explain that the AST test assesses heart and liver function.

- Inform the patient that the test usually requires three venipunctures (one on admission and one each day for the next 2 days).
- Tell him that he doesn't need to restrict food or fluids.
- Explain to the patient that he may experience slight discomfort from the tourniquet and needle puncture.
- Notify the laboratory and practitioner of medications the patient is taking that may affect test results; these medications may need to be restricted.

### Procedure and posttest care
- Confirm the patient's identity using two patient identifiers according to facility policy.
- Perform a venipuncture and collect the sample in a 4-ml clot-activator tube.
- Apply direct pressure to the venipuncture site until bleeding stops.
- If a hematoma develops at the venipuncture site, apply warm soaks. If the hematoma is large, monitor pulses distal to the venipuncture site.
- Instruct the patient to resume medications stopped before the test as ordered.

### Precautions
- To avoid missing peak AST levels, draw serum samples at the same time each day.

# Gamma-glutamyl transferase
### [GGT, gamma-glutamyl transpeptidase]

Gamma-glutamyl transferase (GGT) participates in the transfer of amino acids across cellular membranes and, possibly, in glutathione metabolism. The highest levels of GGT exist in the kidney, but the enzyme also appears in the liver, biliary tract, epithelium, pancreas, lymphocytes, brain, and testes. The GGT test measures serum GGT levels.

Because GGT isn't elevated in bone growth or pregnancy, this test is a somewhat more sensitive indicator of hepatic necrosis than the aspartate aminotransferase assay and is at least as sensitive as the alkaline phosphatase (ALP) assay. The GGT test is nonspecific, providing few data about the type of hepatic disease because increased levels also occur in renal, cardiac, and prostatic disease and with the use of certain medications. GGT is particularly sensitive to the effects of alcohol on the liver, and levels may be elevated after moderate alcohol intake and in chronic alcoholism, even without evidence of hepatic injury.

### Reference values
- For children, GGT levels are 3 to 30 units/L (SI, 0.05 to 0.51 μkat/L).
- For men age 16 and older, GGT levels are 6 to 38 units/L (SI, 0.10 to 0.63 μkat/L).
- For women ages 16 to 45, GGT levels are 4 to 27 units/L (SI, 0.08 to 0.46 μkat/L); for women older than age 45, from 6 to 37 units/L (SI, 0.10 to 0.63 μkat/L).

### Abnormal results
- Serum GGT levels rise in acute hepatic disease because enzyme production increases in response to hepatocellular injury.
- Moderate increases in GGT levels occur in acute pancreatitis, renal disease, prostatic metastases, postoperatively, and in some patients with epilepsy or brain tumors.
- GGT levels also increase after alcohol ingestion because of enzyme induction. The sharpest elevations occur in patients with obstructive jaundice and hepatic metastatic infiltrations.
- GGT levels may also increase 5 to 10 days after acute myocardial infarction, either as a result of tissue granulation

and healing or as an indication of the effects of cardiac insufficiency on the liver.

DRUG CHALLENGE

 Clofibrate and hormonal contraceptives (decrease); aminoglycosides, barbiturates, phenytoin glutethimide, and methaqualone (increase)

### Purpose
■ To provide information about hepatobiliary diseases, to assess liver function, and to detect alcohol ingestion
■ To distinguish between skeletal and hepatic disease when the serum ALP level is elevated (a normal GGT level suggests that such elevation stems from skeletal disease)

### Patient preparation
■ Explain that the GGT test evaluates liver function.
■ Tell the patient that the test requires a blood sample. Explain who will perform the venipuncture and when it will be done.
■ Explain that the patient may experience slight discomfort from the tourniquet and needle puncture.
■ Tell him that he doesn't need to restrict food or fluids.

### Procedure and posttest care
■ Confirm the patient's identity using two patient identifiers according to facility policy.
■ Perform a venipuncture and collect the sample in a 4-ml tube without additives.
■ Apply direct pressure to the venipuncture site until bleeding stops.
■ If a hematoma develops at the venipuncture site, apply warm soaks. If the hematoma is large, monitor pulses distal to the venipuncture site.

# Leucine aminopeptidase
## [LAP]

The leucine aminopeptidase (LAP) test measures serum levels of LAP, an isoenzyme of alkaline phosphatase (ALP) that's widely distributed in body tissues. The greatest LAP levels are in the hepatobiliary tissues, pancreas, and small intestine. Serum LAP levels parallel serum ALP levels in hepatic disease.

### Reference values
■ For men, LAP levels are 80 to 200 units/ml (SI, 80 to 200 kU/L).
■ For women, LAP levels are 75 to 185 units/ml (SI, 75 to 185 kU/L).

### Abnormal results
■ High LAP levels can occur in biliary obstruction, tumors, strictures, atresia, advanced pregnancy, and therapy with drugs containing estrogen or progesterone.

### Purpose
■ To provide information about suspected liver, pancreatic, and biliary diseases
■ To differentiate skeletal disease from hepatobiliary or pancreatic disease
■ To evaluate neonatal jaundice

### Patient preparation
■ Explain that the LAP test evaluates liver and pancreatic function.
■ Tell the patient that the test requires a blood sample. Explain who will perform the venipuncture and when it will be done.
■ Explain that the patient may experience slight discomfort from the tourniquet and needle puncture.
■ Notify the laboratory and practitioner of medications the patient is taking that may affect test results; these medications may need to be restricted.

### Procedure and posttest care

- Confirm the patient's identity using two patient identifiers according to facility policy.
- Perform a venipuncture and collect the sample in a 4-ml clot-activator tube.
- If a hematoma develops at the venipuncture site, apply warm soaks. If the hematoma is large, monitor pulses distal to the venipuncture site.
- Apply direct pressure to the venipuncture site until bleeding stops.
- Instruct the patient to resume his usual diet and medications stopped before the test as ordered.

## ▌5'-nucleotidase
### [5'NT]

The enzyme 5'-nucleotidase (5'NT) is a phosphatase formed almost entirely in the hepatobiliary tract. Unlike alkaline phosphatase (ALP), it hydrolyzes nucleoside 5'-phosphate groups only. Measurement of serum 5'NT levels helps to determine whether ALP elevation is due to skeletal or to hepatic disease. Because 5'NT remains normal in skeletal disease and pregnancy, it's more specific for assessing hepatic dysfunction than ALP or leucine aminopeptidase.

This test, which measures serum 5'NT levels, is technically more difficult than the ALP assay. It hasn't been widely used as a liver function study, although some authorities consider it more sensitive than the ALP test to diagnose cholangitis, biliary cirrhosis, and malignant infiltrations of the liver.

### Reference values

- For adults, 5'NT levels are 2 to 17 units/L (SI, 0.03 to 0.29 µkat/L).
- For children, 5'NT levels may be lower.

### Abnormal results

- Extremely high 5'NT levels occur in common bile duct obstruction by calculi or tumors in diseases that cause severe intrahepatic cholestasis, such as neoplastic infiltrations of the liver.
- Slightly to moderately elevated 5'NT levels may reflect acute hepatocellular damage or active cirrhosis.

#### DRUG CHALLENGE

 Cholestatic drugs, such as phenothiazines, morphine, meperidine, and codeine as well as aspirin, acetaminophen, and phenytoin (increase)

### Purpose

- To distinguish between hepatobiliary and skeletal disease when the source of increased ALP levels is uncertain
- To help differentiate biliary obstruction from acute hepatocellular damage
- To detect hepatic metastasis in the absence of jaundice

### Patient preparation

- Explain that the 5'NT test evaluates liver function.
- Tell the patient that the test requires a blood sample. Explain who will perform the venipuncture and when it will be done.
- Explain that the patient may experience slight discomfort from the tourniquet and needle puncture.
- Tell him that he doesn't need to restrict food or fluids.

### Procedure and posttest care

- Confirm the patient's identity using two patient identifiers according to facility policy.
- Perform a venipuncture and collect the sample in a 4-ml tube without additives.
- Apply direct pressure to the venipuncture site until bleeding stops.

■ If a hematoma develops at the venipuncture site, apply warm soaks. If the hematoma is large, monitor pulses distal to the venipuncture site.

# Pancreatic enzyme tests

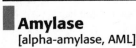

## Amylase
### [alpha-amylase, AML]

An enzyme that's synthesized primarily in the pancreas and salivary glands and is secreted in the GI tract, amylase (AML) helps to digest starch and glycogen in the mouth, stomach, and intestine. In cases of suspected acute pancreatic disease, measurement of AML levels is the most important laboratory test.

### Reference values
■ For adults age 18 and older, AML levels are 25 to 85 units/L (SI, 0.39 to 1.45 µkat/L).
■ Recent peripancreatic surgery may cause falsely high AML levels.
■ Determination of urine levels should follow normal serum AML results to rule out pancreatitis.

### Abnormal results
■ After the onset of acute pancreatitis, AML levels begin to rise within 2 hours, peak within 12 to 48 hours, and return to normal within 3 to 4 days.
■ Moderately elevated serum AML levels may accompany obstruction of the common bile duct, pancreatic duct, or ampulla of Vater; pancreatic injury from a perforated peptic ulcer; pancreatic cancer; and acute salivary gland disease.
■ Increased serum AML levels may indicated impaired kidney function.
■ Slightly elevated serum AML levels may occur in a patient who's asympto-

matic or responding unusually to therapy.
■ Decreased AML levels can occur in chronic pancreatitis, pancreatic cancer, cirrhosis, hepatitis, and toxemia of pregnancy.

### DRUG CHALLENGE

Aminosalicylic acid, asparaginase, azathioprine, corticosteroids, cyproheptadine, narcotic analgesics, hormonal contraceptives, rifampin, sulfasalazine, and thiazide or loop diuretics (possible false-high)

### Purpose
■ To diagnose acute pancreatitis
■ To distinguish between acute pancreatitis and other causes of abdominal pain that require immediate surgery
■ To evaluate possible pancreatic injury caused by abdominal trauma or surgery

### Patient preparation
■ Explain that the AML test assesses pancreatic function.
■ Tell the patient that this test requires a blood sample. Explain who will perform the venipuncture and when it will be done.
■ Inform the patient that he may experience slight discomfort from the tourniquet and needle puncture.
■ Inform him that he doesn't need to fast before the test but he must abstain from alcohol.
■ Notify the laboratory and practitioner of medications the patient is taking that may affect test results; these medications may need to be restricted.

### Procedure and posttest care
■ Confirm the patient's identity using two patient identifiers according to facility policy.
■ Perform a venipuncture and collect the sample in a 4-ml clot-activator tube.

- Apply direct pressure to the venipuncture site until bleeding stops.
- If a hematoma develops at the venipuncture site, apply warm soaks. If the hematoma is large, monitor pulses distal to the venipuncture site.
- Instruct the patient to resume medications stopped before the test as ordered.

## Precautions
DO'S & DON'TS

 If the patient has severe abdominal pain, draw the blood sample before diagnostic or therapeutic intervention. For accurate results, it's important to obtain an early sample.

# Lipase

Lipase is produced in the pancreas and secreted into the duodenum, where it converts triglycerides and other fats into fatty acids and glycerol. The destruction of pancreatic cells that occurs in acute pancreatitis causes large amounts of lipase to be released into the blood. (See *Blocked enzyme pathway*.) The lipase test measures serum lipase levels; it's most useful when performed with a serum or urine amylase test.

## Reference values
- Lipase levels are less than 160 units/L (SI, < 2.72 µkat/L).

## Abnormal results
- High lipase levels suggest acute pancreatitis or pancreatic duct obstruction. After an acute attack, levels remain elevated for up to 14 days.
- Lipase levels may also increase in other pancreatic injuries, such as perforated peptic ulcer with chemical pancreatitis due to gastric juices, and in a patient with high intestinal obstruction, pancreatic cancer, or renal disease with impaired excretion.

## Purpose
- To help diagnose acute pancreatitis

## Patient preparation
- Explain that the lipase test evaluates pancreatic function.
- Tell the patient that the test requires a blood sample. Explain who will perform the venipuncture and when it will be done.
- Inform the patient that he may experience slight discomfort from the tourniquet and needle puncture.
- Instruct him to fast overnight before the test.
- Notify the laboratory of medications the patient is taking that may affect test results; these medications may need to be restricted.

## Procedure and posttest care
- Confirm the patient's identity using two patient identifiers according to facility policy.
- Perform a venipuncture and collect the sample in a 4-ml clot-activator tube.
- Apply direct pressure to the venipuncture site until bleeding stops.
- If a hematoma develops at the venipuncture site, apply warm soaks. If the hematoma is large, monitor pulses distal to the venipuncture site.
- Instruct the patient to resume his usual diet and medications stopped before the test as ordered.

# *Special enzymes*

## Acid phosphatase
[prostatic acid phosphatase, PAP]

Acid phosphatase—a group of phosphatase enzymes most active at a pH of about 5.0—is found primarily in the prostate gland and semen and to a lesser

# Blocked enzyme pathway

The pancreas secretes lipase, amylase, and other enzymes that pass through the pancreatic duct into the duodenum. In pancreatitis and obstruction of the pancreatic duct by a tumor or calculus (shown below), these enzymes can't reach their intended destination. Instead, they're diverted into the bloodstream by a mechanism that isn't fully understood.

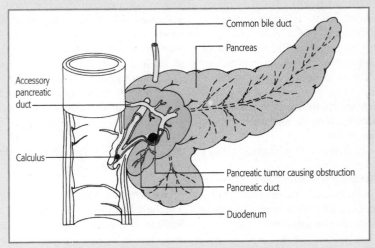

extent in the liver, spleen, red blood cells, bone marrow, and platelets. The acid phosphatase test measures total acid phosphatase and the prostatic fraction in serum.

This group's two major isoenzymes, prostatic and erythrocytic enzymes, can be separated in the laboratory. The prostatic isoenzyme is more specific for prostate cancer. The more widespread the cancer, the more likely that serum acid phosphatase levels will be increased.

### Reference values

- Serum total acid phosphatase levels, which depend on the assay method, are 0 to 3.7 units/L (SI, 0 to 3.7 units/L).

### Abnormal results

- High prostatic acid phosphatase levels usually indicate the presence of a tumor that has spread beyond the prostatic capsule. If the tumor has metastasized to bone, high acid phosphatase levels are accompanied by high alkaline phosphatase (ALP) levels, reflecting increased osteoblastic activity.
- Acid phosphatase levels rise moderately in prostatic infarction, Paget's disease (some cases), Gaucher's disease, and occasionally other conditions such as multiple myeloma. False results may occur if ALP levels are high because acid phosphatase and ALP are similar, differing mainly in their optimum pH ranges.

**D**RUG **CHALLENGE**

 Fluorides, phosphates, and oxalates (possible false-low); clofibrate (possible false-high)

## Purpose

- To detect prostate cancer
- To monitor the patient's response to therapy for prostate cancer (successful treatment decreases acid phosphatase levels)

## Patient preparation

- Explain that the acid phosphatase test evaluates prostate function.
- Tell the patient that the test requires a blood sample. Explain who will perform the venipuncture and when it will be done.
- Explain that he may experience slight discomfort from the tourniquet and needle puncture.
- Tell him that he doesn't need to restrict food or fluids.
- Notify the laboratory and practitioner of medications the patient is taking that may affect test results; these medications may need to be restricted.

## Procedure and posttest care

- Confirm the patient's identity using two patient identifiers according to facility policy.
- Perform a venipuncture and collect the sample in a 4-ml tube without additives.
- Apply direct pressure to the venipuncture site until bleeding stops.
- If a hematoma develops at the venipuncture site, apply warm soaks. If the hematoma is large, monitor pulses distal to the venipuncture site.
- Instruct the patient to resume medications stopped before the test as ordered.

D O ' S  &  D O N ' T S

 Don't draw the blood sample within 48 hours of prostate manipulation, catheterization, or rectal examination.

# Angiotensin-converting enzyme
### [ACE]

The angiotensin-converting enzyme (ACE) test measures serum levels of ACE, which is found in lung capillaries and, in lesser concentrations, in blood vessels and kidney tissue. Its primary function is to help regulate arterial pressure by converting angiotensin I to angiotensin II. Despite ACE's role in blood pressure regulation, this test is of little use in diagnosing hypertension. Instead, it's primarily used to diagnose sarcoidosis because of the high correlation between elevated serum ACE levels and this disease. Presumably, elevated serum ACE levels reflect macrophage activity.

## Reference values

- In the colorimetric assay, serum ACE levels in patients age 20 and older are 8 to 52 units/L (SI, 0.14 to 0.88 µkat/L).

## Abnormal results

- Elevated serum ACE levels may indicate sarcoidosis, Gaucher's disease, or Hansen's disease, but results must be correlated with the patient's clinical condition.
- In some cases, elevated ACE levels may result from hyperthyroidism, diabetic retinopathy, or hepatic disease.
- Serum ACE levels decline as the patient responds to steroid or prednisone therapy for sarcoidosis.

## Purpose

- To help diagnose sarcoidosis, especially pulmonary sarcoidosis
- To monitor the patient's response to therapy in sarcoidosis
- To help confirm Gaucher's or Hansen's disease

## Patient preparation

- Explain that the ACE test helps diagnose sarcoidosis, Gaucher's disease, or Hansen's disease; it may also be used to check the patient's response to sarcoidosis treatment.
- Tell the patient that the test requires a blood sample. Explain who will perform the venipuncture and when it will be done.
- Explain that he may experience slight discomfort from the tourniquet and needle puncture.
- Tell him that he must fast for 12 hours before the test.

 Note the patient's age on the laboratory request. If he's younger than age 20, the test may have to be postponed because of the variable ACE levels in this age-group.

## Procedure and posttest care

- Confirm the patient's identity using two patient identifiers according to facility policy.
- Perform a venipuncture and collect the sample in a 7-ml clot-activator tube.
- Apply direct pressure to the venipuncture site until bleeding stops.
- If a hematoma develops at the venipuncture site, apply warm soaks. If the hematoma is large, monitor pulses distal to the venipuncture site.

# █ Cholinesterase
## [CHS, acetylcholinesterase]

The cholinesterase (CHS) test measures the amounts of two similar enzymes that hydrolyze acetylcholine: acetylcholinesterase and pseudocholinesterase. Acetylcholinesterase is present in nerve tissue, red blood cells of the spleen, and gray matter of the brain. It inactivates acetylcholine at nerve junctions and regulates

muscle contractions. Pseudocholinesterase is produced primarily in the liver and appears in small amounts in the pancreas, intestines, heart, and white matter of the brain. Although the role of pseudocholinesterase is limited, its measurement is significant because certain chemicals that inactivate acetylcholinesterase also affect pseudocholinesterase.

Two groups of anticholinesterase chemicals—organophosphates and muscle relaxants—are important. Organophosphates, which are used by the military as nerve gases and are common ingredients in many insecticides, inactivate acetylcholinesterase directly. Muscle relaxants (such as succinylcholine), which interfere with acetylcholine-mediated transmission across nerve endings, are normally destroyed by pseudocholinesterase.

In suspected poisoning by an organophosphate, levels of either cholinesterase enzyme may be measured. For technical reasons, pseudocholinesterase is usually the enzyme of choice, although this analysis is less sensitive than that of acetylcholinesterase. In suspected poisoning by a muscle relaxant, the patient lacks adequate pseudocholinesterase, which usually inactivates the muscle relaxant. In this scenario, acetylcholinesterase level is measured.

## Reference values

- Pseudocholinesterase levels are 204 to 532 International Units/dl (SI, 2.04 to 5.32 kU/L).
- Pseudocholinesterase levels are usually normal in early extrahepatic obstruction.
- Acetylcholinesterase levels are 30 to 40 units/g hemoglobin.

## Abnormal results

- Severely decreased pseudocholinesterase levels suggest a congenital deficiency or organophosphate insecticide poisoning; levels near 0 necessitate emergency treatment.

- Variably decreased pseudocholinesterase levels occur in hepatocellular diseases, such as hepatitis and cirrhosis (especially cirrhosis with ascites and jaundice).
- Decreased pseudocholinesterase levels may indicate acute infection, chronic malnutrition, anemia, myocardial infarction, obstructive jaundice, and metastasis.
- Increased acetylcholinesterase levels may occur in sickle cell and hemolytic anemias.
- Decreased acetylcholinesterase levels may indicate megaloblastic anemia or organic phosphate poisoning.

#### DRUG CHALLENGE

 Cyclophosphamide, echothiophate iodide, monoamine oxidase inhibitors, succinylcholine, neostigmine, quinine, quinidine, chloroquine, caffeine, theophylline, epinephrine, ether, barbiturates, atropine, morphine, codeine, phenothiazines, vitamin K, and folic acid (possible false-low)

#### Purpose

- To evaluate before surgery or electroconvulsive therapy the patient's potential response to succinylcholine, which is hydrolyzed by cholinesterase
- To screen for adverse reactions to muscle relaxants
- To assess overexposure to insecticides containing organophosphate compounds
- To assess liver function and help diagnose hepatic disease (rarely)

#### Patient preparation

- Explain that the CHS test assesses muscle function or the extent of organophosphate poisoning.

- Tell the patient that the test requires a blood sample. Explain who will perform the venipuncture and when it will be done.
- Explain to the patient that he may experience slight discomfort from the tourniquet and needle puncture.
- Tell him that he doesn't need to restrict food or fluids.
- Notify the laboratory and practitioner of medications the patient is taking that may affect test results; these medications may need to be restricted.

#### Procedure and posttest care

- Confirm the patient's identity using two patient identifiers according to facility policy.
- Perform a venipuncture and collect the sample in a 7-ml clot-activator tube.
- Apply direct pressure to the venipuncture site until bleeding stops.
- If a hematoma develops at the venipuncture site, apply warm soaks. If the hematoma is large, monitor pulses distal to the venipuncture site.
- Instruct the patient to resume medications stopped before the test as ordered.

## Galactose-1-phosphate uridyltransferase
[GPUT]

Galactose-1-phosphate uridyltransferase (GPUT) is involved in the conversion of galactose to glucose during lactose metabolism. Deficiency may lead to galactosemia, a hereditary disorder marked by elevated serum galactose levels and decreased serum glucose levels. Unless detected and treated soon after birth, galactosemia can impair eye, brain, and liver development, causing irreversible cataracts, mental retardation, and cirrhosis.

The qualitative test, a simple screening test for deficiency of GPUT, is required in some facilities for all neonates. If this test yields a positive result, a quantitative test should be ordered as soon as possible. Occasionally this test is ordered for an adult to detect a carrier state. The quantitative test measures the amount of a fluorescent substance generated during a coupled enzyme reaction.

### Reference values

- The qualitative GPUT test result is normally negative.
- Quantitative GPUT test values are 18.5 to 28.5 units/g of hemoglobin (Hb); the normal range should be confirmed with the laboratory in case a different method is used.

### Abnormal results

- A positive qualitative test result may indicate a GPUT deficiency. A follow-up quantitative test should be performed as soon as possible.
- Quantitative test results showing less than 5 units/g of Hb indicate galactosemia.
- GPUT levels between 5 and 18.5 units/ g of Hb may indicate a carrier state.

### Purpose

- To screen an infant for galactosemia
- To identify a heterozygous carrier of galactosemia

### Patient preparation
#### When testing a neonate

- Explain to the parents that the GPUT test screens for galactosemia, a potentially dangerous enzyme deficiency.
- If a blood sample wasn't taken from the umbilical cord at birth, tell the parents that a small amount of blood will be drawn from the infant's heel.

- Explain that the procedure is safe and performed quickly.

### When testing an adult

- Explain that this test identifies carriers of galactosemia, a genetic disorder that may be transmitted to offspring.
- Tell him that the test requires a blood sample. Explain who will perform the venipuncture and when it will be done.
- Explain to the patient that he may experience slight discomfort from the tourniquet and needle puncture.
- Tell the patient that he doesn't need to restrict food or fluids.

### Procedure and posttest care

- Confirm the patient's identity using two patient identifiers according to facility policy.
- For a qualitative (screening) test, collect cord blood, or blood from a heelstick or fingerstick on special filter paper, saturating all three circles.
- For a quantitative test, perform a venipuncture and collect a 4-ml sample in a heparinized or EDTA tube, depending on the laboratory method used.
- Indicate the patient's age on the laboratory request.

Do's & don'ts

 Check the patient's history for a recent exchange transfusion. Note this on the laboratory request or postpone the test.

- Apply direct pressure to the venipuncture site until bleeding stops.
- If a hematoma develops at the venipuncture site, apply warm soaks.
- If test results indicate galactosemia, refer the parents for nutrition counseling and provide a galactose- and lactose-free diet for their infant. A soybean- or meat-based formula may be substituted for formulas based on cow's milk.

## Precautions
- Send the sample to the laboratory on wet ice.

## Hexosaminidase A and B
### [HEX A and B]

This fluorometric test measures the hexosaminidase A and B (HEX A and B) content of serum samples drawn by venipuncture or collected from a neonate's umbilical cord, or of amniotic fluid obtained by amniocentesis. HEX deficiency can also be identified by testing cultured skin fibroblasts; however, this procedure is costly and technically complex. A reference center for congenital disease should be consulted for the preferred screening method and specimen type.

HEX is a group of enzymes that are necessary for metabolism of gangliosides, water-soluble glycolipids found primarily in brain tissue. The HEX A and B test measures the HEX A and B content of serum and amniotic fluid.

Deficiency of HEX A indicates Tay-Sachs disease, which affects people of Eastern European Jewish ancestry about 100 times more often than the general population. Both parents must carry the defective gene to transmit Tay-Sachs disease to their children. Sandhoff's disease, which results from a deficiency of HEX A and B, is uncommon and is not prevalent in any ethnic group.

### Reference values
- Total serum HEX levels are 5 to 12.9 units/L; HEX A accounts for 55% to 76% of the total.

### Abnormal results
- The absence of HEX A indicates Tay-Sachs disease (total HEX levels can be normal).

- The absence of HEX A and B indicates Sandhoff's disease, an uncommon, virulent variant of Tay-Sachs disease, in which deterioration occurs more rapidly.

**DRUG CHALLENGE**

Hormonal contraceptives (false-high); rifampin and isoniazid (increase)

### Purpose
- To confirm or rule out Tay-Sachs disease in the neonate
- To screen for a Tay-Sachs carrier
- To establish prenatal diagnosis of HEX A deficiency

### Patient preparation
- Explain that the HEX A and B test identifies carriers of Tay-Sachs disease.
- Tell the patient that the test requires a blood sample. Explain who will perform the venipuncture and when it will be done.
- Explain that he may experience slight discomfort from the tourniquet and needle puncture.
- Tell him that he doesn't need to restrict food or fluids.
- When testing a neonate, explain to the parents that this test detects Tay-Sachs disease. Tell them that blood will be drawn from the neonate's arm, neck, or umbilical cord; that the procedure is safe and performed quickly; and that the neonate will have a small bandage on the venipuncture site. Inform them that food and fluid restrictions aren't needed.
- If the test is being performed prenatally, advise the patient of preparations for amniocentesis.

### Procedure and posttest care
- Confirm the patient's identity using two patient identifiers according to facility policy.

- Perform a venipuncture, collect cord blood, or assist with amniocentesis, as appropriate. Collect the sample in a 7-ml clot-activator tube.
- Apply direct pressure to the venipuncture site until bleeding stops.
- If a hematoma develops at the venipuncture site, apply warm soaks. If the hematoma is large, monitor pulses distal to the venipuncture site.
- When testing a neonate, follow laboratory procedure for collecting serum samples.

# Lactate dehydrogenase
## [LD, LDH]

Lactate dehydrogenase (LD) catalyzes the reversible conversion of muscle lactic acid into pyruvic acid, an essential step in the metabolic process that ultimately produces cellular energy.

Five tissue-specific isoenzymes can be identified and measured using immunochemical separation and quantitation or electrophoresis. Two of these isoenzymes, $LD_1$ and $LD_2$, appear primarily in the heart, red blood cells (RBCs), and kidneys; $LD_3$ appears primarily in the lungs; and $LD_4$ and $LD_5$ appear in the liver and the skeletal muscles. The midzone fractions ($LD_2$, $LD_3$, $LD_4$) can be elevated in granulocytic leukemia, lymphomas, and platelet disorders.

The specificity of LD isoenzymes and their distribution pattern is useful in diagnosing hepatic, pulmonary, and erythrocyte damage. (See *LD isoenzyme variations in disease,* page 86.)

## Reference values
- Total LD levels are 71 to 207 units/L (SI, 1.20 to 3.52 µkat/L).

- $LD_1$ levels are 14% to 26% (SI, 0.14 to 0.26) of total LD.
- $LD_2$ levels are 29% to 39% (SI, 0.29 to 0.39) of total LD.
- $LD_3$ levels are 20% to 26% (SI, 0.20 to 0.26) of total LD.
- $LD_4$ levels are 8% to 16% (SI, 0.08 to 0.16) of total LD.
- $LD_5$ levels are 6% to 16% (SI, 0.06 to 0.16) of total LD.

## Abnormal results
- Because many common diseases increase total LD levels, isoenzyme electrophoresis is usually necessary for diagnosis.
- In some disorders, total LD levels may be within normal limits, but abnormal proportions of each enzyme indicate specific organ tissue damage.
- Midzone fractions ($LD_2$, $LD_3$, $LD_4$) can be increased in granulocytic leukemia, lymphomas, and platelet disorders.

### DRUG CHALLENGE

 Anabolic steroids, anesthetics, alcohol, opioids, and procainamide (increase)

## Purpose
- To aid in the differential diagnosis of pulmonary infarction, anemias, and hepatic disease
- To monitor the patient's response to some forms of chemotherapy

## Patient preparation
- Explain that the LD test detects tissue alterations.
- Tell the patient that the test requires a blood sample. Explain who will perform the venipuncture and when it will be done.
- Explain that he may experience slight discomfort from the tourniquet and needle puncture.

## LD isoenzyme variations in disease

| Disease | $LD_1$ | $LD_2$ | $LD_3$ | $LD_4$ | $LD_5$ |
|---|---|---|---|---|---|
| **Cardiovascular** | | | | | |
| MI with hepatic congestion | | | | | |
| Rheumatic carditis | | | | | |
| Myocarditis | | | | | |
| Heart failure (decompensated) | | | | | |
| Shock | | | | | |
| Angina pectoris | | | | | |
| **Pulmonary** | | | | | |
| Pulmonary embolism | | | | | |
| Pulmonary infarction | | | | | |
| **Hematologic** | | | | | |
| Pernicious anemia | | | | | |
| Hemolytic anemia | | | | | |
| Sickle cell anemia | | | | | |
| **Hepatobiliary** | | | | | |
| Hepatitis | | | | | |
| Active cirrhosis | | | | | |
| Hepatic congestion | | | | | |

Legend: ▮ Normal ▮ Diagnostic ▮ Not diagnostic

Adapted with permission from Helena Laboratories, 1513 Lindberg Drive, Beaumont, Tex.

- Tell the patient that he doesn't need to restrict food or fluids.

**Procedure and posttest care**
- Confirm the patient's identity using two patient identifiers according to facility policy.

- Perform a venipuncture and collect the sample in a 4-ml clot-activator tube.
- Apply direct pressure to the venipuncture site until bleeding stops.
- If a hematoma develops at the venipuncture site, apply warm soaks. If the hematoma is large, monitor pulses distal to the venipuncture site.

### Precautions

- Draw the blood samples on schedule to avoid missing peak levels and mark the collection time on the laboratory request.
- Handle the sample gently to prevent artifact blood sample hemolysis because RBCs contain $LD_1$.
- Send the sample to the laboratory immediately or, if transport is delayed, keep the sample at room temperature. Changes in temperature reportedly inactivate $LD_5$, thus altering isoenzyme patterns.

## Prostate-specific antigen
### [PSA]

Until recently, digital rectal examination (DRE) and measurement of prostatic acid phosphatase were the primary methods of monitoring the progression of prostate cancer. Now measurement of prostate-specific antigen (PSA) helps track the course of this disease and evaluate the patient's response to treatment.

PSA appears in normal, benign hyperplastic and malignant prostatic tissue as well as in metastatic prostatic carcinoma. Serum PSA levels are measured to monitor the spread or recurrence of prostate cancer and to evaluate the patient's response to treatment. Measurement of serum PSA levels, along with DRE, is now recommended as a screening test for prostate cancer in men over age 50. (See *Controversy over PSA screening*, page 88.) This test is also useful in assessing response to treatment in a patient with stage B3 to D1 prostate cancer and in detecting tumor spread or recurrence.

### Reference values

- For men ages 40 to 50, PSA levels are 2 to 2.8 ng/ml (SI, 2.0 to 2.8 µg/L).
- For men ages 51 to 60, PSA levels are 2.9 to 3.8 ng/ml (SI, 2.9 to 3.8 µg/L).
- For men ages 61 to 70, PSA levels are 4 to 5.3 ng/ml (SI, 4.0 to 5.3 µg/L).
- For men age 71 and older, PSA levels are 5.6 to 7.2 ng/ml (SI, 5.6 to 7.2 µg/L).

### Abnormal results

- About 80% of patients with prostate cancer have pretreatment PSA levels greater than 4 ng/ml.
- About 20% of patients with benign prostatic hyperplasia also have PSA levels greater than 4 ng/ml.
- PSA results alone don't confirm a diagnosis of prostate cancer. Further assessment and testing, including tissue biopsy, are needed to confirm the diagnosis.

DRUG CHALLENGE

 Excessive doses of chemotherapeutic drugs, such as cyclophosphamide, diethylstilbestrol, and methotrexate (possible increase or decrease)

### Purpose

- To screen for prostate cancer in men older than age 50
- To monitor the course of prostate cancer and evaluate treatment

### Patient preparation

- Explain that the PSA test screens for prostate cancer or monitors the course of treatment.
- Tell the patient that the test requires a blood sample. Explain who will perform

## Controversy over PSA screening

Measurement of prostate-specific antigen (PSA) allows earlier detection of prostate cancer than digital rectal examination (DRE) alone. Accordingly, the American Cancer Society and the American Urological Association currently recommend that PSA screening begin at age 40 (in combination with DRE) in black men and any man who has a father or brother with prostate cancer, and at age 50 in all other men.

Does this test actually reduce mortality from prostate cancer? The answer to that question remains unknown. Some specialists question the value of all prostate cancer screening tests because of the costs involved, the uncertain benefits, and the known risks associated with current treatments.

Before undergoing a PSA test, the patient should understand that controversy surrounds nearly every aspect of prostate cancer screening and treatment. The issues he'll face may include:

■ Even if cancer is detected, treatment may not be advisable either because of the patient's advanced age or because the physician believes the tumor is so slow-growing that it won't result in death.

■ The current treatments for prostate cancer—surgery and radiation therapy—may not be as effective as experts formerly believed, and no effective chemotherapy protocol is currently available.

■ Surgery and radiation therapy carry a high risk of impotence, incontinence, and other problems, which the patient must weigh against the uncertain benefits of therapy.

■ Screening tests sometimes yield false-positive results, requiring transrectal ultrasonography or a biopsy to confirm the diagnosis.

■ A mildly elevated PSA level may be the result of normal age-related increases. (Data from a study of more than 9,000 men showed that PSA levels increase by about 30% per year in men younger than age 70 and by more than 40% per year in men age 70 and older.)

In summary, the value of prostate cancer screening in general and PSA testing in particular won't be clearly established until studies show a definitive link between early treatment and reduced mortality.

the venipuncture and when it will be done.
■ Explain that the patient may experience slight discomfort from the tourniquet and needle puncture.
■ Tell him that he doesn't need to restrict food or fluids.

### Procedure and posttest care

■ Confirm the patient's identity using two patient identifiers according to facility policy.
■ Perform a venipuncture and collect the sample in a 7-ml clot-activator tube.
■ Apply direct pressure to the venipuncture site until bleeding stops.

■ If a hematoma develops at the venipuncture site, apply warm soaks. If the hematoma is large, monitor pulses distal to the venipuncture site.

### Precautions

■ Collect the sample either before or at least 48 hours after DRE to avoid falsely elevated PSA levels.

## ▌Pyruvate kinase
### [PK]

An erythrocyte enzyme, pyruvate kinase (PK) takes part in the anaerobic metabolism of glucose. An abnormally low PK level is an inherited autosomal recessive trait that may cause a red blood cell (RBC) membrane defect associated with congenital hemolytic anemia. The PK assay confirms PK deficiency when RBC enzyme deficiency is the suspected cause of anemia.

### Reference values
- Normal serum PK values range from 9 to 22 units/g of hemoglobin (Hb); in the low substrate assay, they range from 1.7 to 6.8 units/g of hemoglobin.

### Abnormal results
- Low serum PK levels confirm a diagnosis of PK deficiency and allow differentiation between PK-deficient hemolytic anemia and other inherited disorders.

### Purpose
- To differentiate PK-deficient hemolytic anemia from other congenital hemolytic anemias or from acquired hemolytic anemia
- To detect PK deficiency in asymptomatic, heterozygous inheritance

### Patient preparation
- Explain that the PK test detects inherited enzyme deficiencies.
- Tell the patient that the test requires a blood sample. Explain who will perform the venipuncture and when it will be done.
- Explain to the patient that he may experience slight discomfort from the tourniquet and needle puncture.
- Tell the patient that he doesn't need to restrict food or fluids.
- Check the patient's history for recent blood transfusions and note it on the laboratory request.

### Procedure and posttest care
- Confirm the patient's identity using two patient identifiers according to facility policy.
- Perform a venipuncture and collect the sample in a 4-ml EDTA tube.
- Apply direct pressure to the venipuncture site until bleeding stops.
- If a hematoma develops at the venipuncture site, apply warm soaks. If the hematoma is large, monitor pulses distal to the venipuncture site.

## Renin activity
### [plasma renin activity, PRA]

Renin secretion from the kidneys is the first stage of the renin-angiotensin-aldosterone cycle, which controls the body's sodium-potassium balance, fluid volume, and blood pressure. Renin is released into the renal veins in response to sodium depletion and blood loss. It catalyzes the conversion of angiotensinogen, an alpha$_2$ globulin plasma protein, to angiotensin I, which in turn is converted by hydrolysis into angiotensin II, a vasoconstrictor that stimulates aldosterone production in the adrenal cortex. (See *Renin-angiotensin feedback system,* page 90.) When present in excessive amounts, angiotensin II causes renal hypertension.

The plasma renin activity (PRA) test is a screening procedure for renovascular hypertension but doesn't unequivocally confirm the diagnosis. When supplemented by other special tests, the PRA test can help establish the cause of hypertension. For instance, sampling blood obtained from the renal veins by renal vein catheterization and analyzing the renal venous renin ratio can identify renovascular disorders. Indexing renin levels against urinary sodium excretion can help identify primary aldosteronism, and a sodium-depleted PRA test can then confirm this diagnosis.

Some experts believe that the type of treatment chosen for essential hypertension should depend on whether renin levels are low, normal, or high; the PRA

# Renin-angiotensin feedback system

The renin-angiotensin-aldosterone system, sometimes known as the juxtaglomerular apparatus, is an important homeostatic device for regulating the body's sodium and water levels and blood pressure. It works this way:

Juxtaglomerular cells (1) in each of the kidney's glomeruli secrete the enzyme renin into the blood. The rate of renin secretion depends on the rate of perfusion in the afferent renal arterioles (2) and on the amount of sodium in the serum. A low sodium load and low perfusion pressure (as in hypovolemia) increase renin secretion; high sodium and high perfusion pressure decrease it.

Renin circulates throughout the body. In the liver, renin converts angiotensinogen to angiotensin I (3), which passes to the lungs. There it's converted by hydrolysis to angiotensin II (4), a potent vasoconstrictor that acts on the adrenal cortex to stimulate production of the hormone aldosterone (5). Aldosterone acts on the juxtaglomerular cells to stimulate or depress renin secretion, completing the feedback cycle that automatically readjusts homeostasis.

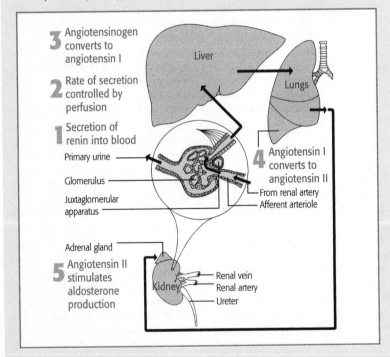

test can therefore categorize the disease to allow for appropriate therapy.

PRA is measured by radioimmunoassay of a peripheral or renal blood sample; results are expressed as the rate of angiotensin I formation per unit of time.

Patient preparation is crucial and may take up to 1 month.

## Reference values

■ PRA and aldosterone levels decrease with age.

### Sodium-depleted, upright, peripheral vein

- For adults ages 18 to 39, normal PRA levels range from 2.9 to 24 ng/ml/hour (mean, 10.8 ng/ml/hour).
- For adults age 40 and older, normal PRA levels range from 2.9 to 10.8 ng/ml/hour (mean, 5.9 ng/ml/hour).

### Sodium-replete, upright, peripheral vein

- For adults ages 18 to 39, normal PRA levels range from less than or equal to 0.6 to 4.3 ng/ml/hour (mean, 1.9 ng/ml/hour).
- For adults age 40 and older, normal PRA levels range from less than or equal to 0.6 to 3.0 ng/ml/hour (mean, 1 ng/ml/hour).

### Renal vein catheterization

- The normal renal venous renin ratio (the renin level in the renal vein compared with the level in the inferior vena cava) is less than 1.5 to 1.

## Abnormal results

- High PRA levels may occur in essential hypertension (uncommon), malignant and renovascular hypertension, cirrhosis, hypokalemia, hypovolemia due to hemorrhage, renin-producing renal tumors (Bartter syndrome), and adrenal hypofunction (Addison's disease).
- High PRA levels may also be found in chronic renal failure with parenchymal disease, end-stage renal disease, and transplant rejection.
- Low PRA levels may indicate hypervolemia due to a high-sodium diet, salt-retaining steroids, primary aldosteronism, Cushing's syndrome, licorice ingestion syndrome, or essential hypertension with low renin levels.
- Low PRA levels with high serum and urine aldosterone levels help identify primary aldosteronism.

- A low PRA level in the sodium-depleted PRA test confirms primary aldosteronism and differentiates it from secondary aldosteronism (characterized by increased renin).

### DRUG CHALLENGE

 Salt intake, hormonal contraceptives, and therapy with diuretics, antihypertensives, or vasodilators (increase); salt-retaining corticosteroid therapy and antidiuretic therapy (decrease)

## Purpose

- To screen for renal origin of hypertension
- To help plan treatment for essential hypertension, a genetic disease commonly aggravated by excess sodium intake
- To help identify hypertension linked to unilateral (sometimes bilateral) renovascular disease by renal vein catheterization
- To help identify primary aldosteronism (Conn's syndrome) resulting from an aldosterone-secreting adrenal adenoma
- To confirm primary aldosteronism (sodium-depleted PRA test)

## Patient preparation

- Explain that the PRA test determines the cause of hypertension.
- Notify the laboratory and practitioner of medications the patient is taking that may affect test results; these medications may need to be restricted.
- Tell the patient to maintain a normal sodium diet (3 g/day) during this period.
- For the sodium-depleted PRA test, tell the patient that he'll receive furosemide (or chlorothiazide, if he has angina or cerebrovascular insufficiency) and follow a specific low-sodium diet for 3 days.

- The patient shouldn't receive radioactive treatments for several days before the test.
- Tell the patient that the test requires a blood sample. Explain who will perform the venipuncture and when it will be done.
- Explain to the patient that he may experience slight discomfort from the tourniquet and needle puncture. Collect a morning blood sample, if possible.
- If a recumbent blood sample is ordered, instruct the patient to remain in bed at least 2 hours before the sample is obtained (posture influences renin secretion). If an upright blood sample is ordered, instruct him to stand or sit upright for 2 hours before the test is performed.
- If renal vein catheterization is ordered, make sure the patient has signed an informed consent form. Tell the patient that the procedure will be done in the X-ray department and that he'll receive a local anesthetic.

### Procedure and posttest care

- Confirm the patient's identity using two patient identifiers according to facility policy.

#### *Peripheral vein sample*

- Perform a venipuncture and collect the sample in a 4-ml EDTA tube.
- Note on the laboratory request if the patient was fasting and whether he was upright or in a supine position during sample collection.
- Apply direct pressure to the venipuncture site until bleeding stops.
- If a hematoma develops at the venipuncture site, apply warm soaks. If the hematoma is large, monitor pulses distal to the venipuncture site.

#### *Renal vein catheterization*

- A catheter is advanced to the kidneys through the femoral vein under fluoro-

scopic control and blood samples are obtained from the renal veins and vena cava.
- After renal vein catheterization, apply pressure to the catheterization site for 10 to 20 minutes, to prevent extravasation.
- Monitor vital signs and check the catheterization site every 30 minutes for 2 hours and then every hour for 4 hours to ensure that the bleeding has stopped. Check the patient's distal pulse for signs of thrombus formation and arterial occlusion (cyanosis, loss of pulse, cool skin).

#### *Both methods*

- Instruct the patient to resume his usual diet and medications stopped before the test as ordered.

### Precautions
**DO'S & DON'TS**

 The blood sample must be drawn into a chilled syringe and collection tube, placed on ice, and sent to the laboratory immediately.

# ▌Total homocysteine
## [tHcy]

Homocysteine (Hcy), a sulfur-containing amino acid, is a transmethylation product of methionine. It's an intermediate in the synthesis of cysteine, which is produced by the enzymatic or acid hydrolysis of proteins. The tHcy test is useful for the biochemical diagnosis of inborn errors of methionine, folate, and vitamin $B_6$ and $B_{12}$ metabolism.

### Reference values
- tHcy values are 4 to 17 µmol/L.

### Abnormal results
- Low tHcy levels are linked to inborn or acquired folate or cobalamin deficien-

cy and with inborn vitamin $B_6$ or $B_{12}$ deficiency.

- High tHcy levels are associated with a higher incidence of atherosclerotic vascular disease.
- In patients with type 2 diabetes mellitus, studies have shown that tHcy levels increase with even a modest deterioration in renal function.

### Purpose

- To aid in the biochemical diagnosis of inborn errors of methionine, folate, and vitamin $B_6$ and $B_{12}$ metabolism .
- To identify acquired folate or cobalamin deficiency
- To evaluate risk factors for atherosclerotic vascular disease
- To evaluate tHcy as a contributing factor in the pathogenesis of neural tube defects
- To evaluate the cause of recurrent spontaneous abortions
- To evaluate delayed child development or failure to thrive in infants

### Patient preparation

- Inform the patient that the tHcy test detects Hcy levels in plasma.
- Advise him to fast for 12 to 14 hours before the test.
- Tell him that this test requires a blood sample. Explain who will perform the venipuncture and when it will be done.
- Explain that he may experience slight discomfort from the tourniquet and needle puncture.

### Procedure and posttest care

- Confirm the patient's identity using two patient identifiers according to facility policy.
- Perform a venipuncture and collect the sample in a 5-ml tube with EDTA added.
- Apply direct pressure to the venipuncture site until bleeding stops.

- If a hematoma develops at the venipuncture site, apply warm soaks. If the hematoma is large, monitor pulses distal to the venipuncture site.

# Uroporphyrinogen I synthase

The uroporphyrinogen I synthase test measures blood levels of uroporphyrinogen I synthase, an enzyme involved in heme biosynthesis. This enzyme is usually present in erythrocytes, fibroblasts, lymphocytes, hepatic cells, and amniotic fluid cells. A hereditary deficiency that can reduce uroporphyrinogen I synthase levels by 50% or more results in acute intermittent porphyria (AIP). This disorder can be latent indefinitely until certain factors (some sex hormones and drugs, a low-carbohydrate diet, or an infection) precipitate active disease.

An improvement over traditional urine tests that can detect AIP only during an acute episode, the uroporphyrinogen I synthase test can detect AIP even during its latent phase. Thus, it can identify an affected individual before an acute episode occurs. Because it's specific for AIP, this test can also differentiate AIP from other types of porphyria.

Enzyme activity is determined by fluorometrically measuring the conversion rate of porphobilinogen to uroporphyrinogen. If uroporphyrinogen I synthase levels are indeterminate, urine and stool tests for aminolevulinic acid (ALA) and porphobilinogen may be ordered to support the diagnosis because excretion of these porphyrin precursors increases substantially during an acute episode of AIP and may increase slightly during the latent phase.

## Reference values
- Normal uroporphyrinogen I synthase levels are greater than or equal to 7 nmol/sec/L.

## Abnormal results
- Decreased uroporphyrinogen I synthase levels generally indicate latent or active AIP; symptoms differentiate these phases.
- Levels that are less than 6 nmol/sec/L confirm AIP.
- Levels between 6 and 6.9 nmol/sec/L are indeterminate, in which case urine and stool tests for the porphyrin precursors ALA and porphobilinogen may be ordered to support the diagnosis.

### DRUG CHALLENGE

 Alcohol and drugs, such as steroid hormones, estrogens, barbiturates, sulfonamides, phenytoin, griseofulvin, chlordiazepoxide, meprobamate, glutethimide, and ergot alkaloids (possible decrease)

## Purpose
- To help diagnose latent or active AIP
- To differentiate AIP from other types of porphyria

## Patient preparation
- Explain that the uroporphyrinogen I synthase test detects a red blood cell disorder.
- Inform the patient that he'll need to fast for 12 to 14 hours before the test and to abstain from alcohol for 24 hours but that he may drink water.
- Tell the patient that the test requires a blood sample. Explain who will perform the venipuncture and when it will be done.
- Explain to the patient that he may experience slight discomfort from the tourniquet and needle puncture.

- If the patient's hematocrit is available, note it on the laboratory request.
- Notify the laboratory and practitioner of medications the patient is taking that may affect test results; these medications may need to be restricted.

## Procedure and posttest care
- Confirm the patient's identity using two patient identifiers according to facility policy.
- Perform a venipuncture and collect the sample in a 10-ml heparinized tube.
- Apply direct pressure to the venipuncture site until bleeding stops.
- If a hematoma develops at the venipuncture site, apply warm soaks. If the hematoma is large, monitor pulses distal to the venipuncture site.
- Instruct the patient to resume his usual diet and medications stopped before the test, as ordered.
- If AIP is present, refer the patient for nutrition and genetic counseling. Advise him to avoid low-carbohydrate diets, alcohol, and drugs that may trigger an acute episode and to seek prompt care for all infections.

# Hormones

## Pituitary hormones

### ■ Alpha-subunit of pituitary glycoprotein hormones

The alpha-subunit of pituitary glycoprotein hormone (alpha-PGH) test uses radioimmunoassay to alpha-PGHs. These hormones—thyroid-stimulating hormone (TSH) and human chorionic gonadotropin (HCG)—contain similar alpha-subunits but differ in their beta-subunits. Alpha-PGH measurement assesses total pituitary production of these hormones.

#### Reference values
- Alpha-PGH level is ≤ 1.2 ng/ml (SI, ≤ 1.2 µg/L).

#### Abnormal results
- Low levels of alpha-PGH appear in the patient with inadequate pituitary hormone production (hypopituitarism). This results in reduced follicle-stimulating hormone (FSH), luteinizing hormone (LH), and TSH levels.
- Elevated levels of alpha-PGH levels indicate recurrent pituitary tumors or ineffective treatment of these tumors.

#### Purpose
- To aid diagnosis of recurrent pituitary tumors in the patient who has undergone pituitary resection

#### Patient preparation
- Explain that this test helps assess pituitary function.
- Inform the patient that he doesn't need to fast.
- Tell him that the test requires a venous blood sample. Explain who will perform the venipuncture and when.
- Explain to the patient that he may experience slight discomfort from the tourniquet and needle puncture.

#### Procedure and posttest care
- Confirm the patient's identity using two patient identifiers according to facility policy.
- Perform a venipuncture, and collect the blood sample in a 5-ml clot-activator tube.
- Send the sample to the laboratory immediately.
- Apply direct pressure to the venipuncture site until bleeding stops.
- If a hematoma develops at the venipuncture site, apply warm soaks.

### ■ Antidiuretic hormone

Antidiuretic hormone (ADH) promotes water reabsorption in response to in-

## ADH release and regulation

Neural impulses signal the supraoptic nuclei of the hypothalamus to produce antidiuretic hormone (ADH). After it's formed, ADH moves along the hypothalamico—hypophysial tract to the posterior pituitary, where it's stored until needed by the kidneys to maintain fluid balance. In the kidneys, ADH acts on the collecting tubules to retain water.

Homeostasis is maintained by a negative feedback mechanism: Ample water or water excess inhibits further ADH secretion by the supraoptic nuclei of the hypothalamus or ADH release from the posterior pituitary. A similar negative feedback mechanism that's vital to hormonal homeostasis prevents oversecretion of other hormones.

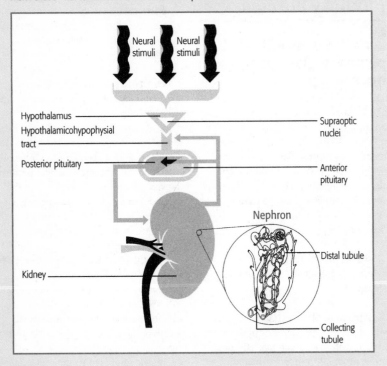

creased osmolality (water deficiency with high concentration of sodium and other solutes). In response to decreased osmolality (water excess), reduced secretion of ADH allows increased excretion of water to maintain fluid balance. (See *ADH release and regulation*.) Along with aldosterone, ADH helps regulate sodium, potassium, and fluid balance. It also stimulates vascular smooth-muscle contraction, causing an increase in arterial blood pressure.

This relatively rare test, a quantitative analysis of serum ADH levels, may identify diabetes insipidus and other causes of severe homeostatic imbalance. It may be ordered as part of dehydration or hypertonic saline infusion testing, which determines the body's response to states of hyperosmolality.

## Reference values

- ADH values range from 1 to 5 pg/ml (SI, 1 to 5 mg/L).
- ADH may also be evaluated in light of serum osmolality; if serum osmolality is less than 285 mOsm/kg, ADH is normally less than 2 pg/ml (SI, < 2 mg/L); if the ADH value is greater than 290 mOsm/kg, ADH may range from 2 to 12 pg/ml (SI, 2 to 12 mg/L).

## Abnormal results

- Absent or below-normal ADH levels indicate pituitary diabetes insipidus, resulting from a neurohypophyseal or hypothalamic tumor, viral infection, metastatic disease, sarcoidosis, tuberculosis, Hand-Schüller-Christian disease, syphilis, neurosurgical procedures, or head trauma.
- Normal ADH levels with signs of diabetes insipidus (such as polydipsia, polyuria, and hypotonic urine) may indicate the nephrogenic form of the disease, marked by renal tubular resistance to ADH; ADH levels may rise, however, if the pituitary gland tries to compensate.
- Elevated ADH levels may also indicate syndrome of inappropriate antidiuretic hormone (SIADH), possibly as a result of bronchogenic carcinoma, acute porphyria, hypothyroidism, Addison's disease, cirrhosis of the liver, infectious hepatitis, severe hemorrhage, or circulatory shock.

### DRUG CHALLENGE

 Anesthetics, carbamazepine, chlorothiazide, chlorpropamide, cyclophosphamide, estrogen, hypnotics, lithium carbonate, morphine, oxytocin, tranquilizers, and vincristine (may interfere with test results)

## Purpose

- To aid in the differential diagnosis of pituitary diabetes insipidus, nephrogenic diabetes insipidus (congenital or familial), and SIADH

## Patient preparation

- Explain that this test, used to measure hormonal secretion levels, may help identify the cause of his symptoms.
- Instruct the patient to fast and limit physical activity for 10 to 12 hours before the test.
- Tell the patient that the test requires a blood sample. Explain who will perform the venipuncture and when.
- Explain to the patient that he may experience slight discomfort from the tourniquet and needle puncture.
- Withhold medications that may cause SIADH before the test as ordered. If the medications must be continued, note this on the laboratory request.
- Advise the patient to lie down and relax for 30 minutes before the test.

## Procedure and posttest care

- Confirm the patient's identity using two patient identifiers according to facility policy.
- Perform a venipuncture, and collect the blood sample in a plastic collection tube (without additives) or a chilled EDTA tube.
- Immediately send the sample to the laboratory, where serum must be separated from the clotted blood within 10 minutes.
- Perform a serum osmolality test at the same time to help interpret the results.
- Apply direct pressure to the venipuncture site until bleeding stops.
- If a hematoma develops at the venipuncture site, apply warm soaks.
- Tell the patient to resume his usual diet, activities, and medications that were stopped before the test, as ordered.

## Precautions

 Make sure you use a plastic syringe and collection tube because the fragile ADH degrades on contact with glass.

---

#  Arginine
## [human growth hormone stimulation]

The arginine test measures human growth hormone (hGH) levels after I.V. administration of arginine, an amino acid that normally stimulates hGH secretion. It's commonly used to identify pituitary dysfunction in infants and children with growth retardation and to confirm hGH deficiency. This test may be performed along with an insulin tolerance test or after administration of other hGH stimulants, such as glucagon, vasopressin, and levodopa.

### Reference values
- The arginine infusion should raise hGH levels to more than 10 ng/ml (SI, > 10 µg/L) in men, more than 15 ng/ml (SI, > 15 µg/L) in women, and more than 48 ng/ml (SI, > 48 µg/L) in children. Such an increase may appear in the first blood sample collected 30 minutes after arginine infusion is discontinued or in the blood samples collected 60 and 90 minutes afterward.

### Abnormal results
- Hormone levels that are elevated during fasting or that rise during sleep help to rule out hGH deficiency.
- Failure of hGH levels to rise after arginine infusion indicates decreased anterior pituitary hGH reserve. In children, this deficiency causes dwarfism; in adults, it can indicate panhypopituitarism. When hGH levels fail to reach 10 ng/ml, retesting is required at the same time of day as the original test.

### Purpose
- To help diagnose pituitary tumors
- To confirm hGH deficiency in infants and children with low baseline levels

### Patient preparation
- Explain to the patient, or his parents if the patient is a child, that this test identifies hGH deficiency.
- Instruct the patient to fast and to limit physical activity for 10 to 12 hours before the test.
- Explain that this test requires I.V. infusion of a drug and collection of several blood samples. Tell him that the test takes at least 2 hours to perform.
- Withhold all steroid medications, including pituitary-based hormones, as ordered. If medications must be continued, record this on the laboratory request.
- Advise the patient to lie down and relax for 90 minutes before the test.

### Procedure and posttest care
- Confirm the patient's identity using two patient identifiers according to facility policy.
- Between 6 a.m. and 8 a.m., perform a venipuncture, and collect 6 ml of blood (basal sample) in a clot-activator tube.
- Use an indwelling venous catheter to avoid repeated venipunctures. Start I.V. infusion of arginine (0.5 g/kg of body weight) in normal saline solution, and continue infusion for 30 minutes.
- Stop the I.V. infusion, and draw three 6-ml blood samples at 30-minute intervals. Collect each sample in a clot-activator tube, and label it appropriately.
- Apply direct pressure to the venipuncture site until bleeding stops.
- If a hematoma develops at the I.V. or venipuncture site, apply warm soaks.

- Monitor the patient for signs and symptoms of hypoglycemia.
- Tell the patient to resume his usual diet, activities, and medications that were stopped before the test as ordered.

### Precautions
- Collect each blood sample at the scheduled time, and specify the collection time on the laboratory request.
- Send each sample to the laboratory immediately because hGH has a half-life of only 20 to 25 minutes.

# Corticotropin
### [ACTH, adrenocorticotropic hormone]

The corticotropin test measures plasma levels of corticotropin by radioimmunoassay. Corticotropin stimulates the adrenal cortex to secrete cortisol and, to a lesser degree, androgens and aldosterone. It also has some melanocyte-stimulating activity, increases the uptake of amino acids by muscle cells, promotes lipolysis by fat cells, stimulates pancreatic beta cells to secrete insulin, and may contribute to the release of growth hormone. Corticotropin levels vary diurnally, peaking between 6 a.m. and 8 a.m. and ebbing between 6 p.m. and 11 p.m. Through a negative feedback mechanism, plasma cortisol levels control corticotropin secretion—for example, high cortisol levels suppress corticotropin secretion. Emotional and physical stress (pain, surgery, insulin-induced hypoglycemia) stimulate secretion and can override the effects of plasma cortisol levels.

The corticotropin test may be ordered for a patient with signs of adrenal hypofunction (insufficiency) or hyperfunction (Cushing's syndrome). Corticotropin suppression or stimulation testing is usually necessary to confirm diagnosis. The instability and unavailability of corticotropin greatly limit this test's diagnostic significance and reliability.

### Reference values
- Mayo Medical Laboratories sets baseline values at less than 120 pg/ml (SI, < 26.4 pmol/L at 6 a.m. to 8 a.m.), but these values may vary, depending on the laboratory.

### Abnormal results
- A higher-than-normal corticotropin level may indicate primary adrenal hypofunction (Addison's disease), in which the pituitary gland attempts to compensate for the unresponsiveness of the target organ by releasing excessive corticotropin. The underlying cause of adrenocortical hypofunction may be idiopathic atrophy of the adrenal cortex or partial destruction of the gland by granuloma, neoplasm, amyloidosis, or inflammatory necrosis.
- A low-normal corticotropin level suggests secondary adrenal hypofunction resulting from pituitary or hypothalamic dysfunction.
- The primary determinant may be panhypopituitarism, absence of corticotropin-releasing hormone in the hypothalamus, or chronic blunting of corticotropin levels by long-term corticosteroid therapy.
- In suspected Cushing's syndrome, an elevated corticotropin level suggests Cushing's disease, in which pituitary dysfunction (from adenoma) causes continuous hypersecretion of corticotropin and, consequently, continuously elevated cortisol levels without diurnal variations.
- Moderately elevated corticotropin levels suggest pituitary-dependent adrenal hyperplasia and nonadrenal tumors, such as oat cell carcinoma of the lungs.
- A low-normal corticotropin level implies adrenal hyperfunction from adrenocortical tumor or hyperplasia.

Corticosteroids, including cortisone and its analogs (corticotropin or cortisol levels decrease); drugs that increase endogenous cortisol secretion, such as estrogens, calcium gluconate, amphetamines, spironolactone, and ethanol (corticotropin or cortisol levels decrease); lithium carbonate (decreases cortisol levels and may interfere with corticotropin secretion)

## Purpose
- To aid in the differential diagnosis of primary and secondary adrenal hypofunction
- To aid in the differential diagnosis of Cushing's syndrome

## Patient preparation
- Explain that this test helps determine if the patient's hormonal secretion is normal.
- Advise the patient to fast and limit his physical activity for 10 to 12 hours before the test.
- Tell the patient that the test requires a blood sample. Explain who will perform the venipuncture and when.
- Explain to the patient that he may experience slight discomfort from the tourniquet and needle puncture.
- Check the patient's history for medications that may affect the accuracy of test results as ordered. Withhold these medications for 48 hours or longer before the test. If they must be continued, note this on the laboratory request.
- Arrange with the dietary department to provide a low-carbohydrate diet for 2 days before the test. This requirement may vary, depending on the laboratory.

## Procedure and posttest care
- Confirm the patient's identity using two patient identifiers according to facility policy.

- For a patient with suspected adrenal hypofunction, perform the venipuncture between 6 a.m. and 8 a.m. (peak secretion) to determine a baseline corticotropin level.
- For a patient with suspected Cushing's syndrome, perform the venipuncture between 6 p.m. and 11 p.m. (low secretion).
- Collect the blood sample in a plastic EDTA tube (corticotropin may adhere to glass). The tube must be full because excess anticoagulant will affect results.
- Pack the sample in ice, and send it to the laboratory immediately, where plasma must be rapidly separated from blood cells at 39.2° F (4° C). The collection technique may vary, depending on the laboratory.
- Apply direct pressure to the venipuncture site until bleeding stops.
- If a hematoma develops at the venipuncture site, apply warm soaks.
- Tell the patient to resume his usual diet, activities, and medications that were stopped before the test as ordered.

## Precautions
DO'S & DON'TS

Because proteolytic enzymes in plasma degrade corticotropin, a temperature of 39.2° F is necessary to retard enzyme activity. Immediate transfer of the sample, packed in ice, to the laboratory is essential for reliable test results.

# Follicle-stimulating hormone
[FSH]

The follicle-stimulating hormone (FSH) test of gonadal function, performed more commonly on women than on men, measures FSH levels and is vital in infertility studies. Its overall diagnostic significance typically depends on the results of related hormone tests (for luteinizing hormone, estrogen, or progesterone, for example).

A glycoprotein secreted by the anterior pituitary gland, FSH stimulates gonadal activity in both sexes. In women, it spurs development of primary ovarian follicles into graafian follicles for ovulation. Secretion varies diurnally and fluctuates during the menstrual cycle, peaking at ovulation. In men, continuous secretion of FSH (and testosterone) stimulates and maintains spermatogenesis. Plasma FSH levels fluctuate widely in women; to obtain a true baseline level, daily testing may be necessary (for 3 to 5 days), or multiple samples may be drawn on the same day.

## Reference values
- Reference values vary greatly, depending on the patient's age, stage of sexual development, and—for a woman— phase of her menstrual cycle.
- For menstruating women, FSH values are
  - follicular phase: 5 to 20 mIU/ml (SI, 5 to 20 International Units/L)
  - ovulatory phase: 15 to 30 mIU/ml (SI, 15 to 30 International Units/L)
  - luteal phase: 5 to 15 mIU/ml (SI, 5 to 15 International Units/L).
- For menopausal women, FSH values are 50 to 100 mIU/ml (SI, 50 to 100 International Units/L).
- For men, FSH values are 5 to 20 mIU/ml (SI, 5 to 20 International Units/L).

## Abnormal results
- Low FSH levels may indicate secondary hypogonadotropic states, possibly resulting from anorexia nervosa, panhypopituitarism, or hypothalamic lesions. Low levels may cause aspermatogenesis in men and anovulation in women.
- In women high FSH levels may indicate ovarian failure associated with Turner's syndrome (primary hypogo-

nadism) or Stein-Leventhal syndrome (polycystic ovary syndrome).
- In men, high FSH levels may indicate destruction of the testes (from mumps orchitis or X-ray exposure), testicular failure, seminoma, or male climacteric.
- High FSH levels may occur in patients with precocious puberty (idiopathic) or with central nervous system lesions and in postmenopausal women.
- High FSH levels may result from congenital absence of the gonads and early stage acromegaly.

### DRUG CHALLENGE

 Ovarian steroid hormones, such as estrogen and progesterone, related compounds, and phenothiazines such as chlorpromazine (possible decrease of FSH)

## Purpose
- To help diagnose and treat infertility and disorders of menstruation, such as amenorrhea
- To help diagnose precocious puberty in girls (before age 9) and in boys (before age 10)
- To aid in the differential diagnosis of hypogonadism

## Patient preparation
- Explain to the patient, or parents if the patient is a child, that this test helps determine if his hormonal secretion is normal.
- Tell the patient that the test requires a blood sample. Explain who will perform the venipuncture and when.
- Explain to the patient that he may experience slight discomfort from the tourniquet and needle puncture.
- Withhold medications that may interfere with accurate determination of test results for 48 hours before the test as ordered. If medications must be continued

(for example, for infertility treatment), note this on the laboratory request.

■ If the patient is female, indicate the phase of her menstrual cycle on the laboratory request. If she's menopausal, note this on the laboratory request.

■ Advise the patient to lie down and relax for 30 minutes before the test.

### Procedure and posttest care

■ Confirm the patient's identity using two patient identifiers according to facility policy.

■ Perform a venipuncture, preferably between 6 a.m. and 8 a.m., and collect the blood sample in a 7-ml clot-activator tube. Send the sample to the laboratory immediately.

■ Apply direct pressure to the venipuncture site until bleeding stops.

■ If a hematoma develops at the venipuncture site, apply warm soaks.

■ Tell the patient to resume medications that were stopped before the test as ordered.

# Growth hormone suppression
### [glucose loading]

The growth hormone suppression test evaluates excessive baseline levels of human growth hormone (hGH) from the anterior pituitary gland. Normally, hGH raises plasma glucose and fatty acid levels. In response, insulin secretion increases to counteract these effects. Consequently, a glucose load should suppress hGH secretions. In a patient with excessive hGH levels, failure of suppression indicates anterior pituitary dysfunction and confirms a diagnosis of acromegaly or gigantism.

### Reference values

■ Glucose suppresses hGH to levels ranging from undetectable to 3 ng/ml

(SI, 3 µg/L) between 30 minutes and 2 hours.

■ In children, rebound stimulation may occur after 2 to 5 hours.

### Abnormal results

■ In patients with active acromegaly, elevated baseline hGH levels (5 ng/ml [SI, 5 µg/L]) aren't suppressed after glucose loading.

■ Unchanged or rising hGH levels after glucose loading indicate hGH hypersecretion and may confirm suspected acromegaly and gigantism. This response may be verified by repeating the test after a 1-day rest.

**DRUG CHALLENGE**

 Corticosteroids and phenothiazines, such as chlorpromazine (possible decrease in hGH secretion); amphetamines, arginine, estrogens, glucagon, levodopa, and niacin (possible increase in hGH secretion)

### Purpose

■ To assess elevated baseline levels of hGH

■ To confirm diagnosis of gigantism in children and acromegaly in adults and adolescents

### Patient preparation

■ Explain to the patient, or the parents if the patient is a child, that this test helps determine the cause of his abnormal growth.

■ Instruct the patient to fast and limit physical activity for 10 to 12 hours before the test.

■ Tell the patient that two blood samples will be drawn. Forewarn him that he may experience nausea after drinking the glucose solution and some discomfort from the tourniquet and needle punctures.

- Withhold all steroids and other pituitary-based hormones. If they or other medications must be continued, note this on the laboratory request.
- Advise the patient to lie down and relax for 30 minutes before the test.

### Procedure and posttest care

- Confirm the patient's identity using two patient identifiers according to facility policy.
- Perform a venipuncture, and collect 6 ml of blood (basal sample) in a 7-ml clot-activator tube between 6 a.m. and 8 a.m.
- Give 100 g of glucose solution by mouth. To prevent nausea, advise the patient to drink the glucose slowly.
- About 1 hour later, draw venous blood into a 7-ml clot-activator tube. Label the tubes appropriately, and send them to the laboratory immediately.
- Apply direct pressure to the venipuncture site until bleeding stops.
- If a hematoma develops at the venipuncture site, apply warm soaks.
- Tell the patient to resume his usual diet, activities, and medications that were stopped before the test as ordered.

# Human growth hormone
### [somatotropin]

Human growth hormone (hGH) is a protein secreted by acidophils of the anterior pituitary gland. It's the primary regulator of human growth. Unlike other pituitary hormones, hGH has no easily defined feedback mechanism or single target gland—it affects many body tissues. Like insulin, hGH promotes protein synthesis and stimulates amino acid uptake by cells. It also raises plasma glucose levels by inhibiting glucose uptake and utilization by cells and increases free fatty acid concentrations by enhancing lipolysis.

Secretion of hGH appears to be regulated by the hypothalamus by means of a growth hormone-releasing factor and a growth hormone release-inhibiting factor (somatostatin). Secretion of hGH is diurnal and varies with such factors as exercise, sleep, stress, and nutritional status. Hyposecretion or hypersecretion of this hormone may induce pathologic states (such as dwarfism or gigantism). Altered hGH levels are common in the patient with pituitary dysfunction.

This test, a quantitative analysis of plasma hGH levels, is usually performed as part of an anterior pituitary stimulation or suppression test. Such testing is crucial because manifestations of an hGH deficiency can rarely be reversed by therapy.

### Reference values

- In men, hGH levels range from undetectable to 5 ng/ml (SI, 5 µg/L); in women, levels range from undetectable to 10 ng/ml (SI, 10 µg/L).
- In children, hGH levels range from undetectable to 16 ng/ml (SI, 16 µg/L) and are usually higher than levels in adults.

### Abnormal results

- Increased hGH levels may indicate a pituitary or hypothalamic tumor, frequently an adenoma, which causes gigantism in children and acromegaly in adults and adolescents.
- Some patients with diabetes mellitus have elevated hGH levels without acromegaly. Suppression testing is needed to confirm diagnosis.
- Pituitary infarction, metastatic disease, and tumors may decrease hGH levels.
- Dwarfism may be due to low hGH levels, although only 15% of all cases of growth failure relate to endocrine dysfunction. Stimulation testing with arginine or insulin is needed to confirm the diagnosis.

Arginine and beta-adrenergic blockers, such as propranolol and estrogens (increase); amphetamines, bromocriptine, levodopa, dopamine, pituitary-based steroids, methyldopa, and histamine (increase); insulin (induced hypoglycemia), glucagon, and nicotinic acid (increase); phenothiazines and corticosteroids (decrease)

## Purpose
- To aid in the differential diagnosis of dwarfism because growth retardation can result from pituitary or thyroid hypofunction
- To confirm diagnosis of acromegaly and gigantism in the adult
- To help diagnose pituitary and hypothalamic tumors
- To help evaluate effect of hGH therapy

## Patient preparation
- Explain to the patient, or his parents if the patient is a child, that this test measures hormone levels and helps determine the cause of abnormal growth.
- Instruct the patient to fast and limit activity for 10 to 12 hours before the test.
- Tell the patient that the test requires a blood sample. Explain who will perform the venipuncture and when. Explain also that another blood sample may have to be drawn the next day for comparison.
- Inform the patient that he may experience slight discomfort from the tourniquet and needle puncture.
- Withhold all medications that affect hGH levels such as pituitary-based steroids. If they must be continued, note this on the laboratory request.
- Advise the patient to lie down and relax for 30 minutes before the test be-

cause stress and activity elevate hGH levels.

## Procedure and posttest care
- Confirm the patient's identity using two patient identifiers according to facility policy.
- Between 6 a.m. and 8 a.m. on 2 consecutive days, or as ordered, perform a venipuncture, and collect at least 7 ml of blood in a clot-activator tube.
- Apply direct pressure to the venipuncture site until bleeding stops.
- If a hematoma develops at the venipuncture site, apply warm soaks.
- Tell the patient to resume his usual diet, activities, and medications that were stopped before the test as ordered.

# ▌Insulin tolerance test

The insulin tolerance test measures serum levels of human growth hormone (hGH) and corticotropin after administration of a loading dose of insulin. This test is more reliable than direct measurement of hGH and corticotropin because many healthy people have undetectable fasting levels of these hormones. Insulin-induced hypoglycemia stimulates hGH and corticotropin secretion in people with an intact hypothalamic-pituitary-adrenal axis. Failure of stimulation indicates anterior pituitary or adrenal hypofunction and helps confirm an hGH or a corticotropin deficiency.

Because the insulin tolerance test stimulates an adrenergic response, it isn't recommended for patients with cardiovascular or cerebrovascular disorders, epilepsy, or low basal plasma cortisol levels.

## Reference values
- Blood glucose level falls to 50% of the fasting glucose level 20 to 30 minutes after insulin administration.

- The decrease in blood glucose level stimulates a 10- to 20-ng/dl (SI, 10 to 20 µg/L) increase in baseline values for hGH and corticotropin, with peak levels occurring between 60 and 90 minutes after insulin administration.

## Abnormal results

- Failure of stimulation or a blunted response suggests dysfunction of the hypothalamic-pituitary-adrenal axis.
- An hGH increase of less than 10 ng/dl (SI, < 10 µg/L) above baseline suggests hGH deficiency. A definitive diagnosis of hGH deficiency requires a supplementary stimulation test such as the arginine test. Additional testing is necessary to determine the site of the abnormality.
- An increase in corticotropin levels of less than 10 ng/dl above baseline suggests adrenal insufficiency. The metyrapone or corticotropin stimulation test then confirms the diagnosis and determines whether the insufficiency is primary or secondary.

### DRUG CHALLENGE

 Corticosteroids and pituitary-based drugs (increase in hGH); beta-adrenergic blockers and glucocorticoids (decrease in hGH); amphetamines, calcium gluconate, estrogens, ethanol glucocorticoids, methamphetamines, and spironolactone (decrease in corticotropin)

## Purpose

- To help diagnose hGH and corticotropin deficiency
- To identify pituitary dysfunction
- To aid in the differential diagnosis of primary and secondary adrenal hypofunction

## Patient preparation

- Explain to the patient that this test evaluates hormonal secretion.
- Instruct the patient to fast and restrict physical activity for 10 to 12 hours before the test.
- Explain that the test involves I.V. infusion of insulin and the collection of multiple blood samples.
- Warn the patient that he may experience an increased heart rate, diaphoresis (profuse sweating), hunger, and anxiety after administration of insulin. Reassure him that these symptoms are transient. If the symptoms become severe, the test will be stopped.
- Advise the patient to lie down and relax for 90 minutes before the test.

## Procedure and posttest care

- Confirm the patient's identity using two patient identifiers according to facility policy.
- Between 6 a.m. and 8 a.m., perform a venipuncture, and collect three 5-ml samples of blood to assess basal levels: one in a gray-top tube (for blood glucose analysis) and two in green-top tubes (for hGH and corticotropin analysis).
- Give an I.V. bolus of U-100 regular insulin (0.15 unit/kg, or as ordered) over 1 to 2 minutes.
- Use an indwelling venous catheter to avoid repeated venipunctures. Collect additional blood samples at 15, 30, 45, 60, 90, and 120 minutes after giving the insulin. At each interval, collect three blood samples: one in a tube with sodium fluoride and potassium oxidate and two in heparinized tubes. Label the tubes appropriately, and send them to the laboratory immediately.
- Apply direct pressure to the venipuncture site until bleeding stops.
- If a hematoma develops at the I.V. or venipuncture site, apply warm soaks.
- Tell the patient to resume his usual diet, activities, and medications that were stopped before the test as ordered.

## Precautions

 Be sure to have concentrated glucose solution readily available in case the patient has a severe hypoglycemic reaction to insulin.

- Label the tubes appropriately; include the collection times on the laboratory request, and send all samples to the laboratory immediately.

# ▌Luteinizing hormone
### [LH, lutropin]

The plasma luteinizing hormone (LH) test, usually ordered for anovulation and infertility studies in women, is a quantitative analysis of plasma LH or interstitial cell-stimulating hormone levels. For accurate diagnosis, results must be evaluated in light of findings obtained from related hormone tests (follicle-stimulating hormone [FSH], estrogen, and testosterone, for example).

LH is a glycoprotein secreted by basophilic cells of the anterior pituitary gland. In women, cyclic LH secretion (with FSH) causes ovulation and transforms the ovarian follicle into the corpus luteum, which in turn secretes progesterone. In men, continuous LH secretion stimulates the interstitial (Leydig) cells of the testes to release testosterone, which stimulates and maintains spermatogenesis (with FSH).

### Reference values
- In menstruating women, the LH values are:
  - follicular phase—5 to 15 mIU/ml (SI, 5 to 15 International Units/L)
  - ovulatory phase—30 to 60 mIU/ml (SI, 30 to 60 International Units/L)
  - luteal phase—5 to 15 mIU/ml (SI, 5 to 15 International Units/L).

- In postmenopausal women, the LH values are 50 to 100 mIU/ml (SI, 50 to 100 International Units/L).
- In men, the LH values are 5 to 20 mIU/ml (SI, 5 to 20 International Units/L).
- In children, the LH values are 4 to 20 mIU/ml (SI, 4 to 20 International Units/L).

### Abnormal results
- In women, absence of a midcycle peak in LH levels may indicate anovulation.
- In women, low or low-normal LH levels may indicate hypogonadism; these findings are commonly associated with amenorrhea. High LH levels may indicate congenital absence of ovaries or ovarian failure associated with Stein-Leventhal syndrome (polycystic ovary syndrome), Turner's syndrome (ovarian dysgenesis), menopause, or early stage acromegaly.
- In men, low LH levels may indicate secondary gonadal dysfunction (of hypothalamic or pituitary origin). High LH levels may indicate testicular failure (primary hypogonadism) or destruction or congenital absence of testes.

DRUG CHALLENGE

 Steroids, including estrogens, progesterone, and testosterone (possible decrease)

### Purpose
- To detect ovulation
- To assess male or female infertility
- To evaluate amenorrhea
- To monitor therapy designed to induce ovulation

### Patient preparation
- Explain that this test helps determine if his secretion of hormones is normal.
- Inform the patient that he doesn't need to restrict food and fluids.

- Tell the patient that this test requires a blood sample. Explain who will perform the venipuncture and when.
- Inform the patient that he may experience slight discomfort from the tourniquet and needle puncture.
- Withhold drugs that may interfere with plasma LH levels, such as corticosteroids (including estrogens and progesterone), for 48 hours before the test as ordered. If they must be continued, note this on the laboratory request.

### Procedure and posttest care
- Confirm the patient's identity using two patient identifiers according to facility policy.
- Perform a venipuncture, and collect the sample in a 7-ml clot-activator tube.
- If the patient is a woman, indicate the phase of her menstrual cycle on the laboratory request. Make a note if the patient is menopausal.
- Apply direct pressure to the venipuncture site until bleeding stops.
- If a hematoma develops at the venipuncture site, apply warm soaks.
- Tell the patient to resume medications stopped before the test as ordered.

# Neonatal thyroid-stimulating hormone

The neonatal thyroid-stimulating hormone (TSH) test is an immunoassay that confirms congenital hypothyroidism after an initial screening test detects low thyroxine ($T_4$) levels. Normally, TSH levels surge after birth, triggering a rise in thyroid hormone that's essential for neurologic development. In primary congenital hypothyroidism, the thyroid gland doesn't respond to TSH stimulation, resulting in diminished thyroid hormone levels and elevated TSH levels. Early detection and treatment of congenital hypothyroidism is critical to prevent mental retardation and cretinism.

### Reference values
- At age 1 to 2 days, TSH levels are 25 to 30 µIU/ml (SI, 25 to 30 mU/L).
- At age 3 days and older, TSH levels are less than 25 µIU/ml (SI, < 25 mU/L).

### Abnormal results
- Neonatal TSH levels must be interpreted in light of the $T_4$ level.
- High TSH levels with low $T_4$ levels indicate primary congenital hypothyroidism (thyroid gland dysfunction).
- Low TSH and $T_4$ levels may indicate secondary congenital hypothyroidism (pituitary or hypothalamic dysfunction).
- Normal TSH levels accompanied by low $T_4$ levels may indicate hypothyroidism due to a congenital defect in $T_4$-binding globulin or transient congenital hypothyroidism due to prematurity or prenatal hypoxia. A complete thyroid workup must be done to confirm the cause of hypothyroidism before treatment can begin.

**DRUG CHALLENGE**

 Corticosteroids, triiodothyronine, and $T_4$ (decrease); excessive topical resorcinol, lithium carbonate, potassium iodide, and TSH injection (increase)

### Purpose
- To confirm diagnosis of congenital hypothyroidism

### Patient preparation
- Explain to the infant's parents that this test helps confirm the diagnosis of congenital hypothyroidism. Emphasize the importance of detecting the disorder early so that prompt therapy can prevent irreversible brain damage.

## Procedure and posttest care

- Confirm the patient's identity using two patient identifiers according to facility policy.

### Filter paper sample

- Assemble the necessary equipment, wash your hands thoroughly, and put on gloves.
- Wipe the infant's heel with an alcohol or povidone-iodine swab, and dry it thoroughly with a gauze pad.
- Perform a heelstick.
- Squeezing the infant's heel gently, fill the circles on the filter paper with blood. Make sure the blood saturates the paper.
- Gently apply pressure with a gauze pad to ensure hemostasis at the puncture site.
- Allow the filter paper to dry, label it appropriately, and send it to the laboratory.

### Serum sample

- Perform a venipuncture, and collect the serum sample in a 3-ml clot-activator tube. Label the tube, and send it to the laboratory immediately.
- Apply direct pressure to the venipuncture site until bleeding stops.
- If a hematoma develops at the venipuncture site, apply warm soaks.

## █ Prolactin
[PRL]

Similar in molecular structure and biological activity to human growth hormone (hGH), prolactin is a polypeptide hormone secreted by the anterior pituitary gland. Prolactin is essential for the development of the mammary glands for lactation during pregnancy and for stimulating and maintaining lactation postpartum. Like hGH, prolactin acts directly on tissues, and its levels rise in re-

sponse to sleep and physical or emotional stress.

This radioimmunoassay is a quantitative analysis of serum prolactin levels, which normally rise 10- to 20-fold during pregnancy, corresponding to elevations in human placental lactogen levels. After delivery, prolactin secretion falls to basal levels in mothers who don't breast-feed. However, prolactin secretion increases during breast-feeding, apparently as a result of a stimulus triggered by suckling that curtails the release of prolactin-inhibiting factor by the hypothalamus. This, in turn, allows transient elevations of prolactin secretion by the pituitary gland.

This test is considered useful in patients suspected of having pituitary tumors, which are known to secrete prolactin in excessive amounts. Another test used to evaluate hypothalamic dysfunction is the thyrotropin-releasing hormone (TRH) stimulation test. (See *TRH stimulation test.*)

## Reference values

- In nonlactating women, prolactin levels range from undetectable to 23 ng/ml (SI, 23 µg/L).
- In pregnant women, prolactin levels rise 10- to 20-fold; after delivery, prolactin levels fall to baseline levels in mothers who don't breast-feed.
- In breast-feeding women, prolactin levels increase.

## Abnormal results

- In nonpregnant nonlactating women, prolactin levels 100 to 300 ng/ml (SI, 100 to 300 µg/L) suggest autonomous prolactin production by a pituitary adenoma, especially when amenorrhea or galactorrhea is present (Forbes-Albright syndrome). Rarely, high prolactin levels may result from severe endocrine disorders such as hypothyroidism. Idiopathic high prolactin levels may be associated with anovulatory infertility. Confirm slight elevations with repeat measurements on two other occasions.

■ Low prolactin levels may indicate empty sella syndrome, in which a flattened pituitary gland makes the pituitary fossa look empty.

■ In a lactating woman, low prolactin levels, which cause failure of lactation, may be associated with postpartum pituitary infarction (Sheehan's syndrome).

### DRUG CHALLENGE

 Estrogens, ethanol, methyldopa, and morphine (increase in prolactin level); apomorphine, ergot alkaloids, and levodopa (decrease in prolactin level)

## Purpose

■ To help diagnose pituitary dysfunction possibly due to pituitary adenoma
■ To help diagnose hypothalamic dysfunction
■ To evaluate the cause of secondary amenorrhea and galactorrhea

## Patient preparation

■ Explain that this test helps evaluate hormonal secretion.
■ Tell the patient the test requires a blood sample. Explain who will perform the venipuncture and when.
■ Explain to the patient that she may experience slight discomfort from the tourniquet and needle puncture.
■ Advise the patient to restrict food and fluids and limit physical activity for 12 hours before the test. Encourage her to relax for about 30 minutes before the test.
■ Withhold drugs that may interfere with test results as ordered. If they must be continued, note this on the laboratory request.

## TRH stimulation test

The thyrotropin-releasing hormone (TRH) stimulation test evaluates hypothalamic dysfunction and pituitary tumors by stimulating the release of prolactin. The procedure is as follows: Perform a venipuncture in the basal state (before I.V. administration of synthetic TRH) to obtain a baseline prolactin level, and then place the patient in the supine position. Administer an I.V. bolus dose (500 mcg) of synthetic TRH over 15 to 30 seconds. Take blood samples at 15-and 30-minute intervals to measure prolactin.

A baseline prolactin reading greater than 200 ng/ml (SI, 200 International Units/L) indicates a pituitary tumor, but levels between 30 and 200 ng/ml (SI, between 30 and 200 International Units/L) are also consistent with this condition. Normally, patients show at least a twofold increase in prolactin after injection with TRH. If the prolactin level fails to rise, hypothalamic dysfunction or adenoma of the pituitary gland is likely.

## Procedure and posttest care

■ Confirm the patient's identity using two patient identifiers according to facility policy.
■ Perform the test by venipuncture at least 3 hours after the patient wakes up; blood samples collected earlier are likely to reflect sleep-induced peak levels. Collect the blood sample in a 7-ml clot-activator tube.
■ Apply direct pressure to the venipuncture site until bleeding stops.
■ If a hematoma develops at the venipuncture site, apply warm soaks.
■ Tell the patient to resume her usual diet, activities, and medications that were stopped before the test as ordered.

# Rapid corticotropin
[cosyntropin, ACTH stimulation, cortisol stimulation]

The rapid corticotropin test is gradually replacing the 8-hour corticotropin stimulation test as the most effective diagnostic tool for evaluating adrenal hypofunction. Using cosyntropin, the rapid corticotropin test provides faster results and causes fewer allergic reactions than the 8-hour test, which uses natural corticotropin from animal sources.

Baseline cortisol levels must be determined before this test to evaluate the effect of cosyntropin administration on cortisol secretion. An unequivocally high morning cortisol level rules out adrenal hypofunction and makes further testing unnecessary.

## Reference values
- Cortisol levels rise after 30 to 60 minutes to a peak of 18 mg/dl (SI, 500 mmol/L) or more after the cosyntropin injection.
- A normal response is usually double the baseline level; normal results rule out adrenal hypofunction (insufficiency).

## Abnormal results
- Cortisol levels that remain low may indicate primary adrenal hypofunction (Addison's disease).
- Subnormal increases in cortisol levels may require prolonged stimulation of the adrenal cortex to distinguish between primary and secondary adrenal hypofunction.

## Purpose
- To help identify primary and secondary adrenal hypofunction

## Patient preparation
- Explain that this test helps determine if the patient's condition is due to a hormonal deficiency.
- Inform the patient that he may have to fast for 10 to 12 hours before the test and that he must be relaxed and resting quietly for 30 minutes before the test.
- Tell him that the test takes at least 1 hour to perform.
- For an inpatient, withhold corticotropin and all steroid medications as ordered. For an outpatient, tell him to refrain from taking these drugs as ordered. If the drugs must be continued, note this on the laboratory request.
- Explain to the patient that he may experience slight discomfort from the tourniquet and needle puncture.

## Procedure and posttest care
- Confirm the patient's identity using two patient identifiers according to facility policy.
- Draw 5 ml of blood for a baseline value. Collect the sample in a 5-ml heparinized tube. Label this sample PREINJECTION, and send it to the laboratory.
- Inject 250 mcg (0.25 mg) of cosyntropin I.V. Direct I.V. injection should take about 2 minutes.
- Draw another 5 ml of blood at 30 and 60 minutes after the cosyntropin injection. Collect the samples in 5-ml heparinized tubes. Label the samples 30 MINUTES POSTINJECTION and 60 MINUTES POSTINJECTION, and send them to the laboratory. Include the collection times on the laboratory request.
- Apply direct pressure to the venipuncture site until bleeding stops.
- If a hematoma develops at the venipuncture site, apply warm soaks.
- Tell the patient to resume his usual diet, activities, and medications that were stopped before the test as ordered.

Observe the patient for signs of a rare allergic reaction to cosyntropin, such as hives, itching, and tachycardia.

# Thyroid-stimulating hormone
## [TSH, thyrotropin]

Thyroid-stimulating hormone (TSH) promotes increases in the size, number, and activity of thyroid cells and stimulates the release of triiodothyronine and thyroxine. These hormones affect total body metabolism and are essential for normal growth and development.

This test measures serum TSH levels by radioimmunoassay. It can detect primary hypothyroidism and determine whether the hypothyroidism results from thyroid gland failure or from pituitary or hypothalamic dysfunction. Normal serum TSH levels rule out primary hypothyroidism. This test may not distinguish between low-normal and subnormal levels, especially in secondary hypothyroidism.

## Reference values
■ TSH level is undetectable to 15 µIU/ml (SI, 15 mU/L).

## Abnormal results
■ TSH levels may be slightly elevated in euthyroid patients with thyroid cancer.
■ TSH levels that exceed 20 µIU/ml (SI, 20 mU/L) suggest primary hypothyroidism or, possibly, endemic goiter.
■ Low or undetectable TSH levels may be normal but occasionally indicate secondary hypothyroidism (with inadequate secretion of TSH or thyrotropin-releasing hormone [TRH]).
■ Low TSH levels may also result from hyperthyroidism (Graves' disease) and thyroiditis; both are marked by hyper-

# TRH challenge test

The thyrotropin-releasing hormone (TRH) challenge test, which evaluates thyroid function and is the first direct test of pituitary reserve, is a reliable diagnostic tool in thyrotoxicosis (Graves' disease). The challenge test requires an injection of TRH.

## How it's done
After a venipuncture is performed to obtain a baseline thyroid-stimulating hormone (TSH) value, synthetic TRH (protirelin) is given by I.V. bolus in a dose of 200 to 500 mcg. As many as five blood samples (5 ml each) are then drawn at 5, 10, 15, 20, and 60 minutes after the TRH injection to assess thyroid response. To facilitate blood collection, an indwelling catheter can be used to obtain the required samples.

## What the test shows
A sudden spike above the baseline TSH value indicates a normally functioning pituitary but suggests hypothalamic dysfunction. If the TSH level fails to rise or remains undetectable, pituitary failure is likely. In thyrotoxicosis and thyroiditis, TSH levels fail to rise when challenged by TRH.

secretion of thyroid hormones, which suppresses TSH release. Provocative testing with TRH is necessary to confirm the diagnosis. (See *TRH challenge test.*)

## Purpose
■ To confirm or rule out primary hypothyroidism and distinguish it from secondary hypothyroidism
■ To monitor drug therapy in the patient with primary hypothyroidism

## Patient preparation
■ Explain that this test helps assess thyroid gland function.

- Tell the patient that the test requires a blood sample. Explain who will perform the venipuncture and when.
- Explain to the patient that he may experience slight discomfort from the tourniquet and needle puncture.
- Withhold steroids, thyroid hormones, aspirin, and other medications that may influence test results as ordered. If they must be continued, note this on the laboratory request.
- Advise the patient to lie down and relax for 30 minutes before the test.

### Procedure and posttest care

- Confirm the patient's identity using two patient identifiers according to facility policy.
- Between 6 a.m. and 8 a.m., perform a venipuncture, and collect the blood sample in a 5-ml clot-activator tube.
- Apply direct pressure to the venipuncture site until bleeding stops.
- If a hematoma develops at the venipuncture site, apply warm soaks.
- Tell the patient to resume medications that were stopped before the test as ordered.

# Thyroid and parathyroid hormones

## ▌Calcitonin
### [thyrocalcitonin]

The plasma calcitonin test is a radioimmunoassay that measures plasma levels of calcitonin. Calcitonin is an antagonist to parathyroid hormone; it also lowers serum calcium levels and inhibits bone resorption by regulating the activity and number of osteoclasts.

The usual clinical indication for this test is suspected medullary carcinoma of the thyroid, which causes hypersecretion of calcitonin (without associated hypocalcemia). Equivocal results require provocative testing with I.V. pentagastrin or calcium to rule out disease. (See *Calcitonin stimulation tests.*)

### Reference values

- Basal serum calcitonin levels are 40 pg/ml (SI, 40 ng/L) for male and 20 pg/ml (SI, 20 ng/L) for female patients.
  - Reference values after 4-hour calcium infusion for male patients are 190 pg/ml (SI, 190 ng/L); for female patients, reference values are 130 pg/ml (SI, 130 ng/L).
  - Reference values after testing with pentagastrin infusion for male patients are 110 pg/ml (SI, 110 ng/L); for female patients, reference values are 30 pg/ml (SI, 30 ng/L).

### Abnormal results

- High calcitonin levels without hypocalcemia usually indicate thyroid medullary carcinoma. Transmitted as an autosomal dominant trait, thyroid medullary carcinoma may be part of multiple endocrine neoplasia.
- High calcitonin levels may be due to ectopic calcitonin production by oat cell carcinoma of the lung or by breast carcinoma.

### Purpose

- To aid diagnosis of thyroid medullary carcinoma and ectopic calcitonin-producing tumors (rare)

### Patient preparation

- Explain that this test helps evaluate thyroid function.
- Instruct the patient to fast overnight because food may interfere with calcium homeostasis and, subsequently, calcitonin levels.

## Calcitonin stimulation tests

Stimulation testing is typically necessary in patients with medullary thyroid carcinoma when baseline calcitonin levels fail to rise high enough to confirm the diagnosis. The most common test is a 4-hour I.V. calcium infusion (15 mg/kg) to provoke calcitonin secretion. Blood samples are taken just before the infusion and at 3 and 4 hours postinfusion. Calci-tonin levels rise rapidly after the infusion in patients with medullary thyroid cancer.

Another test involves I.V. infusion of pentagastrin (0.5 mcg/kg over 5 to 10 seconds). A blood sample is drawn just before the I.V. infusion and at 90 seconds, 5 minutes, and 10 minutes postinfusion. In patients with medullary thyroid carcinoma, calcitonin levels rise markedly over the baseline reading.

■ Tell the patient that the test requires a blood sample. Explain who will perform the venipuncture and when.

■ Explain to the patient that he may experience slight discomfort from the tourniquet and needle puncture.

■ Tell the patient that the laboratory requires several days to complete the analysis.

### Procedure and posttest care

■ Confirm the patient's identity using two patient identifiers according to facility policy.

■ Perform a venipuncture, and collect the sample in a 7-ml heparinized tube.

■ Apply direct pressure to the venipuncture site until bleeding stops.

■ If a hematoma develops at the venipuncture site, apply warm soaks.

■ Tell the patient to resume his usual diet.

## Free thyroxine and free triiodothyronine

The free thyroxine ($FT_4$) and free triiodothyronine ($FT_3$) tests, commonly performed simultaneously, measure serum levels of $FT_4$ and $FT_3$, the minute portions of $T_4$ and $T_3$ not bound to thyroxine-binding globulin (TBG) and other serum proteins. These unbound hormones are responsible for the thyroid's effects on cellular metabolism. Measurement of free hormone levels is the best indicator of thyroid function.

Because of disagreement as to whether $FT_4$ or $FT_3$ is the better indicator, laboratories commonly measure both. The disadvantages of these tests include a cumbersome and difficult laboratory method, inaccessibility, and cost. This test may be useful in the 5% of patients in whom the standard $T_3$ or $T_4$ tests fail to produce diagnostic results.

### Reference values

■ $FT_4$ is 0.9 to 2.3 ng/dl (SI, 10 to 30 nmol/L).

■ $FT_3$ is 0.2 to 0.6 ng/dl (SI, 0.003 to 0.009 nmol/L); values vary depending on the laboratory.

### Abnormal results

■ High $FT_4$ and $FT_3$ levels indicate hyperthyroidism, unless peripheral resistance to thyroid hormone is present.

■ High $FT_3$ levels with normal or low $FT_4$ values indicates $T_3$ toxicosis, a distinct form of hyperthyroidism.

■ Low $FT_4$ levels usually indicate hypothyroidism, except in patients receiving thyroid replacement therapy with $T_3$. These patients may have varying levels of $FT_4$ and $FT_3$, depending on the preparation used and the time of sample collection.

## Purpose

- To measure the metabolically active form of the thyroid hormones
- To help diagnose hyperthyroidism and hypothyroidism when TBG levels are abnormal

## Patient preparation

- Explain that this test helps evaluate thyroid function.
- Tell the patient that the test requires a blood sample. Explain who will perform the venipuncture and when.
- Explain to the patient that he may experience slight discomfort from the tourniquet and needle puncture.

## Procedure and posttest care

- Confirm the patient's identity using two patient identifiers according to facility policy.
- Perform a venipuncture, and collect the blood sample in a 7-ml clot-activator tube.
- Apply direct pressure to the venipuncture site until bleeding stops.
- If a hematoma develops at the venipuncture site, apply warm soaks.

# Parathyroid hormone

[PTH, parathormone]

Parathyroid hormone (PTH) regulates plasma concentration of calcium and phosphorus. Normally, PTH release is regulated by a negative-feedback mechanism involving serum calcium. Normal or elevated circulating calcium levels (especially the ionized form) inhibit PTH release; decreased levels stimulate PTH release. The overall effect of PTH is to raise plasma levels of calcium while lowering phosphorus levels.

Circulating PTH exists in three distinct molecular forms: the intact PTH molecule, which originates in the parathyroid glands, and two smaller circulating forms: N-terminal fragments and C-terminal fragments. Two radioimmunoassays are available to detect intact PTH and the N- and C-terminal fragments. Both tests can be used to confirm diagnosis of hyperparathyroidism and hypoparathyroidism.

Each test has other specific applications as well. The C-terminal PTH assay is more useful in diagnosing chronic disturbances in PTH metabolism, such as secondary and tertiary hyperparathyroidism. The C-terminal PTH assay also better differentiates ectopic from primary hyperparathyroidism. The assay for intact PTH and the N-terminal fragment (measured simultaneously) more accurately reflects acute changes in PTH metabolism and thus is useful in monitoring a patient's response to PTH therapy.

The clinical and diagnostic effects of PTH excess or deficiency are directly related to the effects of PTH on bone and the renal tubules and to its interaction with ionized calcium and biologically active vitamin D. Therefore, measuring serum calcium, phosphorus, and creatinine levels with serum PTH is helpful when trying to understand the causes and effects of pathologic parathyroid function. Suppression or stimulation tests may help confirm findings.

## Reference values

- Serum PTH levels vary, depending on the laboratory, and must be interpreted in association with serum calcium levels.
- Typical values for intact PTH range from 10 to 50 pg/ml (SI, 1.1 to 5.3 pmol/L).

# Clinical implications of abnormal parathyroid secretion

| Conditions | Causes | PTH levels | Ionized calcium levels |
|---|---|---|---|
| Primary hyperparathyroidism | • Parathyroid adenoma or carcinoma | ⬤ High | ⬤ to ⬤ High to Normal |
| Secondary hyperparathyroidism | • Chronic renal disease<br>• Severe vitamin D deficiency<br>• Calcium malabsorption<br>• Pregnancy and lactation | ⬤ High | ◯ Low |
| Tertiary hyperparathyroidism | • Progressive secondary hyperparathyroidism | ⬤ High | ⬤ to ◯ High to Normal |
| Hypoparathyroidism | • Accidental removal of the parathyroid glands<br>• Autoimmune disease | ◯ Low | ◯ Low |
| Malignant tumors | • Squamous cell carcinoma of the lung<br>• Renal, pancreatic, or ovarian carcinoma | ⬤ to ⬤ High to Normal | ⬤ High |

Key: High ⬤  Normal ⬤  Low ◯

– N-terminal fraction is 8 to 24 pg/ml (SI, 0.8 to 2.5 pmol/L).
– C-terminal fraction is 0 to 340 pg/ml (SI, 0 to 35.8 pmol/L).

## Abnormal results

■ Measured along with serum calcium levels, high PTH values may indicate primary, secondary, or tertiary hyperparathyroidism.
■ Low PTH levels may result from hypoparathyroidism and from certain malignant diseases. (See *Clinical implications of abnormal parathyroid secretion*.)

## Purpose

■ To aid in the differential diagnosis of parathyroid disorders

## Patient preparation

■ Explain that this test helps evaluate parathyroid function.
■ Instruct the patient to fast overnight because food may affect PTH levels and interfere with results.
■ Tell the patient that the test requires a blood sample. Explain who will perform the venipuncture and when.
■ Explain to the patient that he may experience slight discomfort from the tourniquet and needle puncture.

## Procedure and posttest care

■ Confirm the patient's identity using two patient identifiers according to facility policy.

- Perform a venipuncture, and collect 3 ml of blood into two separate 7-ml clot-activator tubes.
- Apply direct pressure to the venipuncture site until bleeding stops.
- If a hematoma develops at the venipuncture site, apply warm soaks.
- Tell the patient to resume his usual diet.

# Thyroxine
## [$T_4$]

Thyroxine ($T_4$) is an amine secreted by the thyroid gland in response to thyroid-stimulating hormone (TSH) and, indirectly, thyrotropin-releasing hormone. The rate of secretion is normally regulated by a complex system of negative and positive feedback involving the thyroid, anterior pituitary, and hypothalamus. The suspected precursor, or prohormone, of triiodothyronine ($T_3$), $T_4$ is believed to convert to $T_3$ by monodeiodination, which occurs mainly in the liver and kidneys.

Only a fraction of $T_4$ (about 0.05%) circulates freely in the blood; the rest binds strongly to plasma proteins, primarily thyroxine-binding globulin (TBG). This minute fraction is responsible for the clinical effects of thyroid hormone. TBG binds so tenaciously that $T_4$ survives in the plasma for a relatively long time, with a half-life of about 6 days. This immunoassay, one of the most common thyroid diagnostic tools, measures the total circulating $T_4$ level when TBG is normal. An alternative test is the $T_4$ (D), based on competitive protein binding.

## Reference values

- Circulating $T_4$ level is 5 to 13.5 mcg/dl (SI, 60 to 165 mmol/L). Normal $T_4$ levels don't guarantee euthyroidism; for example, normal levels occur in $T_3$ toxicosis.

## Abnormal results

- High $T_4$ levels are consistent with primary and secondary hyperthyroidism, including excessive $T_4$ (levothyroxine) replacement therapy (factitious or iatrogenic hyperthyroidism).
- Subnormal levels suggest primary or secondary hypothyroidism or $T_4$ suppression by normal, elevated, or replacement $T_3$ levels.
- In doubtful cases of hypothyroidism, measurement of TSH levels may be indicated. Overt signs of hyperthyroidism require further testing.

### D RUG CHALLENGE

 Estrogens, progestins, levothyroxine, and methadone (increase); free fatty acids, heparin, iodides, liothyronine sodium, lithium, methylthiouracil, phenylbutazone, phenytoin, propylthiouracil, salicylates (high doses), steroids, sulfonamides, and sulfonylureas (decrease); clofibrate (possible increase or decrease)

## Purpose

- To evaluate thyroid function
- To help diagnose hyperthyroidism and hypothyroidism
- To monitor the patient's response to antithyroid medication in hyperthyroidism or to thyroid replacement therapy in hypothyroidism (TSH estimates needed to confirm hypothyroidism)

## Patient preparation

- Explain that this test helps evaluate thyroid gland function.
- Inform the patient that he doesn't need to fast or restrict activity.
- Tell the patient that the test requires a blood sample. Explain who will perform the venipuncture and when.
- Explain to the patient that he may experience slight discomfort from the tourniquet and needle puncture.

■ Withhold medications that may interfere with test results as ordered. If they must be continued, note this on the laboratory request. If this test is being performed to monitor thyroid therapy, the patient should continue to receive daily thyroid supplements.

### Procedure and posttest care

■ Confirm the patient's identity using two patient identifiers according to facility policy.
■ Perform a venipuncture, and collect the blood sample in a 7-ml clot-activator tube.
■ Send the blood sample to the laboratory immediately so that the serum can be separated.
■ Apply direct pressure to the venipuncture site until bleeding stops.
■ If a hematoma develops at the venipuncture site, apply warm soaks.
■ Tell the patient to resume medications that were stopped before the test as ordered.

# Thyroxine-binding globulin
[TBG]

The thyroxine-binding globulin (TBG) test measures the serum level of TBG, the predominant protein carrier for circulating thyroxine ($T_4$) and triiodothyronine ($T_3$). TBG values may be identified by saturating the sample for TBG determination with radioactive $T_4$, then subjecting this to electrophoresis and measuring the amount of TBG by the amount of radioactive $T_4$ by radioimmunoassay.

Any condition that affects TBG levels and subsequent binding capacity also affects the amount of free $T_4$ ($FT_4$) in circulation. An underlying TBG abnormality renders tests for total $T_3$ and $T_4$

inaccurate, but doesn't affect the accuracy of tests for free $T_3$ ($FT_3$) and $FT_4$.

### Reference values

■ TBG levels are 16 to 32 mcg/dl (SI, 120 to 180 mg/ml).

### Abnormal results

■ High TBG levels may indicate hypothyroidism or congenital (genetic) excess, some forms of hepatic disease, or acute intermittent porphyria. TBG levels normally rise during pregnancy and are high in neonates.
■ Low TBG levels may indicate hyperthyroidism or congenital deficiency and can occur in active acromegaly, nephrotic syndrome, and malnutrition associated with hypoproteinemia, acute illness, or surgical stress.
■ Patients with high or low TBG levels require additional testing, such as the serum $FT_3$ and $T_4$ tests, to evaluate thyroid function more precisely.

<small>**DRUG CHALLENGE**</small>

 Estrogens, including hormonal contraceptives and phenothiazines, such as perphenazine (increase), androgens, phenytoin, prednisone, and high doses of salicylates (decrease)

### Purpose

■ To evaluate abnormal thyrometabolic states that don't correlate with thyroid hormone ($T_3$ or $T_4$) values (for example, overt signs of hypothyroidism and a low $FT_4$ level with a high total $T_4$ level due to a marked increase of TBG secondary to hormonal contraceptives)
■ To identify TBG abnormalities

### Patient preparation

■ Explain that this test helps evaluate thyroid function.

- Tell the patient that the test requires a blood sample. Explain who will perform the venipuncture and when.
- Explain to the patient that he may experience slight discomfort from the tourniquet and needle puncture.
- Withhold medications that may affect the accuracy of test results, such as anabolic steroids, estrogens, phenytoin, salicylates, or thyroid preparations as ordered. If medications must be continued, note this on the laboratory request. (They may be continued to determine if prescribed drugs are affecting TBG levels.)

### Procedure and posttest care

- Confirm the patient's identity using two patient identifiers according to facility policy.
- Perform a venipuncture, and collect the blood sample in a 7-ml clot activator tube.
- Apply direct pressure to the venipuncture site until bleeding stops.
- If a hematoma develops at the venipuncture site, apply warm soaks.
- Tell the patient to resume medications that were stopped before the test as ordered.

# Triiodothyronine
## $[T_3]$

The triiodothyronine ($T_3$) test is a highly specific radioimmunoassay that measures total (bound and free) serum content of $T_3$ to investigate clinical indications of thyroid dysfunction. $T_3$, the more potent thyroid hormone, is an amine derived primarily from thyroxine ($T_4$) by the process of monodeiodination. At least 50% and as much as 90% of $T_3$ is thought to be derived from $T_4$ as a result of this pivotal transformation, during which $T_4$ loses one of its iodine atoms to become $T_3$. The remaining 10% or more is secreted directly by the thyroid gland. Like $T_4$ secretion, $T_3$ secretion occurs in response to thyroid-stimulating hormone (TSH) and, secondarily, thyrotropin-releasing hormone (TRH).

Although $T_3$ is present in the bloodstream in minute quantities and is metabolically active only briefly, its impact on body metabolism is greater than that of $T_4$. Another significant difference between the two major thyroid hormones is that $T_3$ binds less firmly to thyroxine-binding globulin (TBG). Consequently, $T_3$ persists in the bloodstream for a short time; half disappears in about 1 day, whereas half of $T_4$ disappears in 6 days.

Serum $T_3$ and $T_4$ levels usually rise and fall in tandem. Generally, $T_3$ levels are a more accurate diagnostic indicator of hyperthyroidism. Although $T_3$ and $T_4$ levels are increased in about 90% of patients with hyperthyroidism, there's a disproportionate increase in $T_3$.

### Reference values

- Serum $T_3$ levels are 80 to 200 ng/dl (SI, 1.2 to 3 nmol/L).
- In some patients with hypothyroidism, $T_3$ levels may fall within the normal range and not be diagnostically significant.

### Abnormal results

- High $T_3$ levels with normal $T_4$ levels indicates $T_3$ toxicosis, which occurs in Graves' disease, toxic adenoma, and toxic nodular goiter.
- $T_3$ levels elevated higher than $T_4$ levels are seen in patients receiving thyroid replacement therapy that contains more $T_3$ than $T_4$.
- $T_3$ levels may be higher than $T_4$ levels also in iodine-deficient areas, where the thyroid produces more cellularly active $T_3$ than $T_4$ to try to maintain the euthyroid state.

- High $T_3$ levels normally occur in pregnancy.
- Low $T_3$ levels may appear in the euthyroid patient with systemic illness (especially hepatic or renal disease), severe acute illness, or malnutrition and after trauma or major surgery. (See *Drugs that interfere with $T_3$ tests*.)

### Purpose
- To help diagnose $T_3$ toxicosis
- To help diagnose hypothyroidism and hyperthyroidism
- To monitor the patient's response to thyroid replacement therapy in hypothyroidism

### Patient preparation
- Explain that this test helps to evaluate thyroid gland function and determine the cause of his symptoms.
- Withhold medications, such as steroids, propranolol, and cholestyramine, which may influence thyroid function as ordered. If they must be continued, record this information on the laboratory request.
- Tell the patient that the test requires a blood sample. Explain who will perform the venipuncture and when.
- Explain to the patient that he may experience slight discomfort from the tourniquet and needle puncture.

### Procedure and posttest care
- Confirm the patient's identity using two patient identifiers according to facility policy.
- Perform a venipuncture, and collect the blood sample in a 7-ml clot-activator tube.
- Send the blood sample to the laboratory as soon as possible to avoid stasis and to allow early separation of serum from the clotted blood.
- Apply direct pressure to the venipuncture site until bleeding stops.

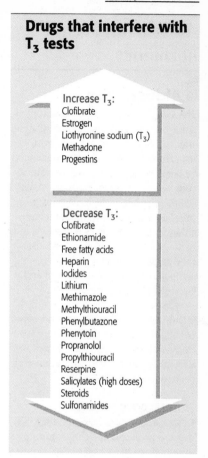

# Drugs that interfere with $T_3$ tests

**Increase $T_3$:**
Clofibrate
Estrogen
Liothyronine sodium ($T_3$)
Methadone
Progestins

**Decrease $T_3$:**
Clofibrate
Ethionamide
Free fatty acids
Heparin
Iodides
Lithium
Methimazole
Methylthiouracil
Phenylbutazone
Phenytoin
Propranolol
Propylthiouracil
Reserpine
Salicylates (high doses)
Steroids
Sulfonamides

- If a hematoma develops at the venipuncture site, apply warm soaks.
- Tell the patient to resume medications that were stopped before the test as ordered.

### Precautions
- If the patient must receive thyroid preparations, such as $T_3$ (liothyronine), note the administration time on the laboratory request. Otherwise, $T_3$ test results aren't reliable.

# Adrenal and renal hormones

## ■ Aldosterone

The aldosterone test measures serum aldosterone levels by quantitative analysis and radioimmunoassay. Aldosterone—the principal mineralocorticoid secreted by the zona glomerulosa of the adrenal cortex—regulates ion transport across cell membranes in the renal tubules to promote reabsorption of sodium and chloride in exchange for potassium and hydrogen ions. Consequently, aldosterone helps to maintain blood pressure and volume and to regulate fluid and electrolyte balance.

Aldosterone secretion is controlled mainly by the renin-angiotensin level of potassium. High serum potassium levels, as well as hyponatremia, hypovolemia, and other disorders, stimulate aldosterone secretion.

### Reference values
- Laboratory values vary with time of day and posture—upright postures produce higher values.
- In upright individuals, normal values are 7 to 30 ng/dl (SI, 190 to 832 pmol/L).
- In supine individuals, values are 3 to 16 ng/dl (SI, 80 to 440 pmol/L).

### Abnormal results
- High aldosterone levels may indicate primary or secondary disease. Primary aldosteronism (Conn's syndrome) may result from adrenocortical adenoma or carcinoma or from bilateral adrenal hyperplasia. Secondary aldosteronism can result from renovascular hypertension, heart failure, cirrhosis of the liver, nephrotic syndrome, idiopathic cyclic edema, and the third trimester of pregnancy.

- Low aldosterone levels may indicate primary hypoaldosteronism, salt-losing syndrome, eclampsia, or Addison's disease.

### DRUG CHALLENGE

Some antihypertensives, such as methyldopa, that promote sodium and water retention (possible decrease); diuretics (possible increase); some corticosteroids, such as fludrocortisone, that mimic mineralocorticoid activity (possible decrease)

### Purpose
- To help diagnose primary and secondary aldosteronism, adrenal hyperplasia, hypoaldosteronism, and salt-losing syndrome

### Patient preparation
- Explain that this test helps determine if his symptoms are due to improper hormonal secretion.
- Tell the patient that the test requires a blood sample. Explain who will perform the venipuncture and when.
- Explain to the patient that he may experience slight discomfort from the tourniquet and needle puncture.
- Instruct the patient to maintain a low-carbohydrate, normal-sodium (135 mEq or 3 g/day) diet for at least 2 weeks or, preferably, for 30 days before the test.
- As ordered, withhold drugs that alter fluid, sodium, and potassium balance—especially diuretics, antihypertensives, steroids, hormonal contraceptives, and estrogens—for at least 2 weeks or, preferably, for 30 days before the test.
- Withhold all renin inhibitors for 1 week before the test as ordered. If they must be continued, note this on the laboratory request.
- Tell the patient to avoid licorice for at least 2 weeks before the test because it produces an aldosterone-like effect.

### Procedure and posttest care

- Confirm the patient's identity using two patient identifiers according to facility policy.
- Perform a venipuncture while the patient is still supine after a night's rest.
- Collect the blood sample in a 7-ml clot-activator tube, and send it to the laboratory immediately.
- Draw another blood sample 4 hours later, while the patient is standing and after he has been up and about, to evaluate the effect of postural change.
- Collect the second sample in a 7-ml clot-activator tube, and send it to the laboratory immediately.
- Apply direct pressure to the venipuncture site until bleeding stops.
- If a hematoma develops at the venipuncture site, apply warm soaks.
- Tell the patient to resume his usual diet and medications that were stopped before the test as ordered.

# Androstenedione

The androstenedione test helps identify disorders related to altered hormone levels, such as female virilization syndromes and polycystic ovary syndrome (Stein-Leventhal syndrome). Androstenedione is a precursor of cortisol, aldosterone, estrogen, and testosterone. Tumors of the ovaries or adrenal glands can secrete excessive amounts of androstenedione, which then converts to testosterone, resulting in virilizing symptoms, such as hirsutism and sterility.

Increased androstenedione production may induce premature sexual development in children. It may produce renewed ovarian stimulation, endometriosis, bleeding, and polycystic ovaries in postmenopausal women. In obese women, increased levels of estrogen can lead to menstrual irregularities. In men, overproduction of androstenedione may cause feminizing signs such as gynecomastia.

### Reference values

- In female patients, normal values by radioimmunoassay are 85 to 275 ng/dl (SI, 3.0 to 9.6 nmol/L).
- In male patients, normal values by radioimmunoassay are 75 to 205 ng/dl (SI, 2.6 to 7.2 nmol/L).

### Abnormal results

- High androstenedione levels suggest polycystic ovary syndrome (Stein-Leventhal syndrome); Cushing's syndrome; ovarian, testicular, and adrenocortical tumors; ectopic corticotropin-producing tumors; late-onset congenital adrenal hyperplasia; and ovarian stromal hyperplasia. High androstenedione levels cause increased estrone levels, leading to premature sexual development in children; menstrual irregularities in premenopausal women; bleeding, endometriosis, and polycystic ovaries in postmenopausal women; and gynecomastia in men.
- Decreased androstenedione levels occur in hypogonadism.

D<small>RUG</small> <small>CHALLENGE</small>

 Steroids and pituitary hormones (possible increase)

### Purpose

- To help determine the cause of gonadal dysfunction, menstrual or menopausal irregularities, virilizing symptoms, and premature sexual development

### Patient preparation

- Explain that this test determines the cause of the patient's symptoms.

▪ Tell the patient that the test requires a blood sample. Explain who will perform the venipuncture and when.
▪ Explain to the patient that slight discomfort may result from the tourniquet and needle puncture.
▪ Explain that the test should be done 1 week before or after a menstrual period and that it may be repeated.
▪ Withhold steroid and pituitary-based hormones as ordered. If they must be continued, note this on the laboratory request.

### Procedure and posttest care
▪ Confirm the patient's identity using two patient identifiers according to facility policy.
▪ Perform a venipuncture, and collect a serum sample in a 7-ml clot-activator tube, or collect a plasma sample in a green-top tube. (If a plasma sample is taken, refrigerate it or place it on ice.) The sample should be drawn at 7 a.m., if possible, because androstenedione production is at its peak then.
▪ Label the plasma sample appropriately, and send it to the laboratory immediately.
▪ Apply direct pressure to the venipuncture site until bleeding stops.
▪ If a hematoma develops at the venipuncture site, apply warm soaks.
▪ Tell the patient to resume medications that were stopped before the test as ordered.

### Precautions
▪ Refrigerate plasma samples or place them on ice.
▪ Record the patient's age, sex, and (if appropriate) phase of the menstrual cycle on the laboratory request.

# Atrial natriuretic factor
### [ANF, atrial natriuretic peptide]
The atrial natriuretic factor (ANF) level is measured by radioimmunoassay. ANF is a potent natriuretic agent and vasodilator that rapidly produces diuresis and increases the glomerular filtration rate. ANF plays a critical role in regulating extracellular fluid volume, blood pressure, and sodium metabolism. It lowers blood pressure by promoting sodium excretion, inhibiting the renin-angiotensin system's effect on aldosterone secretion, and decreasing atrial pressure.

ANF level may be a marker for early asymptomatic left ventricular dysfunction and increased cardiac volume.

### Reference values
▪ ANF level is 20 to 77 pg/ml.

### Abnormal results
▪ High levels of ANF occur in patients with heart failure and in patients with significantly elevated cardiac filling pressure.

DRUG CHALLENGE

 Cardiovascular drugs, including beta-adrenergic blockers, calcium antagonists, cardiac glycosides, diuretics, and vasodilators (may affect test results)

### Purpose
▪ To confirm heart failure
▪ To identify asymptomatic cardiac volume overload

### Patient preparation
▪ As appropriate, explain the purpose of the test to the patient.
▪ Inform the patient that he must fast for 12 hours before the test.

- Tell the patient that the test requires a blood sample. Explain who will perform the venipuncture and when.
- Explain to the patient that he may experience slight discomfort from the tourniquet and needle puncture.
- Explain that the test results will be available within 4 days.
- Check the patient's history for medications that can influence test results.
- Withhold beta-adrenergic blockers, calcium antagonists, cardiac glycosides diuretics, and vasodilators for 24 hours before collection as ordered.

### Procedure and posttest care

- Confirm the patient's identity using two patient identifiers according to facility policy.
- Perform a venipuncture, and collect the blood sample in a prechilled potassium-EDTA tube.
- After chilled centrifugation, the EDTA plasma should be promptly frozen and sent to the laboratory.
- Apply direct pressure to the venipuncture site until bleeding stops.
- If a hematoma develops at the venipuncture site, apply warm soaks.
- Tell the patient to resume his usual diet and medications that were stopped before the test as ordered.

# Catecholamines

The catecholamines test, a quantitative (total or fractionated) analysis of plasma catecholamines, is commonly performed in patients with hypertension and signs of adrenal medullary tumor and in those with a neural tumor that affects endocrine function. Excessive catecholamine secretion by tumors causes hypertension, weight loss, episodic sweating, headache, palpitations, and anxiety. High catecholamine levels necessitate supportive confirmation by urinalysis.

Major catecholamines include the hormones dopamine, epinephrine, and norepinephrine. When secreted into the bloodstream, catecholamines produced in the adrenal medulla prepare the body for the fight-or-flight response. They increase heart rate and contractility, constrict blood vessels and redistribute circulating blood toward the skeletal and coronary muscles, mobilize carbohydrate and lipid reserves, and sharpen alertness.

Catecholamine levels commonly fluctuate in response to temperature, stress, postural change, diet, smoking, anoxia, volume depletion, renal failure, obesity, and many drugs.

### Reference values

- Catecholamine levels range as follows:
  – supine: epinephrine, undetectable to 110 pg/ml (SI, undetectable to 600 pmol/L); norepinephrine, 70 to 750 pg/ml (SI, 413 to 4,432 pmol/L)
  – standing: epinephrine, undetectable to 140 pg/ml (SI, undetectable to 764 pmol/L); norepinephrine, 200 to 1,700 pg/ml (SI, 1,182 to 10,047 pmol/L).

### Abnormal results

- High catecholamine levels may indicate pheochromocytoma, neuroblastoma, ganglioneuroblastoma, or ganglioneuroma; thyroid disorders; hypoglycemia; and cardiac disease. Electroconvulsive therapy, shock resulting from hemorrhage, endotoxins, and anaphylaxis also raise catecholamine levels.
- Fractional analysis helps identify the cause of high catecholamine levels. For example, adrenal medullary tumors secrete epinephrine, whereas ganglioneuromas, ganglioblastomas, and neuroblastomas secrete norepinephrine.
- Normal or low baseline catecholamine levels, with a failure to show an increase

after standing, suggests autonomic nervous system dysfunction.

## Purpose

- To rule out adrenal medullary or extra-adrenal pheochromocytoma in the patient with hypertension
- To help identify neuroblastoma, ganglioneuroblastoma, and ganglioneuroma
- To distinguish between adrenal medullary tumors and other catecholamine-producing tumors through fractional analysis (urinalysis for catecholamine degradation products recommended to support the diagnosis)
- To help diagnose autonomic nervous system dysfunction such as idiopathic orthostatic hypotension

## Patient preparation

- Explain that this test helps determine if hypertension or other symptoms are related to improper hormonal secretion.
- As ordered, instruct the patient to refrain from using self-prescribed medications, especially cold and allergy remedies that may contain sympathomimetics, for 2 weeks before the test.
- Advise the patient to avoid amine-rich foods and beverages, such as bananas, avocados, cheese, coffee, tea, cocoa, beer, and Chianti wine, for 48 hours; to maintain vitamin C intake (needed to form catecholamines); to abstain from smoking for 24 hours; and to fast for 10 to 12 hours before the test.
- Tell the patient that the test requires one or two blood samples. Explain who will perform the venipuncture and when.

- Explain to the patient that he may experience slight discomfort from the tourniquet and needle puncture.
- For inpatients, withhold medications that affect catecholamine levels, such as amphetamines, phenothiazines (chlorpromazine), sympathomimetics, and tricyclic antidepressants, as ordered.
- Insert an indwelling venous catheter (saline lock) 24 hours before the test because the stress of the venipuncture itself may significantly raise catecholamine levels.
- Advise the patient to lie down and relax for 45 to 60 minutes before the test.
- If necessary, provide blankets to keep the patient warm; low temperatures stimulate catecholamine secretion.

## Procedure and posttest care

- Confirm the patient's identity using two patient identifiers according to facility policy.
- Perform a venipuncture between 6 a.m. and 8 a.m.
- Collect the blood sample in a 10-ml chilled EDTA tube (sodium metabisulfite solution), which can be obtained from the laboratory on request.
- If a second blood sample is requested, have the patient stand for 10 minutes, and draw the sample into another tube exactly like the first tube.
- If a saline lock is used, it may be necessary to discard the first 1 or 2 ml of blood. Check with the laboratory for the preferred procedure.
- Apply direct pressure to the venipuncture site until bleeding stops.
- If a hematoma develops at the venipuncture site, apply warm soaks.
- Tell the patient to resume his usual diet and medications that were stopped before the test as ordered.

## Precautions

- Pack the tube in crushed ice to minimize deactivation of catecholamines,

## Diurnal variations in cortisol secretion

Cortisol secretion rises in the early morning, peaking after the patient awakens. Levels decline sharply in the evening and during the early phase of sleep. They rise again during the night and peak by the next morning.

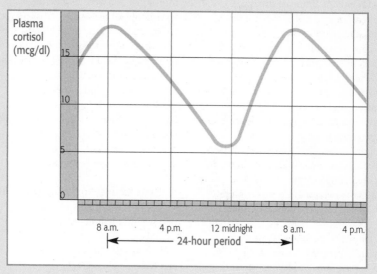

and send it to the laboratory immediately.

• Indicate on the laboratory request whether the patient was supine or standing during the venipuncture; also write the time the blood was drawn.

## ▮ Cortisol

Cortisol—the principal glucocorticoid secreted by the zona fasciculata of the adrenal cortex—helps metabolize nutrients, mediate physiologic stress, and regulate the immune system. Cortisol secretion normally follows a diurnal pattern: Levels rise during the early morning hours and peak around 8 a.m. and then decline to very low levels in the evening and during the early phase of sleep. (See *Diurnal variations in cortisol secretion*.) Intense heat or cold, infection,

trauma, exercise, obesity, and debilitating disease influence cortisol secretion.

This radioimmunoassay test, a quantitative analysis of plasma cortisol levels, is usually ordered for patients with signs of adrenal dysfunction. Dynamic tests, suppression tests for hyperfunction, and stimulation tests for hypofunction are generally required to confirm the diagnosis.

### Reference values

• Cortisol levels are 9 to 35 mcg/dl (SI, 250 to 690 nmol/L) in the morning and 3 to 12 mcg/dl (SI, 80 to 330 nmol/L) in the afternoon.

### Abnormal results

• High cortisol levels may indicate adrenocortical hyperfunction in Cushing's disease (a rare disease caused by basophilic adenoma of the pituitary gland) or Cushing's syndrome (glucocorticoid excess from any cause).

■ In most patients with Cushing's syndrome, the adrenal cortex secretes independently of a diurnal rhythm, so little difference is found between morning and afternoon levels.

■ Low cortisol levels may indicate primary adrenal insufficiency (Addison's disease), usually from idiopathic glandular atrophy. Tuberculosis, fungal invasion, and hemorrhage can cause adrenocortical destruction, leading to low cortisol levels.

■ Low cortisol levels may indicate secondary adrenal insufficiency from impaired corticotropin secretion, as occurs in hypophysectomy, postpartum pituitary necrosis, craniopharyngioma, and chromophobe adenoma.

■ Diurnal variations may be absent in healthy people who are under considerable emotional or physical stress.

### DRUG CHALLENGE

 Androgens and phenytoin (possible decrease); hormonal contraceptives (false-high)

### Purpose

■ To help diagnose Cushing's disease, Cushing's syndrome, Addison's disease, and secondary adrenal insufficiency

### Patient preparation

■ Explain that this test helps determine if his symptoms are due to improper hormonal secretion.

■ Instruct the patient to maintain a normal-sodium (2 to 3 g/day) diet for 3 days before the test and to fast and limit physical activity for 10 to 12 hours before the test.

■ Tell the patient that the test requires a blood sample. Explain who will perform the venipuncture and when.

■ Explain to the patient that he may experience slight discomfort from the tourniquet and needle puncture.

■ Withhold all medications that may interfere with plasma cortisol levels, such as androgens, estrogens, and phenytoin, for 48 hours before the test as ordered. If the patient is receiving replacement therapy and depends on exogenous steroids for survival, note this on the laboratory request as well as other medications that must be continued.

■ Advise the patient to lie down and relax for 30 minutes before the test.

### Procedure and posttest care

■ Confirm the patient's identity using two patient identifiers according to facility policy.

■ Perform a venipuncture between 6 a.m. and 8 a.m.

■ Collect the sample in a 7-ml heparinized tube, label the tube appropriately, and send it to the laboratory immediately.

■ For diurnal variation testing, draw another blood sample between 4 p.m. and 6 p.m.

■ Collect the second sample in a 7-ml heparinized tube, label it appropriately, and send it to the laboratory immediately.

■ Apply direct pressure to the venipuncture site until bleeding stops.

■ If a hematoma develops at the venipuncture site, apply warm soaks.

■ Tell the patient to resume his usual diet, activities, and medications that were stopped before the test as ordered.

### Precautions

■ Pregnancy may cause a false-high test finding because of increase in cortisol-binding plasma proteins.

- Obesity, stress, and severe hepatic or renal disease may cause a possible increase in the cortisol level.

# Erythropoietin
[EPO]

The erythropoietin (EPO) test of renal hormone production measures EPO by immunoassay. The test is used to evaluate anemia, polycythemia, and kidney tumors. It's also used to evaluate abuse of commercially prepared EPO by athletes, who believe that the drug enhances performance by increasing red blood cell (RBC) volume, which conveys additional oxygen-carrying capacity to the blood. Adverse reactions include clotting abnormalities, headache, seizures, hypertension, nausea, vomiting, diarrhea, and rash.

A glycoprotein hormone, EPO is secreted by the liver in fetuses but by the kidneys in adults. The hormone acts on stem cells in the bone marrow to stimulate RBC production. The hormone is regulated by a feedback loop involving RBC volume and oxygen saturation of the blood, especially in the brain.

### Reference values
- EPO level is 5 to 36 mU/ml (SI, 5 to 36 International Units/L).

### Abnormal results
- Low EPO levels suggest anemia, inadequate or no hormone production (possibly congenital), or severe renal disease.
- High EPO levels may indicate anemia, polycythemia, EPO abuse, or EPO-secreting tumors.

### Purpose
- To help diagnose anemia, polycythemia, and other bone marrow disorders
- To help diagnose kidney tumors
- To detect EPO abuse by athletes

### Patient preparation
- Explain that this test determines if hormonal secretion is causing changes in his RBCs.
- Instruct the patient to fast for 8 to 10 hours before the test.
- Tell the patient that the test requires a blood sample. Explain who will perform the venipuncture and when.
- Explain to the patient that he may experience slight discomfort from the tourniquet and needle puncture.
- Advise the patient to lie down and relax for 30 minutes before the test.

### Procedure and posttest care
- Confirm the patient's identity using two patient identifiers according to facility policy.
- Perform a venipuncture, and collect the sample in a 5-ml clot-activator tube.
- If requested, a blood sample to determine the hematocrit value may be drawn at the same time by collecting an additional sample in a 2-ml EDTA tube.
- Apply direct pressure to the venipuncture site until bleeding stops.
- If a hematoma develops at the venipuncture site, apply warm soaks.

# Pancreatic and gastric hormones

# C-peptide

Connecting peptide (C-peptide) is a biologically inactive chain formed during the proteolytic conversion of proinsulin to insulin in the pancreatic beta cells. It has no insulin effect either biologically or immunologically. Circulating insulin is measured by immunologic assay. As insulin is released into the bloodstream, the C-peptide chain splits off from the hormone.

## Reference values
- Serum C-peptide levels usually parallel insulin levels.
- Normal fasting values are 0.78 to 1.89 ng/ml (SI, 0.26 to 0.63 mmol/L).
- Insulin–to–C-peptide ratio test (to differentiate insulinoma from factitious hypoglycemia) results are:
  – 1.0 or less: indicates increased endogenous insulin secretion
  – More than 1.0: indicates exogenous insulin.

## Abnormal results
- High C-peptide levels may indicate endogenous hyperinsulinism (insulinemia), oral hypoglycemic drug ingestion, pancreas or B-cell transplantation, renal failure, or type 2 diabetes mellitus.
- Low C-peptide levels may indicate factitious hypoglycemia (surreptitious insulin administration), radical pancreatectomy, or type 1 diabetes mellitus.

## Purpose
- To determine the cause of hypoglycemia
- To indirectly measure insulin secretion in the presence of circulating insulin antibodies
- To detect residual tissue after total pancreatectomy (for carcinoma)
- To determine beta-cell function in the patient with diabetes mellitus

## Patient preparation
- Explain that this test helps to evaluate pancreatic function and determine the cause of hypoglycemia.
- Instruct the patient to fast for 8 to 12 hours before the test, but water can be consumed.
- Tell the patient that the test requires a blood sample. Explain who will perform the venipuncture and when.
- Explain to the patient that he may experience slight discomfort from the tourniquet and needle puncture.

- If the patient will undergo radioisotope testing, conduct the test after drawing blood for C-peptide measurement. Blood for blood glucose measurement is usually drawn at the same time as blood for C-peptide measurement.
- If the C-peptide stimulation test is performed, give I.V. glucagon as ordered, after drawing a baseline blood sample.
- Withhold medications that may interfere with test results as ordered. If they must be continued, note this on the laboratory request.

## Procedure and posttest care
- Confirm the patient's identity using two patient identifiers according to facility policy.
- Perform a venipuncture, and collect a 1-ml sample in a chilled clot-activator tube. The blood is separated and frozen to be tested later.
- Collect a blood sample to assess glucose level in a tube with sodium fluoride and potassium oxalate if ordered.

### Do's & don'ts
 Pack the blood sample for the C-peptide test in ice, and send it, along with the blood sample for glucose measurement, to the laboratory immediately.

- Apply direct pressure to the venipuncture site until bleeding stops.
- If a hematoma develops at the venipuncture site, apply warm soaks.
- Tell the patient to resume his usual diet, activities, and medications that were stopped before the test as ordered.

# Gastrin

Gastrin is a polypeptide hormone produced and stored primarily in the antrum of the stomach and to a lesser degree in the islets of Langerhans. Mainly it facilitates food digestion by triggering gastric acid secretion. It also stimulates the release of pancreatic enzymes and the gastric enzyme pepsin, increases gastric and intestinal motility, and stimulates bile flow from the liver. Abnormal secretion of gastrin can result from tumors (gastrinomas) and diseases that affect the stomach, pancreas and, less commonly, the esophagus and small bowel.

This radioimmunoassay, a quantitative analysis of gastrin levels, is especially useful for patients suspected of having gastrinomas (Zollinger-Ellison syndrome). In doubtful situations, provocative testing may be necessary.

## Reference values
- Gastrin levels are 50 to 150 pg/ml (SI, 50 to 150 ng/L).

## Abnormal results
- Significantly increased gastrin levels greater than 1,000 pg/ml (SI, > 1,000 ng/L) confirm Zollinger-Ellison syndrome.
- Increased gastrin levels may suggest achlorhydria (with or without pernicious anemia), extensive stomach carcinoma (because of hyposecretion of gastric juices and hydrochloric acid) or, rarely, duodenal ulcer.

### DRUG CHALLENGE

Acetylcholine, amino acids (especially glycine), calcium carbonate, calcium chloride, and ethanol (increase); anticholinergics, such as atropine, hydrochloric acid, and secretin (decrease)

## Purpose
- To confirm a diagnosis of gastrinoma, the gastrin-secreting tumor in Zollinger-Ellison syndrome

- To aid in the differential diagnosis of gastric and duodenal ulcers and pernicious anemia

## Patient preparation
- Explain that this test helps determine the cause of GI symptoms.
- Instruct the patient to abstain from alcohol for at least 24 hours before the test and to fast and avoid caffeinated drinks for 12 hours before the test. Advise the patient that he may drink water.
- Tell the patient that the test requires a blood sample. Explain who will perform the venipuncture and when.
- Explain to the patient that he may experience slight discomfort from the tourniquet and needle puncture.
- Withhold all drugs that may interfere with test results, especially insulin and anticholinergics, such as atropine and belladonna, as ordered. If they must be continued, note this on the laboratory request.
- Advise the patient to lie down and relax for 30 minutes before the test.

## Procedure and posttest care
- Confirm the patient's identity using two patient identifiers according to facility policy.
- Perform a venipuncture, and collect 5 ml of blood in a clot-activator tube.
- Apply direct pressure to the venipuncture site until bleeding stops.
- If a hematoma develops at the venipuncture site, apply warm soaks.
- Tell the patient to resume his usual diet and medications that were stopped before the test as ordered.

## Precautions
- Insulin-induced hypoglycemia may increase the gastrin level.

# Glucagon

Glucagon, a polypeptide hormone secreted by the pancreatic islet cells, promotes glucose production and controls glucose storage. Glucagon is secreted in response to hypoglycemia; secretion is inhibited by the other pancreatic hormones, insulin and somatostatin. Normally, the coordinated release of glucagon, insulin, and somatostatin ensures an adequate and constant fuel supply while keeping blood glucose levels relatively stable.

This test, a quantitative analysis of plasma glucagon by radioimmunoassay, helps detect glucagonoma (alpha cell tumor) or hypoglycemia from idiopathic glucagon deficiency or pancreatic dysfunction. Glucagon is usually measured along with glucose and insulin levels because they influence glucagon secretion.

## Reference values

- Glucagon levels are less than 60 pg/ml (SI, < 60 ng/L).

## Abnormal results

- High fasting glucagon levels (900 to 7,800 pg/ml [SI, 900 to 7,800 ng/L]) can occur in glucagonoma, diabetes mellitus, acute pancreatitis, and pheochromocytoma.
- Low glucagon levels are associated with idiopathic glucagon deficiency and hypoglycemia due to chronic pancreatitis.

## Purpose

- To help diagnose glucagonoma and hypoglycemia due to chronic pancreatitis or idiopathic glucagon deficiency

## Patient preparation

- Explain that this test helps to evaluate pancreatic function.

- Instruct him to fast for 10 to 12 hours before the test.
- Tell the patient that the test requires a blood sample. Explain who will perform the venipuncture and when.
- Explain to the patient that he may experience slight discomfort from the tourniquet and needle puncture.
- Withhold insulin, catecholamines, and other medications that may influence the test results as ordered. If they must be continued, note this on the laboratory request.
- Advise the patient to lie down and relax for 30 minutes before the test.

## Procedure and posttest care

- Confirm the patient's identity using two patient identifiers according to facility policy.
- Perform a venipuncture, and collect the blood sample in a chilled 10-ml EDTA tube.

### Do's & don'ts

 Place the sample on ice, and send it to the laboratory immediately.

- Apply direct pressure to the venipuncture site until bleeding stops.
- If a hematoma develops at the venipuncture site, apply warm soaks.
- Tell the patient to resume his usual diet and medications that were stopped before the test as ordered.

## Precautions

- Exercise, stress, and prolonged fasting may increase glucagon levels.

# Insulin

The insulin test, a radioimmunoassay, is a quantitative analysis of serum insulin levels. Insulin is usually measured along with glucose levels because glucose is the primary stimulus for insulin release from pancreatic islet cells. Insulin regulates the metabolism and transport or mobilization of carbohydrates, amino acids, proteins, and lipids. Stimulated by increased glucose levels, insulin level peaks after meals, when metabolism and food storage are greatest.

### Reference values
- Insulin levels are 0 to 35 µU/ml (SI, 144 to 243 pmol/L).

### Abnormal results
- Insulin levels are interpreted in light of the prevailing glucose concentration. A normal insulin level may be inappropriate for the glucose results.
- High insulin and low glucose levels after a significant fast suggest the presence of an insulinoma. Prolonged fasting or stimulation testing may be required to confirm the diagnosis.
- High insulin levels may indicate insulin-resistant diabetes mellitus.
- Low insulin levels may indicate non–insulin resistant diabetes.

#### DRUG CHALLENGE

Corticosteroids (including hormonal contraceptives), corticotropin, epinephrine, and thyroid hormones (possible increase); use of insulin by the patient with type 2 diabetes mellitus (possible increase)

### Purpose
- To help diagnose hyperinsulinemia and hypoglycemia resulting from a tumor or hyperplasia of pancreatic islet cells, glucocorticoid deficiency, or severe hepatic disease
- To help diagnose diabetes mellitus and insulin-resistant states

### Patient preparation
- Explain that this test helps determine if the pancreas is functioning normally.
- Tell the patient to fast for 10 to 12 hours before the test.
- Explain that the test requires a blood sample. Identify who will perform the venipuncture and when.
- Explain to the patient that he may experience slight discomfort from the tourniquet and needle puncture.
- Explain that questionable results may require repeating the test or performing a simultaneous glucose tolerance test, which requires that the patient drink a glucose solution.
- Withhold corticosteroids (including hormonal contraceptives), corticotropin, epinephrine, thyroid supplements, and other medications that may interfere with test results as ordered. If medications must be continued, note this on the laboratory request.
- Advise the patient to lie down and relax for 30 minutes before the test.

### Procedure and posttest care
- Confirm the patient's identity using two patient identifiers according to facility policy.
- Perform a venipuncture, and collect one blood sample for insulin measurement in a 7-ml EDTA tube.
- Collect a blood sample for glucose measurement in a tube with sodium fluoride and potassium oxalate.

#### DO'S & DON'TS

Pack the insulin sample in ice, and send it, along with the glucose sample, to the laboratory immediately.

- Apply direct pressure to the venipuncture site until bleeding stops.
- If a hematoma develops at the venipuncture site, apply warm soaks.

- Tell the patient to resume his usual diet, activities, and medications that were stopped before the test as ordered.

### Precautions
- In the patient with an insulinoma, fasting for this test may precipitate dangerously severe hypoglycemia. Keep an ampule of dextrose 50% available to counteract possible hypoglycemia.

# Gonadal hormones

## Estrogens

Estrogens (and progesterone) are secreted by the ovaries under the influence of the pituitary gonadotropins, follicle-stimulating hormone (FSH), and luteinizing hormone (LH). Estrogens—in particular, estradiol, the most potent estrogen—interact with the hypothalamic-pituitary axis through negative and positive feedback mechanisms. Slowly rising or sustained high estrogen levels inhibit secretion of FSH and LH, but a rapid rise in estrogen just before ovulation seems to stimulate LH secretion.

Estrogens are responsible for the development of secondary female sexual characteristics and for normal menstruation; levels are usually undetectable in children. These hormones are secreted by ovarian follicular cells during the first half of the menstrual cycle and by the corpus luteum during the luteal phase and during pregnancy. In menopause, estrogen secretion drops to a constantly low level.

This radioimmunoassay measures serum levels of estradiol, estriol, and estrone (the only estrogens that appear in serum in measurable amounts) and has diagnostic significance in evaluating female gonadal dysfunction. (See *Predicting premature labor.*) Tests of hypothalamic-pituitary function may be required to confirm the diagnosis.

### Reference values
- Estrogen levels for premenopausal women are 26 to 149 pg/ml (SI, 90 to 550 pmol/L), depending on the menstrual cycle.
- Estrogen levels for postmenopausal women is 0 to 34 pg/ml (SI, 0 to 125 pmol/L).
- Estrogen levels in men are 12 to 34 pg/ml (SI, 40 to 125 pmol/L).
- Estrogen levels in children younger than age 6 are 3 to 10 pg/ml (SI, 10 to 36 pmol/L).
- Estriol is secreted in large amounts by the placenta during pregnancy. Estriol levels during pregnancy range from 2 ng/ml (SI, 7 nmol/L) by 30 weeks' gestation

---

## Predicting premature labor

A simple saliva test can now help determine whether a pregnant woman is at risk for premature labor, a complication that's detrimental to the health of the fetus. The test, known as the SalEst test, measures salivary levels of estriol, an estrogen that increases a thousandfold during pregnancy. For women determined to be at risk, the SalEst test is 98% accurate in ruling out premature labor and delivery.

The test is performed on women between 22 and 36 weeks' gestation, using their saliva and the SalEst test kit. The estriol level increases 2 to 3 weeks before the spontaneous onset of labor and delivery. A positive test indicates that the patient is at risk for premature labor. With this knowledge and evaluation by a physician, precautions can be instituted to decrease the risk of preterm labor and maintain fetal viability.

to 30 ng/ml (SI, 105 nmol/L) by week 40.

## Abnormal results

- Low estrogen levels may indicate primary hypogonadism, or ovarian failure, as in Turner's syndrome or ovarian agenesis; secondary hypogonadism, such as in hypopituitarism; or menopause.
- High estrogen levels may occur with estrogen-producing tumors, in precocious puberty, in congenital adrenal hyperplasia, and in severe hepatic disease, such as cirrhosis.

### DRUG CHALLENGE

 Pretest use of estrogens such as hormonal contraceptives (possible increase); clomiphene, an estrogen antagonist (possible decrease); steroids and pituitary-based hormones such as dexamethasone (may alter test results)

## Purpose

- To determine sexual maturation and fertility
- To help diagnose gonadal dysfunction, such as precocious or delayed puberty, menstrual disorders (especially amenorrhea), and infertility
- To determine fetal well-being
- To help diagnose tumors known to secrete estrogen

## Patient preparation

- Explain that this test helps determine if secretion of female hormones is normal and that the test may be repeated during the various phases of the menstrual cycle.
- Tell the patient that she doesn't need to restrict food and fluids.
- Inform the patient that the test requires a blood sample. Explain who will perform the venipuncture and when.

- Explain to the patient that she may experience slight discomfort from the tourniquet and needle puncture.
- Withhold all steroid and pituitary-based hormones as ordered. If they must be continued, note this on the laboratory request.

## Procedure and posttest care

- Care may vary slightly, depending on whether plasma or serum is being measured.
- Confirm the patient's identity using two patient identifiers according to facility policy.
- Perform a venipuncture, and collect the sample in a 10-ml clot-activator tube.
- If the patient is premenopausal, indicate the phase of her menstrual cycle on the laboratory request.
- Apply direct pressure to the venipuncture site until bleeding stops.
- If a hematoma develops at the venipuncture site, apply warm soaks.
- Tell the patient to resume medications stopped before the test as ordered.

## ▮ Progesterone

Progesterone, an ovarian steroid hormone secreted by the corpus luteum, causes thickening and secretory development of the endometrium in preparation for implantation of the fertilized ovum. Progesterone levels, therefore, peak during the midluteal phase of the menstrual cycle. If implantation doesn't occur, progesterone (and estrogen) levels drop sharply, and menstruation begins about 2 days later. (See *Understanding the menstrual cycle,* page 134.)

During pregnancy, the placenta releases about 10 times the normal monthly amount of progesterone to maintain the pregnancy. Increased secretion begins toward the end of the first trimester and continues until delivery.

# Understanding the menstrual cycle

The menstrual cycle is divided into three distinct phases.

■ During the *menstrual phase*, which starts on the first day of menstruation, the top layer of the endometrium breaks down and flows out of the body. This flow, the menses, consists of blood, mucus, and unneeded tissue.

■ During the *proliferative (follicular) phase*, the endometrium begins to thicken, and the level of estrogen in the blood increases, surging at midcycle. Then estrogen production decreases, the follicle matures, and ovulation occurs.

■ During the *secretory (luteal) phase*, the endometrium begins to thicken to nourish an embryo should fertilization occur. Without fertilization, the top layer of the endometrium breaks down and the menstrual phase of the cycle begins again.

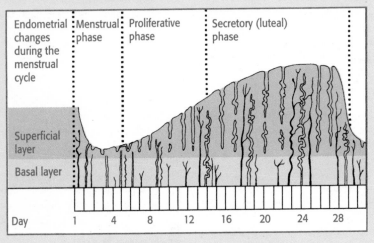

Progesterone prevents abortion by decreasing uterine contractions. Along with estrogen, progesterone helps prepare the breasts for lactation.

This radioimmunoassay is a quantitative analysis of plasma progesterone levels that provides reliable information about corpus luteum function in fertility studies and placental function in pregnancy. Serial determinations are recommended. Although plasma level measurements of progesterone provide accurate information, progesterone can also be monitored by measuring urine pregnanediol, a catabolite of progesterone.

## Reference values

■ During menstruation, progesterone levels are:
  – follicular phase: < 150 ng/dl (SI, < 5 nmol/L)
  – luteal phase: 300 to 1,200 ng/dl (SI, 10 to 40 nmol/L).
■ In pregnant women, progesterone levels are:
  – first trimester: 1,500 to 5,000 ng/dl (SI, 50 to 160 nmol/L)
  – second and third trimesters: 8,000 to 20,000 ng/dl (SI, 250 to 650 nmol/L).
■ In menopausal women, progesterone levels are 10 to 22 ng/dl (SI, 0 to 2 nmol/L).

## Abnormal results

- High progesterone levels may indicate ovulation, luteinizing tumors, ovarian cysts that produce progesterone, or adrenocortical hyperplasia and tumors that produce progesterone and other steroidal hormones.
- Low progesterone levels are associated with amenorrhea from several causes (such as panhypopituitarism and gonadal dysfunction), eclampsia, threatened abortion, and fetal death.

**DRUG CHALLENGE**

 Progesterone or estrogen therapy (may alter test results)

## Purpose

- To assess corpus luteum function as part of infertility studies
- To evaluate placental function in pregnancy
- To help confirm ovulation, in support of basal body temperature readings

## Patient preparation

- Explain that this test helps determine if her progesterone secretion is normal.
- Tell the patient that she doesn't need to restrict food and fluids.
- Tell her that the test requires a blood sample. Explain who will perform the venipuncture and when.
- Explain to the patient that she may experience slight discomfort from the tourniquet and needle puncture.
- Inform the patient that the test may be repeated at specific times coinciding with phases of her menstrual cycle or with each prenatal visit.
- Check the patient's history to determine if she's taking medications that may interfere with test results, including progesterone and estrogen. Note your findings on the laboratory request.

## Procedure and posttest care

- Confirm the patient's identity using two patient identifiers according to facility policy.
- Perform a venipuncture, and collect the blood sample in a 7-ml heparinized tube.
- Apply direct pressure to the venipuncture site until bleeding stops.
- If a hematoma develops at the venipuncture site, apply warm soaks.

## Precautions

- Indicate the date of the patient's last menstrual period and the phase of her cycle on the laboratory request. If the patient is pregnant, also indicate the month of gestation.

# Testosterone

The principal androgen secreted by the interstitial cells of the testes (Leydig cells), testosterone induces puberty in the male and maintains male secondary sex characteristics. Prepubertal levels of testosterone are low. Increased testosterone secretion during puberty stimulates growth of the seminiferous tubules and sperm production; it also contributes to the enlargement of external genitalia, accessory sex organs (such as prostate glands), and voluntary muscles and to the growth of facial, pubic, and axillary hair.

Testosterone production begins to increase at the onset of puberty and continues to rise during adulthood. Production begins to taper off at about age 40 and eventually drops to about one-fifth the peak level by age 80. In women, the adrenal glands and ovaries secrete small amounts of testosterone.

This competitive protein-binding test measures plasma or serum testosterone levels. When combined with measurement of plasma gonadotropin levels (follicle-stimulating hormone and luteinizing hormone), it's a reliable aid in the evaluation of gonadal dysfunction in men and women.

## Reference values

- In men, testosterone levels are 300 to 1,200 ng/dl (SI, 10.4 to 41.6 nmol/L).
- In women testosterone levels are 20 to 80 ng/dl (SI, 0.7 to 2.8 nmol/L).
- In prepubertal children, testosterone levels are lower than adult levels.

## Abnormal results

- High testosterone levels can indicate a benign adrenal tumor or cancer, hyperthyroidism, ovarian tumor, polycystic ovary syndrome, and incipient puberty. In prepubertal boys it may indicate true sexual precocity from excessive gonadotropin secretion or pseudoprecocious puberty from male hormone production by a testicular tumor, congenital adrenal hyperplasia (causing precocious puberty in boys ages 2 to 3), or pseudohermaphroditism; in girls, it may indicate mild virilization.
- Low testosterone levels can indicate primary hypogonadism (as in Klinefelter's syndrome) or secondary hypogonadism (hypogonadotropic eunuchoidism) from hypothalamic-pituitary dysfunction. Low levels can also follow orchiectomy, testicular or prostate cancer, delayed male puberty, estrogen therapy, and cirrhosis of the liver.

### DRUG CHALLENGE

 Estrogens (decrease in free testosterone levels, increasing sex hormone–binding globulin, which binds testosterone); androgens (possible increase)

## Purpose

- To aid in the differential diagnosis in boys younger than age 10 of sexual precocity, distinguishing true precocious puberty from pseudoprecocious puberty
- To aid in the differential diagnosis of hypogonadism, distinguishing primary hypogonadism from secondary hypogonadism
- To evaluate male infertility or other sexual dysfunction
- To evaluate female hirsutism and virilization

## Patient preparation

- Explain that this test helps determine if male sex hormone secretion is normal.
- Inform the patient that he doesn't need to restrict food and fluids.
- Tell the patient that the test requires a blood sample. Explain who will perform the venipuncture and when.
- Explain to the patient that he may experience slight discomfort from the tourniquet and needle puncture.

## Procedure and posttest care

- Confirm the patient's identity using two patient identifiers according to facility policy.
- Perform a venipuncture, and collect a serum sample in a 7-ml clot-activator tube.
- If plasma is to be collected, use a heparinized tube.
- Indicate the patient's age, sex, and history of hormone therapy on the laboratory request.
- Apply direct pressure to the venipuncture site until bleeding stops.
- If a hematoma develops at the venipuncture site, apply warm soaks.

## Precautions

- Exposure to exogenous sources of estrogens and androgens may cause the level to be inaccurate.

## Production of hCG during pregnancy

Production of human chorionic gonadotropin (hCG) increases steadily during the first trimester, peaking around 10 weeks' gestation, as shown below. Levels then fall to less than 10% of first-trimester levels during the rest of the pregnancy.

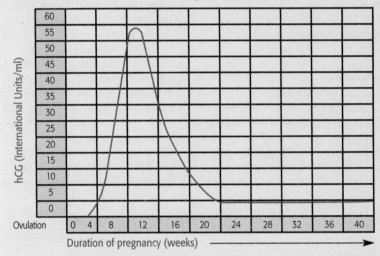

Duration of pregnancy (weeks) ⟶

*Placental hormones*

## █ Human chorionic gonadotropin
### [hCG, pregnancy test]

Human chorionic gonadotropin (hCG) is a glycoprotein hormone produced in the placenta. If conception occurs, a specific assay for hCG—commonly called the beta-subunit assay—may detect this hormone in the blood 9 days after ovulation, when the fertilized ovum would become implanted in the uterine wall. This test is more sensitive (and costlier) than the urine pregnancy test. With progesterone, hCG maintains the corpus luteum during early pregnancy.

Production of hCG increases steadily during the first trimester, peaking around 10 weeks' gestation. Levels then fall to less than 10% of first-trimester peak levels during the remainder of the pregnancy. About 2 weeks after delivery, the hormone may no longer be detectable. (See *Production of hCG during pregnancy*.)

This serum immunoassay, a quantitative analysis of hCG beta-subunit level, is more sensitive (and costlier) than the routine pregnancy test done using a urine sample.

### Reference values

- In nonpregnant women, hCG level is less than 4 International Units/L.
- During pregnancy, hCG levels vary widely, depending partly on the number of days after the last normal menstrual period.

### Abnormal results

- High hCG levels may indicate pregnancy (significantly higher levels are present in a multiple pregnancy); hydatidiform mole, trophoblastic neoplasms of the placenta, and nontrophoblastic carcinomas that secrete hCG (including gastric, pancreatic, and ovarian adenocarcinomas).

- Low hCG levels can occur in ectopic pregnancy or pregnancy of less than 9 days.

### Purpose

- To detect early pregnancy
- To determine adequacy of hormonal production in high-risk pregnancies (for example, habitual abortion)
- To help diagnose trophoblastic tumors, such as hydatidiform mole and choriocarcinoma, and tumors that ectopically secrete hCG
- To monitor treatment for induction of ovulation and conception

### Patient preparation

- Explain the purpose of the test to the patient.
- Tell the patient that she doesn't need to restrict food and fluids.
- Tell her that the test requires a blood sample. Explain who will perform the venipuncture and when.
- Explain to the patient that she may experience slight discomfort from the tourniquet and needle puncture.

### Procedure and posttest care

- Confirm the patient's identity using two patient identifiers according to facility policy.
- Perform a venipuncture, and collect the sample in a 7-ml clot-activator tube.
- Apply direct pressure to the venipuncture site until bleeding stops.
- If a hematoma develops at the venipuncture site, apply warm soaks.

# ▌ Human placental lactogen
### [hPL, human chorionic somatomammotropin]

A polypeptide hormone, human placental lactogen (hPL) helps to prepare the breasts for lactation, provides energy for maternal metabolism and fetal nutrition, and aids protein synthesis and mobilization for fetal growth. Secretion begins at about 5 weeks' gestation and declines rapidly after delivery. According to some evidence, this hormone may not be essential for a successful pregnancy.

This radioimmunoassay measures plasma hPL levels, which are roughly proportional to placental mass. Such assays may be required in high-risk pregnancies (patients with diabetes mellitus or hypertension) and suspected placental tissue dysfunction. Because values vary widely during the latter half of pregnancy, serial determinations over several days provide the most reliable test results. This test, when combined with the measurement of estriol levels, is a reliable indicator of placental function and fetal well-being. It may also be useful as a tumor marker in certain malignant states such as ectopic tumors that secrete hPL.

### Reference values

- For pregnant women, hPL levels are:
  – 5 to 27 weeks' gestation: < 4.6 mcg/ml
  – 28 to 31 weeks' gestation: 2.4 to 6.1 mcg/ml
  – 32 to 35 weeks' gestation: 3.7 to 7.7 mcg/ml
  – 36 weeks' gestation to term: 5 to 8.6 mcg/ml.
- At term, patients with diabetes may have mean levels of 9 to 11 mcg/ml.
- For men and nonpregnant women, hPL levels are < 0.5 mcg/ml.

## Abnormal results

- For reliable interpretation, hPL levels must be correlated with gestational age; for example, after 30 weeks' gestation, levels below 4 mcg/ml may indicate placental dysfunction.
- hPL levels above 6 mcg/ml after 30 weeks' gestation may suggest an unusually large placenta, commonly occurring in a patient with diabetes mellitus, multiple pregnancy, or Rh isoimmunization.
- Declining hPL levels may help differentiate incomplete abortion from threatened abortion.
- Low hPL levels don't confirm fetal distress. The test's usefulness in predicting fetal death in a patient with diabetes mellitus and in managing Rh isoimmunization during pregnancy is limited.
- Low hPL levels may indicate postmaturity syndrome, intrauterine growth retardation, preeclampsia, eclampsia, or trophoblastic neoplastic disease, such as hydatidiform mole and choriocarcinoma.
- High hPL levels have been found in the sera of patients with other neoplastic disorders, including bronchogenic carcinoma, hepatoma, lymphoma, and pheochromocytoma. In these patients, hPL levels are used as tumor markers for evaluating chemotherapy, monitoring tumor growth and recurrence, and detecting residual tissue after excision.

## Purpose

- To assess placental function and fetal well-being (combined with measurement of estriol levels)
- To help diagnose hydatidiform mole and choriocarcinoma
- To help diagnose and monitor treatment of nontrophoblastic tumors that ectopically secrete hPL

## Patient preparation

- Explain that this test helps assess placental function and fetal well-being. If assessing fetal well-being isn't the diagnostic objective, offer an appropriate explanation.
- Tell the patient that the test requires a blood sample. Explain who will perform the venipuncture and when.
- Explain to the patient that she may experience slight discomfort from the tourniquet and needle puncture.
- Inform the pregnant patient that this test may be repeated during her pregnancy.

## Procedure and posttest care

- Confirm the patient's identity using two patient identifiers according to facility policy.
- Perform a venipuncture, and collect the sample in a 7-ml clot-activator tube.
- Apply direct pressure to the venipuncture site until bleeding stops.
- If a hematoma develops at the venipuncture site, apply warm soaks.

# 6

# Lipids and lipoproteins

## Lipid tests

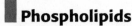

### Phospholipids

The phospholipid test is a quantitative analysis of phospholipids, the major form of lipids in cell membranes. Phospholipids are involved in cellular membrane composition and permeability and help control enzyme activity within the membrane. They help transport fatty acids and lipids across the intestinal barrier and from the liver and other fat stores to other body tissues. Phospholipids are essential for pulmonary gas exchange.

#### Reference values
▪ Phospholipid levels are 180 to 320 mg/dl (SI, 1.8 to 3.2 g/L).
▪ Men usually have higher levels than women; pregnant women have higher levels than men.

#### Abnormal results
▪ High phospholipid levels may indicate hypothyroidism, diabetes mellitus, nephrotic syndrome, chronic pancreatitis, or obstructive jaundice.
▪ Low phospholipid levels may indicate primary hypolipoproteinemia.

DRUG CHALLENGE

Antilipemics (possible decrease); epinephrine, estrogens, and some phenothiazines (increase)

#### Purpose
▪ To assess fat metabolism
▪ To help diagnose hypothyroidism, diabetes mellitus, nephrotic syndrome, chronic pancreatitis, obstructive jaundice, and hypolipoproteinemia

#### Patient preparation
▪ Explain that the phospholipid test determines how the body metabolizes fats.
▪ Tell the patient that the test requires a blood sample. Explain who will perform the venipuncture and when.
▪ Explain to the patient that he may experience slight discomfort from the tourniquet and needle puncture.
▪ Instruct the patient to abstain from drinking alcohol for 24 hours before the test and not to eat or drink anything after midnight before the test.
▪ Notify the laboratory and practitioner of medications the patient is taking that may affect test results; these medications may need to be restricted.

## Procedure and posttest care

- Confirm the patient's identity using two patient identifiers according to facility policy.
- Perform a venipuncture, and collect the blood sample in a 10- to 15-ml tube without additives.
- Apply direct pressure to the venipuncture site until bleeding stops.
- If a hematoma develops at the venipuncture site, apply warm soaks.
- Tell the patient to resume his usual diet and medications stopped before the test as ordered.

### Precautions

- Send the blood sample to the laboratory immediately because spontaneous redistribution of the plasma lipids may occur, rendering them unusable.

# Total cholesterol

The total cholesterol test, the quantitative analysis of serum cholesterol, is used to measure the circulating levels of free cholesterol and cholesterol esters; it reflects the level of the two forms in which this biochemical compound appears in the body. High cholesterol levels may be associated with an increased risk for coronary artery disease (CAD). A 3-minute skin test is now available for use in practitioners' offices. (See *Skin test for cholesterol,* page 142.)

### Reference values

- Total cholesterol values vary with age and sex.
- In men, total cholesterol level should be less than 205 mg/dl (SI, < 5.3 mmol/L).
- In women, total cholesterol level should be less than 190 mg/dl (SI, < 4.9 mmol/L).
- In children ages 12 to 18, total cholesterol level should be less than 170 mg/dl (SI, < 4.4 mmol/L).

## Abnormal results

- High cholesterol levels (hypercholesterolemia) suggest a risk for CAD, as well as incipient hepatitis, lipid disorders, bile duct blockage, nephrotic syndrome, obstructive jaundice, pancreatitis, and hypothyroidism.
- Low cholesterol levels (hypocholesterolemia) are commonly associated with malnutrition, cellular necrosis of the liver, and hyperthyroidism.
- Abnormal cholesterol levels commonly necessitate further testing to pinpoint the cause.

### Drug challenge

 Chlortetracycline, cholestyramine, clofibrate, colestipol, dextrothyroxine, haloperidol, neomycin, and niacin (decrease); chlorpromazine, hormonal contraceptives, epinephrine, trifluoperazine, and trimethadione (increase); androgens (possible variable effect)

### Purpose

- To assess the risk for CAD
- To evaluate fat metabolism
- To aid in diagnosing nephrotic syndrome, pancreatitis, hepatic disease, hypothyroidism, and hyperthyroidism
- To assess the efficacy of lipid-lowering drug therapy

### Patient preparation

- Explain that the total cholesterol test is used to assess the body's fat metabolism.
- Tell the patient that the test requires a blood sample. Explain who will perform the venipuncture and when.
- Inform the patient that he may experience slight discomfort from the tourniquet and needle puncture.
- Instruct the patient not to eat or drink (except water) for 12 hours before the test.

## Skin test for cholesterol

A noninvasive 3-minute test that measures the amount of cholesterol in the skin rather than in the blood is available. It measures how much cholesterol is present in other tissues in the body and provides additional data about a person's risk of heart disease.

The test, which doesn't require patients to fast, involves placing a bandagelike applicator pad on the palm of the hand. Drops of a special solution that reacts to skin cholesterol are then added to the pad; 3 minutes later a handheld computer interprets the information.

Because the test measures the amount of cholesterol that has accumulated in the tissues over time, results don't correlate with blood cholesterol levels; therefore, the test isn't meant to be a substitute or surrogate for a cholesterol test that measures the amount of cholesterol in the blood. The Food and Drug Administration cautions that the test isn't intended for use as a screening tool for heart disease in the general population. Instead, it has been approved for use in adults with severe heart disease—those with at least a 50% blockage of two or more coronary arteries.

■ Notify the laboratory and practitioner of medications the patient is taking that may affect test results; the medications may need to be restricted.

### Procedure and posttest care
■ Confirm the patient's identity using two patient identifiers according to facility policy.
■ Perform a venipuncture, and collect a blood sample in a 4-ml EDTA tube. The patient should be seated for 5 minutes before the blood is drawn. Blood obtained from fingersticks can also be used for initial screening when an automated analyzer is used.
■ Apply direct pressure to the venipuncture site until bleeding stops.
■ Tell the patient to resume his usual diet and medications stopped before the test as ordered.

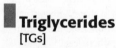

## Triglycerides
[TGs]

Serum triglyceride (TG) analysis provides quantitative analysis of TGs—the main storage form of lipids—which constitute about 95% of fatty tissue. The TG

test permits early identification of hyperlipidemia, which increases the risk for coronary artery disease (CAD).

### Reference values
■ In men, TG levels are 44 to 180 mg/dl (SI, 0.44 to 2.01 mmol/L).
■ In women, TG levels are 10 to 190 mg/dl (SI, 0.11 to 2.21 mmol/L).

### Abnormal results
■ A mild to moderate increase in serum TG levels indicates biliary obstruction, diabetes mellitus, nephrotic syndrome, endocrinopathies, or overconsumption of alcohol.
■ Markedly increased levels without an identifiable cause reflect congenital hyperlipoproteinemia and necessitate lipoprotein phenotyping to confirm the diagnosis.
■ Low TG levels are rare and occur mainly in malnutrition and abetalipoproteinemia.
■ Increased or decreased TG levels require additional tests for a definitive diagnosis.

Antilipemics (decreased serum lipid levels); cholestyramine and colestipol (decreased cholesterol levels, but increased or without effect on triglyceride levels); corticosteroids (long-term use), hormonal contraceptives, estrogen, ethyl alcohol, furosemide, and miconazole (increased cholesterol levels); clofibrate, dextrothyroxine, gemfibrozil, and niacin (decreased cholesterol and triglyceride levels); probucol (decreased cholesterol levels, but variable effect on triglyceride levels)

## Purpose

- To screen for hyperlipidemia or pancreatitis
- To help identify nephrotic syndrome and the individual with poorly controlled diabetes mellitus
- To assess the risk for CAD
- To calculate the low-density lipoprotein (LDL) cholesterol level using the Friedewald equation

## Patient preparation

- Explain that the TG test is used to detect fat metabolism disorders.
- Tell the patient that the test requires a blood sample. Explain who will perform the venipuncture and when.
- Explain to the patient that he may experience slight discomfort from the tourniquet and needle puncture.
- Instruct the patient to fast for at least 12 hours before the test and to abstain from alcohol for 24 hours. Tell him that he can drink water.
- Notify the laboratory and practitioner of medications the patient is taking that may affect test results; these medications may need to be restricted.

## Procedure and posttest care

- Confirm the patient's identity using two patient identifiers according to facility policy.
- Perform a venipuncture, and collect a blood sample in a 4-ml EDTA tube.
- Apply direct pressure to the venipuncture site until bleeding stops.
- If a hematoma develops at the venipuncture site, apply warm soaks.
- Tell the patient to resume his usual diet and medications stopped before the test, as ordered.

# Lipoprotein tests

## Lipoprotein-cholesterol fractionation

Cholesterol fractionation tests are used to isolate and measure the types of cholesterol in serum: low-density lipoproteins (LDLs) and high-density lipoproteins (HDLs). The HDL level is inversely related to the risk of coronary artery disease (CAD); the higher the HDL level, the lower the incidence of CAD. Conversely, the higher the LDL level, the higher the incidence of CAD.

## Reference values

- Lipoprotein values vary by age, sex, geographic area, and ethnic group; check the laboratory for reference values.
- For men, HDL levels are 37 to 70 mg/dl (SI, 0.96 to 1.8 mmol/L); for women, 40 to 85 mg/dl (SI, 1.03 to 2.2 mmol/L). The American College of Cardiology recommends an HDL level of 40 mg/dl or higher in men, 45 mg/dl or higher in women. HDL levels greater than 60 mg/dl are optimal.

# PLAC test

The PLAC test is a blood test that can help determine who might be at risk for coronary artery disease. The FDA based its approval decision on a study of more than 1,300 patients included in a large multicenter study sponsored by the National Heart, Lung, and Blood Institute.

The PLAC test measures lipoprotein-associated phospholipase A2, an enzyme produced by macrophages, a type of white blood cell. When a person has heart disease, macrophages increase production of the phospholipase A2 enzyme. According to the FDA, an elevated PLAC test result, with a low-density-lipoprotein (LDL) cholesterol level under 130 mg/dl, generally indicates that a patient has a two to three times greater risk for coronary artery disease than similar patients with lower PLAC test results.

The study also found that those people with the highest PLAC test results and LDL cholesterol levels lower than 130 mg/dl were at the greatest risk for coronary artery disease.

■ LDL levels are less than 130 mg/dl (SI, < 3.36 mmol/L) in individuals who don't have CAD. Borderline high levels are greater than 160 mg/dl (SI, > 3.3 mmol/L).
■ The American College of Cardiology LDL levels should optimally be less than 100 mg/dl, with levels of 160 mg/dl or more considered high.

## Abnormal results
■ High LDL levels increase the risk for CAD.

■ High HDL levels usually reflect a healthy state but may also indicate chronic hepatitis, early-stage primary biliary cirrhosis, and alcohol consumption.
■ Rarely, a sharp rise (to as high as 100 mg/dl [SI, 2.58 mmol/L]) in a second type of HDL (alpha$_2$-HDL) may signal CAD. (See *PLAC test*.)

### DRUG CHALLENGE

 Antilipemic medications, such as cholestyramine, clofibrate, colestipol, dextrothyroxine, gemfibrozil, niacin, and probucol (decrease in cholesterol level); alcohol, hormonal contraceptives, disulfiram, miconazole, and high doses of phenothiazines (possible increase in cholesterol level); estrogens (possible increase or decrease in cholesterol level)

## Purpose
■ To assess the risk for CAD
■ To assess the efficacy of lipid-lowering drug therapy

## Patient preparation
■ Tell the patient that the lipoprotein-cholesterol fractionation test is used to determine his risk for CAD.
■ Tell the patient that the test requires a blood sample. Explain who will perform the venipuncture and when.
■ Explain to the patient that he may experience slight discomfort from the tourniquet and needle puncture.
■ Instruct the patient to maintain his normal diet for 2 weeks before the test, to abstain from alcohol for 24 hours before the test, and to fast and avoid exercise for 12 to 14 hours before the test.

▪ Notify the laboratory and practitioner of medications the patient is taking that may affect test results; these medications may need to be restricted.

### Procedure and posttest care
▪ Confirm the patient's identity using two patient identifiers according to facility policy.
▪ Perform a venipuncture, and collect a blood sample in a 7-ml EDTA tube.
▪ Apply direct pressure to the venipuncture site until bleeding stops.
▪ If a hematoma develops at the venipuncture site, apply warm soaks.
▪ Tell the patient to resume his usual diet and medications stopped before the test as ordered.

### Precautions
▪ Send the blood sample to the laboratory immediately because spontaneous redistribution of the plasma lipids may occur, rendering them unusable.
▪ The patient's test results may be altered by a concurrent illness, especially if accompanied by fever, recent surgery, or myocardial infarction.

# ▌Lipoprotein phenotyping
[lipoprotein electrophoresis, lipid fractionation]

Lipoprotein phenotyping is used to determine levels of the four major lipoproteins: chylomicrons, very-low-density (prebeta) lipoproteins, low-density (beta) lipoproteins, and high-density (alpha) lipoproteins. (See *Familial hyperlipoproteinemias,* pages 146 and 147.) Detecting altered lipoprotein patterns is essential in identifying hyperlipoproteinemias and hypolipoproteinemias.

### Normal results
▪ Not applicable for this test

### Abnormal results
▪ The types of hyperlipoproteinemias and hypolipoproteinemias are identified by characteristic electrophoretic patterns.
▪ Familial lipoprotein disorders are classified as either hyperlipoproteinemias or hypolipoproteinemias.
▪ There are six types of hyperlipoproteinemias: I, IIa, IIb, III, IV, and V. Types IIa, IIb, and IV are relatively common.
▪ All hypolipoproteinemias are rare, including hypobetalipoproteinemia, betalipoproteinemia, and alphalipoprotein deficiency.

D RUG CHALLENGE

 Recent use of antilipemics (lower levels of the lipids)

### Purpose
▪ To classify hyperlipoproteinemias and hypolipoproteinemias

### Patient preparation
▪ Explain that lipoprotein typing is used to determine how the body metabolizes fats.
▪ Tell the patient that the test requires a blood sample. Explain who will perform the venipuncture and when.
▪ Explain to the patient that he may experience slight discomfort from the tourniquet and needle puncture.
▪ Instruct the patient to abstain from alcohol for 24 hours before the test and to fast after midnight before the test. Provide a low-fat meal the night before the test.
▪ Check the patient's drug history for heparin use. As ordered, withhold antilipemics, such as cholestyramine, about 2 weeks before the test.

# Familial hyperlipoproteinemias

| Type | Causes and incidence | Clinical signs | Laboratory findings |
|---|---|---|---|
| I | • Deficient lipoprotein lipase, resulting in increased chylomicrons<br>• May be induced by alcoholism<br>• Incidence: rare | • Eruptive xanthomas<br>• Lipemia retinalis<br>• Abdominal pain | • Increased chylomicron, total cholesterol, and triglyceride levels<br>• Normal or slightly increased very-low-density lipoprotein (VLDL) levels<br>• Normal or decreased low-density lipoprotein (LDL) and high-density lipoprotein levels<br>• Cholesterol triglyceride ratio < 0.2 |
| IIa | • Deficient cell receptor, resulting in increased LDL and excessive cholesterol synthesis<br>• May be induced by hypothyroidism<br>• Incidence: common | • Premature coronary artery disease (CAD)<br>• Arcus cornea<br>• Xanthelasma<br>• Tendinous and tuberous xanthomas | • Increased LDL level<br>• Normal VLDL level<br>• Cholesterol-triglyceride ratio > 2.0 |
| IIb | • Deficient cell receptor, resulting in increased LDL and excessive cholesterol synthesis<br>• May be induced by dysgammaglobulinemia, hypothyroidism, uncontrolled diabetes mellitus, and nephrotic syndrome<br>• Incidence: common | • Premature CAD<br>• Obesity<br>• Possible xanthelasma | • Increased LDL, VLDL, total cholesterol, and triglyceride levels |

*(continued)*

• Notify the laboratory if the patient is receiving treatment for another condition that might significantly alter lipoprotein metabolism, such as diabetes mellitus, nephrosis, or hypothyroidism.

## Procedure and posttest care

• Confirm the patient's identity using two patient identifiers according to facility policy.
• Perform a venipuncture, and collect the blood sample in a 4-ml EDTA tube.

## Familial hyperlipoproteinemias *(continued)*

| Type | Causes and incidence | Clinical signs | Laboratory findings |
|---|---|---|---|
| III | • Unknown cause, resulting in deficient VLDL-to-LDL conversion<br>• May be induced by hypothyroidism, uncontrolled diabetes mellitus, and paraproteinemia<br>• Incidence: rare | • Premature CAD<br>• Arcus cornea<br>• Eruptive tuberous xanthomas | • Increased total cholesterol, VLDL, and triglyceride levels<br>• Normal or decreased LDL level<br>• Cholesterol-triglyceride ratio > 0.4<br>• Broad beta band observed on electrophoresis |
| IV | • Unknown cause; resulting in decreased levels of lipase<br>• May be induced by uncontrolled diabetes mellitus, alcoholism, pregnancy, steroid or estrogen therapy, dysgammaglobulinemia, and hyperthyroidism<br>• Incidence: common | • Possible premature CAD<br>• Obesity<br>• Hypertension<br>• Peripheral neuropathy | • Increased VLDL and triglycerides<br>• Normal LDL<br>• Cholesterol-triglyceride ratio < 0.25 |
| V | • Unknown cause; resulting in defective tryglyceride clearance<br>• May be induced by alcoholism, dysgammaglobulienmia, uncontrolled diabetes mellitus, nephrotic syndrome, pancreatitis, and steroid therapy<br>• Incidence: rare | • Premature CAD<br>• Abdominal pain<br>• Lipemia retinalis<br>• Eruptive xanthomas<br>• Hepatomegaly | • Increased VLDL, total cholesterol, and triglycerides<br>• Chylomicrons present<br>• Cholesterol-triglyceride ratio < 0.6 |

• If a hematoma develops at the venipuncture site, apply warm soaks.
• Tell the patient to resume his usual diet and medications stopped before the test as ordered.

## Precautions
### DO'S & DON'TS

 When drawing multiple blood samples, collect the sample for lipoprotein phenotyping first because venous obstruction for 2 minutes can affect test results.

# 7

# Proteins, protein metabolites, and pigments

## Protein tests

### Haptoglobin
[Hp, Hapto]

The haptoglobin test measures serum levels of haptoglobin, a glycoprotein produced in the liver. In acute intravascular hemolysis, the haptoglobin level decreases rapidly and may remain low for 5 to 7 days, until the liver synthesizes more glycoprotein. In hemolytic transfusion reactions, haptoglobin levels begin decreasing after 6 to 8 hours and drop to 40% of pretransfusion levels after 24 hours.

### Reference values
- Haptoglobin levels, measured in terms of the protein's hemoglobin-binding capacity, are 40 to 180 mg/dl (SI, 0.4 to 1.8 g/L).
- Nephelometric procedures yield lower results.
- Haptoglobin is absent in 90% of neonates, but levels usually gradually increase to normal by age 4 months.

### Abnormal results
- High haptoglobin levels occur in diseases marked by chronic inflammatory reactions or tissue destruction, such as rheumatoid arthritis and malignant neoplasms.
- Low haptoglobin levels indicate acute and chronic hemolysis, severe hepatocellular disease, infectious mononucleosis, and transfusion reactions.
- In about 1% of the population, including 4% of blacks, haptoglobin is permanently absent; this disorder is known as congenital ahaptoglobinemia.

### DRUG CHALLENGE

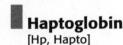 Corticosteroids and androgens (possible increase in haptoglobin; may mask hemolysis in patients with inflammatory disease); hormonal contraceptives, chlorpromazine, diphenhydramine, indomethacin, isoniazid, nitrofurantoin, quinidine, streptomycin (decreased levels of haptoglobin)

### Purpose
- To serve as an index of hemolysis
- To distinguish between hemoglobin and myoglobin in plasma because haptoglobin doesn't bind with myoglobin

- To investigate hemolytic transfusion reactions
- To establish proof of paternity using genetic (phenotypic) variations in haptoglobin structure

### Patient preparation
- Explain that this test is used to determine the condition of red blood cells (RBCs).
- Tell the patient that the test requires a blood sample. Explain who will perform the venipuncture and when.
- Explain to the patient that he may experience slight discomfort from the tourniquet and needle puncture.
- Tell the patient that he doesn't need to restrict food and fluids.
- Notify the laboratory and practitioner of medications the patient is taking that may affect test results; these medications may need to be restricted.

### Procedure and posttest care
- Confirm the patient's identity using two patient identifiers according to facility policy.
- Perform a venipuncture, and collect a blood sample in a 7-ml clot-activator tube.
- Apply direct pressure to the venipuncture site until bleeding stops.
- If a hematoma develops at the venipuncture site, apply warm soaks.
- Tell the patient to resume medications stopped before the test as ordered.

# ▌Protein electrophoresis

Protein electrophoresis measures serum albumin and globulin, the major blood proteins, by separating the proteins into five distinct fractions: albumin and alpha$_1$, alpha$_2$, beta, and gamma globulin proteins.

### Reference values
- Total serum protein levels are 6.4 to 8.3 g/dl (SI, 64 to 83 g/L), and the albumin fraction values are 3.5 to 5 g/dl (SI, 35 to 50 g/L).
- Alpha$_1$-globulin fraction values are 0.1 to 0.3 g/dl (SI, 1 to 3 g/L).
- Alpha$_2$-globulin fraction values are 0.6 to 1 g/dl (SI, 6 to 10 g/L).
- Beta globulin fraction values are 0.7 to 1.1 g/dl (SI, 7 to 11 g/L).
- Gamma globulin ranges from 0.8 to 1.6 g/dl (SI, 8 to 16 g/L).

### Abnormal results
- For common abnormal results, see *Clinical implications of abnormal protein levels,* page 150.

### Purpose
- To help diagnose hepatic disease, protein deficiency, renal disorders, and GI and neoplastic diseases

### Patient preparation
- Explain that protein electrophoresis determines the protein content of the blood.
- Tell the patient that the test requires a blood sample. Explain who will perform the venipuncture and when.
- Explain to the patient that he may experience slight discomfort from the tourniquet and needle puncture.
- Tell the patient that he doesn't need to restrict food and fluids.
- Notify the laboratory and practitioner of medications the patient is taking that may affect test results; these medications may need to be restricted.

### Procedure and posttest care
- Confirm the patient's identity using two patient identifiers according to facility policy.
- Perform a venipuncture, and collect a blood sample in a 7-ml clot-activator tube.

# Clinical implications of abnormal protein levels

## Increased levels

**Total proteins**
- Chronic inflammatory disease (such as rheumatoid arthritis or early stage Laënnec's cirrhosis)
- Dehydration
- Diabetic ketoacidosis
- Fulminating and chronic infections
- Multiple myeloma
- Monocytic leukemia
- Vomiting, diarrhea

**Albumin**
- Multiple myeloma
- Dehydration

**Globulins**
- Chronic syphilis
- Collagen diseases
- Diabetes mellitus
- Hodgkin's disease
- Multiple myeloma
- Rheumatoid arthritis
- Subacute bacterial endocarditis
- Systemic lupus erythematosus (SLE)
- Tuberculosis

## Decreased levels

**Total proteins**
- Benzene and carbon tetrachloride poisoning
- Blood dyscrasias
- Essential hypertension
- Gestational hypertension
- GI disease
- Heart failure
- Hepatic dysfunction
- Hemorrhage
- Hodgkin's disease
- Hyperthyroidism
- Malabsorption
- Malnutrition
- Nephrosis
- Severe burns
- Surgical and traumatic shock
- Uncontrolled diabetes mellitus

**Albumin**
- Acute cholecystitis
- Collagen diseases
- Diarrhea
- Essential hypertension
- Hepatic disease
- Hodgkin's disease
- Hyperthyroidism
- Hypogammaglobulinemia
- Malnutrition
- Metastatic carcinoma
- Nephritis, nephrosis
- Peptic ulcer
- Plasma loss from burns
- Rheumatoid arthritis
- Sarcoidosis
- SLE

**Globulins**
- Benzene and carbon tetrachloride poisoning
- Blood dyscrasias
- Essential hypertension
- Gestational hypertension
- GI disease
- Heart failure
- Hepatic dysfunction
- Hemorrhage
- Hodgkin's disease
- Hyperthyroidism
- Malabsorption
- Malnutrition
- Nephrosis
- Severe burns
- Surgical and traumatic shock
- Uncontrolled diabetes mellitus

- Apply direct pressure to the venipuncture site until bleeding stops.

- If a hematoma develops at the venipuncture site, apply warm soaks.

- Tell the patient to resume medications stopped before the test as ordered.

## Precautions
- This test must be performed on a serum sample to avoid measuring the fibrinogen fraction.

# Transferrin
[siderophilin]

A quantitative analysis of serum transferrin levels is used to evaluate iron metabolism. Transferrin is a glycoprotein formed in the liver. It transports circulating iron obtained from dietary sources or the breakdown of red blood cells (RBCs) by reticuloendothelial cells to bone marrow for use in hemoglobin synthesis or to the liver, spleen, and bone marrow for storage. A serum iron level is usually obtained simultaneously.

## Reference values
- Transferrin levels are 200 to 400 mg/dl (SI, 2 to 4 g/L).

## Abnormal results
- Low transferrin levels may indicate inadequate transferrin production from hepatic damage, excessive protein loss from renal disease, acute or chronic infection, or cancer; low levels may cause impaired hemoglobin synthesis and, possibly, anemia.
- High transferrin levels may indicate severe iron deficiency.

## Purpose
- To determine the iron-transporting capacity of the blood
- To evaluate iron metabolism in iron deficiency anemia

## Patient preparation
- Explain that the transferrin test is used to determine the cause of anemia.

- Tell the patient that the test requires a blood sample. Explain who will perform the venipuncture and when.
- Explain to the patient that he may experience slight discomfort from the tourniquet and needle puncture.
- Tell the patient that he doesn't need to restrict food and fluids.
- Notify the laboratory and practitioner of medications the patient is taking that may affect test results; these medications may need to be restricted.

## Procedure and posttest care
- Confirm the patient's identity using two patient identifiers according to facility policy.
- Perform a venipuncture, and collect a blood sample in a 4-ml clot-activator tube.
- Apply direct pressure to the venipuncture site until bleeding stops.
- If a hematoma develops at the venipuncture site, apply warm soaks.
- Tell the patient to resume medications stopped before the test as ordered.

# Protein metabolite tests

# Amino acid screening

Plasma amino acid screening is a qualitative screen for inborn errors of amino acid metabolism in infants. Amino acids are the chief component of all proteins and polypeptides. The body contains at least 20 amino acids; 10 of these aren't formed in the body and must be acquired by diet. Certain congenital enzyme deficiencies interfere with normal metabolism of these amino acids, resulting in amino acid accumulation or deficiency.

### Normal results
- Chromatography shows a normal plasma amino acid pattern.

### Abnormal results
- Excessive accumulation of amino acids typically produces overflow aminoacidurias.
- Congenital abnormalities of the amino acid transport system in the kidneys produce a second group of disorders called renal aminoacidurias.
- Comparisons of blood and urine chromatography can help distinguish between the two types of aminoacidurias.
- The plasma amino acid pattern is normal in renal aminoacidurias and abnormal in overflow aminoacidurias.

### Purpose
- To screen for inborn errors of amino acid metabolism

### Patient preparation
- Explain to the parents that plasma and amino acid screening is used to determine how well their infant metabolizes amino acids.
- Inform the parents that the infant must fast for 4 hours before the test.
- Tell the parents that a small amount of blood will be drawn from the infant's heel but that collecting the blood sample only takes a few minutes.

### Procedure and posttest care
- Confirm the patient's identity using two patient identifiers according to facility policy.
- Perform a heelstick, and collect 0.1 ml of blood in a heparinized capillary tube.
- Apply direct pressure to the heelstick site until bleeding stops.
- If a hematoma develops at the heelstick site, apply warm soaks.
- Tell the parents to resume their infant's usual diet.

# ■ Ammonia
### [NH₃]

The plasma ammonia test measures plasma levels of ammonia, a nonprotein nitrogen compound that helps maintain acid-base balance. In diseases such as cirrhosis, ammonia can bypass the liver and accumulate in the blood. Plasma ammonia levels may help indicate the severity of hepatocellular damage.

### Reference values
- Plasma ammonia levels in adults are 15 to 56 mcg/dl (SI, 9 to 33 µmol/L).

### Abnormal results
- High ammonia levels are common in severe hepatic disease, such as cirrhosis and acute hepatic necrosis; Reye's syndrome; severe heart failure; GI hemorrhage; and erythroblastosis fetalis.

DRUG CHALLENGE

 Acetazolamide, ammonium salts, furosemide and thiazides, (increase in ammonia level); parenteral nutrition (possible increase in ammonia level); lactulose, neomycin, and kanamycin (decrease in ammonia level)

### Purpose
- To help monitor the progression of severe hepatic disease and the effectiveness of therapy
- To recognize impending or established hepatic coma
- To monitor the patient receiving hyperalimentation therapy

### Patient preparation
- Explain to the patient (or to a family member or legal guardian if the patient is comatose) that the plasma ammonia test is used to evaluate liver function.

■ Tell the patient that the test requires a blood sample. Explain who will perform the venipuncture and when.

■ Inform the patient that he may experience slight discomfort from the tourniquet and needle puncture.

■ Notify the laboratory and practitioner of medications the patient is taking that may affect test results; these medications may need to be restricted.

### Procedure and posttest care

■ Confirm the patient's identity using two patient identifiers according to facility policy.

■ Perform a venipuncture, and collect a blood sample in a 10-ml heparinized tube.

### DO'S & DON'TS

 Immediately place the sample on ice and send to the laboratory

■ Apply direct pressure to the venipuncture site until bleeding stops.

■ If a hematoma develops at the venipuncture site, apply warm soaks.

■ Watch for signs of impending or established hepatic coma if plasma ammonia levels are high.

## ▌Blood urea nitrogen
### [BUN]

The blood urea nitrogen (BUN) test measures the nitrogen fraction of urea, the chief end product of protein metabolism. Formed in the liver from ammonia and excreted by the kidneys, urea constitutes 40% to 50% of the blood's nonprotein nitrogen. The BUN level reflects protein intake and renal excretory capacity, but is a less reliable indicator of uremia than the serum creatinine level.

### Reference values

■ BUN levels are 8 to 20 mg/dl (SI, 2.9 to 7.5 mmol/L).

■ BUN levels are slightly higher in elderly patients.

### Abnormal results

■ High BUN levels occur in renal disease, reduced renal blood flow (from dehydration, for example), urinary tract obstruction, GI bleed, congestive heart failure, and increased protein catabolism (possibly from burns).

■ Low BUN levels indicate severe hepatic damage, malnutrition, low protein diets, and overhydration.

### DRUG CHALLENGE

 Chloramphenicol, streptomycin (possible decrease); allopurinol, aminoglycosides, amphotericin B, furosemide, nonsteroidal anti-inflammatory drugs, thiazide diuretics, and methicillin (increased due to nephrotoxicity)

### Purpose

■ To evaluate renal function and help diagnose renal disease

■ To aid in assessing hydration

### Patient preparation

■ Explain that this test helps evaluate kidney function.

■ Tell the patient that he doesn't have to restrict food and fluids but that he should avoid a diet high in meat.

■ Tell the patient that the test requires a blood sample. Explain who will perform the venipuncture and when.

■ Explain to the patient that he may experience slight discomfort from the tourniquet and needle puncture.

■ Notify the laboratory and practitioner of medications the patient is taking that may affect test results; these medications may need to be restricted.

## Procedure and posttest care

- Confirm the patient's identity using two patient identifiers according to facility policy.
- Perform a venipuncture, and collect a blood sample in a 3- to 4-ml clot-activator tube.
- Apply direct pressure to the venipuncture site until bleeding stops.
- If a hematoma develops at the venipuncture site, apply warm soaks.
- Tell the patient to resume medications stopped before the test as ordered.

# Creatinine

Analysis of serum creatinine levels provides a more sensitive measure of renal damage than blood urea nitrogen levels. Creatinine is a nonprotein end product of creatine metabolism that appears in serum in amounts proportional to the body's muscle mass.

## Reference values

- In male patients, creatinine level is 0.8 to 1.2 mg/dl (SI, 62 to 115 µmol/L).
- In female patients, creatinine level is 0.6 to 0.9 mg/dl (SI, 53 to 97 µmol/L).

## Abnormal results

- High creatinine levels usually indicate renal disease that has seriously damaged 50% or more of the nephrons; high creatinine levels may also suggest gigantism, acromegaly, and rhabdomyolysis.

### DRUG CHALLENGE

Ascorbic acid, barbiturates, cephalosporins, cimetidine, cisplatin, diuretics, and gentamicin (possible increase in creatinine level)

## Purpose

- To assess glomerular filtration
- To screen for renal damage

## Patient preparation

- Explain that the serum creatinine test is used to evaluate kidney function.
- Tell the patient that the test requires a blood sample. Explain who will perform the venipuncture and when.
- Explain to the patient that he may experience slight discomfort from the tourniquet and needle puncture.
- Tell the patient that he doesn't need to restrict food or fluids.
- Notify the laboratory and practitioner of medications the patient is taking that may affect test results; these medications may need to be restricted.

## Procedure and posttest care

- Confirm the patient's identity using two patient identifiers according to facility policy.
- Perform a venipuncture and collect a blood sample in a 3- or 4-ml clot-activator tube.
- Apply direct pressure to the venipuncture site until bleeding stops.
- If a hematoma develops at the venipuncture site, apply warm soaks.
- Tell the patient to resume medications stopped before the test, as ordered.

## Precautions

- Patients with a very large muscle mass may have an increased creatinine level.

# Phenylalanine screening
[Guthrie screening test, PKU test, phenylketonuria test]

The phenylalanine screening test is used to screen infants for elevated serum phenylalanine levels, a possible indication of phenylketonuria (PKU). Phenylalanine is a naturally occurring amino acid essential to growth and nitrogen balance; an accumulation of this amino acid may indicate a serious enzyme deficiency. This test detects abnormal

## Confirming PKU

If phenylalanine screening detects possible phenylketonuria (PKU), serum phenylalanine and tyrosine levels are measured to confirm the diagnosis. Phenylalanine hydroxylase is the enzyme that converts phenylalanine to tyrosine. If this enzyme is absent, increasing phenylalanine levels and falling tyrosine levels indicate PKU.

Blood samples are obtained by venipuncture (femoral or external jugular) and measured by fluorometry. Elevated serum phenylalanine levels (> 4 mg/dl [SI, > 242 µmol/L]) and low tyrosine levels—with urinary excretion of phenylpyruvic acid—confirm the PKU diagnosis.

phenylalanine levels through the growth rate of *Bacillus subtilis*, an organism that needs phenylalanine to thrive. To ensure accurate results, the test must be performed after 3 full days (preferably 4 days) of milk or formula feeding. At birth, a neonate with PKU usually has normal phenylalanine levels, but after milk or formula feeding begins, levels gradually increase because of a deficiency of the liver enzyme that converts phenylalanine to tyrosine.

### Reference values

▪ Phenylalanine levels are less than 2 mg/dl (SI, < 121 µmol/L) (negative test result; no risk of PKU).

### Abnormal results

▪ Phenylalanine levels equal to or greater than 2 mg/dl (SI, 121 µmol/L (positive test result) suggests the possibility of PKU. (A definitive diagnosis requires exact serum phenylalanine measurement and urine testing.)

▪ A positive test result may also indicate hepatic disease, galactosemia, or delayed development of certain enzyme systems. (See *Confirming PKU*.)

### Purpose

▪ To screen infants for PKU

### Patient preparation

▪ Explain to the parents that the test is a routine screening measure for PKU and is required in many states.

▪ Tell the parents that a small amount of blood will be drawn from the infant's heel and collecting the sample only takes a few minutes.

### Procedure and posttest care

▪ Confirm the patient's identity using two patient identifiers according to facility policy.

▪ Perform a heelstick, and collect three drops of blood to deposit on filter paper—one drop for each circle on the filter paper.

▪ Reassure the parents of a child who may have PKU that although this disease is a common cause of congenital mental deficiency, early detection and continuous treatment with a low-phenylalanine diet can prevent permanent mental retardation.

### Precautions

▪ Note the infant's name and birth date and the date of the first milk or formula feeding on the laboratory request.

▪ Performing the test before the infant has received at least 3 full days of milk or formula feeding may yield a false-negative test result.

# Uric acid
[urate]

The uric acid test is used to measure serum levels of uric acid, the major end metabolite of purine. Disorders of purine metabolism, rapid destruction of nucleic acids, and conditions marked by impaired renal excretion characteristically raise serum uric acid levels.

## Reference values
- In men, uric acid levels are 3.4 to 7 mg/dl (SI, 202 to 416 μmol/L).
- In women, uric acid levels are 2.3 to 6 mg/dl (SI, 143 to 357 μmol/L).

## Abnormal results
- High uric acid levels may indicate gout, impaired kidney function, heart failure, glycogen storage disease (type I, von Gierke's disease), infections, hemolytic and sickle cell anemia, polycythemia, neoplasms, and psoriasis.
- Low uric acid levels may indicate defective tubular absorption (such as Fanconi's syndrome) or acute hepatic atrophy.

### DRUG CHALLENGE

 Aspirin in low doses, ethambutol, loop diuretics, pyrazinamide, thiazides, and vincristine (possible increase); acetaminophen, ascorbic acid, and levodopa (possible false-high if using colorimetric method); aspirin in high doses (possible decrease)

## Purpose
- To confirm the diagnosis of gout
- To help detect renal dysfunction

## Patient preparation
- Explain that the uric acid test is used to detect gout and kidney dysfunction.
- Tell the patient that the test requires a blood sample. Explain who will perform the venipuncture and when.
- Explain to the patient that he may experience slight discomfort from the tourniquet and needle puncture.
- Instruct the patient to fast for 8 hours before the test.
- Notify the laboratory and practitioner of medications the patient is taking that may affect test results; these medications may need to be restricted.

## Procedure and posttest care
- Confirm the patient's identity using two patient identifiers according to facility policy.
- Perform a venipuncture, and collect a blood sample in a 3- or 4-ml clot-activator tube.
- Apply direct pressure to the venipuncture site until bleeding stops.
- If a hematoma develops at the venipuncture site, apply warm soaks.
- Tell the patient to resume his usual diet and medications stopped before the test as ordered.

## Precautions
- Starvation, high-purine diet, stress, and alcohol abuse may cause an increase in the uric acid level.

# Pigment tests

## Bilirubin
[total bilirubin]

The bilirubin test measures serum levels of bilirubin, the predominant pigment in bile. Bilirubin is the major product of hemoglobin catabolism. Serum bilirubin measurements are especially significant in neonates because elevated unconjugated bilirubin can accumulate in the brain, causing irreparable damage.

## Reference values

■ Indirect bilirubin levels are 1.1 mg/dl (SI, 19 µmol/L).
■ Direct bilirubin levels are less than 0.5 mg/dl (SI, < 6.8 µmol/L).
■ In neonates, total serum bilirubin levels are 2 to 12 mg/dl (SI, 34 to 205 µmol/L).

## Abnormal results

■ High indirect bilirubin levels usually indicate hepatic damage or severe hemolytic anemia but may also suggest congenital enzyme deficiencies such as Gilbert syndrome.
■ High direct bilirubin levels usually indicate biliary obstruction. If obstruction continues, direct and indirect bilirubin levels may rise.
■ In severe chronic hepatic damage, direct bilirubin levels may return to normal or near-normal levels, but indirect bilirubin levels remain elevated.
■ In neonates, total bilirubin levels of 15 mg/dl (SI, 257 µmol/L) or more indicate the need for an exchange transfusion.

## Purpose

■ To evaluate liver function
■ To aid in the differential diagnosis of jaundice and monitor its progress
■ To help diagnose biliary obstruction and hemolytic anemia
■ To determine whether a neonate requires an exchange transfusion or phototherapy because of dangerously high unconjugated bilirubin levels

## Patient preparation

■ Explain that the bilirubin test is used to evaluate liver function and the condition of red blood cells (RBCs).
■ Tell the adult patient that the test requires a blood sample. Explain who will perform the venipuncture and when.
■ If the patient is an infant, tell the parents that a small amount of blood will be drawn from the child's heel. Tell them who will be performing the heelstick and when.
■ Explain to the patient that he may experience slight discomfort from the tourniquet and needle puncture.
■ Inform the adult patient that he need not restrict fluids, but he should fast for at least 4 hours before the test.
■ Explain that fasting isn't necessary for the neonate.

## Procedure and posttest care

■ Confirm the patient's identity using two patient identifiers according to facility policy.
■ If the patient is an adult, perform a venipuncture, and collect a blood sample in a 3- or 4-ml clot-activator tube.
■ Apply direct pressure to the venipuncture site until bleeding stops.
■ If the patient is an infant, perform a heelstick, and fill the microcapillary tube to the designated level with blood.
■ If a hematoma develops at the venipuncture or heelstick site, apply warm soaks.

## Precautions

■ Protect the blood sample from strong sunlight and ultraviolet light.

# Fractionated erythrocyte porphyrins

The fractionated erythrocyte porphyrin test is used to measure erythrocyte porphyrins (also called erythropoietic porphyrins): protoporphyrin, coproporphyrin, and uroporphyrin. Porphyrins are present in all protoplasm and are significant in energy storage and use. They're produced during heme biosynthesis and usually appear in small amounts in blood, urine, and stool. The production and excretion of porphyrins or their precursors increase in porphyria.

## Reference values
- Total porphyrin levels are 16 to 60 mcg/dl (SI, 0.25 to 1.062 µmol/L) of packed red blood cells (RBCs).
- Protoporphyrin levels are 16 to 60 mcg/dl (SI, 0.25 to 1.062 µmol/L).
- Coproporphyrin and uroporphyrin levels are less than 2 mcg/dl (SI, < 0.035 µmol/L).

## Abnormal results
- Elevated total porphyrin levels suggest the need for further enzyme testing to identify the specific porphyria.
- Elevated protoporphyrin levels may indicate erythropoietic protoporphyria, infection, increased erythropoiesis, thalassemia, sideroblastic anemia, iron deficiency anemia, or lead poisoning.
- Increased coproporphyrin levels may indicate congenital erythropoietic porphyria, erythropoietic protoporphyria or coproporphyria, or sideroblastic anemia.
- Elevated uroporphyrin levels may indicate congenital erythropoietic porphyria or erythropoietic protoporphyria.

## Purpose
- To help diagnose congenital and acquired erythropoietic porphyrias
- To help confirm the diagnosis of disorders affecting RBC activity

## Patient preparation
- Explain that the fractionated erythrocyte porphyrin test is used to detect RBC disorders.
- Tell the patient that the test requires a blood sample. Explain who will perform the venipuncture and when.
- Explain to the patient that he may experience slight discomfort from the tourniquet and needle puncture.

## Procedure and posttest care
- Confirm the patient's identity using two patient identifiers according to facility policy.
- Perform a venipuncture, and collect a blood sample in a 5-ml or larger heparinized tube.
- Label the sample, place it on ice, and send it to the laboratory immediately.
- Apply direct pressure to the venipuncture site until bleeding stops.
- If a hematoma develops at the venipuncture site, apply warm soaks.

# 8

# Carbohydrates

## Carbohydrate metabolism tests

### Fasting plasma glucose
[fasting blood sugar, FBS, glucose, blood sugar]

The fasting plasma glucose test measures plasma glucose levels after a 12- to 14-hour fast. This test is commonly used to screen for diabetes mellitus, in which absent or deficient insulin allows persistently high blood glucose levels.

#### Reference values
- The range for fasting plasma glucose level varies according to the laboratory procedure.
- Values after at least an 8-hour fast are 70 to 110 mg (SI, 3.9 to 6.1 mmol/L) of true glucose per deciliter of blood.

#### Abnormal results
- Confirmation of diabetes mellitus requires fasting plasma glucose levels of 126 mg/dl (SI, 7 mmol/L) or more obtained on two or more occasions. In the patient with borderline or transient elevated levels, a 2-hour postprandial plasma glucose test or oral glucose tolerance test may be performed to confirm the diagnosis.
- High fasting plasma glucose levels can also result from pancreatitis, recent

acute illness (such as myocardial infarction), Cushing's syndrome, acromegaly, pheochromocytoma, hyperlipoproteinemia (especially type III, IV, or V), chronic hepatic disease, nephrotic syndrome, brain tumor, sepsis, gastrectomy with dumping syndrome, eclampsia, anoxia, or seizure disorders.
- Low plasma glucose levels can result from hyperinsulinism, insulinoma, von Gierke's disease, functional and reactive hypoglycemia, myxedema, adrenal insufficiency, congenital adrenal hyperplasia, hypopituitarism, malabsorption syndrome, and some cases of hepatic insufficiency.

#### DRUG CHALLENGE

 Arginine, benzodiazepines, chlorthalidone, hormonal contraceptives, corticosteroids, dextrothyroxine, diazoxide, thiazide diuretics, epinephrine, furosemide, recent I.V. glucose infusions, lithium, large doses of nicotinic acid, phenolphthalein, phenothiazines, phenytoin, and triamterene (increase); ethacrynic acid (may cause hyperglycemia); large doses of ethacrynic acid in patients with uremia (can cause hypoglycemia); oral antidiabetic agents, beta-adrenergic blockers, clofibrate, ethanol, insulin, and monoamine oxidase inhibitors (possible decrease)

## Purpose
- To screen for diabetes mellitus
- To monitor drug or diet therapy in the patient with diabetes mellitus

## Patient preparation
- Explain that this test helps detect disorders of glucose metabolism and helps diagnose diabetes.
- Tell the patient that the test requires a blood sample. Explain who will perform the venipuncture and when.
- Explain to the patient that he may experience slight discomfort from the tourniquet and the needle puncture.
- Instruct the patient to fast for 12 to 14 hours before the test.
- Notify the laboratory and practitioner of medications the patient is taking that may affect test results; these medications may need to be restricted.

Do's & don'ts

Alert the patient to the symptoms of hypoglycemia (weakness, restlessness, nervousness, hunger, and sweating) and tell him to report such symptoms immediately.

## Procedure and posttest care
- Confirm the patient's identity using two patient identifiers according to facility policy.
- Perform a venipuncture, and collect the sample in a 5-ml clot-activator tube.
- Apply direct pressure to the venipuncture site until bleeding stops.
- If a hematoma develops at the venipuncture site, apply warm soaks.
- Provide a balanced meal or a snack.
- Tell the patient to resume medications stopped before the test as ordered.

## Precautions
- A recent infection, illness, or pregnancy may raise blood glucose levels.

- Strenuous exercise may lower blood glucose levels.

# Glycosylated hemoglobin
### [hemoglobin A$_{1c}$, glycohemoglobin]

The glycosylated hemoglobin (HbA$_{1c}$) test is a tool for monitoring diabetes therapy. Measurement of glycosylated Hb value provides information about the patient's average blood glucose level during the preceding 2 to 3 months. This test requires only one venipuncture every 6 to 8 weeks and can therefore be used for evaluating the long-term effectiveness of diabetes therapy.

## Reference values
- HbA$_{1c}$ values are 4% to 7%.

## Abnormal results
- In diabetes, the patient has good control of blood glucose levels when the HbA$_{1c}$ value is less than 8%.
- An HbA$_{1c}$ value greater than 10% indicates poor control.

## Purpose
- To assess control of diabetes mellitus

## Patient preparation
- Explain that the HbA$_{1c}$ test evaluates diabetes therapy.
- Tell the patient that the test requires a blood sample. Explain who will perform the venipuncture and when.
- Explain to the patient that he may experience slight discomfort from the tourniquet and needle puncture.
- Inform the patient that he doesn't need to restrict food and fluids, and tell him to maintain his prescribed medication and diet regimens.

## Procedure and posttest care

- Confirm the patient's identity using two patient identifiers according to facility policy.
- Perform a venipuncture, and collect the sample in a 5-ml EDTA tube.
- Apply direct pressure to the venipuncture site until bleeding stops.
- If a hematoma develops at the venipuncture site, apply warm soaks.
- Schedule the patient for an appointment in 6 to 8 weeks for appropriate follow-up testing.

### Precautions

- Patients with hyperglycemia, thalassemia, or chronic renal failure and those undergoing dialysis may have increased levels.

## Oral glucose tolerance

### [OGTT, glucose tolerance test, GTT]

The oral glucose tolerance test (OGTT) is the most sensitive method of evaluating borderline cases of diabetes mellitus. Plasma and urine glucose levels are monitored for 3 hours after ingestion of a challenge dose of glucose to assess insulin secretion and the body's ability to metabolize glucose.

The OGTT isn't usually used in patients with fasting plasma glucose values greater than 140 mg/dl (SI, > 7.7 mmol/L) or postprandial plasma glucose values greater than 200 mg/dl (SI, > 11 mmol/L).

### Reference values

- Plasma glucose levels peak at 160 to 180 mg/dl (SI, 8.8 to 9.9 mmol/L) within 30 minutes to 1 hour after administration of an oral glucose test dose and return to fasting levels or lower within 2 to 3 hours.

- Urine glucose test results remain negative throughout; no glucose is found in the urine.

### Abnormal results

- Decreased glucose tolerance, in which glucose levels peak sharply before falling slowly to fasting levels, may confirm diabetes mellitus or may result from Cushing's disease, hemochromatosis, pheochromocytoma, or central nervous system lesions.
- Increased glucose tolerance, in which levels may peak at less than normal levels, may indicate insulinoma, malabsorption syndrome, adrenocortical insufficiency (Addison's disease), hypothyroidism, or hypopituitarism.

**DRUG CHALLENGE**

 Arginine, benzodiazepines, caffeine, chlorthalidone, hormonal contraceptives, corticosteroids, dextrothyroxine, diazoxide, thiazide diuretics, epinephrine, furosemide, recent I.V. glucose infusions lithium, large doses of nicotinic acid, phenolphthalein, phenothiazines, phenytoin, and triamterene (possible increase); amphetamines, oral antidiabetic drugs, beta-adrenergic blockers, clofibrate, ethanol, insulin, and monoamine oxidase inhibitors (possible decrease)

### Purpose

- To confirm diabetes mellitus in selected patients
- To help diagnose hypoglycemia and malabsorption syndrome

### Patient preparation

- Explain that the OGTT is used to evaluate glucose metabolism.
- Instruct the patient to maintain a high-carbohydrate diet for 3 days and then to fast for 10 to 16 hours before the test.

■ Advise the patient not to smoke, drink coffee or alcohol, or exercise strenuously for 8 hours before or during the test.
■ Tell the patient that this test requires five blood samples and usually five urine samples. Explain who will perform the venipunctures and when and that the patient may experience slight discomfort from the tourniquet and needle punctures.
■ Suggest to the patient that he bring a book or other quiet diversion with him to the test. The procedure usually takes 3 hours but can last as long as 6 hours.
■ Notify the laboratory and practitioner of medications the patient is taking that may affect test results; these medications may need to be restricted.

### DO'S & DON'TS

Alert the patient to the symptoms of hypoglycemia (weakness, restlessness, nervousness, hunger, and sweating) and tell him to report such symptoms immediately.

### Procedure and posttest care

■ Confirm the patient's identity using two patient identifiers according to facility policy.
■ Between 7 a.m. and 9 a.m., perform a venipuncture to obtain a fasting blood sample. Draw this sample into a 7-ml clot-activator tube. A saline lock may be inserted and used to collect the multiple blood samples needed, according to facility policy.
■ Collect a urine sample at the same time if your facility includes urinalysis as part of the test.
■ After collecting these samples, give the test load of oral glucose and record the time of ingestion. Encourage the patient to drink the entire glucose solution within 5 minutes.
■ Draw blood samples using 7-ml clot-activator tubes 30 minutes, 1 hour, 2

hours, and 3 hours after giving the oral glucose loading dose.
■ Collect urine samples at the same intervals.
■ Tell the patient to lie down if he feels faint from the numerous venipunctures.
■ Encourage the patient to drink water throughout the test to promote adequate urine excretion.
■ Apply direct pressure to the venipuncture site until bleeding stops.
■ If a hematoma develops at the venipuncture site, apply warm soaks.
■ Provide a balanced meal or a snack, also observe for a hypoglycemic reaction.
■ Tell the patient to resume medications stopped before the test as ordered.

### Precautions

■ Send blood and urine samples to the laboratory immediately or refrigerate them.
■ Specify when the patient last ate and the blood and urine sample collection times on the laboratory request.
■ As appropriate, record the time the patient received his last pretest dose of insulin or oral antidiabetic drug.
■ If the patient develops severe hypoglycemia, notify the practitioner. Draw a blood sample, record the time on the laboratory request, and stop the test. Have the patient drink a glass of orange juice with sugar added, or administer I.V. glucose to reverse the reaction.

## Oral lactose tolerance
### [lactose tolerance test, LTT]

The oral lactose tolerance test measures plasma glucose levels after ingestion of a challenge dose of lactose. The test screens for lactose intolerance related to lactase deficiency.

Absence or deficiency of lactase causes undigested lactose to remain in the intestinal lumen, producing such symptoms as abdominal cramps and watery diarrhea. True congenital lactase deficiency is rare. Usually, lactose intolerance is acquired because lactase levels generally decrease with age.

## Reference values
- Plasma glucose levels rise over 20 mg/dl (SI, > 1.1 mmol/L) over fasting levels within 15 to 60 minutes after ingestion of the lactose loading dose.

## Abnormal results
- A rise in plasma glucose of less than 20 mg/dl (SI, < 1.1 mmol/L) indicates lactose intolerance, as does stool acidity (pH of 5.5 or less) and high glucose content (> 1+ on the dipstick).
- Accompanying signs and symptoms provoked by the test also suggest, but don't confirm, the diagnosis because such symptoms may appear in the patient with normal lactase activity after a loading dose of lactose.
- Small-bowel biopsy with lactase assay may be performed to confirm the diagnosis.

### DRUG CHALLENGE
 Benzodiazepines, hormonal contraceptives, thiazide diuretics, propranolol, and insulin (possible false-low plasma glucose level)

## Purpose
- To detect lactose intolerance

## Patient preparation
- Explain that this test determines if the patient's symptoms are due to an inability to digest lactose.
- Instruct the patient to fast and to avoid strenuous activity for 8 hours before the test.
- Tell the patient that this test requires four blood samples. Tell him who will be performing the venipunctures and when.
- Explain to the patient that he may experience slight discomfort from the needle punctures and the tourniquet. Tell him that the entire procedure may take up to 2 hours.
- Notify the laboratory and practitioner of medications the patient is taking that may affect test results; these medications may need to be restricted.

## Procedure and posttest care
- Confirm the patient's identity using two patient identifiers according to facility policy.
- After the patient has fasted for 8 hours, perform a venipuncture, and collect a blood sample in a 4-ml tube with sodium fluoride and potassium oxalate added.
- Give the test load of lactose: for an adult, 50 g of lactose dissolved in 400 ml of water; for a child, 50 g/m² of body surface area. Record the time of ingestion.
- Draw a blood sample 30, 60, and 120 minutes after giving the loading dose. Use a 4-ml tube with sodium fluoride and potassium oxalate added.
- Apply direct pressure to the venipuncture site until bleeding stops.
- If a hematoma develops at the venipuncture site, apply warm soaks.
- If ordered, collect a stool sample 5 hours after giving the loading dose.
- Tell the patient to resume his usual diet, activities, and medications stopped before the test as ordered.

## Precautions
- Watch for symptoms of lactose intolerance—abdominal cramps, nausea, bloating, flatulence, and watery diarrhea—caused by the loading dose.

# 2-hour postprandial plasma glucose
## [2-hour postprandial blood sugar test]

The 2-hour postprandial plasma glucose procedure is a valuable screening tool for detecting diabetes mellitus. The test is performed when the patient demonstrates symptoms of diabetes (polydipsia and polyuria) or when results of the fasting plasma glucose test suggest diabetes.

## Reference values

▪ Two-hour postprandial glucose levels are less than 145 mg/dl (SI, < 8 mmol/L) by the glucose oxidase or hexokinase method.

▪ Levels are slightly higher in people over age 50. (See *2-hour postprandial plasma glucose levels by age*.)

## Abnormal results

▪ Postprandial glucose levels of 200 mg/dl (SI, 11.1 mmol/L) or above indicate diabetes mellitus; they may also indicate pancreatitis, Cushing's syndrome, acromegaly, pheochromocytoma, hyperlipoproteinemia (especially type III, IV, or V), chronic hepatic disease, nephrotic syndrome, brain tumor, sepsis, gastrectomy with dumping syndrome, eclampsia, anoxia, and seizure disorders.

▪ Low postprandial glucose levels suggest hyperinsulinism, insulinoma, von Gierke's disease, functional and reactive hypoglycemia, myxedema, adrenal insufficiency, congenital adrenal hyperpla-

## 2-hour postprandial plasma glucose levels by age

The greatest difference in normal and diabetic insulin responses, and thus in plasma glucose concentration, occurs about 2 hours after a glucose challenge. Test values can fluctuate according to the patient's age. After age 50, for example, normal levels rise markedly and steadily, sometimes reaching 160 mg/dl (SI, 8.82 mmol/L) or higher. In a younger patient, a glucose concentration of more than 145 mg/dl (SI, > 8 mmol/L) suggests incipient diabetes and requires further evaluation.

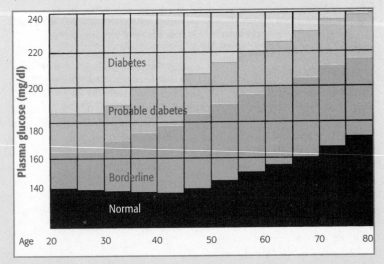

sia, hypopituitarism, malabsorption syndrome, or hepatic insufficiency.

 Chlorthalidone, thiazide diuretics, furosemide, triamterene, hormonal contraceptives, benzodiazepines, phenytoin, phenothiazines, lithium, epinephrine, arginine, phenolphthalein, dextrothyroxine, diazoxide, large doses of nicotinic acid, corticosteroids, and recent I.V. glucose infusions (increase); ethacrynic acid (possible increase); beta-adrenergic blockers, amphetamines, ethanol, clofibrate, insulin, oral antidiabetic drugs, and monoamine oxidase inhibitors (possible decrease)

## Purpose

- To help diagnose diabetes mellitus
- To monitor drug or diet therapy in the patient with diabetes mellitus

## Patient preparation

- Explain that the 2-hour postprandial plasma glucose test evaluates glucose metabolism to detect diabetes.
- Tell the patient that the test requires a blood sample. Explain who will perform the venipuncture and when.
- Explain to the patient that he may experience slight discomfort from the tourniquet and the needle puncture.
- Tell the patient to eat a balanced meal or one containing 100 g of carbohydrates before the test and then fast for 2 hours. Instruct him to avoid smoking and strenuous exercise after the meal.
- Notify the laboratory and practitioner of medications the patient is taking that may affect test results; these medications may need to be restricted.

## Procedure and posttest care

- Confirm the patient's identity using two patient identifiers according to facility policy.

- Perform a venipuncture, and collect the blood sample in a 5-ml clot-activator tube.
- Apply direct pressure to the venipuncture site until bleeding stops.
- If a hematoma develops at the venipuncture site, apply warm soaks.
- Tell the patient to resume his usual diet, activities, and medications stopped before the test as ordered.

## Precautions

- Strenuous exercise or stress may decrease the glucose level.
- Specify on the laboratory request when the patient last ate, the sample collection time, and when the last pretest dose of insulin or oral antidiabetic drug was given.
- If the sample is to be drawn by a technician, tell the patient the exact time the venipuncture must be performed.

# Tissue oxides test

## ■ Lactic acid and pyruvic acid

Lactic acid, present in blood as lactate ion, is derived primarily from muscle cells and erythrocytes. It's an intermediate product of carbohydrate metabolism and is usually metabolized by the liver. Blood lactate concentration depends on the rates of production and metabolism; levels may increase significantly during exercise.

Lactate and pyruvate together form a reversible reaction that's regulated by oxygen supply. When oxygen levels are deficient, pyruvate converts to lactate; when they're adequate, lactate converts to pyruvate. When the hepatic system fails to metabolize lactose sufficiently or when excess pyruvate converts to lactate, lactic acidosis may result. Measurement of blood lactate levels is recommended for all patients with symptoms of lactic acidosis such as Kussmaul's respirations.

Comparison of pyruvate and lactate levels provides reliable information about tissue oxidation, but measurement of pyruvate is technically difficult and infrequently performed.

## Reference values
- Blood lactate values are 0.93 to 1.65 mEq/L (SI, 0.93 to 1.65 mmol/L); pyruvate levels are 0.08 to 0.16 mEq/L (SI, 0.08 to 0.16 mmol/L).
- The lactate-to-pyruvate ratio is less than 10:1.

## Abnormal results
- High blood lactate levels with hypoxia may result from strenuous muscle exercise, shock, hemorrhage, septicemia, myocardial infarction, pulmonary embolism, and cardiac arrest.
- When no reason for diminished tissue perfusion is apparent, increased lactate levels may result from systemic disorders, such as diabetes mellitus, leukemias and lymphomas, hepatic disease, and renal failure, or from enzymatic defects, such as von Gierke's disease (glycogen storage disease) and fructose 1,6-diphosphatase deficiency.
- Lactic acidosis can follow ingestion of large doses of acetaminophen and ethanol as well as I.V. infusion of epinephrine, glucagon, fructose, or sorbitol.

## Purpose
- To assess tissue oxidation
- To help determine the cause of lactic acidosis

## Patient preparation
- Explain that this blood test evaluates the oxygen level in tissues.

- Tell the patient that the test requires a blood sample. Explain who will perform the venipuncture and when.
- Explain to the patient that he may experience slight discomfort from the tourniquet and needle puncture.
- Withhold food overnight, and make sure the patient rests for at least 1 hour before the test.

## Procedure and posttest care
- Confirm the patient's identity using two patient identifiers according to facility policy.
- Perform a venipuncture, and collect a blood sample in a 5-ml tube with sodium fluoride and potassium oxalate added.
- Apply direct pressure to the venipuncture site until bleeding stops.
- If a hematoma develops at the venipuncture site, apply warm soaks.
- Tell the patient to resume his usual diet and activities stopped before the test as ordered.

## Precautions
- Because venostasis may raise blood lactate levels, tell the patient that he must not clench his fist during the venipuncture.
- Avoid using a tourniquet; however, if one must be used, release it at least 2 minutes before collecting the sample so blood can circulate. A lightly inflated blood pressure cuff may be used.

### Do's & don'ts

 Because lactate and pyruvate are extremely unstable, place the sample container in an ice-filled cup, and send it to the laboratory immediately.

# Vitamins and trace elements

## Vitamin assays

### Folic acid
[folate, folacin]

The folic acid test is a quantitative analysis of serum folic acid levels by radioisotope assay of competitive binding. It's commonly performed along with measurement of serum vitamin $B_{12}$ levels. Like vitamin $B_{12}$, folic acid is a water-soluble vitamin that influences hematopoiesis, deoxyribonucleic acid synthesis, and overall body growth.

Normally, diet supplies folic acid in organ meats, such as liver or kidneys, yeast, fruits, leafy vegetables, fortified breads and cereals, eggs, and milk. Inadequate dietary intake may cause a deficiency, especially during pregnancy. Because of folic acid's vital role in hematopoiesis, the usual indication for this test is a suspected hematologic abnormality.

#### Reference values
- Folic acid levels are 1.8 to 20 ng/ml (SI, 4 to 45.3 nmol/L).

#### Abnormal results
- Low folic acid levels may indicate hematologic abnormalities, such as ane-mia (especially megaloblastic anemia), leukopenia, thrombocytopenia, hypermetabolic states (such as hyperthyroidism), inadequate dietary intake, small-bowel malabsorption syndrome, hepatic or renal diseases, chronic alcoholism, or pregnancy.
- The Schilling test, which measures $B_{12}$ absorption, is usually performed to rule out vitamin $B_{12}$ deficiency, which also causes megaloblastic anemia.
- High folic acid levels may indicate excessive dietary intake of folic acid or folic acid supplements. Even when taken in large doses, this vitamin is nontoxic.

**DRUG CHALLENGE**

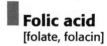 Alcohol; anticonvulsants, such as primidone; antimalarials; antineoplastics; hormonal contraceptives; phenytoin; and pyrimethamine (possible decrease)

#### Purpose
- To aid in the differential diagnosis of megaloblastic anemia, which may result from folic acid or vitamin $B_{12}$ deficiency
- To assess folate stores in pregnancy
- To monitor the response to prolonged parenteral nutrition therapy

### Patient preparation

- Explain that this test determines the folic acid level in the blood.
- Tell the patient that the test requires a blood sample. Explain who will perform the venipuncture and when.
- Explain to the patient that he may experience slight discomfort from the tourniquet and needle puncture.
- Check the patient's history for drugs that may affect test results, such as phenytoin or pyrimethamine; these medications may need to be withheld.

### Procedure and posttest care

- Confirm the patient's identity using two patient identifiers according to facility policy.
- Perform a venipuncture, and collect the blood sample in a 4.5-ml tube without additives.
- Apply direct pressure to the venipuncture site until bleeding stops.
- If a hematoma develops at the venipuncture site, apply warm soaks.
- Advise the patient to resume medications stopped before the test.

## Vitamin A (retinol) and carotene
### [retinol and carotene]

The vitamin A and carotene test measures serum levels of vitamin A and its precursor, carotene. A fat-soluble vitamin normally supplied by diet, vitamin A is important for reproduction, vision (especially night vision), and epithelial tissue and bone growth. Vitamin A is found mostly in fruits, vegetables, eggs, poultry, meat, and fish. Carotene is present in green leafy vegetables and in yellow fruits and vegetables.

### Reference values

- Vitamin A levels are 30 to 80 mcg/dl (SI, 1.05 to 2.8 µmol/L).

- Carotene levels are 10 to 85 mcg/dl (SI, 0.19 to 1.58 µmol/L).

### Abnormal results

- Low vitamin A levels (hypovitaminosis A) may indicate impaired fat absorption, as in celiac disease, infectious hepatitis, cystic fibrosis of the pancreas, obstructive jaundice, protein-calorie malnutrition (marasmic kwashiorkor), or chronic nephritis.
- High vitamin A levels (hypervitaminosis A) usually indicate chronically excessive intake of vitamin A supplements or of foods high in vitamin A, but they may also suggest hyperlipemia and hypercholesterolemia of uncontrolled diabetes mellitus.
- Low carotene levels may indicate impaired fat absorption, pregnancy or, rarely, insufficient dietary intake of carotene.
- High carotene levels indicate grossly excessive dietary intake.

DRUG CHALLENGE

 Cholestyramine, mineral oil, and neomycin (possible decrease); hormonalcontraceptives and glucocorticoids (possible increase)

### Purpose

- To investigate suspected vitamin A deficiency or toxicity
- To help diagnose visual disturbances, especially night blindness and xerophthalmia
- To help diagnose skin diseases, such as keratosis follicularis or ichthyosis
- To screen for malabsorption

### Patient preparation

- Explain that this test measures the vitamin A level in the blood.
- Tell the patient to fast overnight but not to restrict water intake.

- Tell the patient that the test requires a blood sample. Explain who will perform the venipuncture and when.
- Explain to the patient that he may experience slight discomfort from the tourniquet and needle puncture.

### Procedure and posttest care
- Confirm the patient's identity using two patient identifiers according to facility policy.
- Perform a venipuncture, and collect the blood sample in a chilled 7-ml siliconized tube.
- Apply direct pressure to the venipuncture site until bleeding stops.
- If a hematoma develops at the venipuncture site, apply warm soaks.
- Tell the patient to resume his usual diet.

### Precautions
- Protect the blood sample from light because vitamin A characteristically absorbs light.
- Keep the blood sample on ice.

# Vitamin B$_2$
[riboflavin]

The serum vitamin B$_2$ test evaluates serum levels of vitamin B$_2$, a vitamin essential for growth and tissue function. The serum test is considered more reliable than the urine test, which can produce artificially high values in patients after surgery or prolonged fasting.

### Reference values
- Vitamin B$_2$ levels are 3 to 15 mcg/dl.

### Abnormal results
- Marginally low vitamin B$_2$ levels (2 to 3 mcg/dl) indicate vitamin B$_2$ deficiency, resulting from insufficient dietary intake of vitamin B$_2$, malabsorption syndrome, or conditions that increase metabolic demands (such as stress).

- Significantly diminished vitamin B$_2$ levels are less than 2 mcg/dl.

### Purpose
- To detect vitamin B$_2$ deficiency

### Patient preparation
- Explain that this test evaluates vitamin B$_2$ levels.
- Instruct the patient to maintain a normal diet before the test.
- Tell the patient that the test requires a blood sample. Explain who will perform the venipuncture and when.
- Explain to the patient that he may experience slight discomfort from the tourniquet and needle puncture.

### Procedure and posttest care
- Confirm the patient's identity using two patient identifiers according to facility policy.
- Perform a venipuncture and collect a blood sample in a 4.5-ml siliconized tube.
- Apply direct pressure to the venipuncture site until bleeding stops.
- If a hematoma develops at the venipuncture site, apply warm soaks.
- Inform the patient with vitamin B$_2$ deficiency that good dietary sources of vitamin B$_2$ include milk products, organ meats (liver and kidneys), fish, green leafy vegetables, legumes, and fortified breads and cereals.

# Vitamin B$_{12}$
[cyanocobalamin, antipernicious anemia factor, extrinsic factor]

The vitamin B$_{12}$ radioisotope assay of competitive binding is a quantitative analysis of serum levels of vitamin B$_{12}$. This test is usually performed concurrently with measurement of serum folic acid levels.

# Cobalt: Critical trace element

A trace element found mainly in the liver, cobalt is an essential component of vitamin $B_{12}$ and therefore is a critical factor in hematopoiesis. A balanced diet supplies sufficient cobalt to maintain hematopoiesis, primarily through foods containing vitamin $B_{12}$.

However, excessive ingestion of cobalt may have toxic effects. Toxicity has occurred, for example, in individuals who consumed large quantities of beer containing cobalt as a stabilizer, with heart failure from cardiomyopathy the result. Because quantitative analysis of cobalt alone is difficult because of the minute amount found in the body, cobalt is commonly measured by bioassay as part of vitamin $B_{12}$ testing.

Normal cobalt concentration in human plasma is 60 to 80 pg/ml.

$B_{12}$; hypermetabolic states, such as hyperthyroidism; pregnancy; and CNS damage (for example, posterolateral sclerosis or funicular degeneration).

- High vitamin $B_{12}$ levels may result from excessive dietary intake; hepatic disease, such as cirrhosis or acute or chronic hepatitis; and myeloproliferative disorders such as myelocytic leukemia.

### DRUG CHALLENGE

 Anticonvulsants, ethanol, metformin, and neomycin, (possible decrease); hormonal contraceptives (increase)

## Purpose

- To aid in the differential diagnosis of megaloblastic anemia, which may be due to a vitamin $B_{12}$ or folic acid deficiency
- To aid in the differential diagnosis of CNS disorders that affect peripheral and spinal myelinated nerves

## Patient preparation

- Explain to the patient that this test determines the amount of vitamin $B_{12}$ in the blood.
- Instruct the patient to fast overnight before the test.
- Tell the patient that the test requires a blood sample. Explain who will perform the venipuncture and when.
- Explain to the patient that he may experience slight discomfort from the tourniquet and needle puncture.
- Check the patient's history for drugs that may alter test results, and identify them on the laboratory request.

A water-soluble vitamin containing cobalt, vitamin $B_{12}$ is essential to hematopoiesis, deoxyribonucleic acid (DNA) synthesis and growth, myelin synthesis, and central nervous system (CNS) integrity. This vitamin is found almost exclusively in animal products, such as meat, shellfish, milk, and eggs. (See *Cobalt: Critical trace element.*)

## Reference values

- Vitamin $B_{12}$ levels are 200 to 900 pg/ml (SI, 148 to 664 pmol/L).

## Abnormal results

- Low vitamin $B_{12}$ levels may indicate inadequate dietary intake, especially if the patient is a strict vegetarian. Low levels are also associated with malabsorption syndromes, such as celiac disease; isolated malabsorption of vitamin

## Procedure and posttest care

- Confirm the patient's identity using two patient identifiers according to facility policy.

- Perform a venipuncture, and collect a blood sample in a 4.5-ml siliconized tube.
- Apply direct pressure to the venipuncture site until bleeding stops.
- If a hematoma develops at the venipuncture site, apply warm soaks.
- Instruct the patient to resume his usual diet.

# Vitamin C
## [ascorbic acid]

Vitamin C chemical assay measures plasma levels of vitamin C, a water-soluble vitamin required for collagen synthesis and cartilage and bone maintenance. Vitamin C also promotes iron absorption, influences folic acid metabolism, and may be necessary for withstanding the stresses of injury and infection.

This vitamin is present in generous amounts in citrus fruits, berries, tomatoes, raw cabbage, green peppers, green leafy vegetables, and fortified juices. Severe vitamin C deficiency, or scurvy, causes capillary fragility, joint abnormalities, and multisystemic symptoms.

### Reference values
- Vitamin C levels are 0.2 to 2 mg/dl (SI, 11 to 114 μmol/L).

### Abnormal results
- Vitamin C levels less than 0.3 mg/dl (< 16.5 μmol/L) indicate significant deficiency, possibly from pregnancy or infection, fever, and anemia; severe deficiencies result in scurvy.
- High vitamin C levels can indicate increased ingestion of vitamin C, which may eventually lead to production of urinary calculi.

### Purpose
- To help diagnose scurvy, scurvylike conditions, and metabolic disorders, such as malnutrition and malabsorption syndromes

### Patient preparation
- Explain that this test detects the amount of vitamin C in the blood.
- Instruct the patient to fast overnight before the test.
- Tell the patient that the test requires a blood sample. Explain who will perform the venipuncture and when.
- Explain to the patient that he may experience slight discomfort from the tourniquet and the needle puncture.

### Procedure and posttest care
- Confirm the patient's identity using two patient identifiers according to facility policy.
- Perform a venipuncture, and collect the blood sample in a 4.5-ml heparinized tube.
- Apply direct pressure to the venipuncture site until bleeding stops.
- If a hematoma develops at the venipuncture site, apply warm soaks.
- Tell the patient to resume his usual diet.

# Vitamin D₃
## [cholecalciferol]

Vitamin D₃, the major form of vitamin D, is endogenously produced in the skin by the sun's ultraviolet rays and occurs naturally in fish liver oils, egg yolks, liver, and butter.

This competitive protein-binding assay determines serum levels of 25-hydroxycholecalciferol after chromatography has separated it from other vitamin D metabolites and contaminants. The test is commonly combined with measurement of serum calcium and alkaline phosphatase levels.

### Reference values
- Vitamin $D_3$ levels are 10 to 60 ng/ml (SI, 25 to 150 nmol/L).

### Abnormal results
- Low or undetectable levels may result from vitamin D deficiency from poor diet; decreased exposure to the sun; impaired absorption of vitamin D (caused by hepatobiliary disease, pancreatitis, celiac disease, cystic fibrosis, or gastric or small-bowel resection); hepatic, parathyroid, and renal diseases that directly affect vitamin D metabolism. This deficiency can cause rickets or osteomalacia.
- High vitamin $D_3$ levels (over 100 ng/ml [SI, > 250 nmol/L]) may indicate toxicity from excessive self-medication or prolonged therapy; high levels along with hypercalcemia may be due to hypersensitivity to vitamin D, as in sarcoidosis.

**DRUG CHALLENGE**

Aluminum hydroxide, anticonvulsants, cholestyramine, colestipol, corticosteroids, isoniazid, and mineral oil (possible decrease)

### Purpose
- To evaluate skeletal disease, such as rickets and osteomalacia
- To help diagnose hypercalcemia
- To detect vitamin D toxicity
- To monitor therapy with vitamin $D_3$

### Patient preparation
- Explain that this test measures the amount of vitamin D in the body.
- Tell the patient that the test requires a blood sample. Explain who will perform the venipuncture and when.
- Explain to the patient that he may experience slight discomfort from the tourniquet and needle puncture.
- Check for medications that may alter test results. If the medications must be continued, note this on the laboratory request.

### Procedure and posttest care
- Confirm the patient's identity using two patient identifiers according to facility policy.
- Perform a venipuncture, and collect a blood sample in a 4.5-ml siliconized tube.
- Apply direct pressure to the venipuncture site until bleeding stops.
- If a hematoma develops at the venipuncture site, apply warm soaks.
- Tell the patient to resume medications stopped before the test as ordered.

## *Trace elements assays*

 **Manganese**

The manganese test, an analysis by atomic absorption spectroscopy, measures serum levels of manganese, a trace element. Although its function is only partially understood, manganese is known to activate several enzymes—including cholinesterase, thyroxine, and arginase—that are essential to metabolism. Manganese is also necessary for vitamin K production. Dietary sources of manganese include unrefined cereals, green leafy vegetables, and nuts.

Manganese toxicity may result from the inhalation of manganese dust or fumes—a hazard in the steel and dry-cell battery industries—or from ingestion of contaminated water.

### Reference values
- Manganese levels are 0.4 to 1.4 mcg/ml (SI, 7.28 to 25.5 nmol/L).

## Abnormal results

 Significantly high manganese levels indicate manganese toxicity, which requires prompt medical attention to prevent central nervous system deterioration.

■ Low manganese levels may indicate deficient dietary intake, although deficiency hasn't been linked to disease.

DRUG CHALLENGE

 Estrogen (increase); glucocorticoids (increase or decrease due to altered distribution of manganese in the body)

### Purpose
■ To detect manganese toxicity

### Patient preparation
■ Explain that this test determines the level of manganese in the blood.
■ Inform the patient that he need not restrict food and fluids.
■ Tell the patient that the test requires a blood sample. Explain who will perform the venipuncture and when.
■ Explain to the patient that he may experience slight discomfort from the tourniquet and the needle puncture.
■ Check the patient's history for medications that may influence serum manganese levels, such as estrogens and glucocorticoids.

### Procedure and posttest care
■ Confirm the patient's identity using two patient identifiers according to facility policy.
■ Perform a venipuncture, and collect a blood sample in a metal-free collection tube. Laboratories will supply a special kit for this test on request.

■ Apply direct pressure to the venipuncture site until bleeding stops.
■ If a hematoma develops at the venipuncture site, apply warm soaks.

### Precautions
■ Be sure to use a metal-free tube for collection of the blood sample or test results may be altered.

# Zinc
[Zn]

The zinc test, an analysis by atomic absorption spectroscopy, measures serum zinc levels. An important trace element, zinc is an integral component of more than 80 enzymes and proteins and plays a critical role in enzyme catalytic reactions.

Zinc occurs naturally in water and in most foods; high concentrations are found in meat, seafood, dairy products, whole grains, nuts, and legumes. Zinc deficiency can seriously impair body metabolism, growth, and development.

### Reference values
■ Zinc levels are 70 to 120 mcg/dl (SI, 10.7 to 18.4 µmol/L).

### Abnormal results
■ Low zinc levels may indicate an acquired deficiency (from insufficient dietary intake or from an underlying disease) or a hereditary deficiency.
■ Low zinc levels occur in leukemia and may be related to impaired zinc-dependent enzyme systems.
■ Low zinc levels are commonly associated with alcoholic cirrhosis of the liver, myocardial infarction, ileitis, chronic renal failure, rheumatoid arthritis, and anemia (such as hemolytic or sickle cell anemia).

- High and potentially toxic serum zinc levels may result from accidental ingestion or industrial exposure.

### DRUG CHALLENGE

 Zinc-chelating agents, such as penicillinase, and corticosteroids (decrease); antimetabolites; antineoplastics, such as cisplatin; diuretics; estrogens; and penicillamine (possible decrease)

## Purpose
- To detect zinc deficiency or toxicity

## Patient preparation
- Explain to the patient that this test determines the concentration of zinc in the blood.
- Inform the patient that he doesn't need to restrict food and fluids.
- Tell the patient that the test requires a blood sample. Explain who will perform the venipuncture and when.
- Explain to the patient that he may experience slight discomfort from the tourniquet and needle puncture.

## Procedure and posttest care
- Confirm the patient's identity using two patient identifiers according to facility policy.
- Perform a venipuncture, and collect a 7- to 10-ml blood sample in a zinc-free collection tube.
- Apply direct pressure to the venipuncture site until bleeding stops.
- If a hematoma develops at the venipuncture site, apply warm soaks.

## Precautions
- Send the blood sample to the laboratory immediately. Reliable analysis must begin before platelet disintegration can alter test results.

# Immunohematology

## Agglutination tests

### ABO blood typing
[blood typing]

ABO blood typing classifies blood according to the presence of major antigens A and B on red blood cell (RBC) surfaces and according to serum antibodies anti-A and anti-B. ABO blood typing, using forward and reverse methods, is required before transfusion to prevent a lethal reaction.

In forward typing, the patient's RBCs are mixed with anti-A serum, then with anti-B serum; the presence or absence of agglutination determines the blood group. In reverse typing, the results of the forward method are verified by mixing the patient's serum with known group A and group B cells. Blood group determination is confirmed when the results of forward and reverse typing match perfectly.

#### Reference values
- In forward typing:
  - If agglutination occurs when the patient's RBCs are mixed with anti-A serum, the A antigen is present, and the blood is typed A.
  - If agglutination occurs when the patient's RBCs are mixed with anti-B serum, the B antigen is present, and the blood is typed B.
  - If agglutination occurs in both mixes, A and B antigens are present, and the blood is typed AB.
  - If agglutination doesn't occur in either mix, no antigens are present, and the blood is typed O.
- In reverse typing:
  - If agglutination occurs when B cells are mixed with the patient's serum, anti-B is present, and the blood is typed A.
  - If agglutination occurs when A cells are mixed, anti-A is present, and the blood is typed B.
  - If agglutination occurs when A and B cells are mixed, anti-A and anti-B are present, and the blood is typed O.
  - If agglutination doesn't occur when A and B cells are mixed, neither anti-A nor anti-B is present, and the blood is typed AB.

**ALERT**

 Donor blood may be transfused only when ABO compatibility has been confirmed with the recipient's blood. The transfusion of blood containing either A or B antigens to a recipient whose RBCs lack these antigens can cause a potentially fatal reaction.

#### Abnormal results
Not applicable to this test.

## Purpose

- To establish blood group according to the ABO system
- To check compatibility of donor and recipient blood before transfusion

## Patient preparation

- Explain that this test determines the patient's blood group.
- If the patient is scheduled for a transfusion, explain that after his blood group is known, it can be matched with the right donor blood.
- Tell the patient that he doesn't need to restrict food and fluids.
- Tell him that the test requires a blood sample. Explain who will perform the venipuncture and when.
- Explain to the patient that he may experience slight discomfort from the tourniquet and needle puncture.
- Check the patient's history for recent administration of blood, dextran, or I.V. contrast agents, and note this on the laboratory request.

## Procedure and posttest care

- Confirm the patient's identity using two patient identifiers according to facility policy.
- Perform a venipuncture, and collect a blood sample in a 10-ml tube without additives.
- Apply direct pressure to the venipuncture site until bleeding stops.
- If a hematoma develops at the venipuncture site, apply warm soaks.

## Precautions

- Label the blood sample with the patient's name, the hospital or blood bank number, the date, and the phlebotomist's initials.
- A recent blood transfusion or pregnancy within the last 3 months may cause lingering antibodies.

# Antibody screening
### [indirect Coombs' test]

The antibody screening test detects unexpected circulating antibodies in the patient's serum. After incubating the serum with group O red blood cells (RBCs), which are unaffected by anti-A or anti-B antibodies, an antiglobulin (Coombs') serum is added. Agglutination occurs if the patient's serum contains an antibody to one or more antigens on the RBCs.

The antibody screening test detects 95% to 99% of the circulating antibodies. After this screening procedure detects them, the antibody identification test can determine the specific identity of the antibodies present.

## Normal results

- Agglutination doesn't occur, indicating that the patient's serum contains no circulating antibodies other than anti-A or anti-B.

## Abnormal results

- A positive test result indicates the presence of unexpected circulating antibodies to RBC antigens. Such a reaction demonstrates donor and recipient incompatibility.
- A positive test result in a pregnant patient with Rh-negative blood may indicate the presence of antibodies to the Rh factor from an earlier transfusion with incompatible blood or from a previous pregnancy with an Rh-positive fetus.
- A positive test result indicates that the fetus may develop hemolytic disease of the neonate. As a result, repeated testing throughout the pregnancy is necessary to evaluate progressive development of circulating antibody levels.

## Purpose
- To detect unexpected circulating antibodies to RBC antigens in the recipient's or donor's serum before transfusion
- To detect anti-D antibody in maternal blood
- To evaluate the need for $Rh_o(D)$ immune globulin
- To help diagnose acquired hemolytic anemia

### Patient preparation
- Explain to the prospective blood recipient that the antibody screening test helps evaluate the possibility of a transfusion reaction or determine if fetal antibodies are in the patient's blood and if treatment is needed, as appropriate.
- If the test is being performed because the patient is anemic, explain to him that the test helps identify the specific type of anemia.
- Tell the patient that he doesn't need to restrict food and fluids.
- Tell him that the test requires a blood sample. Explain who will perform the venipuncture and when.
- Inform the patient that he may experience slight discomfort from the tourniquet and needle puncture.
- Check the patient's history for recent administration of blood, dextran, or I.V. contrast agents, and note this on the laboratory request.

### Procedure and posttest care
- Confirm the patient's identity using two patient identifiers according to facility policy.
- Perform a venipuncture, and collect a blood sample in two 10-ml tubes. If the antibody screen is positive, antibody identification is performed on the blood.
- Apply direct pressure to the venipuncture site until bleeding stops.
- If a hematoma develops at the venipuncture site, apply warm soaks.

### Precautions
- Label the sample with the patient's name, the hospital or blood bank number, the date, and the phlebotomist's initials. Be sure to include on the laboratory request the patient's diagnosis and pregnancy status, history of transfusions, and current drug therapy.

# Crossmatching
### [compatibility testing]

Crossmatching establishes compatibility or incompatibility of a donor's and a recipient's blood. It's the best antibody detection test available for avoiding lethal transfusion reactions. After the donor's and the recipient's ABO and Rh-factor type are determined, major crossmatching determines compatibility between the donor's red blood cells (RBCs) and the recipient's serum. Minor crossmatching determines compatibility between the donor's serum and the recipient's RBCs. Because the antibody-screening test is routinely performed on all blood donors, minor crossmatching is commonly omitted.

Because a complete crossmatch may take from 45 minutes to 2 hours, an incomplete (10-minute) crossmatch may be performed in an emergency such as severe blood loss resulting from trauma. In an emergency, transfusion can begin with limited amounts of group O packed RBCs while crossmatching is completed. Incomplete typing and crossmatching increase the risk of complications. After crossmatching, compatible units of blood are labeled, and a compatibility record is completed.

**ALERT**

 The most carefully performed crossmatch may not detect all the possible sources of patient-donor incompatibility.

## Normal results

■ Absence of agglutination indicates compatibility between the donor's and the recipient's blood, which means that the transfusion of donor blood can proceed. Note that this doesn't guarantee a safe transfusion.

## Abnormal results

■ A positive crossmatch indicates incompatibility between the donor's blood and the recipient's blood, which means that the donor's blood can't be transfused to the recipient. The sign of a positive crossmatch is agglutination, or clumping, when the donor's RBCs and the recipient's serum are correctly mixed and incubated.
■ Agglutination indicates an undesirable antigen-antibody reaction.
■ The donor's blood must be withheld and the crossmatch continued to determine the cause of the incompatibility and identify the antibody.

## Purpose

■ To serve as the final check for compatibility between a donor's and a recipient's blood

## Patient preparation

■ Explain that this test is to make sure that the blood the patient receives matches his own, to prevent a transfusion reaction.
■ Tell the patient that he doesn't need to restrict food and fluids.
■ Tell him that the test requires a blood sample. Explain who will perform the venipuncture and when.
■ Explain to the patient that he may experience slight discomfort from the tourniquet and the needle puncture.
■ Check the patient's history for recent administration of blood, dextran, or I.V. contrast agents, and note this on the laboratory request.

## Procedure and posttest care

■ Confirm the patient's identity using two patient identifiers according to facility policy.
■ Perform a venipuncture, and collect a blood sample in a 10-ml tube without additives or EDTA. ABO typing, Rh typing, and crossmatching are all performed together.
■ Apply direct pressure to the venipuncture site until bleeding stops.
■ If a hematoma develops at the venipuncture site, apply warm soaks.

## Precautions

■ Handle the sample gently to prevent hemolysis, which can mask hemolysis of the donor's RBCs.
■ Label the blood sample with the patient's name, the hospital or blood bank number, the date, and the phlebotomist's initials.
■ Indicate on the laboratory request the amount and type of blood component needed.
■ If more than 72 hours have elapsed since an earlier transfusion, previously crossmatched donor blood must be re-crossmatched with a new recipient serum sample to detect newly acquired incompatibilities before transfusion.
■ If the patient is scheduled for surgery and has received blood during the past 3 months, be aware that his blood needs to be crossmatched again if his surgery is rescheduled to detect recently acquired incompatibilities.

# Fetal-maternal erythrocyte distribution

Some transfer of red blood cells (RBCs) from the fetal to the maternal circulation occurs during most spontaneous or elective abortions and most normal deliveries. Usually, the amount of blood transferred is minimal and has no clinical significance. However, transfer of significant amounts of blood from an Rh-positive fetus to an Rh-negative mother can result in maternal immunization to the D antigen and the development of anti-D antibodies in the maternal circulation.

During a subsequent pregnancy, the maternal immunization subjects an Rh-positive fetus to potentially fatal hemolysis and erythroblastosis. This test measures the number of fetal RBCs in the maternal circulation.

$Rh_o(D)$ immune globulin is given to an unsensitized Rh-negative mother as soon as possible (no later than 72 hours) after the birth of an Rh-positive infant or after a spontaneous or elective abortion, to prevent complications in subsequent pregnancies. Most practitioners now give $Rh_o(D)$ immune globulin prophylactically at 28 weeks' gestation to women who are Rh-negative but have no detectable Rh antibodies.

The following patients should be screened for Rh isoimmunization or irregular antibodies: Rh-negative mothers during their first prenatal visit and at 28 weeks' gestation and Rh-positive mothers with histories of transfusion, a jaundiced infant, stillbirth, cesarean delivery, or induced or spontaneous abortion.

### Normal results

- Maternal whole blood contains no fetal RBCs.

### Abnormal results

- An elevated fetal RBC volume in the maternal circulation necessitates administration of more than one dose of $Rh_o(D)$ immune globulin. The number of vials of $Rh_o(D)$ immune globulin needed is determined by dividing the calculated fetomaternal hemorrhage by 30. A single vial of $Rh_o(D)$ immune globulin provides protection against a 30-ml fetomaternal hemorrhage.

### Purpose

- To detect and measure fetal-maternal blood transfer
- To determine the amount of $Rh_o(D)$ immune globulin needed to prevent maternal immunization to the D antigen

### Patient preparation

- Explain that this test determines the amount of fetal blood transferred to the maternal circulation and helps determine the appropriate treatment if necessary.
- Tell the patient that she doesn't need to restrict food and fluids.
- Tell her that the test requires a blood sample. Explain who will perform the venipuncture and when.
- Explain to the patient that she may experience slight discomfort from the tourniquet and needle puncture.
- Check the patient's history for recent administration of blood, dextran, or I.V. contrast agents and note this on the laboratory request.

### Procedure and posttest care

- Confirm the patient's identity using two patient identifiers according to facility policy.
- Perform a venipuncture, and collect a blood sample in a 7-ml EDTA tube.
- Apply direct pressure to the venipuncture site until bleeding stops.
- If a hematoma develops at the venipuncture site, apply warm soaks.

### Precautions

- Label the blood sample with the patient's name, the hospital or blood bank number, the date, and the phlebotomist's initials.
- Send the blood sample to the laboratory immediately with a properly completed laboratory request.

# Leukoagglutinins
## [WBC antibodies, human leukocyte antigen antibodies]

This test detects leukoagglutinins—antibodies that react with white blood cells (WBCs) and may cause a transfusion reaction. These antibodies usually develop after exposure to foreign WBCs through transfusions, pregnancies, and allografts.

If a blood recipient has these antibodies, a febrile nonhemolytic reaction may occur 1 to 4 hours after the start of whole blood, red blood cell, platelet, or granulocyte transfusion. This nonhemolytic reaction (marked by fever and severe chills, sometimes with nausea, headache, and transient hypertension) must be distinguished from a true hemolytic reaction before further transfusion can proceed.

The technique used to detect leukoagglutinins is the microlymphocytotoxicity test. In this test, the recipient serum is tested against donor lymphocytes or against a panel of lymphocytes of known human leukocyte antigen (HLA) phenotype. The antibodies in the recipient serum bind to the corresponding antigen present in the lymphocytes and cause cell membrane injury when the complement is added to the test system. Cell injury is detected by examining the lymphocytes under a microscope. If the lymphocytes don't absorb an added dye, the test finding is negative. If the lymphocytes show dye uptake, the test finding is positive.

## Normal results

- Test results are negative: agglutination doesn't occur because the serum contains no antibodies.

## Abnormal results

- A positive result in a transfusion recipient indicates that he has leukoagglutinins in his blood, identifying his transfusion reaction as a febrile nonhemolytic reaction to these antibodies.
- Recipients who test positive for HLA antibodies may need HLA-matched platelets to control bleeding episodes caused by thrombocytopenia.

## Purpose

- To detect leukoagglutinins in blood recipients who develop transfusion reactions, thus differentiating between hemolytic and febrile nonhemolytic transfusion reactions
- To detect leukoagglutinins in blood donors after transfusion of donor blood causes a reaction

## Patient preparation

- Explain that this test helps determine the cause of the patient's transfusion reaction.
- Tell him that the test requires a blood sample. Explain who will perform the venipuncture and when.
- Explain to the patient that he may experience slight discomfort from the tourniquet and the needle puncture.
- Check the patient's history for recent administration of blood, dextran, or I.V. contrast agents and note this on the laboratory request.

## Procedure and posttest care

- Confirm the patient's identity using two patient identifiers according to facility policy.
- Perform a venipuncture, and collect a blood sample in a 10-ml clot-activator tube. The laboratory requires 3 to 4 ml of serum for testing.
- Apply direct pressure to the venipuncture site until bleeding stops.
- If a hematoma develops at the venipuncture site, apply warm soaks.

## Do's & don'ts

 If a transfusion recipient tests positive for leukoagglutinin, know that continued transfusions require premedication with acetaminophen 1 to 2 hours before the transfusion, specially prepared leukocyte-poor blood, or use of leukocyte-removal blood filters to prevent further reactions.

### Precautions

- Label the blood sample with the patient's name, the hospital or blood bank number, the date, and the phlebotomist's initials.
- Be sure to include on the laboratory request the patient's suspected diagnosis and history of blood transfusions, pregnancies, and drug therapy.
- Note that tests for these antibodies aren't useful in deciding which patient should receive leukocyte-poor blood components; the decision must be based on clinical experience.

# Immune response

## 11

---

## *General cellular tests*

### Lymphocyte transformation

Transformation tests evaluate lymphocyte competency without injection of antigens into the patient's skin. These in vitro tests eliminate the risk of adverse effects but can still accurately assess the ability of lymphocytes to proliferate and to recognize and respond to antigens.

The mitogen assay evaluates the mitotic response of T and B lymphocytes to a foreign antigen. The antigen assay uses specific substances, such as purified protein derivative, *Candida,* mumps, tetanus toxoid, and streptokinase, to stimulate lymphocyte transformation. The mixed lymphocyte culture (MLC) assay helps match transplant recipients and donors and test immunocompetence.

The neutrophils' ability to engulf and destroy bacteria and foreign particles can also be determined. (See *Neutrophil function tests.*)

#### Reference values
- Results depend on the mitogens used. Reference ranges accompany test results. In general, a positive test result is normal.

### Abnormal results
- A negative test result indicates a deficiency. In the mitogen and antigen assays, a low stimulation index or unresponsiveness indicates a depressed or defective immune system. Serial testing can be performed to monitor the effectiveness of therapy in a patient with an immunodeficiency disease.
- In the MLC test, the stimulation index is a measure of compatibility. A high index indicates poor compatibility, whereas a low stimulation index indicates good compatibility.
- A high stimulation index, in response to the relevant pathogen, can also demonstrate exposure to malaria, hepatitis, mycoplasmal pneumonia, periodontal disease, and certain viral infections in a patient who no longer has detectable serum antibodies.

#### DRUG CHALLENGE

 Use of hormonal contraceptives, depressing lymphocyte response to phytohemagglutinin (low stimulation index); chemotherapy (unless pretherapy baseline values are available for comparison)

#### Purpose
- To assess and monitor genetic and acquired immunodeficiency states
- To provide histocompatibility typing of tissue transplant recipients and donors

- To detect exposure to various pathogens, such as those that cause malaria, hepatitis, and mycoplasmal pneumonia

### Patient preparation

- Explain that this test evaluates lymphocyte function, which is crucial to immune system function.
- Tell the patient that the test monitors his response to therapy, if appropriate.
- For histocompatibility typing, explain that this test helps determine the best match for a transplant procedure.
- Inform the patient that he doesn't need to restrict food and fluids.
- Tell the patient that the test requires a blood sample. Explain who will perform the venipuncture and when.
- Explain to the patient that he may experience slight discomfort from the tourniquet and the needle puncture.

**DO'S & DON'TS**

 If a radioisotope scan is scheduled, make sure to draw the serum sample for this test first.

### Procedure and posttest care

- Confirm the patient's identity using two patient identifiers according to facility policy.
- Perform a venipuncture. If the patient is an adult, collect the blood sample in a 7-ml heparinized tube; for a child, use a 5-ml heparinized tube.
- Because the patient may have a compromised immune system, take special care to keep the venipuncture site clean and dry.
- Apply direct pressure to the venipuncture site until bleeding stops.
- If a hematoma develops at the venipuncture site, apply warm soaks.

## Neutrophil function tests

Neutrophil function tests may reveal the inability of neutrophils to kill a target bacteria or to migrate to the bacterial site (chemotaxis). The killing ability can be evaluated by the nitroblue tetrazolium (NBT) test, which relies on neutrophil generation of bactericidal enzymes and toxins during killing. This action increases oxygen consumption and glucose metabolism, which reduces colorless NBT to blue formazan. The reduced dye is then extracted with pyridine and measured photometrically; the level of reduction indicates phagocytic activity.

Neutrophil killing activity can also be evaluated by noting the neutrophil's chemiluminescence (its ability to emit light). After a neutrophil phagocytizes a microorganism, oxygen-containing substances form within phagocytic vacuoles. As the cell is stimulated, it emits light in proportion to the amount of oxygen-containing substances that are formed, thereby providing an indirect measurement of phagocytosis.

Chemotaxis can be assessed *in vitro* by placing bacteria in the lower half of a two-part chamber and phagocytic neutrophils in the upper half. After incubation, migrating cells are counted microscopically and compared with standard values.

## Terminal deoxynucleotidyl transferase
### [TdT]

Using indirect immunofluorescence, the terminal deoxynucleotidyl transferase (TdT) test measures levels of TdT. The test differentiates certain types of leukemias and lymphomas marked by primitive cells that can't be identified by cell studies alone. Measurement of TdT may also help determine the prognosis for these diseases and may detect early relapse.

## Reference values

■ TdT is present in less than 2% of marrow cells and is undetectable in normal peripheral blood.

## Abnormal results

■ Positive cells are present in more than 90% of patients with acute lymphocytic leukemia (ALL), in 33% of patients with chronic myelogenous leukemia in blast crisis, and in 5% of patients with non-lymphocytic leukemias.
■ TdT-positive cells are absent in patients with ALL that is in remission.

## Purpose

■ To help differentiate ALL from acute nonlymphocytic leukemia
■ To help differentiate lymphoblastic lymphomas from malignant lymphomas
■ To monitor the patient's response to therapy, help determine his prognosis, or detect early relapse

## Patient preparation

■ Explain to the patient that this test detects an enzyme that can help classify the origin of his cancer.

### Blood test

■ Tell the patient to fast for 12 to 14 hours before the test.
■ Inform him that the test requires a blood sample. Explain who will perform the venipuncture and when.
■ Explain to the patient that he may experience slight discomfort from the tourniquet and the needle puncture.

### Bone marrow aspiration

■ Describe the procedure to the patient, and answer his questions.
■ Inform the patient that he doesn't need to restrict food and fluids.
■ Tell the patient who will obtain the specimen for biopsy; inform him that the test usually takes 5 to 10 minutes.
■ Make sure the patient or a responsible family member has signed an informed consent form.
■ Check the patient's history for hypersensitivity to the local anesthetic.
■ After checking with the practitioner, tell the patient which bone will provide the specimen for biopsy.
■ Tell the patient that he'll receive a local anesthetic but will feel pressure on insertion of the biopsy needle and a brief, pulling pain when the marrow is withdrawn.
■ Give a mild sedative 1 hour before the test as ordered.

### Procedure and posttest care

■ Confirm the patient's identity using two patient identifiers according to facility policy.
■ If a blood test is scheduled, perform a venipuncture, and collect the sample in one 10-ml heparinized blood tube and one EDTA tube.
■ If assisting with bone marrow aspiration, inject 1 ml of bone marrow into a 7-ml heparinized tube, and dilute it with 5 ml of normal saline solution, or submit four air-dried marrow smears.
■ Send the sample to the laboratory immediately.
■ Because the patient may have a compromised immune system, take special care to keep the venipuncture site clean and dry.
■ Because a patient with leukemia may bleed excessively, apply pressure to the venipuncture site until bleeding stops.
■ If a hematoma develops at the venipuncture site, apply warm soaks.

- Check the bone marrow aspiration site for bleeding and inflammation, and observe the patient for signs of hemorrhage and infection.

### Precautions
- Before performing the venipuncture, contact the laboratory to make sure it can process the blood sample and verify how much blood to draw.
- Because the patient with leukemia is more susceptible to infection, clean the skin thoroughly before performing the venipuncture.
- A false-positive test result may occur from a child's bone-marrow aspirate because of TdT-positive bone marrow produced during proliferation of prelymphocytes.
- Bone marrow regeneration, idiopathic thrombocytopenic purpura, and neuroblastomas may cause TdT-positive bone marrow and a possible false-positive test result.

# General humoral tests

## ▌Complement assays

Complement is a collective term for a system of at least 20 serum proteins designed to destroy foreign cells and help remove foreign materials. The system may be triggered by contact with antigen-antibody complexes or by clotting factor XIIa. A cascade of events follows, resulting in the formation of a complex that ruptures cell membranes.

Complement components are numerically designated as C1 through C9, with C1 having three subcomponents: C1q, C1r, and C1s. These components constitute 3% to 4% of total serum globulins and play a key role in antibody-mediated immune reactions.

Complement can function as a defense by promoting the removal of infectious agents or as a threat by triggering destructive reactions in host tissues. Complement deficiency can increase susceptibility to infection and predispose a person to other diseases. Complement assays are indicated in patients with known or suspected immune-mediated disease or a repeatedly abnormal response to infection.

Various laboratory methods are used to evaluate and measure total complement and its components. Hemolytic assay, laser nephelometry, and radial immunodiffusion are the most common.

Although complement assays provide valuable information about the patient's immune system, the results must be considered in light of serum immunoglobulin and autoantibody tests for a definitive diagnosis of immune-mediated disease or an abnormal response to infection.

### Reference values
- Total complement levels are 25 to 110 units/ml (SI, 0.25 to 1.1 g/L).
- C3 levels are 70 to 150 mg/dl (SI, 0.7 to 1.5 g/L).
- C4 levels are 15 to 45 mg/dl (SI, 0.15 to 0.45 g/L).

### Abnormal results
- Complement abnormalities may be genetic or acquired; acquired abnormalities are most common.
- Low total complement levels (which are clinically more significant than high levels) may result from excessive formation of antigen-antibody complexes, insufficient complement synthesis, inhibitor formation, or increased complement catabolism and are characteristic in such conditions as systemic lupus erythematosus (SLE), acute poststreptococcal glomerulonephritis, acute serum sickness, advanced cirrhosis of the liver,

multiple myeloma, hypogammaglobulinemia, or rapidly rejecting allografts.

■ High total complement levels may occur in obstructive jaundice, thyroiditis, acute rheumatic fever, rheumatoid arthritis, acute myocardial infarction, ulcerative colitis, and diabetes.

■ C1 esterase inhibitor deficiency is characteristic in hereditary angioedema, the most common genetic abnormality associated with complement.

■ C3 deficiency is characteristic in recurrent pyogenic infection and disease activation in SLE.

■ C4 deficiency is found in SLE and rheumatoid arthritis; its level is increased in autoimmune hemolytic anemia.

#### DRUG CHALLENGE

Recent heparin therapy (may inactivate complement)

### Purpose

■ To help detect immune-mediated disease and genetic complement deficiency
■ To monitor the effectiveness of therapy

### Patient preparation

■ Explain that this test measures a group of proteins that fight infection.
■ Inform the patient that he doesn't need to restrict food and fluids.
■ Tell the patient that the test requires a blood sample. Explain who will perform the venipuncture and when.
■ Explain to the patient that he may experience slight discomfort from the tourniquet and the needle puncture.
■ If the patient is scheduled for C1q assay, check his history for recent heparin therapy. Report heparin therapy to the laboratory.

### Procedure and posttest care

■ Confirm the patient's identity using two patient identifiers according to facility policy.
■ Perform a venipuncture, and collect the blood sample in a 7-ml tube without additives.
■ Because many patients with complement defects have a compromised immune system, keep the venipuncture site clean and dry.
■ Apply direct pressure to the venipuncture site until bleeding stops.
■ If a hematoma develops at the venipuncture site, apply warm soaks.

## Human leukocyte antigens
### [HLA]

The human leukocyte antigen (HLA) test identifies a group of antigens that appear on the surface of all nucleated cells, but which are most easily detected on lymphocytes. The four types of HLA are HLA-A, HLA-B, HLA-C, and HLA-D. These antigens are essential to immunity and determine the degree of histocompatibility between transplant recipients and donors. Numerous antigenic determinants are present for each site (more than 60, for instance, at the HLA-B locus); one set of each antigen is inherited from each parent.

A high incidence of specific HLA types has been linked to specific diseases, such as rheumatoid arthritis and multiple sclerosis, but these findings have little diagnostic significance.

### Normal results

■ In HLA-A, HLA-B, and HLA-C testing, lymphocytes that react with the test antiserum undergo lysis; they're detected by phase microscopy.
■ In HLA-D testing, leukocyte incompatibility is marked by blast formation, de-

oxyribonucleic acid (DNA) synthesis, and proliferation.

### Abnormal results

- Incompatible HLA-A, HLA-B, HLA-C, and HLA-D groups may cause unsuccessful tissue transplantation.
- Many diseases have a strong association with certain types of HLAs. For example, HLA-DR5 is associated with Hashimoto's thyroiditis. B8 and Dw3 are associated with Graves' disease, whereas B8 alone is associated with chronic autoimmune hepatitis, celiac disease, and myasthenia gravis.
- Dw3 alone is associated with Addison's disease, Sjögren's syndrome, dermatitis herpetiformis, and systemic lupus erythematosus.
- In paternity testing, a putative father who presents a phenotype (two haplotypes: one from the father and one from the mother) with no haplotype or antigen pair identical to one of the child's is excluded as the father. A putative father with one haplotype identical to one of the child's may be the father; the probability varies with the incidence of the haplotype in the population.

### Purpose

- To provide histocompatibility typing of transplant recipients and donors
- To aid in genetic counseling
- To aid in paternal identity

### Patient preparation

- Explain that this test detects antigens on white blood cells.
- Inform the patient that he doesn't need to restrict food and fluids.
- Tell the patient that the test requires a blood sample. Explain who will perform the venipuncture and when.
- Explain to the patient that he may experience slight discomfort from the tourniquet and the needle puncture.

- Check the patient's history for recent blood transfusions. HLA testing may need to be postponed if he recently had a transfusion.

### Procedure and posttest care

- Confirm the patient's identity using two patient identifiers according to facility policy.
- Perform a venipuncture; collect the blood sample in a tube containing anticoagulant acid citrate dextrose solution.
- Apply direct pressure to the venipuncture site until bleeding stops.
- If a hematoma develops at the venipuncture site, apply warm soaks.

# Immune complex assays

When immune complexes are produced faster than they can be cleared by the lymphoreticular system, immune complex disease, such as postinfectious syndromes, serum sickness, drug sensitivity, rheumatoid arthritis, and systemic lupus erythematosus (SLE), may occur. Immune complexes can develop when a certain ratio of antigen reacts with antibody of isotopes immunoglobulin (Ig) G 1, 2, 3, or IgM in tissues. These complexes can fix the first component of complement (C1) and activate the complement cascade. Subsequent complement-mediated activity leads to inflammation and local tissue necrosis. In the blood, soluble circulating immune complexes may also activate complement and eventually cause damage, usually in the renal glomeruli, the aorta, and other large blood vessels.

Histologic examination of tissue obtained by biopsy and the use of fluorescence or peroxidase staining with antibodies specific for immunologic types generally detect immune complexes. However, tissue biopsies can't provide information about titers of complexes still in circulation; therefore, serum assays, which detect circulating immune complexes indirectly, may be required. Because of the inherent variability of these complexes, several serum test methods may be appropriate using C1, rheumatoid factor (RF), or cellular substrates, such as Raji cells, as reagents.

Most immune complex assays haven't been standardized, so more than one test may be required to achieve accurate results.

## Normal results
- Immune complexes aren't detectable in serum.

## Abnormal results
- Detectable immune complexes in serum have etiologic importance in many autoimmune diseases, such as SLE and rheumatoid arthritis.
- For definitive diagnosis, the presence of these complexes must be considered with the results of other studies. For example, in SLE, immune complexes are associated with high titers of antinuclear antibodies and circulating antinative deoxyribonucleic acid antibodies.
- Because of their filtering function, renal glomeruli seem vulnerable to immune complex deposition, although blood vessel walls and choroid plexuses (vascular folds in the ventricles of the brain) can be affected.
- Renal biopsy to detect immune complexes can provide conclusive evidence for immune complex (type III) glomerulonephritis, differentiating it from other types of glomerulonephritis.

## Purpose
- To demonstrate circulating immune complexes in serum
- To monitor the patient's response to therapy
- To estimate disease severity

## Patient preparation
- Explain that these tests help evaluate the immune system.
- Inform the patient that the test may be repeated to monitor his response to therapy, if appropriate.
- Inform the patient that he doesn't need to restrict food and fluids.
- Tell him that the test requires a blood sample. Explain who will perform the venipuncture and when.
- Explain to the patient that he may experience slight discomfort from the tourniquet and needle puncture.
- If the patient is scheduled for C1q assay (a component of C1), check his history for recent heparin therapy. Report recent heparin therapy to the laboratory.

## Procedure and posttest care
- Confirm the patient's identity using two patient identifiers according to facility policy.
- Perform a venipuncture, and collect the blood sample in a 7-ml clot-activator tube.
- Because many patients with immune complexes have a compromised immune system, keep the venipuncture site clean and dry.
- Apply direct pressure to the venipuncture site until bleeding stops.
- If a hematoma develops at the venipuncture site, apply warm soaks.

## Precautions
- Send the blood sample to the laboratory immediately to prevent deterioration of immune complexes.

# Quantitative immunoglobulins G, A, and M

Immunoglobulins, proteins that can function as specific antibodies in response to antigen stimulation, are responsible for the humoral aspects of immunity. They are classed in five groups—immunoglobulin (Ig) G, IgA, IgM, IgD, and IgE—that are normally present in serum in predictable percentages.

IgG constitutes about 75% of serum immunoglobulins and includes the warm-temperature type; IgA, about 15% of the total; IgM, 5% to 7%, including cold agglutinins, rheumatoid factor, and ABO blood group isoagglutinins; and IgD and allergen-specific IgE, less than 2%. Deviations from normal immunoglobulin percentages are characteristic in many immune disorders, including cancer, hepatic disorders, rheumatoid arthritis, and systemic lupus erythematosus.

Immunoelectrophoresis identifies IgG, IgA, and IgM in a serum sample; the level of each is measured by radial immunodiffusion or nephelometry. Some laboratories detect immunoglobulin by indirect immunofluorescence and radioimmunoassay.

### Reference values
- With nephelometry:
  - IgG level is 800 to 1,800 mg/dl (SI, 8 to 18 g/L).
  - IgA level is 100 to 400 mg/dl (SI, 1 to 4 g/L).
  - IgM level is 55 to 150 mg/dl (SI, 0.55 to 1.5 g/L).

### Abnormal results
- See *Serum immunoglobulin levels in various disorders,* page 190, for IgG, IgA, and IgM levels in various disorders.
- In congenital and acquired hypogammaglobulinemias, myelomas, and macroglobulinemia, abnormal results confirm the diagnosis.
- In hepatic and autoimmune diseases, leukemias, and lymphomas, such findings are less important, but they can support the diagnosis based on other

tests, such as biopsies and white blood cell differential, and on the physical examination.

### DRUG CHALLENGE

Aminophenazone, anticonvulsants, asparaginase, hydralazine, hydantoin derivatives, hormonal contraceptives, and phenylbutazone (possible increase); methotrexate and severe hypersensitivity to bacille Calmette-Guérin vaccine (possible decrease); dextrans and methylprednisolone (decrease in IgM levels); dextrans and high doses of methylprednisolone and phenytoin (decrease in IgG and IgA levels); methadone (increase in IgA levels)

### Purpose
- To diagnose paraproteinemias, such as multiple myeloma and Waldenström's macroglobulinemia
- To detect hypogammaglobulinemia and hypergammaglobulinemia as well as nonimmunologic diseases, such as cirrhosis and hepatitis, that are associated with abnormally high immunoglobulin levels
- To assess the effectiveness of chemotherapy and radiation therapy

### Patient preparation
- Explain that this test measures antibody levels.
- If appropriate, tell the patient that the test evaluates the effectiveness of treatment.
- Instruct the patient to restrict food and fluids (except water), for 12 to 14 hours before the test.
- Tell the patient that the test requires a blood sample. Explain who will perform the venipuncture and when.
- Explain to the patient that he may experience slight discomfort from the tourniquet and needle puncture.

# Serum immunoglobulin levels in various disorders

| Disorder | IgG | IgA | IgM |
|---|---|---|---|
| **Immunoglobulin disorders** | | | |
| Lymphoid aplasia | D | D | D |
| Agammaglobulinemia | D | D | D |
| Type I dysgammaglobulinemia (selective immunoglobulin [Ig] G and IgA deficiency) | D | D | N or I |
| Type II dysgammaglobulinemia (absent IgA and IgM) | N | D | D |
| IgA globulinemia | N | D | N |
| Ataxia-telangiectasia | N | D | N |
| **Multiple myeloma, macroglobulinemia, lymphomas** | | | |
| Heavy chain disease (Franklin's disease) | D | D | D |
| IgG myeloma | I | D | D |
| IgA myeloma | D | I | D |
| Macroglobulinemia | D | D | I |
| Acute lymphocytic leukemia | N | D | N |
| Chronic lymphocytic leukemia | D | D | D |
| Acute myelocytic leukemia | N | N | N |
| Chronic myelocytic leukemia | N | D | N |
| Hodgkin's disease | N | N | N |
| **Hepatic disorders** | | | |
| Hepatitis | I | I | I |
| Laënnec's cirrhosis | I | I | N |
| Biliary cirrhosis | N | N | I |
| Hepatoma | N | N | D |
| **Other disorders** | | | |
| Rheumatoid arthritis | I | I | I |
| Systemic lupus erythematosus | I | I | I |
| Nephrotic syndrome | D | D | N |
| Trypanosomiasis | N | N | I |
| Pulmonary tuberculosis | I | N | N |

Key: N = normal; I = increased; D = decreased

■ Check the patient's history for drugs that may affect test results.
■ Be aware that alcohol or opioid drug abuse may affect results.

## Procedure and posttest care
■ Confirm the patient's identity using two patient identifiers according to facility policy.
■ Perform a venipuncture and collect the blood sample in a 7-ml clot-activator tube.

- Advise the patient with abnormally low immunoglobulin levels (especially IgG or IgM) to protect himself against bacterial infection. When caring for such a patient, watch for signs of infection, such as fever, chills, rash, and skin ulcers.
- Instruct the patient with abnormally high immunoglobulin levels and symptoms of monoclonal gammopathies to report bone pain and tenderness. Such a patient has numerous antibody-producing malignant plasma cells in bone marrow, which hamper production of other blood components. Watch for signs of hypercalcemia, renal failure, and spontaneous pathologic fractures.
- Apply direct pressure to the venipuncture site until bleeding stops.
- If a hematoma develops at the venipuncture site, apply warm soaks.
- Tell the patient to resume his usual diet and medications stopped before the test as ordered.

### Precautions

- Send the blood sample to the laboratory immediately to prevent immunoglobulin deterioration.
- Radiation therapy or chemotherapy may decrease Ig levels because of its suppressive effects on the bone marrow.

# ▪ Radioallergosorbent test
### [RAST]

The radioallergosorbent test (RAST) measures immunoglobulin (Ig) E antibodies in serum by radioimmunoassay and identifies specific allergens that cause rash, asthma, hay fever, drug reactions, and other atopic complaints. The RAST is easier to perform and more specific than skin testing; it's also less painful for and less dangerous to the patient. Careful selection of specific aller-

gens, based on the patient's history, is crucial for effective testing.

Although skin testing is still the preferred means of diagnosing IgE-mediated hypersensitivities, the RAST may be more useful when a skin disorder makes accurate reading of skin tests difficult, when a patient requires continual antihistamine therapy, or when skin tests are negative but the patient's history supports IgE-mediated hypersensitivity.

In the RAST, a sample of the patient's serum is exposed to a panel of allergen particle complexes (APCs) on cellulose disks. The patient's IgE complexes mixes with those APCs to which it's sensitive. Radiolabeled anti-IgE antibody is then added, and this binds to the IgE-APC complexes. After centrifugation, the amount of radioactivity in the particulate material is directly proportional to the amount of IgE antibodies present. Test results are compared with control values and represent the patient's reactivity to a specific allergen.

### Reference values

- Results are interpreted in relation to a control or reference serum that differs among laboratories.

### Abnormal results

- High serum IgE levels suggest hypersensitivity to the specific allergen or allergens used.

### Purpose

- To identify allergens to which the patient has an immediate (IgE-mediated) hypersensitivity
- To monitor the patient's response to therapy

### Patient preparation

- Explain that this test may detect the cause of allergy or monitor the effectiveness of allergy treatment.

- Inform the patient that he doesn't need to restrict food and fluids.
- Tell the patient that the test requires a blood sample. Explain who will perform the venipuncture and when.
- Explain to the patient that he may experience slight discomfort from the tourniquet and needle puncture.
- If the patient is scheduled for a radioactive scan, make sure the blood sample is collected before the scan.

### Procedure and posttest care

- Confirm the patient's identity using two patient identifiers according to facility policy.
- Perform a venipuncture, and collect the blood sample in a 7-ml clot-activator tube. Usually, 1 ml of serum is sufficient for five allergen assays.
- Note on the laboratory request the specific allergens to be tested.
- Apply direct pressure to the venipuncture site until bleeding stops.
- If a hematoma develops at the venipuncture site, apply warm soaks.

# *Autoantibody tests*

## Acetylcholine receptor antibodies
### [AChR]

The acetylcholine receptor (AChR) antibodies test is the most useful immunologic test for confirming acquired (autoimmune) myasthenia gravis (MG), a disorder of neuromuscular transmission. In MG, antibodies block and destroy AChR sites, causing muscle weakness that can be either generalized or localized to the ocular muscles.

Two test methods—a binding assay and a blocking assay—are now available to determine the relative concentration of AChR antibodies in serum. Determi-

nation of AChR antibodies by either method also helps monitor immunosuppressive therapy for MG, although antibody levels don't usually parallel the severity of disease.

### Normal results

- Serum test results are negative for AChR-binding antibodies and AChR-blocking antibodies.

### Abnormal results

- Positive results for AChR antibodies in symptomatic adults confirm the diagnosis of MG.
- Patients who have only ocular symptoms have lower antibody titers than those with generalized symptoms.

### Purpose

- To confirm the diagnosis of MG
- To monitor the effectiveness of immunosuppressive therapy for MG

### Patient preparation

- Explain that this test helps confirm the diagnosis of MG.
- Tell the patient that the test assesses the effectiveness of treatment, if appropriate.
- Inform the patient that he doesn't need to restrict food and fluids.
- Tell the patient that the test requires a blood sample. Explain who will perform the venipuncture and when.
- Explain to the patient that he may experience slight discomfort from the tourniquet and the needle puncture.
- Check the patient's history for immunosuppressive drugs that may affect test results and identify the drugs on the laboratory request.

### Procedure and posttest care

- Confirm the patient's identity using two patient identifiers according to facility policy.

- Perform a venipuncture and collect the blood sample in a 7-ml tube without additives.
- Because a patient with an autoimmune disease has a compromised immune system, check the venipuncture site for infection, and promptly report changes.
- Keep a clean, dry bandage over the site for at least 24 hours.
- Apply direct pressure to the venipuncture site until bleeding stops.
- If a hematoma develops at the venipuncture site, apply warm soaks.

### Precautions

- In a patient who had a thymectomy, thoracic duct drainage, or recent plasmapheresis, the AChR level may be decreased.
- Amyotrophic lateral sclerosis may cause a false-positive test result.

## ▌Anti-deoxyribonucleic acid antibodies
### [anti-DNA antibodies, anti-ds-DNA antibodies]

About two-thirds of patients with active systemic lupus erythematosus (SLE) have measurable levels of autoantibodies to double-stranded (native) deoxyribonucleic acid (known as anti-ds-DNA). These antibodies are rarely detected in patients with other connective tissue diseases.

In autoimmune diseases such as SLE, native DNA is thought to be the antigen that forms a complex with antibody and complement, causing local tissue damage where these complexes are deposited. Serum anti-ds-DNA levels are directly related to the extent of renal or vascular damage caused by the disease.

The anti-ds-DNA antibody test measures and differentiates these antibody levels in a serum sample, using radioimmunoassay, agglutination, complement fixation, or immunoelectrophoresis. If anti-ds-DNA antibodies are present, they combine with native DNA and form complexes that are too large to pass through a membrane filter. The test counts these oversized complexes.

### Reference values

- An anti-ds-DNA antibody level less than 25 International Units/ml (SI, < 25 kIU/L) is considered negative for SLE.
- Low anti-ds-DNA antibody levels may follow immunosuppressive therapy, demonstrating effective treatment of SLE.

### Abnormal results

- High anti-ds-DNA antibody levels may indicate SLE.
  – Antibody levels of 25 to 30 International Units/ml (SI, 25 to 30 kIU/L) are considered borderline positive.
  – Antibody levels of 31 to 200 International Units/ml (SI, 31 to 200 kIU/L) are positive, and those greater than 200 International Units/ml (SI, >200 kIU/L) are strongly positive.

### Purpose

- To confirm a diagnosis of SLE
- To monitor the SLE patient's response to therapy and determine his prognosis

### Patient preparation

- Explain that this test helps diagnose and determine the appropriate therapy for SLE.
- Inform the patient that he doesn't need to restrict food and fluids.
- Tell him that the test requires a blood sample. Explain who will perform the venipuncture and when.
- Explain to the patient that he may experience slight discomfort from the tourniquet and needle puncture.
- Ask the patient if he has had a recent test that used a radioactive substance

such as an isotope. If so, note this on the laboratory request.

### Procedure and posttest care
■ Confirm the patient's identity using two patient identifiers according to facility policy.
■ Perform a venipuncture, and collect the blood sample in a 7-ml tube without additives. (Some laboratories may specify a tube with EDTA or sodium fluoride and potassium oxalate added.)
■ Apply direct pressure to the venipuncture site until bleeding stops.
■ If a hematoma develops at the venipuncture site, apply warm soaks.

# Anti-insulin antibodies

Some patients with diabetes form antibodies to the insulin they take. These antibodies bind with some of the insulin, making less insulin available for glucose metabolism and necessitating increased insulin dosages. This phenomenon is known as insulin resistance.

Performed on the blood of a patient with diabetes who takes insulin, the anti-insulin antibody test detects insulin antibodies.

### Normal results
■ Less than 3% of the patient's serum binds with labeled beef, human, and pork insulin.

### Abnormal results
■ Elevated levels may occur in insulin allergy or resistance and in factitious hypoglycemia.

### Purpose
■ To determine insulin allergy
■ To confirm insulin resistance
■ To determine if hypoglycemia is caused by insulin overuse

### Patient preparation
■ Explain to the patient that this test determines the most appropriate treatment for his diabetes and if he has insulin resistance or an allergy to insulin.
■ Tell the patient that the test requires a blood sample. Explain who will perform the venipuncture and when.
■ Explain to the patient that he may experience slight discomfort from the tourniquet and needle puncture.
■ Inform the patient that he doesn't need to restrict food and fluids.
■ Ask the patient if he has had a test that uses radioactive agents recently; if so, note this on the laboratory request.

### Procedure and posttest care
■ Confirm the patient's identity using two patient identifiers according to facility policy.
■ Perform a venipuncture, and collect the sample in a 7-ml tube without additives.
■ Apply direct pressure to the venipuncture site until bleeding stops.
■ If a hematoma develops at the venipuncture site, apply warm soaks.

# Antimitochondrial antibodies
### [AMA]

Usually performed with the test for anti-smooth-muscle antibodies, the antiitochondrial antibodies test detects antimitochondrial antibodies in serum by indirect immunofluorescence. These autoantibodies are present in several hepatic diseases. Their role in disease pathogenesis is unknown, and there's no evidence that they cause hepatic damage. Most commonly, they're associated with primary biliary cirrhosis and, sometimes, with chronic active hepatitis and drug-induced jaundice. Antimitochondrial antibodies are also associated with autoimmune diseases, such as sys-

# Incidence of serum antibodies in various disorders

The table below shows the percentage of patients with certain disorders who have antimitochondrial or anti-smooth-muscle antibodies in the serum. When these antibodies are present, further testing is needed to confirm the diagnosis. (In up to 1% of healthy people antimitochondrial antibodies also appear.)

| Disorder | Antimitochondrial antibodies | Anti-smooth-muscle antibodies |
|---|---|---|
| Primary biliary cirrhosis | 75% to 95% | 0% to 50% [a] |
| Chronic active hepatitis | 0% to 30% | 50% to 80% |
| Extrahepatic biliary obstruction | 0% to 5% | 0% |
| Cryptogenic cirrhosis | 0% to 25% | 0% to 1% |
| Viral (infectious) hepatitis | 0% | 1% to 2% [b] |
| Drug-induced jaundice | 50% to 80% | |
| Intrinsic asthma | | 20% |
| Rheumatoid arthritis and other collagen diseases | 1% to 2% | |
| Systemic lupus erythematosus | 3% to 5% [c] | 0% |

[a] In chronic disease, values fall at the upper end of the range.
[b] Much higher incidence occurs with hepatic damage.
[c] Much higher incidence occurs with renal involvement.

temic lupus erythematosus, rheumatoid arthritis, pernicious anemia, and idiopathic Addison's disease.

### Normal results

- Serum is negative for antimitochondrial antibodies. Positive results are titered.

### Abnormal results

- Although antimitochondrial antibodies appear in 79% to 94% of patients with primary biliary cirrhosis, this test alone doesn't confirm the diagnosis. Further tests, such as serum alkaline phosphatase, serum bilirubin, aspartate aminotransferase, alanine aminotransferase

and, possibly, liver biopsy or cholangiography, may also be necessary.
- The autoantibodies also appear in some patients with chronic active hepatitis, drug-induced jaundice, and cryptogenic cirrhosis. (See *Incidence of serum antibodies in various disorders*.)
- Antimitochondrial antibodies seldom appear in patients with extrahepatic biliary obstruction, and a positive test result helps rule out this condition.

### Purpose

- To help diagnose primary biliary cirrhosis

■ To distinguish between extrahepatic jaundice and biliary cirrhosis

## Patient preparation
■ Explain that this test evaluates liver function.
■ Inform the patient that he doesn't need to restrict food and fluids.
■ Tell the patient that the test requires a blood sample. Explain who will perform the venipuncture and when.
■ Explain to the patient that he may experience slight discomfort from the tourniquet and needle puncture.

## Procedure and posttest care
■ Confirm the patient's identity using two patient identifiers according to facility policy.
■ Perform a venipuncture, and collect a blood sample in a 7-ml tube with no additives.
■ Because the patient with hepatic disease may bleed excessively, apply pressure to the venipuncture site until bleeding stops.
■ If a hematoma develops at the venipuncture site, apply warm soaks.

# Antinuclear antibodies
## [ANA]

In such conditions as systemic lupus erythematosus (SLE), scleroderma, and certain infections, the body's immune system may perceive portions of its own cell nuclei as foreign and may produce antinuclear antibodies (ANAs). Specific ANAs include antibodies to deoxyribonucleic acid (DNA), nucleoprotein, histones, nuclear ribonucleoprotein, and other nuclear constituents.

Because they don't penetrate living cells, ANAs are harmless, but they sometimes form antigen-antibody complexes that cause tissue damage (as in SLE). Because of multiorgan involve-

ment, test results aren't diagnostic and can only partially confirm clinical evidence. (See *Comparative incidence of antinuclear antibodies.*)

This test measures the relative concentration of ANAs in a serum sample through indirect immunofluorescence. Serial dilutions of serum are mixed with either Hep-2 or mouse kidney substrate. Serum containing ANA forms antigen-antibody complexes with the substrate. After the preparation is mixed with fluorescein-labeled antihuman serum, it's examined under an ultraviolet microscope. If ANAs are present, the complex glows (fluoresces). The greatest dilution that shows the reaction is taken as the titer.

## Normal results
■ Test results are negative.

## Abnormal results
■ Low titers may occur in patients with viral diseases, chronic hepatic disease, collagen vascular disease, and autoimmune diseases and in some healthy adults; the incidence increases with age.
■ The higher the titer, the more specific the test is for SLE (titer typically exceeds 1:256).
■ The pattern of nuclear fluorescence helps identify the type of immune disease. A peripheral pattern is almost exclusively associated with SLE because it indicates anti-DNA antibodies. Sometimes anti-DNA antibodies are measured by radioimmunoassay if ANA titers are high or if a peripheral pattern is observed.
■ A homogeneous, or diffuse, pattern is also associated with SLE as well as with related connective tissue disorders; a nucleolar pattern, with scleroderma; and a speckled, irregular pattern, with infectious mononucleosis and mixed connective tissue disorders (for example, SLE and scleroderma).

## Comparative incidence of antinuclear antibodies

| Condition | Incidence of positive antinuclear antibodies |
|---|---|
| Systemic lupus erythematosus (SLE) | 95% to 100% |
| Lupoid hepatitis | 95% to 100% |
| Felty's syndrome | 95% to 100% |
| Progressive systemic sclerosis (scleroderma) | 75% to 80% |
| Drugs associated with SLE-like syndrome (hydralazine, procainamide, isoniazid) | About 50% |
| Sjögren's syndrome | 40% to 75% |
| Rheumatoid arthritis | 25% to 60% |
| Healthy family member of patient with SLE | About 25% |
| Chronic discoid lupus erythematosus | 15% to 50% |
| Juvenile rheumatoid arthritis | 15% to 30% |
| Polyarteritis nodosa | 15% to 25% |
| Miscellaneous disorders | 10% to 50% |
| Dermatomyositis, polymyositis | 10% to 30% |
| Rheumatic fever | About 5% |

■ A single serum sample, especially one collected from a patient with collagen vascular disease, may contain antibodies to several parts of the cell's nucleus.
■ As serum dilution increases, the fluorescent pattern may change because different antibodies are reactive at different titers.

### DRUG CHALLENGE

 Most commonly hydralazine, isoniazid, and procainamide, but also chlorpromazine, clofibrate, contraceptives (hormonal), ethosuximide, gold salts, griseofulvin, mephenytoin, methyldopa, methysergide, para-aminosalicylic acid, penicillin, phenylbutazone, phenytoin, primidone, propylthiouracil, quinidine, reserpine, streptomycin, sulfonamides, tetracyclines, and trimethadione (possible production of a syndrome resembling SLE)

### Purpose
■ To screen for SLE (failure to detect ANAs essentially rules out active SLE)
■ To monitor the effectiveness of immunosuppressive therapy for SLE

## Patient preparation

- Explain that this test evaluates the immune system and that further testing is usually required for diagnosis.
- Inform the patient that the test will be repeated to monitor his response to therapy, if appropriate.
- Inform the patient that he doesn't need to restrict food and fluids.
- Tell the patient that the test requires a blood sample. Explain who will perform the venipuncture and when.
- Explain to the patient that he may experience slight discomfort from the tourniquet and the needle puncture.
- Check the patient's history for drugs that may affect test results, such as isoniazid and procainamide. Note findings on the laboratory request.

## Procedure and posttest care

- Confirm the patient's identity using two patient identifiers according to facility policy.
- Perform a venipuncture, and collect a blood sample in a 7-ml tube without additives.
- Because a patient with an autoimmune disease has a compromised immune system, observe the venipuncture site for signs of infection. Report changes to the physician immediately.
- Apply direct pressure to the venipuncture site until bleeding stops.
- If a hematoma develops at the venipuncture site, apply warm soaks.
- Keep a clean, dry bandage over the site for at least 24 hours.

# Anti-smooth-muscle antibodies

Using indirect immunofluorescence, the anti-smooth-muscle antibodies test measures the relative concentration of anti-smooth-muscle antibodies in serum. This test is usually performed along with the test for antimitochondrial antibodies. The serum sample is exposed to a thin section of smooth muscle and incubated; then a fluorescent-labeled antiglobulin is added. This antiglobulin binds only to antibodies that have formed a complex with smooth muscle and that appear fluorescent when viewed through the microscope under ultraviolet light.

Anti-smooth-muscle antibodies appear in several hepatic diseases, especially chronic active hepatitis and, less commonly, primary biliary cirrhosis. Although anti-smooth-muscle antibodies are usually associated with hepatic diseases, their role is unknown, and there's no evidence that they cause hepatic damage.

## Normal results

- No anti-smooth-muscle antibodies appear.

## Abnormal results

- Positive findings are titered.
- The test for anti-smooth-muscle antibodies isn't specific; these antibodies appear in many patients with chronic active hepatitis and in fewer patients with primary biliary cirrhosis.
- Anti-smooth-muscle antibodies may also be present in patients with infectious mononucleosis, acute viral hepatitis, a malignant tumor of the liver, and intrinsic asthma.

## Purpose

- To help diagnose active chronic hepatitis and primary biliary cirrhosis

## Patient preparation

- Explain that this test helps evaluate liver function.
- Inform the patient that he doesn't need to restrict food and fluids.
- Tell the patient that the test requires a blood sample. Explain who will perform the venipuncture and when.

- Explain to the patient that he may experience slight discomfort from the tourniquet and needle puncture.

### Procedure and posttest care
- Confirm the patient's identity using two patient identifiers according to facility policy.
- Perform a venipuncture, and collect the blood sample in a 7-ml tube without additives.
- If a hematoma develops at the venipuncture site, apply warm soaks.

# Antithyroid antibodies

In autoimmune disorders—such as Hashimoto's thyroiditis and Graves' disease (hyperthyroidism)—thyroglobulin, the major colloidal storage compound, is released into the blood. Because thyroxine usually separates from thyroglobulin before its release into the blood, thyroglobulin doesn't normally enter the circulation. When it does, antithyroglobulin antibodies are formed to attack this foreign substance; the ensuing autoimmune response damages the thyroid gland. The serum of a patient whose autoimmune system produces antithyroglobulin antibodies usually contains antimicrosomal antibodies, which react with the microsomes of the thyroid epithelial cells.

The tanned red cell hemagglutination test detects antithyroglobulin and antimicrosomal antibodies. Another laboratory technique, indirect immunofluorescence, can detect antimicrosomal antibodies.

### Reference values
- The normal titer value is less than 1:100 for antithyroglobulin and antimicrosomal antibodies.

### Abnormal results
- Antithyroglobulin or antimicrosomal antibodies in serum can indicate subclinical autoimmune thyroid disease, Graves' disease, or idiopathic myxedema.
- Titer values of 1:400 or greater strongly suggest Hashimoto's thyroiditis.
- Antithyroglobulin antibodies may also occur in some patients with other autoimmune disorders, such as systemic lupus erythematosus (SLE), rheumatoid arthritis, and autoimmune hemolytic anemia.

### Purpose
- To detect circulating antithyroglobulin antibodies when clinical evidence indicates Hashimoto's thyroiditis, Graves' disease, or other thyroid diseases

### Patient preparation
- Explain that this test evaluates thyroid function.
- Inform the patient that he doesn't need to restrict food and fluids.
- Tell the patient that the test requires a blood sample. Explain who will perform the venipuncture and when.
- Explain to the patient that he may experience slight discomfort from the tourniquet and the needle puncture.

### Procedure and posttest care
- Confirm the patient's identity using two patient identifiers according to facility policy.
- Perform a venipuncture, and collect the blood sample in a 7-ml tube without additives.
- Apply direct pressure to the venipuncture site until bleeding stops.
- If a hematoma develops at the venipuncture site, apply warm soaks.

# Cardiolipin antibodies
[ACA]

The cardiolipin antibodies test measures serum concentrations of immunoglobulin (Ig) G and IgM antibodies in relation to the phospholipid cardiolipin. These antibodies appear in some patients with systemic lupus erythematosus (SLE) whose serum also contains a coagulation inhibitor (lupus anticoagulant). They also appear in some patients who don't fulfill all the diagnostic criteria for LE, but who experience recurrent episodes of spontaneous thrombosis, fetal loss, or thrombocytopenia. Serum cardiolipin antibody levels are measured by enzyme-linked immunosorbent assay.

### Reference values
- Cardiolipin antibody results are negative.

### Abnormal results
- A positive result is titered.
- A positive result along with a history of recurrent spontaneous thrombosis, fetal loss, or thrombocytopenia suggests cardiolipin antibody syndrome. Treatment may involve anticoagulant or platelet inhibitor therapy.

### Purpose
- To help diagnose cardiolipin antibody syndrome in the patient with or without LE who experiences recurrent episodes of spontaneous thrombosis, fetal loss, or thrombocytopenia

### Patient preparation
- Explain that this test helps diagnose cardiolipin antibody syndrome and LE.
- Inform the patient that he doesn't need to restrict food and fluids.
- Tell the patient that the test requires a blood sample. Explain who will perform the venipuncture and when.
- Explain to the patient that he may experience slight discomfort from the tourniquet and needle puncture.

### Procedure and posttest care
- Confirm the patient's identity using two patient identifiers according to facility policy.
- Perform a venipuncture, and collect the blood sample in a 5-ml tube without additives.
- Apply direct pressure to the venipuncture site until bleeding stops.
- If a hematoma develops at the venipuncture site, apply warm soaks.

# Cold agglutinins

Cold agglutinins are antibodies, usually of the immunoglobulin M type, that cause red blood cells (RBCs) to aggregate at low temperatures. They may occur in small amounts in healthy people. Transient elevations of these antibodies develop during certain infectious diseases, notably primary atypical pneumonia. This test reliably detects such pneumonia within 1 to 2 weeks after its onset.

Patients with high cold agglutinin titers, such as those with primary atypical pneumonia, may develop acute transient hemolytic anemia after repeated exposure to cold; patients with persistently high titers may develop chronic hemolytic anemia.

### Reference values
- Results are reported as negative or positive.
- A positive result, indicating the presence of cold agglutinin, is titered.
- A normal titer is less than 1:16.

### Abnormal results
- High titers may occur as primary phenomena or secondary to infections or lymphoreticular cancer. They may be

present in infectious mononucleosis, cytomegalovirus infection, hemolytic anemia, multiple myeloma, scleroderma, malaria, cirrhosis of the liver, congenital syphilis, peripheral vascular disease, pulmonary embolism, trypanosomiasis, tonsillitis, staphylococcemia, scarlatina, influenza and, occasionally, pregnancy.
- Chronically elevated titers are most commonly associated with pneumonia and lymphoreticular cancer; an acute transient elevation typically accompanies many viral infections.
- In primary atypical pneumonia, cold agglutinins appear in serum in one-half to two-thirds of all patients during the first week of acute infection, even before antimycoplasmal antibodies can be detected by complement fixation or metabolic inhibition tests. Thus, titers usually become positive at 7 days, peak above 1:32 in 4 weeks, and subside rapidly after 6 weeks. When sequential titers verify this pattern and clinical evidence of pneumonia exists, the diagnosis is confirmed.
- Extremely high titers (> 1:2,000) can occur with idiopathic cold agglutinin disease that precedes lymphoma development. Patients with titers this high are susceptible to intravascular agglutination, which causes significant clinical problems.

**DRUG CHALLENGE**

 Antimicrobial drugs (false negative)

## Purpose
- To help confirm primary atypical pneumonia
- To provide additional diagnostic evidence for cold agglutinin disease associated with many viral infections and lymphoreticular cancer

- To detect cold agglutinins in the patient with suspected cold agglutinin disease

## Patient preparation
- Explain to the patient that this test detects antibodies in the blood that attack RBCs after exposure to low temperatures.
- Tell the patient that the test will be repeated to monitor his response to therapy, if appropriate.
- Tell the patient that he doesn't need to restrict food and fluids.
- Tell the patient that the test requires a blood sample. Explain who will perform the venipuncture and when.
- Explain to the patient that he may experience slight discomfort from the tourniquet and needle puncture.
- If the patient is receiving antimicrobial drugs, note this on the laboratory request because the use of such drugs may interfere with the development of cold agglutinins.

## Procedure and posttest care
- Confirm the patient's identity using two patient identifiers according to facility policy.
- Perform a venipuncture, and collect a blood sample in a 7-ml tube without additives that has been prewarmed to 98.6° F (37° C).
- If cold agglutinin disease is suspected, keep the patient warm. If he's exposed to low temperatures, agglutination may occur within peripheral vessels, possibly leading to frostbite, anemia, Raynaud's phenomenon and, rarely, focal gangrene.
- Watch for signs of vascular abnormalities, such as mottled skin, purpura, jaundice, pallor, pain or swelling of extremities, and cramping of fingers and toes. Hemoglobinuria may result from severe intravascular hemolysis on exposure to severe cold.

- Apply direct pressure to the venipuncture site until bleeding stops.
- If a hematoma develops at the venipuncture site, apply warm soaks.

## Precautions

 Don't refrigerate the sample; cold agglutinins will coat the RBCs, leaving none in the serum for testing.

# Cryoglobulins

Cryoglobulins are abnormal serum proteins that precipitate at low laboratory temperatures (39.2° F [4° C]) and redissolve after being warmed. In the blood (cryoglobulinemia), they are usually associated with immunologic disease, but they can also occur without known immunopathology. (See *Diseases associated with cryoglobulinemia.*) If patients with cryoglobulinemia are subjected to cold, they may experience Raynaud-like symptoms (pain, cyanosis, and cold fingers and toes), which generally result from cryoglobulin precipitation in cooler parts of the body.

The cryoglobulin test involves refrigerating a serum sample at 33.8° F (1° C) for 24 hours and observing for formation of a heat-reversible precipitate. Such a precipitate requires further study by immunoelectrophoresis or double diffusion to identify cryoglobulin components.

## Normal results
- Normally, serum is negative for cryoglobulins.
- Positive results are reported as a percentage based on the amount of sample cryoprecipitation.

## Abnormal results
- Cryoglobulins in the blood confirm cryoglobulinemia.

## Purpose
- To detect cryoglobulinemia in the patient with Raynaud-like vascular symptoms

## Patient preparation
- Explain that this test detects antibodies in blood that may cause sensitivity to low temperatures.
- Instruct the patient to fast for 4 to 6 hours before the test.
- Tell the patient that the test requires a blood sample. Explain who will perform the venipuncture and when.
- Explain to the patient that he may experience slight discomfort from the tourniquet and needle puncture.

## Procedure and posttest care
- Confirm the patient's identity using two patient identifiers according to facility policy.
- Perform a venipuncture, and collect the blood sample in a prewarmed 10-ml tube without additives.
- Tell the patient to resume his usual diet.
- Tell the patient to avoid cold temperatures or contact with cold objects if the test finding shows cryoglobulins in the blood as ordered.
- Apply direct pressure to the venipuncture site until bleeding stops.
- If a hematoma develops at the venipuncture site, apply warm soaks.
- Observe for signs of intravascular coagulation, such as decreased color and temperature in distal extremities, and increased pain.

## Precautions

 Warm the syringe and collection tube to 98.6° F (37° C) before venipuncture, and keep the tube at that temperature to prevent cryoglobulin loss.

# Diseases associated with cryoglobulinemia

This chart indicates typical serum levels and diseases associated with the three types of cryoglobulins.

| Type of cryoglobulin | Serum level | Associated diseases |
|---|---|---|
| **Type I** | | |
| Monoclonal cryoglobulin | > 5 mg/ml | ▪ Myeloma<br>▪ Waldenström's macroglobulinemia<br>▪ Chronic lymphocytic leukemia |
| **Type II** | | |
| Mixed cryoglobulin | > 1 mg/ml | ▪ Rheumatoid arthritis<br>▪ Sjögren's syndrome<br>▪ Mixed essential cryoglobulinemia |
| **Type III** | | |
| Mixed polyclonal cryoglobulin | < 1 mg/ml<br>(50% below<br>80 mcg/ml) | ▪ Systemic lupus erythematosus<br>▪ Rheumatoid arthritis<br>▪ Sjögren's syndrome<br>▪ Infectious mononucleosis<br>▪ Cytomegalovirus infection<br>▪ Acute viral hepatitis<br>▪ Chronic active hepatitis<br>▪ Primary biliary cirrhosis<br>▪ Poststreptococcal glomerulonephritis<br>▪ Infective endocarditis<br>▪ Leprosy<br>▪ Kala-azar<br>▪ Tropical splenomegaly syndrome |

# Extractable nuclear antigen antibodies
## [ENA]

Extractable nuclear antigen (ENA) is a complex of at least four antigens. One of them—ribonucleoprotein (RNP—is susceptible to degradation by ribonuclease. The second—Smith (Sm) antigen—is an acidic nuclear protein that resists ribonuclease degradation. The third and fourth antigens that are sometimes included in this group—Sjögren's syndrome A (SS-A) antigen and Sjögren's syndrome B (SS-B) antigen—form a precipitate when an antibody is present.

Antibodies to these antigens are associated with certain autoimmune disorders. Tests to detect ENA antibodies help differentiate autoimmune disorders with similar signs and symptoms.

The RNP antibody test detects RNP autoantibodies, which are associated with systemic lupus erythematosus (SLE), progressive systemic sclerosis, and other rheumatic disorders. This test aids in the differential diagnosis of systemic rheumatic disease and is a useful follow-up test for collagen vascular autoimmune disease.

The anti-Sm antibody test detects Sm autoantibodies, which are a specific marker for SLE; thus, positive results strongly suggest SLE. This test also helps monitor collagen vascular autoimmune disease. The Sjögren's antibody test detects the SS-B autoantibodies produced by Sjögren's syndrome, an immunologic abnormality sometimes associated with rheumatic arthritis and SLE. However, this test doesn't confirm a Sjögren's syndrome diagnosis.

### Reference values

- Serum is negative for anti-RNP, anti-Sm, and SS-B antibodies.

### Abnormal results

- Anti-RNP antibodies are elevated in SLE (35% to 40% of cases) and in mixed connective tissue disease.
- Anti-Sm antibodies are specific for SLE.
- Anti-SS-A and anti-SS-B antibodies are elevated in Sjögren's syndrome (40% to 45% of cases).
- Anti-SS-B antibodies are also elevated in SLE.

### Purpose

- To aid in the differential diagnosis of autoimmune disease
- To distinguish between anti-RNP and anti-Sm antibodies
- To screen for anti-RNP antibodies (common in mixed connective tissue disease)
- To screen for anti-Sm antibodies (common in SLE)
- To support the diagnosis of collagen vascular autoimmune diseases
- To monitor the patient's response to therapy

### Patient preparation

- Explain that this test detects certain antibodies and that the test results help determine diagnosis and treatment.
- Explain that the test assesses the effectiveness of treatment, when appropriate.
- Inform the patient that he doesn't need to restrict food and fluids.
- Tell the patient that the test requires a blood sample. Explain who will perform the venipuncture and when.
- Explain to the patient that he may experience slight discomfort from the tourniquet and needle puncture.

### Procedure and posttest care

- Confirm the patient's identity using two patient identifiers according to facility policy.
- Perform a venipuncture, and collect the blood sample in a 7-ml tube without additives.
- Because a patient with an autoimmune disease has a compromised immune system, check the venipuncture site for infection, and report changes promptly.
- Apply direct pressure to the venipuncture site until bleeding stops.
- If a hematoma develops at the venipuncture site, apply warm soaks.
- Keep a clean, dry bandage over the site for at least 24 hours.

## Lupus erythematosus cell preparation

Lupus erythematosus (LE) cell preparation is an in vitro procedure used in diagnosing systemic lupus erythematosus (SLE). Although this test is less sensitive and reliable than either the antinuclear antibody (ANA) or the anti–deoxyribonucleic acid (DNA) antibody test, it's commonly used because it requires minimal equipment and reagents.

In this test, a blood sample is mixed with laboratory-treated nucleoprotein (the antigen). A sample containing

ANAs reacts with the nucleoprotein, causing swelling and rupture. Phagocytes from the serum then engulf the extruded nuclei, forming LE cells, which are then detected by microscopic examination of the sample.

## Normal results
- No LE cells are present in serum.
- About 60% of successfully treated patients fail to show LE cells after 4 to 6 weeks of therapy.

## Abnormal results
- The presence of at least two LE cells may indicate SLE. Although these cells occur primarily in SLE, they may also appear in chronic active hepatitis, rheumatoid arthritis, scleroderma, and certain drug reactions. Up to 25% of patients with SLE demonstrate no LE cells. In addition to supportive signs and symptoms, a definitive diagnosis of SLE may require a confirming ANA or anti-DNA test.
- The ANA test detects autoantibodies in the serum of many patients with SLE who have negative LE cell tests.
- Anti-DNA antibodies appear in two-thirds of all patients with SLE but are rare in other conditions; thus, the presence of these antibodies is strong evidence of SLE.

### DRUG CHALLENGE

 Hydralazine, isoniazid, and procainamide (may produce a syndrome resembling SLE); acetazolamide, chlorothiazide, chlorpromazine, chlorprothixene, clofibrate, contraceptives (hormonal), ethosuximide, gold salts, griseofulvin, mephenytoin, methyldopa, methysergide, para-aminosalicylic acid, penicillin, phenylbutazone, phenytoin, primidone, propylthiouracil, quinidine, reserpine, streptomycin, sulfonamides, tetracyclines, and trimethadione

## Purpose
- To help diagnose SLE
- To monitor treatment of SLE

## Patient preparation
- Explain to the patient that this test helps detect antibodies to his own tissue. (See *Understanding autoantibodies in autoimmune disease,* pages 206 and 207.)
- If appropriate, tell him that the test will be repeated to monitor his response to therapy and that certain test results (such as those that indicate SLE) may require further testing to determine or to monitor treatment.
- Inform the patient that he doesn't need to restrict food and fluids.
- Tell him that the test requires a blood sample. Explain who will perform the venipuncture and when.
- Explain to the patient that he may experience slight discomfort from the tourniquet and needle puncture.
- Check the patient's medication history for drugs that may affect test results, such as isoniazid, hydralazine, and procainamide. If such drugs must be continued, be sure to note this on the laboratory request.

## Procedure and posttest care
- Confirm the patient's identity using two patient identifiers according to facility policy.
- Perform a venipuncture, and collect the sample in a 7-ml red-top tube.
- Apply direct pressure to the venipuncture site until bleeding stops.
- If a hematoma develops at the venipuncture site, apply warm soaks.
- Because the patient with SLE may have a compromised immune system, keep a clean, dry bandage over the venipunc-

*(Text continues on page 208.)*

# Understanding autoantibodies in autoimmune disease

When the immune system produces autoantibodies against the antigenic determinants on and in cells, two types of autoimmune disease can result. *Organ-specific diseases,* such as pernicious anemia, occur when the targeted antigenic determinants are specific to an organ or tissue or to certain cells or cell types. Lymphocytes invade the target organ, tissue, or cell and destroy targeted cells. *Non–organ-specific diseases,* such as myasthenia gravis, occur when the targeted antigenic determinants are shared with other cells (self-antigens). This causes deposition of immune complexes (type III hypersensitivity) with subsequent lesions anywhere in the body.

Various diagnostic techniques are used to detect antibodies in autoimmune disease, including radioimmunoassay, hemagglutination, complement fixation, and immunofluorescence. The chart below lists common test methods and findings in various autoimmune diseases.

| Disease | Affected area |
|---------|---------------|
| Hashimoto's thyroiditis | Thyroid gland |
| Pernicious anemia | Hematopoietic system |
| Pemphigus vulgaris | Skin |
| Myasthenia gravis | Neuromuscular system |
| Autoimmune hemolytic anemia | Hematopoietic system |
| Primary biliary cirrhosis | Small bile ducts in liver |
| Rheumatoid arthritis | Joints, blood vessels, skin, muscles, lymph nodes |
| Goodpasture's syndrome | Lungs and kidneys |
| Systemic lupus erythematosus | Skin, joints, muscles, lungs, heart, kidneys, brain, eyes |

| Antigen | Antibody | Diagnostic technique |
|---------|----------|----------------------|
| Thyroglobulin, second colloid antigen, cytoplasmic microsomes, cell-surface antigens | Antibodies to thyroglobulin and to microsomal antigens | Radioimmunoassay, hemagglutination, complement fixation, immunofluorescence |
| Intrinsic factor | Antibodies to gastric parietal cells and vitamin $B_{12}$ binding site of intrinsic factor | Immunofluorecence, radioimmunoassay |
| Desmosomes between prickle cells in the epidermis | Antibodies to intercellular substances of the skin and mucous membranes | Immunofluorescence |
| Acetylcholine receptors of skeletal and heart muscle | Antiacetylcholine antibodies | Immunoprecipitation radioimmunoassay |
| Red blood cells (RBCs) | Anti-RBC antibodies | Direct and indirect Coombs' test |
| Mitochondria | Antimitochondrial antibodies | Immunofluorescence of mitochondrial-rich cells (kidney biopsy) |
| Immunoglobulin (Ig) G | Antigammaglobulin antibodies | Sheep RBC agglutination, latex immunoglobulin agglutination, radioimmunoassay, immunofluorescence, immunodiffusion |
| Glomerular and lung basement membranes | Anti-basement membrane antibodies | Immunofluorescence of kidney biopsy sample, radioimmunoassay |
| Deoxyribonucleic acid (DNA), nucleoprotein, blood cells, clotting factors, IgG, Wasserman antigen | Antinuclear antibodies, anti-DNA antibodies, Anti-ds-DNA antibodies, anti-SS-DNA antibodies, anti-ribonucleoprotein antibodies, antigammaglobulin antibodies, anti-RBC antibodies, antilymphocyte antibodies, antiplatelet antibodies, antineuronal cell antibodies, anti-Sm antibodies | Counterelectrophoresis, hemagglutination, radioimmunoassay, immunofluorescence, Coombs' test |

ture site for at least 24 hours and check for infection.

# Rheumatoid factor
[RF]

The rheumatoid factor (RF) test is the most useful immunologic test for confirming rheumatoid arthritis (RA). In this disease, "renegade" immunoglobulin (Ig) G antibodies, produced by lymphocytes in the synovial joints, react with IgM antibody to produce immune complexes, complement activation, and tissue destruction. How IgG molecules become antigenic is still unknown, but they may be altered by aggregating with viruses or other antigens. Techniques for detecting RF include the sheep cell agglutination test and the latex fixation test.

### Reference values
▪ The normal RF titer is less than 1:20; a normal rheumatoid screening test finding is nonreactive.

### Abnormal results
▪ Non-RA and RA populations aren't clearly separated with regard to the presence of RF: 25% of patients with RA have a nonreactive titer; 8% of non-RA patients are reactive at greater than 39 International Units/ml, and only 3% of non-RA patients are reactive at greater than 80 International Units/ml.
▪ Patients with various non-RA diseases characterized by chronic inflammation may test positive for RF. These diseases include systemic lupus erythematosus, polymyositis, tuberculosis, infectious mononucleosis, syphilis, viral hepatic disease, and influenza.

### Purpose
▪ To confirm RA, especially when clinical diagnosis is doubtful

### Patient preparation
▪ Explain to the patient that this test helps confirm RA.
▪ Inform the patient that he doesn't need to restrict food and fluids.
▪ Tell the patient that the test requires a blood sample. Explain who will perform the venipuncture and when.
▪ Explain to the patient that he may experience slight discomfort from the tourniquet and needle puncture.

### Procedure and posttest care
▪ Confirm the patient's identity using two patient identifiers according to facility policy.
▪ Perform a venipuncture, and collect the sample in a 7-ml clot-activator tube.
▪ Because a patient with RA may be immunologically compromised, keep the venipuncture site clean and dry for 24 hours.
▪ Check regularly for signs of infection.
▪ Apply direct pressure to the venipuncture site until bleeding stops.
▪ If a hematoma develops at the venipuncture site, apply warm soaks.

### Precautions
▪ A patient with high serum IgG levels may have a false-negative test result because the IgG will compete with the latex particles or sheep RBCs used as substrate.

# Thyroid-stimulating immunoglobulin
[TSI]

Thyroid-stimulating immunoglobulin (TSI) appears in the blood of most patients with Graves' disease. This autoantibody reacts with the cell-surface receptors that usually combine with thyroid-stimulating hormone (TSH). TSI reacts with these receptors, activates intracellular enzymes, and promotes epithelial cell activity that functions outside the normal feedback regulation mechanism for TSH. It stimulates the thyroid gland to produce and excrete excessive amounts of thyroid hormone.

Reportedly, 90% of people with Graves' disease have elevated TSI levels. Positive results of this test strongly suggest Graves' disease, despite normal routine thyroid tests in patients still suspected of having Graves' disease or progressive exophthalmos.

### Reference values
▪ TSI doesn't appear in serum usually, but levels equal to or greater than 1.3 index (130% of basal activity) are considered normal.

### Abnormal results
▪ Increased TSI levels are associated with exophthalmos, Graves' disease (thyrotoxicosis), and recurrence of hyperthyroidism.

### Purpose
▪ To help evaluate suspected thyroid disease
▪ To help diagnose suspected thyrotoxicosis, especially in patients with exophthalmos
▪ To monitor treatment of thyrotoxicosis

### Patient preparation
▪ Explain that this test evaluates thyroid function, as appropriate.
▪ Tell the patient that the test requires a blood sample. Explain who will perform the venipuncture and when.
▪ Explain to the patient that he may experience slight discomfort from the tourniquet and needle puncture.

### Procedure and posttest care
▪ Confirm the patient's identity using two patient identifiers according to facility policy.
▪ Perform a venipuncture, and collect the sample in a 5-ml clot-activator tube.

▪ Apply direct pressure to the venipuncture site until bleeding stops.
▪ If a hematoma develops at the venipuncture site, apply warm soaks.
▪ If the patient had a radioactive iodine scan within 48 hours of the test, note this on the laboratory request.

# Viral tests

## Cytomegalovirus antibodies
### [CMV]

After primary infection, cytomegalovirus (CMV) remains latent in white blood cells (WBCs). The presence of CMV antibodies indicates past infection with this virus. In an immunocompromised patient, CMV can be reactivated to cause active infection. Administration of blood or tissue from a seropositive donor may cause active CMV infection in a CMV-seronegative organ transplant recipient or neonate, especially one born prematurely.

Antibodies to CMV can be detected by several methods, including passive hemagglutination, latex agglutination, enzyme immunoassay, and indirect immunofluorescence. The complement fixation test is only 60% sensitive compared with other assays and shouldn't be used to screen for CMV antibodies. Screening tests for CMV antibodies are qualitative; they detect the antibody at a single low dilution. In quantitative methods, several dilutions of the serum sample are tested to detect acute CMV infection.

### Reference values
▪ The patient who has never been infected with CMV has no detectable antibodies to the virus.

■ Immunoglobulin (Ig) G and IgM are normally negative.

## Abnormal results
■ A serum sample collected early during the acute CMV phase or late in the convalescent stage may not contain detectable IgG or IgM antibodies to CMV. Therefore, a negative result doesn't preclude recent infection. More than a single sample is needed to ensure accurate results.
■ A serum sample that tests positive for antibodies at this single dilution indicates that the patient has been infected with CMV and that his WBCs contain latent virus capable of being reactivated in an immunocompromised host.

## Purpose
■ To detect CMV infection in donors and recipients of organs and blood and in immunocompromised patients
■ To screen for CMV infection in infants who require blood transfusions or tissue transplants

## Patient preparation
■ Explain the purpose of the test to the patient or the parents of an infant, as appropriate.
■ Tell the patient that the test requires a blood sample. Explain who will perform the venipuncture and when.
■ Explain to the patient that he may experience slight discomfort from the tourniquet and the needle puncture.

## Procedure and posttest care
■ Confirm the patient's identity using two patient identifiers according to facility policy.
■ Perform a venipuncture, and collect the blood sample in a 5-ml tube designated by the laboratory.
■ Allow the blood to clot for at least 1 hour at room temperature.

■ Apply direct pressure to the venipuncture site until bleeding stops.
■ Because the patient may have a compromised immune system, keep the venipuncture site clean and dry.
■ If a hematoma develops at the venipuncture site, apply warm soaks.

## Precautions
■ Patients with a compromised immune system may not be able to generate antibodies against CMV, resulting in false-negative test results.
■ Immunosuppressed patients without antibodies to CMV should receive blood products or organ transplants from seronegative donors.
■ Patients with CMV antibodies don't require seronegative blood products.

# ▮ Epstein-Barr virus antibodies

Epstein-Barr virus (EBV), a member of the herpesvirus group, causes heterophil-positive infectious mononucleosis, Burkitt's lymphoma, and nasopharyngeal carcinoma. Although the virus doesn't replicate in standard cell cultures, most EBV infections can be recognized by testing the patient's serum for heterophil antibodies (monospot test), which usually appear within the first 3 weeks of illness and then decline rapidly within a few weeks.

In about 10% of adults and a larger percentage of children, the monospot test findings are negative despite primary infection with EBV. Further, EBV has been associated with lymphoproliferative processes in immunosuppressed patients. These disorders occur with reactivated, rather than primary, EBV infections and therefore are also known as monospot-negative. (Most cases of monospot-negative infectious mononucleosis are caused by cytomegalovirus infections.)

Alternatively, EBV-specific antibodies, which develop in response to several antigens of the virus during active infection, can be measured with a high level of sensitivity and specificity by indirect immunofluorescence.

## Normal results

- Sera from patients who have never been infected with EBV have no detectable antibodies to the virus as measured by either the monospot test or the indirect immunofluorescence test.
- The monospot test is positive only during the acute phase of infection with EBV; the indirect immunofluorescence test detects and discriminates between acute and past infection with the virus.

## Abnormal results

- A positive monospot test or an indirect immunofluorescence test that's either immunoglobulin M (IgM)–positive or Epstein-Barr nuclear antigen (EBNA)–negative indicates acute EBV infection.
- A monospot-negative result doesn't necessarily rule out acute or past infection with EBV. Conversely, IgG class antibody to viral capsid antigen and EBNA antigens (IgM-negative) indicates remote (more than 2 months past) infection with EBV.

## Purpose

- To provide a laboratory diagnosis of heterophil- (or monospot-) negative cases of infectious mononucleosis
- To determine the antibody-to-EBV status of immunosuppressed patients with lymphoproliferative processes

## Patient preparation

- Explain the purpose of the test to the patient.
- Tell the patient that the test requires a blood sample. Explain who will perform the venipuncture and when.

- Explain to the patient that he may experience slight discomfort from the tourniquet and needle puncture.

## Procedure and posttest care

- Confirm the patient's identity using two patient identifiers according to facility policy.
- Perform a venipuncture, and collect 5 ml of sterile blood in a clot-activator tube.
- Allow the blood to clot for at least 1 hour at room temperature.
- Apply direct pressure to the venipuncture site until bleeding stops.
- If a hematoma develops at the venipuncture site, apply warm soaks.

# Hepatitis B surface antigen
### [HBsAg, Australian antigen]

Hepatitis B surface antigen (HBsAg) appears in the serum of the patient with hepatitis B virus. It can be detected by radioimmunoassay or, less commonly, reverse passive hemagglutination during the extended incubation period and usually during the first 3 weeks of acute infection or if the patient is a carrier.

Because hepatitis transmission is one of the gravest complications associated with blood transfusion, all donors must be screened for hepatitis B before their blood is stored. This screening, required by the Food and Drug Administration's Bureau of Biologics, has helped reduce the incidence of hepatitis. This test doesn't screen for hepatitis A virus (infectious hepatitis).

For information on related tests, see *Viral hepatitis test panel,* page 212.

## Normal results

- Normal serum is negative for HBsAg.

# Viral hepatitis test panel

The six types of viral hepatitis produce similar symptoms, but differ in transmission mode, course of treatment, prognosis, and carrier status. When the clinical history is insufficient for differentiation, serologic tests can aid in a diagnosis. Testing helps to identify antibodies specific to the causative virus and establish the type of hepatitis:

■ Type A: Detection of an antibody to hepatitis A confirms the diagnosis.

■ Type B: The presence of hepatitis B surface antigens and hepatitis B antibodies confirms the diagnosis.

■ Type C: Diagnosis depends on serologic testing for the specific antibody 1 or more months after the onset of acute illness: until then, diagnosis is established principally by obtaining negative test results for hepatitis A, B, and D.

■ Type D: Detection of intrahepatic delta antigens or immunoglobulin (Ig) M antidelta antigens in acute disease (or IgM and IgG in chronic disease) establishes the diagnosis.

■ Type E: Detection of hepatitis E antigens supports the diagnosis and possibly rules out hepatitis C.

■ Type G: Detection of hepatitis G ribonucleic acid supports the diagnosis (serologic assays are being developed).

Additional findings from liver function studies that support the diagnosis include:

■ Serum aspartate aminotransferase and serum alanine aminotransferase levels increased in the prodromal stage of acute viral hepatitis

■ Serum alkaline phosphatase levels slightly increased

■ Serum bilirubin levels elevated, with levels possibly remaining elevated late in the disease, especially with severe disease

■ Prothrombin time (PT) prolonged (PT of more than 3 seconds longer than normal, indicating severe liver damage)

■ White blood cell counts commonly revealing transient neutropenia and lymphopenia followed by lymphocytosis.

## Abnormal results

■ HBsAg in patients with hepatitis confirms hepatitis B.

■ In chronic carriers and in people with chronic active hepatitis, HBsAg may be present in the serum several months after the onset of acute infection.

■ HBsAg may also appear in the serum of more than 5% of patients with certain diseases other than hepatitis, such as hemophilia, Hodgkin's disease, and leukemia.

■ If HbsAg is found in donor blood, that blood must be discarded because it may transmit hepatitis.

■ Blood samples that test positive for HBsAg should be retested because inaccurate results do occur.

### DRUG CHALLENGE

 Hepatitis B vaccine (possible positive test result)

## Purpose

■ To screen blood donors for hepatitis B

■ To screen people at high risk for contracting hepatitis B; for example, hemodialysis health care workers

■ To aid in the differential diagnosis of viral hepatitis

## Patient preparation

■ Explain that this test helps identify a type of viral hepatitis.

■ Inform the patient that he doesn't need to restrict food and fluids.

- Tell the patient that the test requires a blood sample. Explain who will perform the venipuncture and when.
- Explain to the patient that he may experience slight discomfort from the tourniquet and needle puncture.
- Check the patient's history for administration of hepatitis B vaccine.
- If the patient is giving blood, explain the donation procedure to him.

### Procedure and posttest care
- Confirm the patient's identity using two patient identifiers according to facility policy.
- Perform a venipuncture, and collect the sample in a 10-ml clot-activator tube.
- Apply direct pressure to the venipuncture site until bleeding stops.
- If a hematoma develops at the venipuncture site, apply warm soaks.
- Report confirmed viral hepatitis to public health authorities. This is a reportable disease in most states.

### Precautions
- Wash your hands carefully after the procedure.
- Remember to wear gloves when drawing blood and to dispose of the needle properly.

# Herpes simplex virus antibodies
[HSV]

Herpes simplex virus (HSV), a member of the herpesvirus group, causes various severe manifestations, including genital lesions, keratitis or conjunctivitis, generalized dermal lesions, and pneumonia. Severe involvement is associated with intrauterine or neonatal infections and encephalitis; such infections are most severe in immunosuppressed patients. Of the two closely related antigenic types, type 1 usually causes infections above the waistline; type 2 infections predominantly involve the external genitalia. Primary contact with this virus occurs in early childhood as acute stomatitis or, more commonly, as an inapparent infection. More than 50% of adults have antibodies to HSV.

Sensitive assays, such as indirect immunofluorescence and enzyme immunoassay, are used to demonstrate immunoglobulin (Ig) M class antibodies to HSV or to detect a fourfold or greater increase in IgG class antibodies between acute- and convalescent-phase sera.

### Reference values
- Sera from patients who have never been infected with HSV have no detectable antibodies (less than 1:5). HSV infection can be ruled out in patients whose serum shows no detectable antibodies to the virus.

### Abnormal results
- The presence of IgM or a fourfold or greater increase in IgG antibodies indicates active HSV infection.

### Purpose
- To confirm infections caused by HSV
- To detect recent or past HSV infection

### Patient preparation
- Explain the purpose of the test to the patient.
- Tell the patient that the test requires a blood sample. Explain who will perform the venipuncture and when.
- Explain to the patient that he may experience slight discomfort from the tourniquet and needle puncture.

### Procedure and posttest care
- Confirm the patient's identity using two patient identifiers according to facility policy.

■ Perform a venipuncture, and collect 5 ml of sterile blood in a tube designated by the laboratory.

■ Allow the blood to clot for at least 1 hour at room temperature.

■ Apply direct pressure to the venipuncture site until bleeding stops.

■ If a hematoma develops at the venipuncture site, apply warm soaks.

■ Because the patient may have a compromised immune system, keep the venipuncture site clean and dry.

■ If the patient's immune system is compromised, check the venipuncture site for changes, and report them promptly.

## Precautions

■ A patient infected within the last 3 months may not have developed an antibody response and may have a false-negative test result.

## Heterophil antibodies

Heterophil antibody tests detect and identify two immunoglobulin (Ig) M antibodies in human serum that react against foreign red blood cells (RBCs): Epstein-Barr virus (EBV) antibodies and Forssman antibodies.

In the Paul-Bunnell test—also called the presumptive test—EBV antibodies, found in the sera of patients with infectious mononucleosis, agglutinate with sheep RBCs in a test tube. Forssman antibodies, present in the sera of some healthy people as well as in the sera of patients with such conditions as serum sickness, also agglutinate with sheep RBCs, thus rendering test results inconclusive for infectious mononucleosis.

If the Paul-Bunnell test establishes a presumptive titer, the Davidsohn differential absorption test can then distinguish between EBV and Forssman antibodies. (See *Monospot test for infectious mononucleosis.*)

## Normal results

■ The titer is less than 1:56, but it may be higher in elderly people.

## Abnormal results

■ Although heterophil antibodies are present in the sera of about 80% of patients with infectious mononucleosis 1 month after the disease's onset, a positive finding—a titer higher than 1:56—doesn't confirm this disorder.

■ A high titer can also result from systemic lupus erythematosus, syphilis, cryoglobulinemia, or antibodies to nonsyphilitic treponemata (yaws, pinta, bejel).

■ A gradual increase in the titer during week 3 or 4 followed by a gradual decrease during weeks 4 to 8 proves most conclusive for infectious mononucleosis.

■ A negative titer doesn't always rule out infectious mononucleosis; occasionally, the titer becomes reactive 2 weeks later. Therefore, if symptoms persist, the test should be repeated in 2 weeks.

■ Confirming infectious mononucleosis depends on heterophil agglutination and hematologic tests that show absolute lymphocytosis, with 10% or more atypical lymphocytes.

### DRUG CHALLENGE

 Opioid use and phenytoin therapy (false-positive test results)

## Purpose

■ To aid in the differential diagnosis of infectious mononucleosis

## Patient preparation

■ Explain that this test helps detect infectious mononucleosis.

■ Tell the patient that the test requires a blood sample. Explain who will perform the venipuncture and when.

## Monospot test for infectious mononucleosis

Several screening tests can detect the heterophil infectious mononucleosis (IM) antibody. One of these tests—the monospot—converts the Paul-Bunnell and the Davidsohn differential absorption tests into one rapid slide test without titration. The monospot test relies on agglutination of horse red blood cells (RBCs) by heterophil antibodies.

### Distinguishing antibodies
Because horse RBCs contain Forssman and IM antigens, differential absorption of the patient's serum is necessary to distinguish between them. This is done by mixing the serum sample with guinea pig kidney antigen (containing only Forssman antigen) on one end of a slide and with beef RBC stroma (containing only IM antigen) on the other end of the slide. Each absorbs only the heterophil antibody specific to it. After addition of horse RBCs to each spot, agglutination on the beef cell end of the slide indicates the presence of the IM heterophil antibody and confirms IM.

The monospot test rivals the classic heterophil agglutination test for sensitivity. False-positive results may occur in patients with lymphoma, hepatitis A and B, leukemia, and pancreatic cancer.

▪ Explain to the patient that he may experience slight discomfort from the tourniquet and needle puncture.

### Procedure and posttest care
▪ Confirm the patient's identity using two patient identifiers according to facility policy.
▪ Perform a venipuncture, and collect the sample in a 7-ml clot-activator tube.
▪ Apply direct pressure to the venipuncture site until bleeding stops.
▪ If a hematoma develops at the venipuncture site, apply warm soaks.
▪ If the titer is positive and infectious mononucleosis is confirmed, teach the patient about the treatment plan.
▪ If the titer is positive but infectious mononucleosis isn't confirmed, or if the titer is negative but symptoms persist, explain that additional testing will be necessary in a few days or weeks to confirm the diagnosis and plan effective treatment.

### Precautions
▪ The patient with lymphoma, leukemia, and hepatitis may have a false-positive result.

# Human immunodeficiency virus antibodies
[HIV test]

The human immunodeficiency virus (HIV) antibodies test detects antibodies to HIV in serum. HIV is the virus that causes acquired immunodeficiency syndrome (AIDS). Transmission occurs by direct exposure of a person's blood to body fluids containing the virus. The virus may be transmitted from one person to another through exchange of contaminated blood and blood products, during sexual intercourse with an infected partner, when I.V. drugs are shared, and from an infected mother to her child during pregnancy or breast-feeding.

Initial identification of HIV is usually achieved through enzyme-linked immunosorbent assay. Positive results are confirmed by Western blot test and immunofluorescence. Other available tests may be performed to detect antibodies. (See *Testing for HIV,* page 216.)

# Testing for HIV

More and newer tests are available to help identify human immunodeficiency virus (HIV)–infected antibodies quicker and more conveniently, including a test to identify genetic changes that may alter the patient's course of treatment.

The Centers for Disease Control and Prevention and American Medical Association recommend HIV testing for all patients between the ages of 13 and 64.

## OraQuick rapid HIV-1 antibody test

For the many people each year who don't check back for test results, rapid HIV testing may be performed in any outpatient setting. The OraQuick rapid HIV-1 antibody test, approved by the Food and Drug Administration (FDA), allows results to be obtained in less than 20 minutes using 1 drop of blood. A color indicator similar to a home pregnancy test is used. If the test result is positive, another test must be done to confirm the results.

## Nucleic acid test

The FDA has also approved a nucleic acid test to screen plasma donation for HIV and hepatitis C. This test has dramatically reduced the waiting time involved until blood and blood products may be used.

## Gene-based test

Spikes of HIV virus in the bloodstream commonly mean that the individual being treated for HIV is growing resistant to his current drug treatment. The government has approved the first gene-based test to help determine if an HIV-infected person's virus is mutating, thereby causing therapy to fail. This test can help the physician select more appropriate treatment.

## Normal results

- Test results are negative.

## Abnormal results

- Although the test detects previous exposure to HIV, it doesn't identify a patient who has been exposed to HIV but hasn't yet made antibodies.
- In most cases, the patient with AIDS has antibodies to HIV.
- A positive test for the HIV antibody can't determine whether a patient harbors actively replicating virus or when the patient will show signs and symptoms of AIDS.
- Many apparently healthy people have been exposed to HIV and have circulating antibodies. The test results for such people aren't considered false-positives.
- Patients in the later stages of AIDS may exhibit no detectable antibody in their sera because they can no longer mount an antibody response.

## Purpose

- To screen for HIV in the high-risk patient
- To screen donated blood for HIV

## Patient preparation

- Explain to the patient that this test detects HIV infection.
- Provide adequate counseling about the reasons for performing the test, which is usually requested by the patient's practitioner.
- If the patient has questions about his condition, be sure to provide full and accurate information.
- Tell the patient that the test requires a blood sample. Explain who will perform the venipuncture and when.
- Explain to the patient that he may experience slight discomfort from the tourniquet and needle puncture.

## Procedure and posttest care

- Confirm the patient's identity using two patient identifiers according to facility policy.
- Perform a venipuncture, and collect the sample in a 10-ml barrier tube. Barrier tubes help prevent contamination when pouring out the serum in the laboratory.
- Apply direct pressure to the venipuncture site until bleeding stops.
- Because the patient may have a compromised immune system, keep the venipuncture site clean and dry.
- If a hematoma develops at the venipuncture site, apply warm soaks.
- Keep test results confidential.
- When the patient receives the results, give him another opportunity to ask questions.
- Encourage the patient who tests positive for HIV to seek medical follow-up care, even if he's asymptomatic.
- Give the patient with positive results information regarding counseling or support groups if he is interested
- Tell the patient to report early signs of AIDS, such as fever, weight loss, axillary or inguinal lymphadenopathy, rash, and persistent cough or diarrhea. Women should also report gynecologic symptoms.
- Tell the patient to assume that he can transmit HIV to others until conclusively proved otherwise. To prevent possible virus transmission, advise him about safer sex practices.
- Instruct the patient not to share razors, toothbrushes, or utensils (which may be contaminated with blood) and to clean such items with household bleach: one part bleach to ten parts water.
- Advise the patient against donating blood, tissues, or an organ.
- Warn the patient to inform his practitioner and dentist about his condition so that they can take proper precautions.

# Parvovirus B19 antibodies

Parvovirus B19, a small, single-stranded deoxyribonucleic acid (DNA) virus belonging to the family *Parvoviridae*, destroys red blood cell (RBC) precursors and interferes with normal RBC production. The virus is also associated with erythema infectiosum (a self-limiting, low-grade fever and rash in young children) and aplastic crisis (in patients with chronic hemolytic anemia and immunodeficient patients with bone marrow failure). Immunoglobulin (Ig) G and IgM antibodies can be detected by enzyme-linked immunosorbent assay and immunofluorescence.

## Normal results

- Test results are negative for IgM- and IgG-specific antibodies to parvovirus B19.

## Abnormal results

- About 50% of all adults lack immunity to parvovirus B19, with as many as 20% of susceptible adults becoming infected after exposure.
- Positive test findings are associated with joint arthralgia, hydrops fetalis, fetal loss, transient aplastic anemia, chronic anemia in immunocompromised patients, and bone marrow failure.
- Abnormal results for parvovirus B19 should be confirmed using the Western blot test.

## Purpose

- To detect parvovirus B19 antibody, especially in prospective organ donors
- To diagnose erythema infectiosum, parvovirus B19 aplastic crisis, and related parvovirus B19 diseases

## Patient preparation

- Explain the test purpose and procedure to the patient. To a potential organ donor, explain that the test is part of a panel of tests performed before organ donation to protect the organ recipient from potential infection.

- Tell the patient that the test requires a blood sample. Explain who will perform the venipuncture and when.
- Explain to the patient that he may experience slight discomfort from the tourniquet and needle puncture.

### Procedure and posttest care

- Confirm the patient's identity using two patient identifiers according to facility policy.
- Perform a venipuncture, and collect the blood sample in a 5-ml clot-activator tube.

D O ' S  &  D O N ' T S

Place the sample on ice immediately after collection.

- Apply direct pressure to the venipuncture site until bleeding stops.
- If a hematoma develops at the venipuncture site, apply warm soaks.

## Rubella antibodies
### [German measles]

Although rubella is usually a mild viral infection in children and young adults, it can produce severe infection in the fetus, resulting in spontaneous abortion, stillbirth, or congenital rubella syndrome. Because rubella infection normally induces immunoglobulin (Ig) G and IgM antibody production, measuring rubella antibodies can determine present infection as well as immunity resulting from past infection. The hemagglutination inhibition test is the most commonly used serologic test for rubella antibodies.

Suspected cases of congenital rubella may be confirmed if rubella-specific IgM antibodies are present in the infant's serum. Immune status in adults can be confirmed by an existing IgG-specific titer.

Exposure risk (when the immunity status is unknown) may be evaluated using two serum samples. The first serum sample should be drawn in the acute phase of clinical symptoms. If clinical symptoms aren't apparent, the sample should be drawn as soon as possible after the suspected exposure. The second sample should be drawn 3 to 4 weeks later during the convalescent phase.

### Reference values

- An IgG titer of 1:8 or less indicates little or no immunity against rubella; titer more than 1:10 indicates adequate protection against rubella.
- IgM results are reported as positive or negative.

### Abnormal results

- The presence of rubella-specific IgM antibodies indicates recent infection in an adult and congenital rubella in an infant.

### Purpose

- To diagnose rubella infection, especially congenital infection
- To determine susceptibility to rubella in children and in women of childbearing age

### Patient preparation

- Explain that this test diagnoses or evaluates susceptibility to rubella.
- Inform the patient that she doesn't need to restrict food and fluids.
- Tell the patient that this test requires a blood sample and that if a current infection is suspected, a second blood sample will be needed in 2 to 3 weeks to identify a rise in the titer.

- Explain who will perform the venipuncture and when.
- Explain to the patient that she may experience slight discomfort from the tourniquet and needle puncture.

### Procedure and posttest care

- Confirm the patient's identity using two patient identifiers according to facility policy.
- Perform a venipuncture, and collect the blood sample in a 7-ml clot-activator tube.
- Apply direct pressure to the venipuncture site until bleeding stops.
- If a hematoma develops at the venipuncture site, apply warm soaks.
- Instruct the patient to return for an additional blood test, when appropriate.
- If a woman of childbearing age is found to be susceptible to rubella, explain that vaccination can prevent rubella and that she must wait at least 3 months after the vaccination to become pregnant or risk permanent damage or death to the fetus.
- If the pregnant patient is found to be susceptible to rubella, instruct her to return for follow-up rubella antibody tests to detect possible subsequent infection.
- If the test confirms rubella in a pregnant patient, provide emotional support. As needed, refer her for appropriate counseling.

## Bacterial and fungal tests

### ▍Antistreptolysin-O

The antistreptolysin-O test measures the relative serum concentrations of the antibody to streptolysin-O (known as ASO). A serum sample is diluted with a commercial preparation of streptolysin-O and incubated. After the addition of human red blood cells, the tube is reincubated and examined visually. Failure of hemolysis to develop indicates recent streptococcal infection. The end point is read in Todd units, the reciprocal of the highest dilution (titer) that inhibits hemolysis.

### Reference values

- Even healthy people have some detectable ASO titers from previous minor streptococcal infections.
- Normal ASO titer for school-age children is 170 Todd units/ml; for preschoolers and adults it is 85 Todd units/ml.

### Abnormal results

- High ASO titers usually occur only after prolonged or recurrent infections.
- Usually, a titer higher than 166 Todd units/ml is considered a definite elevation. A higher titer doesn't necessarily mean that rheumatic fever or glomerulonephritis is present; however, it does indicate a streptococcal infection.
- Low ASO titers is good evidence of the absence of active rheumatic fever.
- Serial titers, determined at 10- to 14-day intervals, provide more reliable information than a single titer. An increase in titer 2 to 5 weeks after the acute infection, which peaks 4 to 6 weeks after the initial increase, confirms poststreptococcal disease.

**DRUG CHALLENGE**

 Antibiotic or corticosteroid therapy (possible suppression of the streptococcal antibody response)

### Purpose

- To confirm recent or ongoing streptococcal infection
- To help diagnose rheumatic fever and poststreptococcal glomerulonephritis in

## Test for anti-DNase B

The antideoxyribonuclease B (anti-DNase B) test, a process similar to the antistreptolysin-O (ASO) test, detects antibodies to DNase B, a potent antigen produced by all group A streptococci.

For adults, normal anti-DNase B titer is less than 85 Todd units/ml; for school-age children, it's less than 170 Todd units/ml; and for pre-schoolers, it's less than 60 Todd units/ml.

Elevated anti-DNase B titers appear in 80% of patients with acute rheumatic fever, in 75% of those with poststreptococcal glomerulonephritis (following streptococcal pharyngitis), and in 60% of those with glomerulonephritis (following group A streptococcal pyoderma). This is a much higher percentage than those with ASO titer elevations (25%), making the test for anti-DNase B especially valuable in detecting a reaction to group A streptococcal pyoderma.

Other streptococcal antigens are of limited diagnostic value, or their use is controversial.

the presence of clinical symptoms (See *Test for anti-DNase B*, for information about another method of diagnosing these two diseases.)

- To distinguish between rheumatic fever and rheumatoid arthritis when patient reports joint pain

### Patient preparation

- Explain that this test detects an immunologic response to certain bacteria (streptococci).
- Inform the patient that he doesn't need to restrict food and fluids.
- Tell the patient that the test requires a blood sample. Explain who will perform the venipuncture and when.

- Explain to the patient that he may experience slight discomfort from the tourniquet and needle puncture.
- If the test will be repeated at regular intervals to identify active and inactive states of rheumatic fever or to confirm acute glomerulonephritis, tell the patient that measuring changes in antibody levels helps determine the effectiveness of therapy.
- Check the patient's history for drugs that may suppress the streptococcal antibody responses. If the drug therapy must continue, note this on the laboratory request.

### Procedure and posttest care

- Confirm the patient's identity using two patient identifiers according to facility policy.
- Perform a venipuncture, and collect the sample in a 7-ml tube without additives.
- Apply direct pressure to the venipuncture site until bleeding stops.
- If a hematoma develops at the venipuncture site, apply warm soaks.

### Precautions

- Streptococcal skin infection will seldom produce an abnormal ASO titer even with post-streptococcal disease (false-negative).

# Bacterial meningitis antigen

The bacterial meningitis antigen test can detect specific antigens of *Streptococcus pneumoniae, Neisseria meningitidis,* and *Haemophilus influenzae* type B, the principal agents causing meningitis. The test can be performed on samples of serum, cerebrospinal fluid (CSF), urine, pleural fluid, and joint fluid, but CSF and urine are preferred.

## Normal results
- Results are negative for bacterial antigens.

## Abnormal results
- Positive results identify the specific bacterial antigen: *S. pneumoniae, N. meningitidis, H. influenzae* type B, or group B streptococci.

**DRUG CHALLENGE**

 Previous antimicrobial therapy

## Purpose
- To identify the agent causing meningitis
- To help diagnose bacterial meningitis
- To help diagnose meningitis when results of the Gram stain smear and culture are negative

## Patient preparation
- Explain the purpose of the test to the patient as appropriate.
- Inform the patient that this test requires a specimen of urine or CSF. Explain who will perform the procedure and when.
- If a CSF specimen is required, describe how it will be obtained by lumbar puncture.
- Explain to the patient that he may experience discomfort from the needle puncture.
- Advise the patient that a headache is the most common complication of lumbar puncture, but that his cooperation during the test minimizes such an effect.
- Make sure the patient or a responsible family member has signed an informed consent form.

## Procedure and posttest care
- Confirm the patient's identity using two patient identifiers according to facility policy.
- Collect a 10-ml urine specimen or a 1-ml CSF specimen in a sterile container.

## Precautions
- Maintain specimen sterility during collection.
- Place the specimen on a refrigerated coolant, and send it to the laboratory immediately.

# Febrile agglutination

Sometimes bacterial infections (such as tularemia, brucellosis, and the disorders caused by *Salmonella*) and rickettsial infections (such as Rocky Mountain spotted fever and typhus) cause puzzling fevers, called fevers of undetermined origin (FUO). In these infections and others in which microorganisms are difficult to isolate from blood or excreta, febrile agglutination tests can provide important diagnostic information.

The Weil-Felix test for rickettsial disease, Widal's test for *Salmonella*, and tests for brucellosis and tularemia are essentially the same. In these tests, a serum sample is mixed with a few drops of prepared antigens in normal saline solution on a slide, and the reaction is observed.

The Weil-Felix test establishes rickettsial antibody titers. It uses three forms of Proteus antigens (OX-19, OX-2, and OX-K) that cross-react with the various strains of rickettsiae. Antibodies to certain rickettsial strains react with more than one Proteus antigen, whereas antibodies to other strains fail to react with any Proteus antigens.

Widal's test establishes the titers for flagellar (H) and somatic (O) antigens,

which may indicate *Salmonella* gastroenteritis and extraintestinal focal infections, caused by *S. enteritidis*, or enteric
(typhoid) fever, caused by *S. typhosa*. A
third antigen, the Vi or envelope antigen, may indicate typhoid carrier status,
which commonly tests negative for H
and O antigens. Widal's test isn't recommended for diagnosing *Salmonella* gastroenteritis.

Slide agglutination and tube dilution
tests, using killed suspensions of the
disease organisms as antigens, establish
titers for the gram-negative coccobacilli
*Brucella* and *Francisella tularensis*, which
cause brucellosis and tularemia, respectively.

### Reference values
- Normal dilutions are:
  - Salmonella antibody: < 1:80
  - Brucellosis antibody: < 1:80
  - Tularemia antibody: < 1:40
  - Rickettsial antibody: < 1:40.

### Abnormal results
- Observed rise and fall of titers is crucial for detecting active infection. If this
isn't possible, certain titer levels can suggest the disorder.
- For all febrile agglutinins, a fourfold
increase in titers is strong evidence of
infection.
- The Weil-Felix test is positive for rickettsiae with antibodies to Proteus 6 to
12 days after infection; titers peak in 1
month and usually drop to negative in 5
or 6 months. This test can't be used to
diagnose rickettsialpox or Q fever because the antibodies of these diseases
don't cross-react with Proteus antigens;
the test shows positive titers in Proteus
infections and, in such cases, is nonspecific for rickettsiae.
- In *Salmonella* infection, H and O agglutinins usually appear in serum after 1
week, and titers rise for 3 to 6 weeks. O
agglutinins usually fall to insignificant

levels in 6 to 12 months. Agglutinin
titers may remain elevated for years.
- In brucellosis, titers usually rise after 2
to 3 weeks and reach their highest levels
between 4 and 8 weeks. The absence of
*Brucella* agglutinins doesn't rule out brucellosis.
- In tularemia, titers usually become
positive during week 2 of infection, exceed 1:320 by week 3, peak within 4 to
7 weeks, and usually decline gradually 1
year after recovery.

**DRUG CHALLENGE**

 Antibiotics (low titers early in
the course of infection)

### Purpose
- To support clinical findings in diagno-
sis of disorders caused by *Salmonella*,
*Rickettsia*, *F. tularensis*, and *Brucella* or-
ganisms
- To identify the cause of FUO

### Patient preparation
- Explain that this test detects and quan-
tifies microorganisms that may cause
fever and other symptoms.
- Inform the patient that he doesn't need
to restrict food and fluids.
- Tell the patient that the test requires a
blood sample. Explain who will perform
the venipuncture and when.
- Explain to the patient that he may experience slight discomfort from the
tourniquet and needle puncture.
- Explain to the patient that this test requires a series of blood samples to detect a pattern of titers characteristic of
the suspected disorder if appropriate.
Reassure him that a positive titer only
suggests a disorder.
- Note on the laboratory request when
antimicrobial therapy began if appropriate.

## Procedure and posttest care

- Confirm the patient's identity using two patient identifiers according to facility policy.
- Perform a venipuncture, and collect the sample in a 7-ml clot-activator tube.
- Apply direct pressure to the venipuncture site until bleeding stops.
- If a hematoma develops at the venipuncture site, apply warm soaks.
- In FUO and suspected infection, contact the facility's infection control department. Isolation may be necessary.

## Precautions

- Vaccination or continuous exposure to bacterial or rickettsial infection may result in immunity or high titer levels.
- An immunocompromised patient may have negative titers despite symptomatic infection due to inability to form antibodies.
- Hepatic disease or excessive drug use may cause high *Salmonella* titers.

# Fungal serology

Most fungal organisms enter the body as spores inhaled into the lungs or infiltrated through wounds in the skin or mucosa. If the body's defenses can't destroy the organisms initially, the fungi multiply to form lesions; blood and lymph vessels may then spread the mycoses throughout the body. Most healthy people easily overcome initial mycotic infection, but elderly people and others with a deficient immune system are more susceptible to acute or chronic mycotic infection and to disorders secondary to such infection. Mycosis may be deep-seated or superficial. Deep-seated mycosis occurs primarily in the lungs; superficial mycosis, in the skin or mucosal linings.

Although cultures are usually performed to diagnose mycoses by identifying the causative organism, serologic tests occasionally provide the sole evidence for mycosis. Such serologic tests use immunodiffusion, complement fixation, precipitin, latex agglutination, or agglutination methods to demonstrate the presence of specific mycotic antibodies. (See *Serum test methods for fungal infections,* pages 224 and 225.)

## Normal results

- Depending on the test method, a negative finding, or normal titer, usually indicates the absence of mycosis.

## Abnormal results

- *Serum test methods for fungal infections* explains the significance of findings for specific organisms.

## Purpose

- To rapidly detect antifungal antibodies, aiding in the diagnosis of mycoses
- To monitor the effectiveness of therapy for mycoses

## Patient preparation

- Explain that this test aids in diagnosing certain fungal infections. If appropriate, tell him that this test monitors his response to antimycotic therapy and that it may be necessary to repeat the test.
- Instruct him to restrict food and fluids for 12 to 24 hours before the test.
- Tell the patient that the test requires a blood sample. Explain who will perform the venipuncture and when.
- Explain to the patient that he may experience slight discomfort from the tourniquet and needle puncture.

## Procedure and posttest care

- Confirm the patient's identity using two patient identifiers according to facility policy.
- Perform a venipuncture, and collect the sample in a 10-ml sterile clot-activator tube.

# Serum test methods for fungal infections

| Disease and normal values | Clinical significance of abnormal results |
|---|---|
| **Aspergillosis** | |
| Complement fixation: titers < 1:8 | Titers > 1:8 suggest infection; 70% to 90% of patients with known pulmonary aspergillosis or aspergillus allergy present antibodies. This test can't detect invasive aspergillosis because patients with this disease don't have antibodies; biopsy is required. |
| Immunodiffusion: negative | One or more precipitin bands suggests infection. The number of bands is related to complement fixation titers; the more precipitin bands, the higher the titer. |
| **Blastomycosis** | |
| Complement fixation: titers < 1:8 | Titers ranging from 1:8 to 1:16 suggest infection; titers > 1:32 denote active disease. A rising titer in serial samples taken every 3 to 4 weeks indicates disease progression; a falling titer indicates regression. This test has limited diagnostic value because of a high percentage of false-negatives. |
| Immunodiffusion: negative | A more sensitive test for blastomycosis; detects 80% of infected people. |
| **Coccidioidomycosis** | |
| Complement fixation: titers < 1:2 | Most sensitive test for this fungus. Titers ranging from 1:2 to 1:4 suggest active infection; titers > 1:16 usually denote active disease. Test may remain active in mild infections. |
| Immunodiffusion: negative | Most useful for screening, followed by complement fixation test for confirmation. |
| Precipitin: titers < 1:16 | Good screening test; titers > 1:16 usually indicate infection. About 80% of infected people show positive titers by 2 weeks; most revert to negative by 6 months. Early primary disease is shown by positive precipitin and negative complement fixation test. A positive complement fixation and negative precipitin test indicate chronic disease. |

## Serum test methods for fungal infections (continued)

| Disease and normal values | Clinical significance of abnormal results |
|---|---|
| **Cryptococcosis** | |
| Latex agglutination for cryptococcal antigen: negative | About 90% of patients with cryptococcal meningitis exhibit positive latex agglutination in cerebrospinal fluid (CSF). (Serum is less frequently positive than CSF.) Culturing is definitive because false-positives do occur. (Presence of rheumatoid factor may cause a positive reaction.) Serum antigen tests are positive in 33% of patients with pulmonary cryptococcosis; biopsy is usually required. |
| **Histoplasmosis** | |
| Complement fixation (histoplasmin): titers < 1:8 | Titers ranging from 1:8 to 1:16 suggest infection; titers > 1:32 indicate active disease. Antibodies generally appear 10 to 21 days after initial infection. Test is positive in 10% to 15% of cases. |
| Complement fixation: titers < 1:18 | Titers ranging from 1:8 to 1:16 suggest infection; titers > 1:32 indicate active disease. More sensitive than histoplasmin complement fixation test; gives positive results in 75% to 80% of cases. (Histoplasmin and yeast antigens are positive in 10% of cases.) A rising titer in serial samples taken every 2 to 3 weeks indicates progressive infection; a decreasing titer indicates regression. |
| Immunodiffusion (histoplasmin): negative | Appearance of H and M bands indicates active infection. If the M band appears first and lasts longer than the H band, the infection may be regressing. The M band alone may indicate early infection, chronic disease, or a recent skin test. |
| **Sporotrichosis** | |
| Agglutination: titers < 1:40 | Titers > 1:80 usually indicate active infection. The test usually is negative in cutaneous infections and positive in extracutaneous infections. |

- Apply direct pressure to the venipuncture site until bleeding stops.
- If a hematoma develops at the venipuncture site, apply warm soaks.

### Precautions
- Recent skin testing with fungal antigens may cause high titers.
- Mycosis-caused immunosuppression may cause low titers or a false-negative result.

# Helicobacter pylori antibodies
## [H. pylori test]

Helicobacter pylori is a spiral, gram-negative bacterium associated with chronic gastritis and idiopathic chronic duodenal ulceration. Although a gastric specimen can be obtained by endoscopy and cultured for H. pylori, the H. pylori antibody blood test is a more useful noninvasive screening procedure and may be performed using the enzyme-linked immunosorbent assay. (See Additional tests for Helicobacter pylori.)

## Normal results
- No antibodies to H. pylori are seen.

## Abnormal results
- A positive H. pylori test result indicates that the patient has antibodies to the bacterium.
- The serologic results should be interpreted in light of the clinical findings.

## Purpose
- To help diagnose H. pylori infection in the patient with GI symptoms

## Patient preparation
- Explain that this test is used to diagnose the infection that may cause ulcers.
- Inform the patient that he doesn't need to restrict food and fluids.
- Tell the patient that the test requires a blood sample. Explain who will perform the venipuncture and when.
- Explain to the patient that he may experience slight discomfort from the tourniquet and needle puncture.

---

## Additional tests for Helicobacter pylori

Helicobacter pylori is diagnosed through blood, breath, stool, and tissue tests. Blood tests are the most common. They detect antibodies to H. pylori bacteria.

Urea breath tests are an effective diagnostic tool for H. pylori. They are also used after treatment to see whether treatment was effective. In the physician's office, the patient drinks a urea solution that contains a special carbon atom. If H. pylori is present, it breaks down the urea, releasing the carbon. The blood carries the carbon to the lungs, where the patient exhales it. The breath test is 96% to 98% accurate.

Stool tests may be used to detect H. pylori infection in the patient's stool. Studies show that this test, called the H. pylori stool antigen (HpSA) test is accurate for diagnosing H. pylori.

Tissue tests are usually performed using the biopsy sample taken with the endoscope. There are three types:
- The rapid urease detects the enzyme disease produced by H. pylori.
- A histology test allows the physician to find and examine the actual bacteria.
- A culture test involves allowing H. pylori to grow in the tissue sample.

In diagnosing H. pylori, blood, breath, and stool tests are commonly done before tissue tests because they are less invasive. However, blood tests aren't used to detect H. pylori following treatment because a patient's blood can show positive results even after H. pylori has been eliminated.

Source: U.S. National Institute of Diabetes & Digestive & Kidney Diseases of the National Institutes of Health, 2003.

## Procedure and posttest care

- Confirm the patient's identity using two patient identifiers according to facility policy.
- Perform a venipuncture, and collect the blood sample in a 7-ml clot-activator tube.
- Send the blood sample to the laboratory immediately.
- Apply direct pressure to the venipuncture site until bleeding stops.
- If a hematoma develops at the venipuncture site, apply warm soaks.

### Precautions

- This test should be performed only on a patient with GI symptoms because of the large number of healthy people who have *H. pylori* antibodies.

# ▌Lyme disease serology

Lyme disease is a multisystem disorder characterized by dermatologic, neurologic, cardiac, and rheumatic manifestations in various stages. Epidemiologic and serologic studies implicate a common tickborne spirochete, *Borrelia burgdorferi*, as the causative agent. Serologic tests for Lyme disease, both indirect immunofluorescent and enzyme-linked immunosorbent assays, measure antibody response to this spirochete and indicate current infection or past exposure. Serologic tests can identify 50% of patients with early-stage Lyme disease and all patients with later complications of carditis, neuritis, and arthritis or patients in remission.

In an indirect immunofluorescent assay, *B. burgdorferi* is grown in culture, fixed to a microscope slide, and then incubated with a human serum sample. A fluorescein-labeled antiglobulin is then introduced into the antigen-antibody complex. Any human antibody that binds to the spirochete is detected by viewing (under an ultraviolet microscope) the fluorescent antiglobulin that attaches to it.

### Reference values

- Normal serum values are nonreactive.

### Abnormal results

- A positive result can help confirm the diagnosis but isn't definitive.
- Other treponemal diseases and high rheumatoid factor titers can cause false-positive results.
- More than 15% of patients with Lyme disease fail to develop antibodies.

### Purpose

- To confirm a Lyme disease diagnosis

### Patient preparation

- Explain that this test helps determine whether the patient's symptoms are caused by Lyme disease.
- Instruct the patient to fast for 12 hours before the blood sample is drawn, but to drink fluids as usual.
- Tell the patient that the test requires a blood sample. Explain who will perform the venipuncture and when.
- Explain to the patient that he may experience slight discomfort from the tourniquet and needle puncture.

### Procedure and posttest care

- Confirm the patient's identity using two patient identifiers according to facility policy.
- Perform a venipuncture, and collect the sample in a 7-ml clot-activator tube.
- Apply direct pressure to the venipuncture site until bleeding stops.
- If a hematoma develops at the venipuncture site, apply warm soaks.

# Syphilis tests

## Fluorescent treponemal antibody absorption
### [FTA-ABS, FTA]

The fluorescent treponemal antibody absorption test uses indirect immunofluorescence to detect antibodies to the spirochete *Treponema pallidum* in serum. This spirochete causes syphilis.

In this test, prepared *T. pallidum* is fixed on a slide, and the patient's serum is added after the addition of an absorbed preparation of Reiter treponema. This addition to the test serum prevents interference by antibodies from nonsyphilitic treponemas; Reiter treponema combines with most nonsyphilitic antibodies, making the FTA-ABS test specific for *T. pallidum*.

If syphilitic antibodies are present in the test serum, they will coat the treponemal organisms. The slide is then stained with fluorescein-labeled antiglobulin. This antiglobulin attaches to the coated spirochetes, which fluoresce when viewed under an ultraviolet microscope.

Although the FTA-ABS test is generally performed on a serum sample to detect primary or secondary syphilis, a cerebrospinal fluid (CSF) specimen is required to detect tertiary syphilis. Because antibody levels remain constant for long periods, the FTA-ABS test isn't recommended for monitoring the patient's response to therapy. (See *Two tests for* Treponema pallidum.)

### Normal results
- No treponemal antibodies are found in the serum—a nonreactive test result.
- A nonreactive test result doesn't necessarily rule out syphilis. *T. pallidum* causes no detectable immunologic changes in the blood for 14 to 21 days after initial infection. Darkfield microscopy of exudate from suspicious lesions can provide early diagnosis by identifying the causative spirochetes.

### Abnormal results
- Treponemal antibodies are detected in the serum—a reactive test result. This doesn't indicate the stage or severity of infection. (These antibodies identified in the CSF provides strong evidence of tertiary neurosyphilis.)
- High antibody levels appear in most patients with primary syphilis and in almost all patients with secondary syphilis. High antibody levels persist for several years, with or without treatment.
- Low antibody levels and other nonspecific factors produce borderline findings. In such cases, repeated testing and a thorough review of the patient's history may be productive.

---

### Two tests for *Treponema pallidum*

The microhemagglutination assay for the *Treponema pallidum* antibody increases the specificity of syphilis testing by eliminating methodologic interference. In this assay, tanned sheep red blood cells are coated with *T. pallidum* antigen and combined with absorbed test serum. Hemagglutination occurs when specific anti-*T. pallidum* antibodies are in the serum.

In the enzyme-linked immunosorbent assay, tubes coated with *T. pallidum* are washed and then treated with enzyme-labeled antihuman globulin. After the substrate for the enzymes is added to the tubes, the enzymatic activity is measured by quantitating the product formed by the reaction.

- Although the FTA-ABS test is specific, some patients with nonsyphilitic conditions, such as systemic lupus erythematosus, genital herpes, and increased or abnormal globulins, or those who are pregnant may show minimally reactive levels.
- The FTA-ABS test doesn't always distinguish between *T. pallidum* and certain other treponemas, such as those that cause pinta, yaws, and bejel.

### Purpose
- To confirm primary and secondary syphilis
- To screen for suspected false-positive results of Venereal Disease Research Laboratories tests

### Patient preparation
- Explain that this test can confirm or rule out syphilis.
- Inform the patient that he doesn't need to restrict food and fluids.
- Tell the patient that the test requires a blood sample. Explain who will perform the venipuncture and when.
- Inform the patient that he may experience slight discomfort from the tourniquet and the needle puncture.

### Procedure and posttest care
- Confirm the patient's identity using two patient identifiers according to facility policy.
- Perform a venipuncture, and collect the sample in a 7-ml clot-activator tube.
- Apply direct pressure to the venipuncture site until bleeding stops.
- If a hematoma develops at the venipuncture site, apply warm soaks.
- If the test result is reactive, explain the nature of syphilis, and stress the importance of proper treatment and the need to find and treat the patient's sexual contacts.
- Provide the patient with additional information about syphilis and how it's

spread; emphasize the need for antibiotic therapy, if appropriate. Report positive results to state public health authorities, and prepare the patient for mandatory inquiries.
- If the test result is nonreactive or findings are borderline, but syphilis hasn't been ruled out, instruct the patient to return for follow-up testing. Explain that inconclusive results don't necessarily mean that he's free of disease.

## VDRL test

The Venereal Disease Research Laboratory (VDRL) test, a flocculation test, is widely used to screen for primary and secondary syphilis. Although the test has diagnostic significance during the first two stages of syphilis, transient or permanent biologic false-positive reactions can make accurate interpretation difficult. A biologic false-positive reaction can result from viral or bacterial infection, chronic systemic illness, or nonsyphilitic treponemal disease. Usually, a serum sample is used in the VDRL test, but this test may also be performed on a cerebrospinal fluid (CSF) specimen obtained by lumbar puncture to test for tertiary syphilis. The VDRL test of CSF is less sensitive than the fluorescent treponemal antibody absorption test.

The rapid plasma reagin test can also be used to diagnose syphilis. (See *Rapid plasma reagin test,* page 230.)

### Normal results
- Normal serum shows no flocculation and is reported as nonreactive.
- A nonreactive test doesn't rule out syphilis because *T. pallidum* causes no detectable immunologic changes in the serum for 14 to 21 days after infection. Darkfield microscopy of exudate from suspicious lesions can provide early diagnosis by identifying the causative spirochetes.

# Rapid plasma reagin test

The rapid plasma reagin (RPR) test is a rapid, macroscopic serologic test that's an acceptable substitute for the VDRL test in diagnosing syphilis. The RPR test, available as a kit, uses a cardiolipin antigen to detect reagin, the antibody relatively specific for *Treponema pallidum*, the agent that causes syphilis.

In the RPR test, the patient's serum is mixed with cardiolipin on a plastic-coated card, rotated mechanically, and then examined with the unaided eye. If flocculation occurs, the test sample is diluted until no visible reaction occurs. The last dilution to show visible flocculation is the titer of the reagin antibody.

In the RPR test, like the VDRL test, normal serum shows no flocculation.

## Abnormal results

- Definite flocculation is reported as a reactive test result; slight flocculation is reported as a weakly reactive test result.
- A reactive VDRL test occurs in about 50% of patients with primary syphilis and in nearly all patients with secondary syphilis.
- If syphilitic lesions exist, a reactive VDRL test is diagnostic. If no lesions are evident, a reactive VDRL test necessitates repeated testing.
- Biologic false-positive reactions can be caused by conditions unrelated to syphilis; for example, infectious mononucleosis, malaria, leprosy, hepatitis, systemic lupus erythematosus, rheumatoid arthritis, and nonsyphilitic treponemal diseases, such as pinta and yaws.
- A reactive VDRL test using a CSF specimen indicates neurosyphilis, which can follow the primary and secondary stages in patients who remain untreated.

## Purpose

- To screen for primary and secondary syphilis
- To confirm primary or secondary syphilis in patients with syphilitic lesions
- To monitor the patient's response to treatment

## Patient preparation

- Explain to the patient that this test detects syphilis.
- Inform the patient that the disease usually goes undetected in the general population because infected people remain untreated.
- Tell the patient that he doesn't need to restrict food, fluids, or medications but should abstain from alcohol for 24 hours before the test.
- Tell the patient that the test requires a blood sample. Explain who will perform the venipuncture and when.
- Explain to the patient that he may experience slight discomfort from the tourniquet and needle puncture.

## Procedure and posttest care

- Confirm the patient's identity using two patient identifiers according to facility policy.
- Perform a venipuncture, and collect the sample in a 7-ml clot-activator tube.
- Apply direct pressure to the venipuncture site until bleeding stops.
- If a hematoma develops at the venipuncture site, apply warm soaks.
- If the test result is nonreactive or borderline but syphilis hasn't been ruled out, instruct the patient to return for follow-up testing. Explain that borderline test results don't necessarily mean that he's free of disease.
- If the test is reactive, explain the importance of proper treatment. Provide the patient with further information about sexually transmitted diseases and how they're spread, and stress the need

for antibiotic therapy. Report the results to state public health authorities, and prepare the patient for mandatory inquiries.

■ If the test is reactive but the patient shows no clinical signs of syphilis, explain that many uninfected people show false-positive reactions. Stress the need for further specific tests to rule out syphilis.

### Precautions

■ An immunosuppressed patient may have a false-negative test result.

# Fetal antigen tests

## Alpha-fetoprotein
### [AFP]

Alpha-fetoprotein (AFP) is a glycoprotein produced by fetal tissue and tumors that differentiate from midline embryonic structures. During fetal development, AFP levels in serum and amniotic fluid rise. AFP crosses the placenta and appears in maternal serum.

High maternal serum AFP levels may suggest fetal neural tube defects, such as spina bifida and anencephaly, but positive confirmation requires amniocentesis and ultrasonography. Other congenital anomalies, such as Down syndrome and other chromosomal disorders, may be associated with low maternal serum AFP levels.

Elevated AFP levels in the patient who isn't pregnant may occur in cancers, such as hepatocellular carcinoma, or certain nonmalignant conditions such as ataxia-telangiectasia. In these conditions, AFP assays are more useful for monitoring the patient's response to therapy than for diagnosis. AFP levels are best determined by enzyme immunoassay on amniotic fluid or serum.

### Reference values

■ In men and nonpregnant women, when testing by immunoassay, AFP levels are less than 15 ng/ml (SI, < 15 mg/L).

■ In pregnant women, AFP levels are less than 25 ng/ml (SI, < 25 mg/L). At 15 to 18 weeks' gestation, values range from 10 to 150 ng/ml (SI, 10 to 150 mg/L).

### Abnormal results

■ High AFP levels in pregnant women may suggest neural tube defects or other tube anomalies. Maternal AFP levels rise sharply in the maternal blood of about 90% of women carrying a fetus with anencephaly and in 50% of those carrying a fetus with spina bifida. Definitive diagnosis requires ultrasonography and amniocentesis.

■ High AFP levels may indicate intrauterine death. Sometimes high levels indicate other anomalies, such as duodenal atresia, omphalocele, tetralogy of Fallot, and Turner's syndrome.

■ High AFP levels occur in 70% of nonpregnant patients with hepatocellular carcinoma.

■ High AFP levels are also related to germ cell tumor of gonadal, retroperitoneal, or mediastinal origin.

■ High AFP levels may suggest ataxia-telangiectasia; cancer of the pancreas, stomach, or biliary system; or nonseminiferous testicular tumors.

■ Transient high AFP levels can occur in nonneoplastic hepatocellular disease, such as alcoholic cirrhosis and acute or chronic hepatitis.

■ In hepatocellular carcinoma, a gradual decrease in AFP levels indicates a favorable response to therapy. In germ cell tumors, serum AFP levels and serum human chorionic gonadotropin levels should be measured concurrently.

■ High AFP levels after remission suggests tumor recurrence.

## Purpose
- To monitor the effectiveness of therapy in malignant conditions, such as hepatomas and germ cell tumors, and certain nonmalignant conditions, such as ataxia-telangiectasia
- To assess the need for amniocentesis or high-resolution ultrasonography in a pregnant woman

## Patient preparation
- Explain that this test helps in monitoring fetal development, screens for a need for further testing, helps detect possible congenital defects in the fetus, and monitors the patient's response to therapy by measuring a specific blood protein, as appropriate.
- Inform the patient that she doesn't need to restrict food, fluids, or medications.
- Tell the patient that the test requires a blood sample. Explain who will perform the venipuncture and when.
- Explain to the patient that she may experience slight discomfort from the tourniquet and needle puncture.

## Procedure and posttest care
- Confirm the patient's identity using two patient identifiers according to facility policy.
- Perform a venipuncture, and collect the blood sample in a 7-ml clot-activator tube.
- Record the patient's age, race, weight, and gestational period on the laboratory request.
- Apply direct pressure to the venipuncture site until bleeding stops.
- If a hematoma develops at the venipuncture site, apply warm soaks.

## Precautions
- A female with a multiple pregnancy may have a false-positive test result.

# Carcinoembryonic antigen
### [CEA]

Carcinoembryonic antigen (CEA) is a protein normally found in embryonic entodermal epithelium and fetal GI tissue. Production of CEA stops before birth, but it may begin again later if a neoplasm develops. Because CEA levels are also raised by biliary obstruction, alcoholic hepatitis, chronic heavy smoking, and other conditions, this test can't be used as a general indicator of cancer. The measurement of enzyme CEA levels by immunoassay is useful for staging and monitoring treatment of certain cancers. (See *Using CEA to monitor cancer treatment.*)

## Reference values
- CEA level is less than 5 ng/ml (SI, < 5 mg/L).

## Abnormal results
- Persistent elevation of CEA levels suggests residual or recurrent tumor. If levels exceed normal before surgical resection, chemotherapy, or radiation therapy, their return to normal within 6 weeks suggests successful treatment.
- High CEA levels are characteristic in various malignant conditions, particularly entodermally derived neoplasms of the GI organs and lungs, and in certain nonmalignant conditions, such as benign hepatic disease, hepatic cirrhosis, alcoholic pancreatitis, and inflammatory bowel disease.
- Elevated CEA concentrations may occur in nonendodermal carcinomas, such as breast and ovarian cancers.

## Purpose
- To monitor the effectiveness of cancer therapy
- To assist in preoperative staging of colorectal cancers, assess the adequacy of

# Using CEA to monitor cancer treatment

Because many patients in the early stages of colorectal cancer have normal or low levels of carcinoembryonic antigen (CEA), the CEA test doesn't screen successfully for early cancer. It's a good tool, however, for monitoring response to cancer therapy.

After a patient's serum CEA level drops after surgery, chemotherapy, or other treatment, an increase suggests recurrence of cancer or diminished effectiveness of treatment.

Both charts below illustrate CEA levels in patients during and after treatment for colorectal cancer. In the left chart, initial results show the usual dramatic drop in response to treatment; the subsequent rise in CEA indicates a diminishing response to chemotherapy. In the right chart, the progressive rise in CEA signals a recurrence of cancer 8 months before clinical symptoms or radiologic evidence.

CEA levels

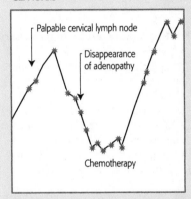

CEA levels

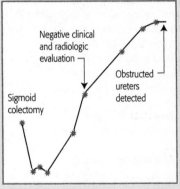

surgical resection, and test for the recurrence of colorectal cancers

## Patient preparation

- Explain that this test detects and measures a special protein that isn't normally present in adults.
- Inform the patient that the test will be repeated to monitor the effectiveness of therapy, if appropriate.
- Inform the patient that he doesn't need to restrict food, fluids, or medications.
- Tell the patient that the test requires a blood sample. Explain who will perform the venipuncture and when.

- Explain to the patient that he may experience slight discomfort from the tourniquet and the needle puncture.

## Procedure and posttest care

- Confirm the patient's identity using two patient identifiers according to facility policy.
- Perform a venipuncture, and collect the sample in a 7-ml tube without additives.
- Apply direct pressure to the venipuncture site until bleeding stops.
- If a hematoma develops at the venipuncture site, apply warm soaks.

### Precautions
- CEA levels may be increased in patients who smoke cigarettes.

# Miscellaneous tests

## ▌TORCH test

The TORCH test helps detect exposure to pathogens involved in congenital and neonatal infections. TORCH is an acronym for TOxoplasmosis, Rubella, Cytomegalovirus, and Herpes simplex antibodies. These pathogens are commonly associated with congenital and neonatal infections that aren't clinically apparent and may cause severe central nervous system impairment. This test detects specific immunoglobulin M-associated antibodies in infant blood.

### Normal results
- Negative for TORCH agents

### Abnormal results
- Toxoplasmosis is diagnosed by sequential examination that shows rising antibody titers, changing titers, and serologic conversion from negative to positive; a titer of 1:256 suggests recent Toxoplasma infection.
- In infants less than 6 months old, rubella infection is associated with a marked and persistent rise in complement-fixing antibody titer over time.
- Persistence of rubella antibody in an infant after age 6 months strongly suggests congenital infection. Congenital rubella is associated with cardiac anomalies, neurosensory deafness, growth retardation, and encephalitic symptoms.
- Detection of herpes antibodies in cerebrospinal fluid with signs of herpetic encephalitis and persistent herpes simplex virus type 2 antibody levels confirms

herpes simplex infection in a neonate without obvious herpetic lesions.

### Purpose
- To help diagnose acute, congenital, and intrapartum infections

### Patient preparation
- Explain to the infant's parents the purpose of the test, and mention that the test requires a blood sample.
- Tell the parents who will perform the venipuncture and when.
- Explain that the infant may experience slight discomfort from the tourniquet and the needle puncture.

### Procedure and posttest care
- Confirm the patient's identity using two patient identifiers according to facility policy.
- Obtain a 3-ml sample of venous or cord blood.
- Apply direct pressure to the venipuncture site until bleeding stops.
- If a hematoma develops at the venipuncture site, apply warm soaks.

## ▌Tuberculin skin tests
### [TB test, PPD skin test]

Tuberculin skin tests are used to screen for previous infection by the tubercle bacillus. They're routinely performed in children, young adults, and patients with radiographic findings that suggest this infection. In the purified protein derivative (PPD) test, intradermal injection of the tuberculin antigen causes a delayed hypersensitivity reaction in patients with active or dormant tuberculosis (TB).

The Mantoux test uses a single-needle intradermal injection of PPD, permitting precise measurement of the dose. Multipuncture tests, such as the tine test, MonoVacc tests, and Aplitest, use intradermal injections with tines impregnated with PPD. Because they require less skill and are more rapidly administered, multipuncture tests are generally used for screening. A positive multipuncture test result usually requires a Mantoux test for confirmation.

### Normal results

- In tuberculin skin tests, Normal results show negative or minimal reactions.
- In the Mantoux test, no induration may appear, or the patient may develop induration less than 5 mm in diameter.
- In the tine and Aplitest tests, no vesiculation or induration may appear, or the patient may develop induration less than 2 mm in diameter.
- In the MonoVacc tests, no induration appears.

### Abnormal results

- A positive tuberculin reaction indicates previous infection by tubercle bacilli. It doesn't distinguish between an active and a dormant infection or provide a definitive diagnosis.
- If a positive reaction occurs, sputum smear and culture and chest radiography are necessary for further information.
- In the Mantoux test, induration 5 to 9 mm in diameter indicates a borderline reaction; larger induration, a positive reaction.
- Because patients infected with atypical mycobacteria other than tubercle bacilli may have borderline reactions, repeated testing is necessary.
- In the tine or Aplitest tests, vesiculation indicates a positive reaction; induration 2 mm in diameter without vesiculation requires confirmation by the Mantoux test. Any induration in the MonoVacc test indicates a positive reaction; however, the diagnosis requires confirmation by the Mantoux test.

**DRUG CHALLENGE**

 Corticosteroids, other immunosuppressants, and live vaccine viruses, such as measles, mumps, rubella, and polio, within 4 to 6 weeks before the test (possible suppression of skin reaction)

### Purpose

- To distinguish TB from blastomycosis, coccidioidomycosis, and histoplasmosis
- To identify people who need diagnostic investigation for TB because of possible exposure

### Patient preparation

- Explain to the patient that this test helps detect TB.
- Tell the patient that the test requires an intradermal injection, which may cause him discomfort.
- Check the patient's history for active TB, the results of previous skin tests, and hypersensitivities.
- If the patient has had TB, don't perform a skin test.
- If the patient has had a positive reaction to previous skin tests, consult the physician or follow facility policy.
- If you're performing a tuberculin test on an outpatient, instruct him to return at the specified time so that you can read the test results.
- Inform the patient that a positive reaction to a skin test appears as a red, hard, raised area at the injection site. Although the area may itch, instruct him not to scratch it.
- Stress that a positive reaction doesn't always indicate active TB.

### Procedure and posttest care

- Confirm the patient's identity using two patient identifiers according to facility policy.

- Ask the patient to sit and support his extended arm on a flat surface.
- Clean the volar surface of the upper forearm with alcohol, and allow the area to dry completely.

### Mantoux test
- Perform an intradermal injection.

### Multipuncture test
- Remove the protective cap on the injection device to expose the four tines.
- Hold the patient's forearm in one hand, stretching the skin of the forearm tightly. Then, with your other hand, firmly depress the device into the patient's skin without twisting it.
- Hold the device in place for at least 1 second before removing it.
- If you've applied sufficient pressure, you'll see four puncture sites and a circular depression made by the device on the patient's skin.

### Both tests
- Record where the test was given, the date and time, and when the results are to be read. Tuberculin skin tests are generally read 48 to 72 hours after injection; the MonoVacc test can be read 48 to 96 hours after the test.
- If ulceration or necrosis develops at the injection site, apply cold soaks or a topical steroid.

### Precautions
- Tuberculin skin tests are contraindicated in the patient with current reactions to smallpox vaccinations, a rash, a skin disorder, or active TB.
- Don't perform a skin test in areas with excessive hair, acne, or insufficient subcutaneous tissue, such as over a tendon or bone.
- If fewer than 10 weeks pass between the time of infection and the time of

the test, the test result may be a false-negative.
- If the patient is known to be hypersensitive to skin tests, use a first-strength dose in the Mantoux test to avoid necrosis at the puncture site.

ACTION STAT!

 Have epinephrine available to treat a possible anaphylactic or acute hypersensitivity reaction.

# Tumor markers
[CA 15-3 (CA 27.29); CA 19-9; CA-125; and CA-50]

Tumor markers are substances produced and secreted by tumor cells to help determine tumor activity. They can be found in the serum of the cancer patient. Specific tests are ordered depending on the type of cancer the patient has. The CA 15-3 antigen may be used in conjunction with CEA and is helpful particularly in the breast cancer patient (CA 27.29, a newer test, measures the same marker as CA 15-3). CA 19-9 carbohydrate antigen may be ordered in the patient with pancreas, hepatobiliary, or lung cancer. The CA-125 glycoprotein antigen and serum carbohydrate antigen is commonly associated with types of ovarian cancers. The CA-50 may be ordered in the patient with GI or pancreatic cancer.

A combination of markers may be used due to low sensitivity and specificity of the markers. Few tumor markers meet Food and Drug Administration approval due to the controversy over their role in cancer diagnosis and treatment.

## Reference values

- Normal values are:
  - CA 15-3 (CA 27.29): < 30 units/ml
  - CA 19-9: < 70 units/ml
  - CA-125: < 34 units/ml
  - CA-50: < 17 units/ml.

## Abnormal results

- CA 15-3 (CA 27.29) greatly increases in metastatic breast cancer; it also increases in pancreas, lung, colorectal, ovarian, and liver cancers. It decreases with therapy; an increase after therapy suggests progressive disease.
- CA 19-9 increases in pancreatic, hepatobiliary, and lung cancers. It may be mildly increased in gastric and colorectal cancers.
- CA-125 increases in epithelial ovary, fallopian tube, endometrial, endocervix, pancreas, and liver cancers. CA-125 increases less in colon, breast, lung, and GI cancers.
- CA-50 increases in GI and pancreatic cancers.

## Purpose

- To assist tumor staging and identify possible metastasis
- To monitor and detect disease recurrence
- To assess the patient's response to therapy

## Patient preparation

- Explain the purpose of the particular test ordered and that it may be helpful in evaluating the patient's disease, as appropriate.
- Specific directions from the laboratory or cancer center should be followed for the particular test ordered. Fasting may be involved, and factors may be identified that may interfere with test results. Note interfering factors on the appropriate laboratory requests.
- Tell the patient that the test requires a blood sample. Explain who will perform the venipuncture and when.
- Explain to the patient that he may experience slight discomfort from the tourniquet and the needle puncture.

## Procedure and posttest care

- Confirm the patient's identity using two patient identifiers according to facility policy.
- Obtain a 10-ml venous blood sample, as ordered, in the tube specified by the laboratory or cancer center, and transport the sample as directed.
- Apply direct pressure to the venipuncture site until bleeding stops.
- If a hematoma develops at the venipuncture site, apply warm soaks.
- Provide emotional support to the patient.

## Precautions

- Consult the laboratory or cancer center as to specific patient preparation required (fasting, identifying interfering factors). Interfering factors may include:
  - CA 15-3 (CA 27.29) is increased in benign breast or ovarian disease.
  - CA 19-9 is increased in pancreatitis, cholecystitis, cirrhosis, gallstones, and cystic fibrosis (minimal elevations).
  - CA-125 is increased in pregnancy, endometriosis, pelvic inflammatory disease, menstruation, acute and chronic hepatitis, ascites, peritonitis, pancreatitis, GI disease, Meig's syndrome, pleural effusion, and pulmonary disease.

# II

# Urine tests

# Urinalysis

## Physical and chemical tests

### Routine urinalysis
[UA]

A routine urinalysis tests for urinary and systemic disorders. This test evaluates physical characteristics (color, odor, turbidity, and opacity) of urine; determines specific gravity and pH; detects and measures protein, glucose, and ketone bodies; and examines sediment for blood cells, casts, and crystals.

Diagnostic laboratory methods include visual examination, reagent strip screening, refractometry for specific gravity, and microscopic inspection of centrifuged sediment.

#### Normal results
- See *Normal findings in routine urinalysis*.

#### Abnormal results
- Nonpathologic variations in normal values may result from diet, nonpathologic conditions, specimen collection time, medications, and other factors. (See *Drugs that influence routine urinalysis results*, pages 242 and 243.)
- An alkaline pH (above 7.0)—characteristic of a vegetarian diet—causes turbidity and the formation of phosphate, carbonate, and amorphous crystals; it

may indicate Fanconi's syndrome, urinary tract infection from urea-splitting bacteria (*Proteus* and *Pseudomonas*), and metabolic or respiratory alkalosis.
- An acid pH (below 7.0)—typical of a high-protein diet—produces turbidity and the formation of oxalate, cystine, leucine, tyrosine, amorphous urate, and uric acid crystals. Acid urine pH is associated with renal tuberculosis, pyrexia, phenylketonuria, alkaptonuria, and acidosis.
- Turbid urine may contain red or white cells, bacteria, fat, or chyle and may indicate renal infection.
- Transient nonpathologic proteinuria may result from fever, exposure to cold, emotional stress, strenuous exercise, or a benign condition known as orthostatic (postural) proteinuria; protein in the urine may also indicate lymphoma, hepatitis, diabetes mellitus, toxemia, hypertension, lupus erythematosus, renal failure or disease (including nephrosis, glomerulosclerosis, glomerulonephritis, nephrolithiasis, nephrotic syndrome, and polycystic kidney disease), or multiple myeloma.
- Glycosuria (glucose in the urine) usually indicates diabetes mellitus but may result from pheochromocytoma, Cushing's syndrome, impaired tubular reabsorption, advanced renal disease, and increased intracranial pressure. I.V. solutions or total parenteral nutrition containing glucose can also lead to glycos-

## Normal findings in routine urinalysis

| Element | Findings |
|---|---|

**Macroscopic**

| | |
|---|---|
| Color | ■ Straw to dark yellow |
| Odor | ■ Slightly aromatic |
| Appearance | ■ Clear |
| Specific gravity | ■ 1.005 to 1.035 |
| pH | ■ 4.5 to 8.0 |
| Protein | ■ None |
| Glucose | ■ None |
| Ketone bodies | ■ None |
| Bilirubin | ■ None |
| Urobilinogen | ■ Normal |
| Hemoglobin | ■ None |
| Erythrocytes (red blood cells [RBCs]) | ■ None |
| Nitrites (bacteria) | ■ None |
| Leukocytes (white blood cells [WBCs]) | ■ None |

**Microscopic**

| | |
|---|---|
| RBCs | ■ 0 to 2/high-power field |
| WBCs | ■ 0 to 5/high-power field |
| Epithelial cells | ■ 0 to 5/high-power field |
| Casts | ■ None, except 1 to 2 hyaline casts/low-power field |
| Crystals | ■ Present |
| Bacteria | ■ None |
| Yeast cells | ■ None |
| Parasites | ■ None |

uria. Transient nonpathologic glycosuria may result from emotional stress or pregnancy and may follow ingestion of a high-carbohydrate meal.

■ Fructosuria, galactosuria, and pentosuria usually suggest rare hereditary metabolic disorders, but lactosuria can occur during pregnancy and breast-feeding, and an alimentary form of pentosuria and fructosuria may follow excessive ingestion of pentose or fructose.

■ Centrifuged urine sediment contains cells, casts, crystals, bacteria, yeast, and parasites.

■ Hematuria (red blood cells [RBCs] in urine) indicates bleeding within the genitourinary tract and may result from infection, obstruction, inflammation, trauma, tumors, glomerulonephritis, renal hypertension, lupus nephritis, renal tuberculosis, renal vein thrombosis, renal calculi, hydronephrosis, pyelonephritis, scurvy, malaria, parasitic infection of the bladder, subacute bacterial endocarditis, polyarteritis nodosa, and hemorrhagic disorders. Strenuous exercise or exposure to toxic chemicals may also cause hematuria.

# Drugs that influence routine urinalysis results

## Drugs that change urine color
Chlorzoxazone (orange to purple-red)
Deferoxamine mesylate (red)
Fluorescein sodium I.V. (yellow-orange)
Furazolidone (brown)
Iron salts (black)
Levodopa (dark)
Methylene blue (blue-green)
Metronidazole (dark)
Nitrofurantoin (brown)
Oral anticoagulants, indandione derivatives (orange)
Phenazopyridine (orange, red, or orange-brown)
Phenothiazines (dark)
Quinacrine (deep yellow)
Riboflavin (yellow)
Rifabutin (red-orange)
Rifampin (red-orange)
Sulfasalazine (orange-yellow)

## Drugs that cause urine odor
Antibiotics
Paraldehyde
Vitamins

## Drugs that increase specific gravity
Albumin
Dextran
Glucose
Radiopaque contrast media

## Drugs that decrease pH
Ammonium chloride
Ascorbic acid
Diazoxide
Metolazone

## Drugs that increase pH
Amphotericin B
Carbonic anhydrase inhibitors
Mafenide
Potassium citrate
Sodium bicarbonate

## Drugs that cause false-positive results for proteinuria
Acetazolamide (Combistix)
Aminosalicylic acid (sulfosalicylic acid or Extons method)
Methazolamide
Nafcillin (sulfosalicylic acid method)
Sodium bicarbonate
Tolbutamide (sulfosalicylic acid method)
Tolmetin (sulfosalicylic acid method)

## Drugs that cause true proteinuria
Aminoglycosides
Amphotericin B
Bacitracin
Cephalosporins
Cisplatin
Gold preparations
Isotretinoin
Nonsteroidal anti-inflammatory drugs
Polymyxin B
Sulfonamides

## Drugs that cause either true proteinuria or false-positive results
Penicillin in large doses (except with Ames reagent strips); however, some penicillins cause true proteinuria
Sulfonamides (sulfosalicylic acid method)

## Drugs that cause false-positive results for glycosuria
Aminosalicylic acid (Benedict's test)
Ascorbic acid (Clinistix, Diastix, Tes-Tape)
Ascorbic acid in large doses (Clinitest tablets)
Cephalosporins (Clinitest tablets)
Chloral hydrate (Benedict's test)
Isoniazid (Benedict's test)
Levodopa (Clinistix, Diastix, Tes-Tape)
Levodopa in large doses (Clinitest tablets)
Methyldopa (Tes-Tape)
Nalidixic acid (Benedict's test or Clinitest tablets)
Nitrofurantoin (Benedict's test)

## Drugs that influence routine urinalysis results *(continued)*

Penicillin G in large doses (Benedict's test)

Phenazopyridine (Clinistix, Diastix, Tes-Tape)

Probenecid (Benedict's test, Clinitest tablets)

Salicylates in large doses (Clinitest tablets, Clinistix, Diastix, Tes-Tape)

Streptomycin (Benedict's test)

Tetracycline (Clinistix, Diastix, Tes-Tape)

Tetracyclines, due to ascorbic acid buffer (Benedict's test, Clinitest tablets)

### Drugs that cause true glycosuria
Ammonium chloride
Asparaginase
Carbamazepine
Corticosteroids
Lithium carbonate
Nicotinic acid (large doses)
Phenothiazines (long-term)
Thiazide diuretics

### Drugs that cause false-positive results for ketonuria
Levodopa (Ketostix, Labstix)
Phenazopyridine (Ketostix or Gerhardt's reagent strip shows atypical color)
Phenothiazines (Gerhardt's reagent strip shows atypical color)
Salicylates (Gerhardt's reagent strip shows reddish color)

### Drugs that cause true ketonuria
Ether (anesthesia)
Insulin (excessive doses)
Isoniazid (intoxication)
Isopropyl alcohol (intoxication)

### Drugs that increase white blood cell count
Allopurinol
Ampicillin
Aspirin (toxicity)
Kanamycin
Methicillin

### Drugs that cause hematuria
Amphotericin B
Coumarin derivatives
Methicillin
Sulfonamides

### Drugs that cause casts
Amphotericin B
Aspirin (toxicity)
Bacitracin
Ethacrynic acid
Furosemide
Gentamicin
Isoniazid
Kanamycin
Neomycin
Penicillin
Radiographic agents
Streptomycin
Sulfonamides

### Drugs that cause crystals (if urine is acidic)
Acetazolamide
Aminosalicylic acid
Ascorbic acid
Nitrofurantoin
Theophylline
Thiazide diuretics

■ An excess of white blood cells (WBCs) in urine usually implies urinary tract inflammation, especially cystitis or pyelonephritis.

■ Numerous epithelial cells suggest renal tubular degeneration, such as heavy metal poisoning, eclampsia, and kidney transplant rejection.

■ Color change can result from diet (especially beets, berries, and rhubarb), drugs, and many diseases. For example, yellow urine can be caused by liver disease with increased bilirubin level; brown urine may also be caused by liver disease, as well as by multiple myeloma or copper poisoning. Blue urine may be caused by a pseudomonas bacterial infection.

- Odor change can indicate different conditions.
  - A fruity odor suggests formation of ketone bodies, as occurs in diabetes mellitus, starvation, and dehydration.
  - A fetid odor in urinary tract infections (UTIs) is associated with *Escherichia coli*.
  - Maple syrup odor and a "mousy" odor may cause maple syrup disorder and phenylketonuria, respectively.
- Ketonuria occurs in diabetes mellitus when cellular energy needs exceed available cellular glucose. In the absence of glucose, cells metabolize fat for energy. Ketone bodies—the end products of incomplete fat metabolism—are excreted in the urine. Ketonuria may also occur in starvation states, in low- or no-carbohydrate diets, and following diarrhea or vomiting.
- Low specific gravity (< 1.005) is characteristic of diabetes insipidus, nephrogenic diabetes insipidus, acute tubular necrosis, and pyelonephritis. Fixed specific gravity, in which values remain 1.010 regardless of fluid intake, occurs in chronic glomerulonephritis with severe renal damage. High specific gravity (> 1.035) occurs in nephrotic syndrome, dehydration, acute glomerulonephritis, heart failure, liver failure, and shock.
- Bilirubin in urine may occur in liver disease resulting from obstructive jaundice or hepatotoxic drugs or toxins or from fibrosis of the biliary canaliculi (which may occur in cirrhosis).
- Increased urobilinogen levels in urine may indicate liver damage, hemolytic disease, or severe infection. Decreased urobilinogen levels may occur with biliary obstruction, inflammatory disease, antimicrobial therapy, severe diarrhea, or renal insufficiency.

- Excessive casts (plugs of gelled proteinaceous material) in urine indicate renal disease.
  - Hyaline casts suggest renal parenchymal disease, inflammation, trauma to the glomerular capillary membrane, and some physiologic states (such as after exercise).
  - Epithelial casts indicate renal tubular damage, nephrosis, eclampsia, amyloidosis, and heavy metal poisoning.
  - Coarse and fine granular casts suggest acute or chronic renal failure, pyelonephritis, and chronic lead intoxication.
  - Fatty and waxy casts are associated with nephrotic syndrome, chronic renal disease, and diabetes mellitus
  - RBC casts indicate renal parenchymal disease (especially glomerulonephritis), renal infarction, subacute bacterial endocarditis, vascular disorders, sickle cell anemia, scurvy, blood dyscrasias, malignant hypertension, collagen disease, and acute inflammation.
  - WBC casts indicate acute pyelonephritis and glomerulonephritis, nephrotic syndrome, pyogenic infection, and lupus nephritis.
- Excessive calcium oxalate crystals suggest hypercalcemia or ethylene glycol ingestion. Cystine crystals (cystinuria) reflect an inborn error of metabolism.
- Bacteria, yeast cells, and parasites in urine sediment reflect genitourinary tract infection or contamination of external genitalia. Yeast cells, which may be mistaken for RBCs, are identifiable by their ovoid shape, lack of color, variable size and, frequently, signs of budding. The most common parasite in sediment is *Trichomonas vaginalis*, which causes vaginitis, urethritis, and prostatovesiculitis.

## Purpose
- To screen the patient's urine for renal or urinary tract disease
- To help detect metabolic or systemic disease unrelated to renal disorders
- To detect substances (drugs)

## Patient preparation
- Explain that this test aids in the diagnosis of renal or urinary tract disease and helps evaluate overall body function.
- Inform the patient that he doesn't need to restrict food and fluids.
- Notify the laboratory and practitioner of medications the patient is taking that may affect laboratory results; these medications may need to be restricted.
- Explain how to collect a clean-catch specimen

## Procedure and posttest care
- Confirm the patient's identity using two patient identifiers according to facility policy.
- Collect a random clean-catch urine specimen of at least 15 ml.
- Obtain a first-voided morning specimen if possible.
- Tell the patient to resume his usual diet and medications stopped before the test, as ordered.

## Precautions
- Strenuous exercise before routine urinalysis may cause transient myoglobulinuria or hematuria.
- Foods such as beets, berries, and rhubarb may cause the urine to change color.

# ▌Urinary calculi screening

Urinary calculi (urolithiasis or, more commonly, urinary stones) are insoluble substances most commonly formed of the mineral salts—calcium oxalate, calcium phosphate, magnesium ammonium phosphate, urate, or cystine. They may appear anywhere in the urinary tract and range in size from microscopic to several centimeters. Calculi usually possess well-defined nuclei composed of bacteria, fibrin, blood clots, or epithelial cells that are enclosed in a protein matrix. Mineral salts accumulate around this matrix in layers, causing progressive enlargement.

Formation of calculi can result from reduced urinary volume, increased excretion of mineral salts, urinary stasis, pH changes, and decreased protective substances. Calculi commonly form in the kidney, pass into the ureter, and are excreted in the urine. Because not all calculi pass spontaneously, they may require surgical extraction or pulverization using extracorporeal shock-wave lithotripsy. Calculi don't always cause symptoms, but when they do, hematuria is most common. If calculi obstruct the ureter, they may cause hematuria, severe flank pain, dysuria, and urinary retention, frequency, and urgency.

To test for urinary calculi, the patient must have all his urine carefully strained to remove any calculi. Qualitative chemical analysis then reveals the calculi's composition, which helps to identify their causes.

## Normal results
- Calculi aren't present in urine.

## Abnormal results
- More than one-half of all calculi in urine are of mixed composition, containing two or more mineral salts; calcium oxalate is the most common component.
- Determining the calculi's composition helps identify various metabolic disorders, guiding proper treatment and prevention measures. (See *Types and causes of calculi,* page 246.)

# Types and causes of calculi

**A**

*Calcium oxalate calculi* usually result from idiopathic hypercalciuria, a condition that reflects absorption of calcium from the bowel.

**B**

*Calcium phosphate calculi* usually result from primary hyperparathyroidism, which causes excessive reabsorption of calcium from bone.

**C**

*Cystine calculi* result from primary cystinuria, an inborn error of metabolism that prevents renal tubular reabsorption of cystine.

**D**

*Urate calculi* result from gout, dehydration (causing elevated uric acid levels), acidic urine, or hepatic dysfunction.

**E**

*Magnesium ammonium phosphate calculi* result from the presence of urea-splitting organisms, such as *Proteus,* which raises ammonia concentration and makes urine alkaline.

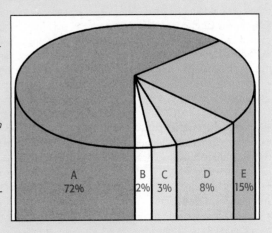

A 72% | B 2% | C 3% | D 8% | E 15%

## Purpose
- To detect and analyze calculi in the urine

## Patient preparation
- Explain that this test detects urinary calculi and that laboratory analysis will reveal their composition.
- Tell the patient that his urine will be collected and strained.
- Inform the patient that he doesn't need to restrict food and fluids.
- Inform the patient that medication to control pain will be administered.

## Procedure and posttest care
- Confirm the patient's identity using two patient identifiers according to facility policy.
- Have the patient void into the strainer.
- Inspect the strainer carefully because calculi may be minute, looking like gravel or sand.
- If calculi are found, document the appearance of the calculi and the number, if possible. Place the calculi in a properly labeled container and send the container to the laboratory immediately for prompt analysis.

- Observe the patient throughout the test for severe flank pain, dysuria, and urinary retention, frequency, or urgency.
- Hematuria should subside.

### Precautions
- Keep the strainer and urinal or bedpan within the patient's reach if he has received analgesics because he may be drowsy and unable to get out of bed to void.

# *Tubular function tests*

## ▌Tubular reabsorption of phosphate

The test for tubular reabsorption of phosphate is an indirect measure of parathyroid hormone (PTH) levels. PTH helps maintain optimum blood levels of ionized calcium and controls renal excretion of calcium and phosphate. Specifically, PTH stimulates reabsorption of calcium and inhibits reabsorption of phosphate from the glomerular filtrate. A regulatory feedback mechanism results in diminished PTH secretion as ionized calcium levels return to normal. In primary hyperparathyroidism, excessive secretion of PTH disrupts this calcium-phosphate balance. This test measures urine and serum phosphate and creatinine levels. These values are then used to calculate the tubular reabsorption of phosphate.

### Normal results
- Renal tubules normally reabsorb 80% or more of phosphate.

### Abnormal results
- Reabsorption of less than 74% of phosphate strongly suggests primary hyperparathyroidism.
- Hypercalcemia is the most common sign of primary hyperparathyroidism, but a patient with hypercalcemia may need additional testing to confirm primary hyperparathyroidism as the cause.

### DRUG CHALLENGE
 Furosemide and gentamicin (possible increase); amphotericin B and thiazide diuretics (possible decrease)

### Purpose
- To evaluate parathyroid gland function
- To aid in the diagnosis of primary hyperparathyroidism
- To aid in the differential diagnosis of hypercalcemia

### Patient preparation
- Explain that this test evaluates parathyroid gland function.
- Advise the patient that the test requires a blood sample and urine collection over a 24-hour period.
- Tell the patient who will perform the venipuncture and when.
- Advise the patient that he may experience slight discomfort from the needle puncture and the tourniquet.
- Instruct the patient to maintain a normal phosphate diet for 3 days before the test because low phosphate intake (< 500 mg/day) may elevate tubular reabsorption values and a high-phosphate diet (3,000 mg/day) may lower them. Common nutritional sources of phosphorus include legumes, nuts, milk, egg

yolks, meat, poultry, fish, cereals, and cheese. These foods should be eaten in moderate amounts.

▪ Instruct the patient to fast after midnight the night before the test.

▪ Notify the laboratory and practitioner of medications the patient is taking that may affect test results; they may need to be restricted. If they must be continued, note this on the laboratory request.

### Procedure and posttest care

▪ Confirm the patient's identity using two patient identifiers according to facility policy.

▪ Perform a venipuncture and collect the blood sample in a 10-ml clot-activator tube.

▪ Instruct the patient to empty his bladder and discard the urine; record this as time zero.

▪ Collect the patient's urine over a 24-hour period with the first sample discarded and the last sample retained; occasionally, a 4-hour collection or a random collection is ordered instead.

▪ Allow the patient to eat and encourage fluid intake to maintain adequate urine flow after the venipuncture.

▪ Apply direct pressure to the venipuncture site until bleeding stops. Apply warm soaks if a hematoma develops at the venipuncture site.

▪ Tell the patient to resume his usual diet and medications stopped before the test, as ordered.

### Precautions

▪ Keep the urine specimen container refrigerated or on ice during the collection period.

▪ Uremia, renal tubular disease, osteomalacia, myeloma, and sarcoidosis may cause a possible increase in reabsorption.

# Urine enzymes

## General tests

### Arylsulfatase A

Arylsulfatase A (ARSA), a lysosomal enzyme found in every cell except the mature erythrocyte, is principally active in the liver, pancreas, and kidneys, where exogenous substances are detoxified into ester sulfates.

Urine ARSA levels rise in transitional bladder cancer, colorectal cancer, and leukemia. Whether high ARSA levels help to cause malignant growths or are simply an enzymatic response to them isn't known.

#### Reference values
- Random values are 1.6 to 42 units/g creatinine; 24-hour urine values are 0.37 to 3.60 units/day creatinine; 1-hour test values are 2 to 19 units/ 1 hour (SI, 2 to 19 units/h); 2-hour test values are 4 to 37 units/2 hours (SI, 4 to 37 units/2 hours); 24-hour test values are 170 to 2,000 units/24 hours (SI, 170 to 2,000 units/24 hours).

#### Abnormal results
- High ARSA levels may be present in cancer of the bladder, colon, or rectum or myeloid leukemia.
- Low ARSA levels can result from metachromatic leukodystrophy. In a patient with this condition, urine studies show metachromatic granules in the urinary sediment.

#### Purpose
- To help diagnose bladder, colon, or rectal cancer; myeloid (granulocytic) leukemia; and metachromatic leukodystrophy (an inherited lipid storage disease)

#### Patient preparation
- Explain that this test measures an enzyme that's present throughout the body.
- Inform the patient that he doesn't need to restrict food and fluids.
- Tell the patient that the test requires urine collection over a 24-hour period and teach him how to collect a timed specimen.

#### Procedure and posttest care
- Confirm the patient's identity using two patient identifiers according to facility policy.
- Collect the patient's urine over a 24-hour period, discarding the first sample and retaining the last sample in the appropriate container.

DO'S & DON'TS

Keep the collection container refrigerated or on ice during the collection period.

## Precautions

- If a female patient is menstruating, anticipate possible test rescheduling.
- If the patient has an indwelling urinary catheter in place, keep the collection bag on ice for the duration of the test.
- Begin the test period with a new, unused continuous urinary drainage apparatus.

# ▌Cyclic adenosine monophosphate
## [cAMP]

Formed from adenosine triphosphate by the action of the enzyme adenylate cyclase, the nucleotide cyclic adenosine monophosphate (cAMP) influences the protein synthesis rate within cells. Measurement of the urinary excretion of cAMP after an I.V. infusion of a standard dose of parathyroid hormone (PTH) can show renal tubular resistance in a patient with hypoparathyroid symptoms and high levels of PTH. Such findings suggest type I pseudohypoparathyroidism, a rare inherited disorder. (Urinary cAMP levels respond normally with type II pseudohypoparathyroidism because the defect is beyond the level of cAMP generation.)

## Reference values

- Levels of cAMP are normally 0.3 to 3.6 mg/day or 0.29 to 2.1 mg/g creatinine.

## Abnormal results

- Failure to respond to PTH, indicated by normal urinary excretion of cAMP, suggests type I pseudohypoparathyroidism.

## Purpose

- To aid in the differential diagnosis of hypoparathyroidism and pseudohypoparathyroidism

## Patient preparation

- Explain that this test evaluates parathyroid function.
- Tell the patient that the test requires a 15-minute I.V. infusion of PTH and a 3-to 4-hour urine specimen collection.

<u>**A**LERT</u>

Perform a skin test to detect an allergy to PTH; keep epinephrine or a histamine-1-receptor antagonist, such as diphenhydramine or glucocorticoids (methylprednisolone), readily available in case of an adverse reaction.

- Just before the procedure is performed, instruct the patient not to touch the I.V. line or exert pressure on the arm receiving the infusion.
- Tell the patient that he may experience discomfort from the needle puncture. Tell him to notify you if he feels severe burning or if the site becomes inflamed or swollen.

## Procedure and posttest care

- Confirm the patient's identity using two patient identifiers according to facility policy.
- Instruct the patient to empty his bladder.
- If the patient has an indwelling urinary catheter in place, replace the collection apparatus with an unused one.
- Send this specimen to the laboratory, if ordered; otherwise, discard it.
- Prepare the PTH for infusion, as directed, using sterile water for dilution.
- Start the infusion with dextrose 5% in water and infuse the PTH over 15 minutes. Record the start of the infusion as time zero.
- Collect a urine specimen 3 to 4 hours after the infusion.
- Stop the I.V. infusion, as ordered.
- Observe the patient for symptoms of hypercalcemia, including lethargy,

anorexia, nausea, vomiting, vertigo, and abdominal cramps.
- Apply warm soaks if a hematoma or irritation develops at the venipuncture site.

### Precautions
- The cAMP test is contraindicated in the patient with a positive PTH test as well as one with high calcium levels because PTH further raises calcium levels. It should be performed cautiously in the patient receiving a cardiac glycoside and in the patient with sarcoidosis or renal or cardiac disease.
- Keep the collection bag on ice if the patient has a catheter in place.

# Lysozyme
[muramidase]

Lysozyme, a low-molecular-weight enzyme, is present in mucus, saliva, tears, skin secretions, and various internal body cells and fluids. This enzyme splits, or lyses, the cell walls of gram-positive bacteria and, with complement and other blood factors, acts to destroy them. Lysozyme seems to be synthesized in granulocytes and monocytes, first appearing in serum after the destruction of such cells. When the serum lysozyme level exceeds three times the normal level, the enzyme appears in the urine. Because renal tissue also contains lysozyme, renal injury alone can cause measurable excretion of this enzyme.

This test measures urine lysozyme levels with a turbidimeter. Serum lysozyme determinations, using the same method, confirm the results of urine testing.

### Reference values
- Urine lysozyme values are 0 to 3 mg/ 24 hours.

### Abnormal results
- Elevated urine lysozyme levels are characteristic of impaired renal proximal tubular reabsorption, acute pyelonephritis, nephrotic syndrome, tuberculosis of the kidney, severe extrarenal infection, rejection or infarction of kidney transplantation (levels normally increase during the first few days after transplantation), and polycythemia vera.
- Urine levels rise markedly after the acute onset or relapse of monocytic or myelomonocytic leukemia and rise moderately after acute onset or relapse of granulocytic (myeloid) leukemia.
- Urine lysozyme levels remain normal or decrease in lymphocytic leukemia and remain normal in myeloblastic and myelocytic leukemias.

### Purpose
- To aid in the diagnosis of acute monocytic or granulocytic leukemia and to monitor the progression of these diseases
- To evaluate proximal tubular function and to diagnose renal impairment
- To detect rejection or infarction of kidney transplantation

### Patient preparation
- Explain that this test evaluates renal function and the immune system.
- Inform him that he doesn't need to restrict food and fluids.
- Tell the patient that the test requires collection of urine over a 24-hour period and teach him how to collect the specimen correctly.

### Procedure and posttest care
- Confirm the patient's identity using two patient identifiers according to facility policy.
- Collect the patient's urine over a 24-hour period, discarding the first specimen and retaining the last specimen in the appropriate container.

Do's & don'ts

 Cover and refrigerate the specimen throughout the collection period.

## Precautions
- If a female patient is menstruating, anticipate possible test rescheduling.
- Keep the collection bag on ice if the patient has an indwelling urinary catheter in place.

# Urine hormones and metabolites

## Urine hormone tests

### Catecholamines, urine

The test for catecholamines uses spectrophotofluorimetry to measure urine levels of the major catecholamines—epinephrine, norepinephrine, and dopamine. Catecholamines help regulate metabolism and prepare the body for the fight-or-flight response to stress. Certain tumors can also secrete catecholamines.

A 24-hour urine specimen is preferred because catecholamine secretion fluctuates diurnally and in response to pain, heat, cold, emotional stress, physical exercise, hypoglycemia, injury, hemorrhage, asphyxia, and drugs. A random specimen may be useful for evaluating catecholamine levels after a hypertensive episode.

For a complete diagnostic workup of catecholamine secretion, urine levels of catecholamine metabolites are also measured.

#### Reference values
- Values for catecholamine fractionalization range as follows:

– Epinephrine: 0 to 20 mcg/24 hours (SI, 0 to 109 nmol/24 hours)
– Norepinephrine: 15 to 80 mcg/24 hours (SI, 89 to 473 nmol/24 hours)
– Dopamine: 65 to 400 mcg/24 hours (SI, 425 to 2,610 nmol/24 hours)

#### Abnormal results
- In a patient with undiagnosed hypertension, elevated urine catecholamine levels following a hypertensive episode usually indicate a pheochromocytoma.
- If tests indicate a pheochromocytoma, the patient may also be tested for multiple endocrine neoplasia.
- With the exception of homovanillic acid (HVA)—a dopamine metabolite—catecholamine metabolites may also be elevated.
- Abnormally high HVA levels rule out a pheochromocytoma because this tumor mainly secretes epinephrine, whose primary metabolite is vanillylmandelic acid, not HVA.
- Elevated catecholamine levels, without marked hypertension, may be due to a neuroblastoma or a ganglioneuroma, although HVA levels reflect these conditions more accurately.
- Elevated levels are also seen in severe systemic situations (burns, peritonitis, shock, and septicemia), cor pulmonale,

manic depressive disorders, or depressive neurosis.

- Myasthenia gravis and progressive muscular dystrophy commonly cause urine catecholamine levels to rise above normal, but this test is rarely performed to diagnose these disorders.
- Consistently low-normal catecholamine levels may indicate dysautonomia marked by orthostatic hypotension.

### DRUG CHALLENGE

 Caffeine, insulin, nitroglycerin, aminophylline, sympathomimetics, methyldopa, tricyclic antidepressants, chloral hydrate, quinidine, quinine, tetracycline, B-complex vitamins, isoproterenol, levodopa, and monoamine oxidase inhibitors (possible increase); clonidine, reserpine, and iodine-containing contrast media (possible decrease); phenothiazines, erythromycin, and methenamine compounds (possible increase or decrease)

### Purpose

- To help diagnose pheochromocytoma in a patient with unexplained hypertension
- To help diagnose neuroblastoma, ganglioneuroma, and dysautonomia

### Patient preparation

- Explain to the patient that the urine catecholamine test evaluates adrenal function.
- Inform the patient that he should avoid chocolate, coffee, and bananas for 7 hours before the test, and he should avoid stressful situations and excessive physical activity during the collection period.
- Tell the patient that the test requires either the collection of urine over 24 hours or a random specimen, and explain the collection procedure.

- Notify the laboratory and practitioner of medications the patient is taking that may affect test results; they may need to be restricted.

### Procedure and posttest care

- Confirm the patient's identity using two patient identifiers according to facility policy.
- Collect the patient's urine over a 24-hour period. Use a bottle containing a preservative to keep the specimen acidified to a pH of 3.0 or less. (If a random specimen is ordered, collect it immediately after a hypertensive episode.)
- Refrigerate a 24-hour specimen or place it on ice during the collection period.
- Instruct the patient that he may resume his usual activities, diet, and medications, as ordered.

### Precautions

- Excessive physical exercise or emotional stress may cause increased levels.

## Free cortisol, urine

Used as a screen for adrenocortical hyperfunction, the free cortisol test measures urine levels of the portion of cortisol not bound to the corticosteroid-binding globulin transcortin. It's one of the best diagnostic tools for detecting Cushing's syndrome.

Unlike a single measurement of plasma cortisol, radioimmunoassay determinations of free cortisol levels in a 24-hour urine specimen reflect overall secretion levels instead of diurnal variations. Concurrent measurements of plasma cortisol and corticotropin, with urine 17-hydroxycorticosteroids and the dexamethasone suppression test, may be used to confirm the diagnosis.

## Reference values
▪ Normal reference values are less than 50 mcg/24 hours (SI, < 138 mmol/24 hours).

## Abnormal results
▪ Elevated free cortisol levels may indicate Cushing's syndrome resulting from adrenal hyperplasia, adrenal or pituitary tumor, or ectopic corticotropin production.
▪ Hepatic disease and obesity, which can raise plasma cortisol levels, generally don't appreciably raise urine levels of free cortisol.
▪ Low levels have little diagnostic significance and don't necessarily indicate adrenocortical hypofunction.

### DRUG CHALLENGE

 Reserpine, phenothiazines, morphine, amphetamines, hormonal contraceptives, danazol, aldactone, and prolonged steroid therapy (possible increase); dexamethasone, ethacrynic acid, thiazides, and ketoconazole (decrease)

## Purpose
▪ To help diagnose Cushing's syndrome
▪ To evaluate adrenocortical function

## Patient preparation
▪ Explain that the urine-free cortisol test helps evaluate adrenal gland function.
▪ Inform the patient that he doesn't need to restrict food and fluids, but he should avoid stressful situations and excessive physical exercise during the collection period.
▪ Tell him that the test requires collection of urine over a 24-hour period.
▪ Teach the patient the proper collection technique for a 24-hour urine specimen.
▪ Notify the laboratory and practitioner of medications the patient is taking that may affect test results; they may need to be restricted.

## Procedure and posttest care
▪ Confirm the patient's identity using two patient identifiers according to facility policy.
▪ Collect the patient's urine over a 24-hour period, discarding the first specimen and retaining the last specimen. Use a bottle containing a preservative to keep the specimen at a pH of 4.0 to 4.5.

### DO'S & DON'TS

 Refrigerate the specimen or place it on ice during the collection period.

▪ Instruct the patient that he may resume his usual activities and medications, as ordered.

## Precautions
▪ Pregnancy may cause an increased urine-free cortisol level.

# ▮ Human chorionic gonadotropin, urine
### [hCG, pregnancy test]

Qualitative analysis of urine levels of human chorionic gonadotropin (hCG) allows for the detection of pregnancy as early as 14 days after ovulation. Production of hCG, a glycoprotein, which prevents degeneration of the corpus luteum at the end of the normal menstrual cycle, begins after conception. During the first trimester, hCG levels rise steadily and rapidly, peaking around 10 weeks' gestation, subsequently tapering off to less than 10% of peak levels.

The most common method of evaluating hCG in urine is hemagglutination inhibition. This laboratory procedure can provide qualitative and quantitative information. The qualitative urine test is easier and less expensive than the serum hCG test (beta-subunit assay); therefore, it's used more commonly to detect pregnancy.

## Normal results

■ In a qualitative immunoassay analysis, results are reported as negative (non-pregnant) or positive (pregnant) for hCG.
■ In quantitative analysis, urine hCG levels in the first trimester of a normal pregnancy may be as high as 500,000 International Units/24 hours; in the second trimester, they range from 10,000 to 25,000 International Units/24 hours; and in the third trimester, from 5,000 to 15,000 International Units/24 hours.
■ Measurable hCG levels don't normally appear in the urine of men or nonpregnant women.

## Abnormal results

■ During pregnancy, elevated urine hCG levels may indicate multiple pregnancy or erythroblastosis fetalis; depressed urine hCG levels may indicate threatened abortion or ectopic pregnancy.
■ Measurable levels of hCG in males and nonpregnant females may indicate choriocarcinoma, ovarian or testicular tumors, melanoma, multiple myeloma, or gastric, hepatic, pancreatic, or breast cancer.

### DRUG CHALLENGE

Phenothiazines (possible false-negative or false-positive)

## Purpose

■ To detect and confirm pregnancy
■ To help diagnose hydatidiform mole or hCG-secreting tumors, threatened abortion, or dead fetus

## Patient preparation

■ If appropriate, explain to the patient that the urine hCG test determines whether she's pregnant or the status of her pregnancy. Alternatively, explain how the test functions as a screen for some types of cancer.
■ Tell the patient that she doesn't need to restrict food, but she should restrict fluids for 8 hours before the test.
■ Inform the patient that the test requires a first-voided morning specimen or urine collection over a 24-hour period, depending on whether the test is qualitative or quantitative.
■ Notify the laboratory and practitioner of medications the patient is taking that may affect test results; they may need to be restricted.

## Procedure and posttest care

■ Confirm the patient's identity using two patient identifiers according to facility policy.
■ For verification of pregnancy (qualitative analysis), collect a first-voided morning specimen. If this isn't possible, collect a random specimen.
■ For quantitative analysis of hCG, collect the patient's urine over a 24-hour period in the appropriate container, discarding the first specimen and retaining the last.

### DO'S & DON'TS

Refrigerate the 24-hour specimen or keep it on ice during the collection period.

■ Specify the date of the patient's last menstrual period on the laboratory request.
■ Instruct the patient that she may resume her usual diet and medications, as ordered.

## Precautions

- Be sure the test is performed at least 5 days after a missed period to avoid a false-negative result.
- Ectopic pregnancy or a threatened abortion may cause a possible false-negative result.

# Urine metabolite tests

## ▉ 17-hydroxycortico-steroids
### [17-OHCS]

The 17-hydroxycorticosteroid (17-OHCS) test measures urine levels of 17-OHCS—metabolites of the hormones that regulate glyconeogenesis. More than 80% of all urinary 17-OHCS are metabolites of cortisol, the primary adrenocortical steroid. Test findings thus reflect cortisol secretion and, indirectly, adrenocortical function.

Urine 17-OHCS levels are most accurately determined from a 24-hour specimen because cortisol secretion varies diurnally and in response to stress and many other factors. Column chromatography and spectrophotofluorimetry with the Porter-Silber reagent are used to measure 17-OHCS levels.

Levels of plasma cortisol, urine-free cortisol, and urine 17-ketosteroids may be measured and corticotropin stimulation and suppression testing performed to confirm test results.

### Reference values

- Normal reference values in men are 4.5 to 12 mg/24 hours (SI, 12.4 to 33.1 µmol/d).
- Normal reference values in women are 2.5 to 10 mg/24 hours (SI, 6.9 to 27.6 µmol/d).

- In children ages 8 to 12, levels are less than 4.5 mg/24 hours (SI, < 12.4 µmol/d).
- In children younger than age 8, levels are normally less than 1.5 mg/24 hours (SI, < 4.14 µmol/d).

### Abnormal results

- Elevated urine 17-OHCS levels may indicate Cushing's syndrome, an adrenal carcinoma or adenoma, or a pituitary tumor. Increased levels may also occur in the patient with virilism, hyperthyroidism, or severe hypertension. Extreme stress induced by such conditions as acute pancreatitis and eclampsia also causes urine 17-OHCS levels to rise above normal.
- Low urine 17-OHCS levels may indicate Addison's disease, hypopituitarism, or myxedema.

**DRUG CHALLENGE**

 Meprobamate, phenothiazines, spironolactone, ascorbic acid, chloral hydrate, chlordiazepoxide, penicillin G, hydroxyzine, quinidine, quinine, iodides, and methenamine (possible increase); hydralazine, phenytoin, thiazide diuretics, estrogens, hormonal contraceptives, phenothiazines, nalidixic acid, and reserpine (possible decrease)

### Purpose

- To assess adrenocortical function

### Patient preparation

- Explain to the patient that this test evaluates how his adrenal glands are functioning.
- Inform the patient that he should restrict food and fluids that will alter test results (coffee, tea) and avoid excessive physical exercise and stressful situations during the collection period.

- Tell the patient that the test requires collection of urine over a 24-hour period and instruct him in the proper collection technique.
- Notify the laboratory and practitioner of medications the patient is taking that may affect test results; they may need to be restricted.

### Procedure and posttest care

- Confirm the patient's identity using two patient identifiers according to facility policy.
- Collect the patient's urine over a 24-hour period, discarding the first specimen and retaining the last. Use a bottle containing a preservative to prevent deterioration of the specimen. Label the specimen appropriately, including the patient's gender on the request forms.

D O ' S  &  D O N ' T S

 Refrigerate the specimen or place it on ice during the collection period.

- Instruct the patient that he may resume his usual activities, diet, and medications, as ordered.

## ▌17-ketogenic steroids
[17-KGS]

Using spectrophotofluorimetry, the 17-ketogenic steroids (17-KGS) test determines urine levels of 17-KGS, which consist of the 17-hydroxycorticosteroids—cortisol and its metabolites, for example—and other adrenocortical steroids, such as pregnanetriol, that can be oxidized in the laboratory to 17-ketosteroids. Because 17-KGS represent such a large group of steroids, this test provides an excellent overall assessment of adrenocortical function. For accurate diagnosis of a specific disease, 17-KGS levels must be compared with results of other tests, including plasma corti-cotropin, plasma cortisol, corticotropin stimulation, single-dose metyrapone, and dexamethasone suppression.

### Reference values

- Normal reference values are 4 to 14 mg/24 hours (SI, 14 to 49 μmol/d) in men.
- Normal reference values are 2 to 12 mg/24 hours (SI, 7 to 42 μmol/d) in women.
- Children ages 11 to 14 excrete 2 to 9 mg/24 hours (SI, 7 to 31 μmol/d).
- Younger children and infants excrete 0.1 to 4 mg/24 hours (SI, 0.3 to 14 μmol/d).

### Abnormal results

- Elevated urine 17-KGS levels indicate hyperadrenalism, which may occur in Cushing's syndrome, adrenogenital syndrome (congenital adrenal hyperplasia), and adrenal carcinoma or adenoma. Levels also rise with severe physical stress (burns, infections, or surgery, for example) or emotional stress.
- Low levels may reflect hypoadrenalism, which may occur in Addison's disease and may also be associated with panhypopituitarism, cretinism, and general wasting.

D R U G  C H A L L E N G E

 Corticotropin, meprobamate, phenothiazines, spironolactone, penicillin, and hydralazine (possible increase); estrogens, quinine, reserpine, thiazide diuretics, and long-term corticosteroid therapy (possible decrease); nalidixic acid, dexamethasone, and carbamazepine (possible increase or decrease)

### Purpose

- To evaluate adrenocortical and testicular function

- To help diagnose Cushing's syndrome and Addison's disease

### Patient preparation

- Explain to the patient that the urine 17-KGS test evaluates adrenal function.
- Inform the patient that he doesn't need to restrict food and fluids, but he should avoid excessive physical exercise and stressful situations during the collection period.
- Tell the patient that the test requires urine collection over a 24-hour period and teach him how to collect the specimen correctly.
- Notify the laboratory and practitioner of medications the patient is taking that may affect test results; they may need to be restricted.

### Procedure and posttest care

- Confirm the patient's identity using two patient identifiers according to facility policy.
- Collect the patient's urine over a 24-hour period, discarding the first specimen and retaining the last. Use a bottle containing a preservative to keep the specimen at a pH of 4.0 to 4.5. Appropriately label the specimen and laboratory requisition requests with the patient's gender.

DO'S & DON'TS

Refrigerate the specimen or place it on ice during the collection period.

- Instruct the patient that he may resume his usual activities and medications, as ordered.

## ▌17-ketosteroids
[17-KS]

The 17-ketosteroids (17-KS) is a fractionation test that uses the spectrophotofluorimetric technique to measure urine levels of 17-KS. Steroids and steroid metabolites characterized by a ketone group on carbon 17 in the steroid nucleus, 17-KS originate primarily in the adrenal glands, but also in the testes and ovaries.

Although not all 17-KS are androgens, they cause androgenic effects. For example, excessive secretion of 17-KS may result in hirsutism and may increase clitoral or phallic size; in utero, elevated 17-KS levels may cause a female fetus to develop a male urogenital tract. Because 17-KS doesn't include all the androgens (testosterone, for example, the most potent androgen), these levels provide only a rough estimate of androgenic activity. To provide additional information about androgen secretion, plasma testosterone levels may be measured concurrently.

### Reference values

- Normal reference values are 10 to 25 mg/24 hours (SI, 35 to 87 µmol/d) in men.
- Normal reference values are 4 to 6 mg/24 hours (SI, 4 to 21 µmol/d) in women.
- Children between ages 10 and 14 excrete 1 to 6 mg/24 hours (SI, 2 to 21 µmol/d).
- Children younger than age 10 excrete less than 3 mg/24 hours (SI, <10 µmol/d).
- For more information about specific steroids in the 17-KS group, the 17-KS fractionation test may be performed. (See *Normal values for the 17-ketosteroid fractionation test,* pages 260 and 261.)

### Abnormal results

- Elevated urine 17-KS levels may result from adrenal hyperplasia, carcinoma or adenoma, or adrenogenital syndrome.
- In women, elevated levels may also indicate ovarian dysfunction, such as polycystic ovary disease (Stein-Leventhal

## Normal values for the 17-ketosteroid fractionation test

Through gas-liquid chromatography, the 17-ketosteroid (17-KS) fractionation test shows which specific steroids in the 17-KS group are elevated or suppressed and thus aids differential diagnosis of conditions suggested by abnormal 17-KS levels. Note that 17-KS levels are measured in milligrams per 24 hours.

| Steroid | Adult male | Adult female | Male ages 10 to 15 |
|---|---|---|---|
| Androsterone | 0.9 to 6.1 | 0 to 3.1 | 0.2 to 2 |
| Dehydroepiandrosterone | 0 to 3.1 | 0 to 1.5 | < 0.4 |
| Etiocholanolone | 0.9 to 5.2 | 0.1 to 3.5 | 0.1 to 1.6 |
| 11-hydroxyandrosterone | 0.2 to 1.6 | 0 to 1.1 | 0.1 to 1.1 |
| 11-hydroxyetiocholanolone | 0.1 to 0.9 | 0.1 to 0.8 | < 0.3 |
| 11-ketoandrosterone | 0 to 0.5 | 0 to 0.3 | < 0.1 |
| 11-ketoetiocholanolone | 0 to 1.6 | 0 to 1 | < 0.3 |
| Pregnanetriol | 0.2 to 2 | 0 to 1.4 | 0.2 to 0.6 |

syndrome), lutein cell tumor of the ovary, or androgenic arrhenoblastoma.

■ In men, elevated 17-KS levels may indicate interstitial cell tumor of the testis.

■ Characteristically, 17-KS levels also rise during pregnancy, severe stress, chronic illness, or debilitating disease.

■ Depressed urine 17-KS levels may result from Addison's disease, panhypopituitarism, eunuchoidism, or castration and may occur in cretinism, myxedema, and nephrosis.

■ When this test is used to monitor cortisol therapy for adrenogenital syndrome, 17-KS levels typically return to normal with adequate cortisol administration.

**D RUG CHALLENGE**

 Meprobamate, phenothiazines, corticotropin, antibiotics, dexamethasone, and spironolactone (possible increase); estrogens, penicillin, ethacrynic acid, and phenytoin (possible decrease); nalidixic acid and quinine (possible increase or decrease)

### Purpose

■ To help diagnose adrenal and gonadal dysfunction

■ To help diagnose adrenogenital syndrome (congenital adrenal hyperplasia)

■ To monitor cortisol therapy in the treatment of adrenogenital syndrome

| Female ages 10 to 15 | Both sexes ages 6 to 9 | Both sexes ages 3 to 5 | Both sexes ages 1 to 2 | Both sexes birth to age 1 |
|---|---|---|---|---|
| 0.5 to 2.5 | 0.1 to 1 | < 0.3 | < 0.3 | < 0.1 |
| < 0.4 | < 0.2 | < 0.1 | < 0.1 | < 0.1 |
| 0.7 to 3.1 | 0.3 to 1 | < 0.7 | < 0.4 | < 0.1 |
| 0.2 to 1 | 0.4 to 1 | < 0.4 | < 0.3 | < 0.3 |
| 0.1 to 0.5 | 0.1 to 0.5 | < 0.4 | < 0.1 | < 0.1 |
| < 0.1 | < 0.1 | < 0.1 | < 0.1 | < 0.1 |
| 0.1 to 0.5 | 0.1 to 0.5 | < 0.4 | < 0.1 | < 0.1 |
| 0.1 to 0.6 | < 0.3 | < 0.1 | < 0.1 | < 0.1 |

## Patient preparation

- Explain to the patient that the urine 17-KS test evaluates hormonal balance.
- Inform the patient that he doesn't need to restrict food and fluids, but he should avoid excessive physical exercise and stressful situations during the collection period.
- Tell the patient that the test requires urine collection over a 24-hour period and instruct him in the proper collection technique.
- Notify the laboratory and practitioner of medications the patient is taking that may affect test results; they may need to be restricted.

## Procedure and posttest care

- Confirm the patient's identity using two patient identifiers according to facility policy.
- Collect the patient's urine over a 24-hour period, discarding the first sample and retaining the last. Use a bottle containing a preservative to keep the specimen at a pH of 4.0 to 4.5. Appropriately label the specimen and laboratory requisition requests with the patient's gender.

### DO'S & DON'TS

 Refrigerate the specimen or place it on ice during the collection period.

- Instruct the patient that he may resume his usual activities and medications, as ordered.

# Pregnanediol, urine

Using gas chromatography or radioimmunoassay, this test measures urine levels of pregnanediol, the chief metabolite of progesterone. Although biologically inert, pregnanediol has diagnostic significance because it reflects about 10% of the endogenous production of its parent hormone.

Normally, urine levels of pregnanediol reflect variations in progesterone secretion during the menstrual cycle and during pregnancy. Direct measurement of plasma progesterone levels by radioimmunoassay may also be done.

## Normal findings

- In nonpregnant females, urine pregnanediol values normally range from 0.5 to 1.5 mg/24 hours during the follicular phase of the menstrual cycle.
- In pregnant females:
  - first trimester: 10 to 30 mg/24 hours
  - second trimester: 35 to 70 mg/24 hours
  - third trimester: 70 to 100 mg/24 hours.
- Normal postmenopausal values range from 0.2 to 1 mg/24 hours.
- In males, urine pregnanediol levels are 0 to 1 mg/24 hours.

## Abnormal results

- During pregnancy, a marked decrease in urine pregnanediol levels based on a single 24-hour urine specimen or a steady decrease in pregnanediol levels in serial measurements may indicate placental insufficiency and requires immediate investigation.
- A precipitous drop in pregnanediol values may suggest fetal distress—for example, threatened abortion or pre-eclampsia—or fetal death.
- Pregnanediol measurements aren't reliable indicators of fetal viability because levels can remain normal even after fetal

death, as long as maternal circulation to the placenta remains adequate.
- In nonpregnant females, abnormally low urine pregnanediol levels may occur with anovulation, amenorrhea, or other menstrual abnormalities.
- Low to normal pregnanediol levels may be associated with hydatidiform mole.
- Elevations may indicate luteinized granulosa or theca cell tumors, diffuse thecal luteinization, or metastatic ovarian cancer.
- Adrenal hyperplasia or biliary tract obstruction may elevate urine pregnanediol values in males or females.
- Some forms of primary hepatic disease produce abnormally low levels in both sexes.

### DRUG CHALLENGE

 Methenamine mandelate, methenamine hippurate, progestogens, combination hormonal contraceptives, and drugs containing corticotropin (possible increase or decrease)

## Purpose

- To evaluate placental function in pregnant females
- To evaluate ovarian function in nonpregnant females
- To help diagnose menstrual disorders

## Patient preparation

- Explain to the patient that the urine pregnanediol test evaluates placental or ovarian function.
- Inform the patient that she doesn't need to restrict food and fluids.
- Tell the patient that the test requires collection of urine over a 24-hour period and teach her the proper collection technique.

■ Advise the pregnant patient that this
test may be repeated several times to obtain serial measurements.
■ Notify the laboratory and practitioner
of medications the patient is taking that
may affect test results; they may need to
be restricted.

### Procedure and posttest care
■ Confirm the patient's identity using
two patient identifiers according to facility policy.
■ Collect the patient's urine over a 24-
hour period, discarding the first specimen and retaining the last.

D o ' s   &   d o n ' t s

 Refrigerate the specimen or
place it on ice during the collection period.

■ Instruct the patient that she may resume her usual medications, as ordered.

### Precautions
■ If the patient is pregnant, note the approximate week of gestation on the laboratory request.
■ For premenopausal women who aren't
pregnant, note the stage of the menstrual cycle on the laboratory request.

# Urine protein, protein metabolites, and pigments

## Protein tests

### Bence Jones protein

Bence Jones proteins are abnormal light-chain immunoglobulins of low molecular weight that are derived from the clone of a single plasma cell. This globulin appears in the urine of 50% to 80% of patients with multiple myeloma and in most patients with Waldenström's macroglobulinemia.

Screening tests, such as thermal coagulation and Bradshaw's test, can detect Bence Jones proteins, but urine immunoelectrophoresis is usually the method of choice for quantitative studies. Serum immunoelectrophoresis, which is sometimes used, is less sensitive than other tests. Nevertheless, urine and serum studies are usually used when multiple myeloma is suspected.

#### Normal results
- No Bence Jones proteins are present.

#### Abnormal results
- The presence of Bence Jones proteins in urine suggests multiple myeloma or Waldenström's macroglobulinemia.

- Very low levels of Bence Jones proteins with no other symptoms may result from benign monoclonal gammopathy.

#### Purpose
- To confirm the presence of multiple myeloma in patients with characteristic signs, such as bone pain (especially in the back and the thorax) and persistent anemia and fatigue

#### Patient preparation
- Explain that the Bence Jones protein test can detect an abnormal protein in the urine.
- Tell the patient that the test requires an early-morning urine specimen; teach him how to collect a midstream clean-catch specimen.
- If a 24-hour urine specimen is being used, instruct the patient on proper collection of a 24-hour urine specimen.

#### Procedure and posttest care
- Confirm the patient's identity using two patient identifiers according to facility policy.
- Collect an early-morning urine specimen of at least 50 ml.
- If performing a 24-hour urine collection, collect the patient's urine over a

24-hour period, discarding the first specimen and retaining the last.

### Precautions
- Keep a 24-hour specimen on ice or in the refrigerator during the collection period.
- Send the specimen to the laboratory immediately after collection or refrigerate it if transport is delayed. If a refrigerated specimen isn't analyzed within 24 hours or it must be discarded.
- Connective tissue disease, renal insufficiency, and certain cancers may cause possible false-positive readings.

# Protein metabolite tests

## Amino acid screening, urine

Urine amino acid tests screen for aminoaciduria—elevated urine amino acid levels—a condition that may result from inborn errors of metabolism due to the absence of specific enzymatic activities. Abnormal metabolism causes an excess of one or more amino acids to appear in plasma and, as the renal threshold is exceeded, in urine. (See *Chromatographic identification of amino acid disorders,* pages 266 and 267.) Aminoacidurias may be classified as primary (overflow) aminoacidopathies or secondary (renal) aminoacidopathies. The latter type is found in conditions marked by defective tubular reabsorption from congenital disorders. A more specific defect, such as cystinuria, may cause one or more amino acids to appear in urine.

To screen neonates, children, and adults for congenital aminoacidurias, plasma or urine specimens may be used. The plasma test is the better indicator of overflow aminoacidurias, whereas the urine test is used to confirm and monitor certain amino acid disorders and to screen for renal aminoacidurias.

Chromatography is the preferred method to screen for aminoacidurias. Positive findings on chromatography can be elaborated by fractionation, showing specific amino acid levels. Testing for specific amino acid levels is also necessary for infants or young children with acidosis, severe vomiting and diarrhea, and abnormal urine odor. Such testing is especially important in neonates because early diagnosis and prompt treatment of aminoacidurias may prevent mental retardation.

### Normal results
- Results are age-dependent and are indicated as normal or abnormal.

### Abnormal results
- Gross changes or abnormal patterns found by thin-layer chromatography, indicating the need for blood and 24-hour urine quantitative column chromatography to be performed to identify specific amino acid abnormalities and differentiate overflow from renal aminoacidurias.

### Purpose
- To screen for renal aminoacidurias
- To follow up on plasma test findings when results of these tests suggest overflow aminoacidurias

### Patient preparation
- Explain to the patient (or the parents if the patient is an infant or a child) that the urine amino acid screening test helps detect amino acid disorders. Advise him that additional tests may be necessary.
- Tell the patient that he doesn't need to restrict food or fluids.

(Text continues on page 268.)

# Chromatographic identification of amino acid disorders

In chromatography—the preferred method for screening aminoacidurias—amino acids migrate into multicolored bands. The sequence of amino acids and their corresponding band numbers, as listed below, reflect these standard migratory patterns. When congenital enzyme deficiencies and subsequent metabolic disorders increase plasma and urine amino acid levels, these bands intensify.

| Chromatographic band number | Amino acids | Metabolic amino acid disorders | | | | | |
| --- | --- | --- | --- | --- | --- | --- | --- |
| | | Phenyl-ketonuria | | Maple syrup urine disease | | Cystinuria | |
| | | Plasma | Urine | Plasma | Urine | Plasma | Urine |
| 1 | Leucine, isoleucine | | | + | + | | + |
| 2 | Phenylalanine | + | + | | | | |
| 3 | Valine, methionine | | | + | + | | |
| 4 | Tryptophan, beta-aminoisobutyric acid | | | | | | |
| 5 | Tyrosine | | | | | | |
| 6 | Proline | | | + | | | |
| 7 | Alanine, ethanolamine | | | | | | |
| 8 | Threonine, glutamic acid | | | | | | |
| 9 | Homocitrulline, glycine, serine, hydroxyproline, aspartic acid, glutamine, citrulline | | | + | | | |
| 10 | Homocystine, asparagine | | | | | | |
| 11 | Argininosuccinic acid, histidine, arginine, lysine, ornithine, cystathionine, cystine, cysteine, hydroxylysine | | | | | | + |

Key: + = increased amino acids in plasma or urine

| | Homo-cystinuria | | Hartnup disease | | Argininosuc-cinicaciduria | | Histidinemia | | Hyperprolin-emia type A | | Citrullinuria | |
|---|---|---|---|---|---|---|---|---|---|---|---|---|
| | Plasma | Urine | Plasma | Urine | Plasma | Urine | Plasma | Urine | Plasma | Urine | Plasma | Urine |
| | | | | + | | | | | | | | |
| | | | | + | | | | | | | | |
| | + | | | + | | | | | | | + | |
| | | | | + | | | | | | | | |
| | | | | + | | | | | | | | |
| | | | | | | | | | + | + | | |
| | | | | + | | | | + | | | | + |
| | | | | | | | | + | | | | + |
| | | | | + | | + | | | | + | + | + |
| | | + | | | | | | | | | | |
| | | | | + | | + | + | + | | | | + |

- Tell the patient that the test requires a urine specimen.
- Notify the laboratory and practitioner of medications the patient is taking that may affect test results; the medications may need to be restricted. If such drugs must be continued, note this on the laboratory request. (If the patient is a breast-fed infant, record any drugs the mother is taking.)

### Procedure and posttest care

- Confirm the patient's identity using two patient identifiers according to facility policy.
- If the patient is an infant, clean and dry the genital area, attach the collection device, and observe for voiding. Transfer urine—at least 20 ml—to a specimen container. Remove the collection device carefully to prevent skin irritation and remove all adhesive residues.
- If the patient is an adult or a child, collect a fresh random specimen.

### Precautions

- If the patient is an infant, apply the adhesive flanges of the collection device securely to the skin to prevent leakage.

## ▌Creatinine clearance

An anhydride of creatine, creatinine is formed and excreted in constant amounts by an irreversible reaction and functions solely as the main end product of creatine. Creatinine production is proportional to total muscle mass and is relatively unaffected by urine volume or normal physical activity or diet.

An excellent diagnostic indicator of renal function, the creatinine clearance test determines how efficiently the kidneys are clearing creatinine from the blood. The rate of clearance is expressed in terms of the volume of blood (in milliliters) that can be cleared of creatinine in 1 minute. This is also known as the glomerular filtration rate (GFR) and is the standard by which kidney function is assessed. Creatinine levels become abnormal when more than 50% of the nephrons have been damaged.

### Reference values

- In males, normal reference values range from 94 to 140 ml/min/1.73 m² (SI, 0.91 to 1.35 ml/s/m²).
- In females, normal reference values range from 72 to 110 ml/min/1.73 m² (SI, 0.69 to 1.06 ml/s/m²).

### Abnormal results

- Low creatinine clearance may result from reduced renal blood flow (associated with shock or renal artery obstruction), acute tubular necrosis, acute or chronic glomerulonephritis, advanced bilateral chronic pyelonephritis, advanced bilateral renal lesions (which may occur in polycystic kidney disease, renal tuberculosis, and cancer), nephrosclerosis, heart failure, Wilms' tumor, or severe dehydration.
- High creatinine clearance can suggest poor hydration.

D**RUG CHALLENGE**

Amphotericin B, thiazide diuretics, furosemide, and aminoglycosides (possible decrease)

### Purpose

- To assess renal function (primarily glomerular filtration)
- To monitor progression of renal insufficiency

### Patient preparation

- Explain that the creatinine clearance test assesses kidney function.
- Inform the patient that he may need to avoid meat, poultry, fish, tea, or coffee for 6 hours before the test.

- Advise the patient that he should avoid strenuous physical exercise during the collection period.
- Tell the patient that the test requires a timed urine specimen and at least one blood sample.
- Tell the patient how the urine specimen will be collected.
- Inform him who will perform the venipuncture and when and that he may feel some discomfort from the needle puncture.
- Explain that more than one venipuncture may be necessary.
- Notify the laboratory and practitioner of medications the patient is taking that may affect test results; the medications may need to be restricted.

### Procedure and posttest care

- Confirm the patient's identity using two patient identifiers according to facility policy.
- Collect a timed urine specimen at 2, 6, 12, or 24 hours in a bottle containing a preservative to prevent creatinine degradation.

##### Do's & don'ts

Refrigerate the urine specimen or keep it on ice during the collection period.

- Perform a venipuncture anytime during the collection period and collect the sample in a 7-ml tube without additives.
- Apply direct pressure to the venipuncture site until bleeding stops.
- If a hematoma develops at the venipuncture site, apply warm soaks.
- Tell the patient to resume his usual diet, activities, and medications, as ordered.

# ▌Creatinine, urine

The creatinine test measures urine levels of creatinine, the chief metabolite of creatine. Produced in amounts proportional to total body muscle mass, creatinine is removed from the plasma primarily by glomerular filtration and is excreted in the urine. Because the body doesn't recycle it, creatinine has a relatively high, constant clearance rate, making it an efficient indicator of renal function. A standard method for determining urine creatinine levels is based on Jaffe's reaction, in which creatinine treated with an alkaline picrate solution yields a bright orange-red complex.

The creatinine clearance test, which measures urine and plasma creatinine clearance, is a more precise index than this test.

### Reference values

- In males, the level is 14 to 26 mg/kg body weight/24 hours (SI, 124 to 230 µmol/kg body weight/d).
- In females, the level is 11 to 20 mg/kg body weight/24 hours (SI, 97 to 177 µmol/kg body weight/d).

### Abnormal results

- Low urine creatinine levels may result from impaired renal perfusion (associated with shock, for example), renal disease due to urinary tract obstruction, chronic bilateral pyelonephritis, acute or chronic glomerulonephritis, or polycystic kidney disease.
- High urine creatinine levels usually have little diagnostic significance.

##### Drug challenge

Corticosteroids, gentamicin, tetracyclines, diuretics, and amphotericin B (possible decrease)

## Purpose
- To help assess glomerular filtration
- To check the accuracy of 24-hour urine collection based on the relatively constant levels of creatinine excretion

### Patient preparation
- Explain that the urine creatinine test helps evaluate kidney function.
- Tell the patient that he doesn't need to restrict fluids but that he shouldn't eat an excessive amount of meat before the test.
- Advise the patient that he should avoid strenuous physical exercise during the collection period.
- Tell the patient that the test usually requires urine collection over a 24-hour period and teach him the proper collection technique.
- Notify the laboratory and practitioner of medications the patient is taking that may affect test results; the medications may need to be restricted.

### Procedure and posttest care
- Confirm the patient's identity using two patient identifiers according to facility policy.
- Collect the patient's urine over a 24-hour period, discarding the first specimen and retaining the last. Use a specimen bottle that contains a preservative to prevent creatinine degradation.

DO'S & DON'TS

 Refrigerate the urine specimen or keep it on ice during the collection period.

- Tell the patient to resume his usual diet, activities, and medications, as ordered.

# ◼ Hydroxyproline

Total urine levels of hydroxyproline, an amino acid found mainly in collagen (a component of skin and bone), are a good index of bone matrix turnover because levels increase when collagen breaks down during bone resorption. Bone matrix turnover and hydroxyproline levels normally rise in children during periods of rapid skeletal growth. They also rise in disorders that increase bone resorption, such as Paget's disease, metastatic bone tumors, and certain endocrine disorders.

Hydroxyproline levels are typically determined colorimetrically on a timed urine sample; they may also be determined by ion-exchange or gas-liquid chromatography. A collagen-restricted diet is essential for this test because hydroxyproline levels reflect collagen intake. Free hydroxyproline, a small component of total hydroxyproline and a sensitive indicator of dietary collagen intake, may be measured to validate results.

### Reference values
- Hydroxyproline levels are 1 to 9 mg/24 hours (SI, 1.0 to 3.4 International Units/d).

### Abnormal results
- High hydroxyproline levels may indicate bone disease, metastatic bone tumors, or endocrine disorders that stimulate hormonal secretion.
- Hydroxyproline levels should decrease slowly during therapy for bone resorption disorders.

DRUG CHALLENGE

 Ascorbic acid, vitamin D, aspirin, glucocorticoids, antineoplastic agents, calcium gluconate, corticosteroids, estradiol, propranolol, calcitonin (possible decrease); growth hormone, parathyroid hormone, phenobarbital, and sulfonylureas (increase)

## Purpose
▪ To monitor treatment for disorders characterized by bone resorption, including Paget's disease, metastatic bone tumors, certain endocrine disorders (hyperthyroidism), rheumatoid arthritis, and osteoporosis
▪ To help diagnose disorders characterized by bone resorption

## Patient preparation
▪ Explain that the urine hydroxyproline test helps monitor treatment or detect an amino acid disorder related to bone formation.
▪ Inform the patient that he must follow a collagen-free diet and avoid eating ice cream, candy, meat, fish, poultry, jelly, and any foods containing gelatin for 24 hours before the test and during the test period itself.
▪ Tell the patient that the test requires urine collection over a 2-hour or 24-hour period and teach him the correct collection technique.
▪ Note the patient's age and sex on the laboratory request.
▪ Notify the laboratory and practitioner of medications the patient is taking that may affect test results; the medications may need to be restricted.

## Procedure and posttest care
▪ Confirm the patient's identity using two patient identifiers according to facility policy.
▪ Collect the patient's urine over a 2-hour or 24-hour period. In a 24-hour collection, discard the first sample and retain the last. Use a container that has a preservative to prevent hydroxyproline degradation.

**DO'S & DON'TS**

 Refrigerate the urine specimen or keep it on ice during the collection period.

▪ Tell the patient to resume his usual diet, activities, and medications, as ordered.

## Precautions
▪ Psoriasis and burns may increase hydroxyproline levels because of collagen turnover.

# Urea clearance
The urea clearance test is a quantitative analysis of urine levels of urea, the main nitrogenous component in urine and the end product of protein metabolism. (See *How urea is formed,* page 272.) After filtration by the glomeruli, roughly 40% of the urea is reabsorbed by the renal tubules. Because of this reabsorption, urea clearance was once considered a precise fraction (60%) of the glomerular filtration rate (GFR); however, because the reabsorption rate of urea varies with the amount of water reabsorbed, this test actually assesses overall renal function; the creatinine clearance test provides a more accurate evaluation of the GFR.

In urea clearance, blood urea content and the total amount of urea excreted in the urine are proportional only when the rate of urine flow is 2 ml/minute or higher (maximal clearance). At lower flow rates, the test's accuracy decreases. The equation for determining urea clearance is $C = (U \times V) \, P$; it's similar to the equation used for creatinine clearance.

## Reference values
▪ If the urine flow rate is 2 ml/minute or higher, urea clearance rate is 64 to 99 ml/minute.

## How urea is formed

Urea, the main nitrogenous component in urine, is the final product of protein metabolism. Amino acids absorbed by the intestinal villi pass from the portal vein into the liver. Because the liver stores only small amounts of amino acids—which are later returned to the blood for use in the synthesis of enzymes, hormones, or new protoplasm—the excess is converted into other substances, such as glucose, glycogen, and fat.

Before this conversion, the amino acids are deaminated—they lose their nitrogenous amino groups. These amino groups are then converted to ammonia. Because ammonia is very toxic, especially to the brain, it must be removed as quickly as it's formed. (Serious liver disease causes elevated blood ammonia levels and eventually leads to hepatic coma.)

In the liver, ammonia combines with carbon dioxide to form urea, which is released into the blood and ultimately secreted in urine.

■ If the urine flow rate is less than 2 ml/minute, urea clearance rate is 41 to 68 ml/minute.
■ If the urine flow rate is less than 1 ml/minute, this test shouldn't be performed.

### Abnormal results
■ Low urea clearance rates may indicate decreased renal blood flow (due to shock or renal artery obstruction), acute or chronic glomerulonephritis, advanced bilateral chronic pyelonephritis, acute tubular necrosis, nephrosclerosis, advanced bilateral renal lesions (as in polycystic kidney disease, renal tuberculosis, or cancer), bilateral ureteral obstruction, heart failure, or dehydration.

■ High urea clearance rates usually aren't diagnostically significant.

**Drug challenge**

 Caffeine, milk, or small doses of epinephrine (increase); antidiuretic hormone or large doses of epinephrine (decrease); corticosteroids, amphotericin B, thiazide diuretics, and streptomycin

### Purpose
■ To assess overall renal function

### Patient preparation
■ Explain that the urea clearance test evaluates kidney function.
■ Instruct the patient to fast from midnight before the test and to abstain from exercise before and during the test.
■ Tell the patient that the test requires two timed urine specimens and one blood sample.
■ Tell him how the urine specimens will be collected, who will perform the venipuncture and when, and that he may experience slight discomfort from the needle puncture and the tourniquet.
■ Notify the laboratory and practitioner of medications the patient is taking that may affect test results; the medications may need to be restricted.

### Procedure and posttest care
■ Confirm the patient's identity using two patient identifiers according to facility policy.
■ Instruct the patient to empty his bladder and discard the urine. Then give him water to drink to ensure adequate urine output.
■ Collect two specimens 1 hour apart and mark the collection time on the laboratory request.

- Perform a venipuncture anytime during the collection period and collect the sample in a 7-ml red-top tube.
- If a hematoma develops at the venipuncture site, apply warm soaks.
- Tell the patient to resume his usual diet, activities, and medications, as ordered.

### Precautions
- Because this is a clearance test, make sure the patient empties his bladder completely and that the total amount of urine is collected from each hour's specimen.
- If the patient is catheterized, empty the drainage bag before beginning the specimen collection.

# Pigment tests

## Hemoglobin, urine

An abnormal finding, free hemoglobin (Hb) in the urine may occur in hemolytic anemias, infection, strenuous exercise, or severe intravascular hemolysis from a transfusion reaction. Contained in red blood cells (RBCs), Hb consists of an iron-protoporphyrin complex (heme) and a polypeptide (globin). Usually, RBC destruction occurs within the reticuloendothelial system. When RBC destruction occurs within the circulation, free Hb enters the plasma and binds with haptoglobin. If the plasma level of Hb exceeds that of haptoglobin, the excess of unbound Hb is excreted in the urine (hemoglobinuria).

Heme proteins act like enzymes that catalyze oxidation of organic substances. This reaction produces a blue coloration; the intensity of color varies with the amount of Hb present. Microscopic examination is required to identify intact RBCs in urine (hematuria), which can occur in the presence of unbound Hb.

### Normal results
- Hb isn't present in the urine.

### Abnormal results
- Hemoglobinuria may result from severe intravascular hemolysis due to a blood transfusion reaction, burns, or a crush injury; acquired hemolytic anemias caused by chemical or drug intoxication or malaria; congenital hemolytic anemias, such as hemoglobinopathies or enzyme defects; paroxysmal nocturnal hemoglobinuria (another type of hemolytic anemia); or cystitis, ureteral calculi, or urethritis
- Hemoglobinuria and hematuria occur in renal epithelial damage (which may result from acute glomerulonephritis or pyelonephritis), renal tumor, and tuberculosis.

**DRUG CHALLENGE**

 Nephrotoxic drugs and anticoagulants (positive results); large doses of vitamin C or drugs that contain vitamin C as a preservative (false-negative)

### Purpose
- To help diagnose hemolytic anemias, infection, or severe intravascular hemolysis from a transfusion reaction

### Patient preparation
- Explain that the urine hemoglobin test detects excessive RBC destruction.
- Tell the patient that he doesn't need to restrict food or fluids.
- Tell the patient that the test requires a random urine specimen and teach him the proper collection technique.

## Bedside testing for urine blood pigments

To test a patient's urine for blood pigments at the bedside, use one of these methods.

### Dipstick, Multistix, or Chemstrip
- Collect a urine specimen.
- Dip the stick into the specimen and withdraw it.
- After 30 seconds, compare the stick to the color chart. Blue indicates a positive reaction; the intensity of color indicates pigment concentration.

### Occult tablet
- Collect a urine specimen.
- Put one drop of urine on the filter paper. Place the tablet on the urine and then put two drops of water on the tablet.
- After 2 minutes inspect the filter paper around the tablet. Blue indicates a

positive reaction; the intensity of color indicates pigment concentration.

### Occult solution
- Collect a urine specimen.
- After placing one drop of urine on the filter paper, close the package and turn it over. Open the opposite ends and place two drops of solution on the filter paper.
- After 30 seconds inspect the filter paper. Blue indicates a positive reaction; the intensity of color indicates pigment concentration.

### Distinguishing hemoglobin
- Because these methods detect only blood pigments, immunochemical studies are necessary to differentiate hemoglobin from other blood pigments such as myoglobin.

---

- If a female patient is menstruating, reschedule the test because menstruation can alter test results.
- Notify the laboratory and practitioner of medications the patient is taking that may affect test results; the medications may need to be restricted.

### Procedure and posttest care
- Confirm the patient's identity using two patient identifiers according to facility policy.
- Collect a random urine specimen. (See *Bedside testing for urine blood pigments.*)
- Tell the patient to resume his medications, as ordered.

## Porphyrins, urine

The test for porphyrins is a quantitative analysis of urine porphyrins (most notably, uroporphyrins and coproporphyrins) and their precursors (porphyrinogens such as porphobilinogen [PBG]). Tests for porphyrins may include PBG and urine aminolevulinic acid. Porphyrins are red-orange fluorescent compounds consisting of four pyrrole rings that are produced during heme biosynthesis. They're present in all protoplasm, figure in energy storage and usage, and are normally excreted in urine in small amounts. High urine levels of porphyrins or porphyrinogens reflect impaired heme biosynthesis. Such impairment may result from inherited enzyme deficiencies (congenital porphyrias) or from defects caused by such disorders as hemolytic anemias and hepatic disease (acquired porphyrias).

Determination of the specific porphyrins and porphyrinogens found in a urine specimen can help identify the impaired metabolic step in heme biosynthesis. Occasionally, a preliminary qualitative screening is performed on a random specimen; however, a positive finding on the screening test must be confirmed by the quantitative analysis of a 24-hour specimen. For correct diagnosis of a specific porphyria, urine porphyrin levels should be correlated with plasma and fecal porphyrin levels.

## Reference values

- Uroporphyrin levels are normally 27 to 52 mcg/24 hours (SI, 32 to 63 nmol/d).
- Coproporphyrin levels are normally 34 to 230 mcg/24 hours (SI, 52 to 351 nmol/d).

## Abnormal results

- High levels of porphyrins and porphyrin precursors in urine are characteristic of porphyria, infectious hepatitis, Hodgkin's disease, central nervous system disorders, cirrhosis, or heavy metal, benzene, or carbon tetrachloride toxicity. (See *Urine porphyrin levels in porphyria*, pages 276 and 277.)

DRUG CHALLENGE

Barbiturates, chloral hydrate, sulfonamides, meprobamate, and chlordiazepoxide (induce porphyria or porphyrinuria); hormonal contraceptives and griseofulvin (increase); rifampin (elevated urine urobilinogen)

## Purpose

- To help diagnose congenital or acquired porphyrias
- To help diagnose suspected lead poisoning

## Patient preparation

- Explain that the urine porphyrin test detects abnormal hemoglobin formation.
- Tell the patient that he doesn't need to restrict food or fluids.
- Tell the patient that the test requires urine collection over a 24-hour period and teach him the proper collection technique.
- Notify the laboratory and practitioner of medications the patient is taking that may affect test results; the medications may need to be restricted.

## Procedure and posttest care

- Confirm the patient's identity using two patient identifiers according to facility policy.
- Collect the patient's urine over a 24-hour period, discarding the first specimen and retaining the last. Use a light-resistant specimen bottle containing a preservative to prevent degradation of the light-sensitive porphyrins and their precursors.

DO'S & DON'TS

Refrigerate the urine specimen or keep it on ice during the collection period.

- Tell the patient to resume his medications, as ordered.

# Urine porphyrin levels in porphyria

In porphyria, defective heme biosynthesis increases urinary porphyrins and their corresponding precursors.

| Porphyria | Porphyrins | |
|---|---|---|
| | *Uroporphyrins* | *Coproporphyrins* |
| Acute intermittent porphyria | Variable | Variable |
| Coproporphyria | Not applicable | May be highly increased during acute attack |
| Erythropoietic porphyria | Highly increased | Increased |
| Erythropoietic protoporphyria | Normal | Normal |
| Porphyria cutanea tarda | Highly increased | Increased |
| Variegate porphyria | Normal or slightly increased; may be highly increased during acute attack | Normal or slightly increased; may be highly increased during acute attack |

| Porphyrin precursors | |
| --- | --- |
| *D-amino-* *levulinic acid* | *Porpho-* *bilinogens* |
| Highly increased | Highly increased |
| Increased during acute attack | Increased during acute attack |
| Normal | Normal |
| Normal | Normal |
| Variable | Variable |
| Highly increased during acute attack | Normal or slightly increased; highly increased during acute attack |

## Precautions

- Be aware that pregnancy or menstruation may affect the accuracy of test results.
- Protect the specimen from light exposure if a light-resistant container isn't available.
- Put the collection bag in a dark plastic bag if an indwelling urinary catheter is in place.

# 16

# Urine sugars, ketones, and mucopolysaccharides

## Carbohydrate and fat metabolism tests

### ▌Glucose oxidase

The glucose oxidase test—which involves the use of commercial, plastic-coated reagent strips (Clinistix, Diastix) or Tes-Tape—is a specific, qualitative test for glycosuria. The test is used primarily to monitor urine glucose in patients with diabetes. Patients can perform this test at home because of its simplicity and convenience.

#### Normal results
- No glucose is present in urine.

#### Abnormal results
- Glycosuria occurs in diabetes mellitus, adrenal and thyroid disorders, hepatic and central nervous system diseases, conditions involving low renal threshold (such as Fanconi's syndrome), toxic renal tubular disease, heavy metal poisoning, glomerulonephritis, and nephrosis; in pregnant women; and in those receiving total parenteral nutrition.

- Glycosuria also occurs with the administration of large amounts of glucose and of certain drugs.

#### Purpose
- To detect glycosuria and determine the renal threshold for glucose
- To monitor urine glucose levels during insulin therapy

#### Patient preparation
- Explain that the glucose oxidase test determines urine glucose concentration.
- If the patient is newly diagnosed with diabetes, teach him how to perform a reagent strip test.

- If the patient is taking levodopa, ascorbic acid, phenazopyridine, or salicylates, use Clinitest tablets instead.

### Procedure and posttest care

- Confirm the patient's identity using two patient identifiers according to facility policy.
- Have the patient void, then give him a drink of water.
- Collect a second-voided specimen after 30 to 45 minutes.

### Clinistix test

- Dip the test area of the reagent strip in the specimen for 2 seconds.
- Remove excess urine by tapping the strip against a clean surface or the side of the container and begin timing.
- Hold the strip in the air and "read" the color exactly 10 seconds after taking the strip out of the urine by comparing it with the reference color blocks on the label of the container.
- Record the results.
- Ignore color changes that develop after 10 seconds.

### Diastix test

- Dip the reagent strip in the specimen for 2 seconds.
- Remove excess urine by tapping the strip against the container and begin timing.
- Hold the strip in the air and compare the color to the color chart exactly 30 seconds after taking the strip out of the urine.
- Record the results.
- Ignore color changes that develop after 30 seconds.

### Tes-Tape

- Withdraw about 1″ (2.5 cm) of the reagent tape from the dispenser; dip ¼″ (0.6 cm) in the specimen for 2 seconds.

- Remove excess urine by tapping the strip against the side of the container and begin timing.
- Hold the tape in the air and compare the color of the darkest part of the tape to the color chart exactly 60 seconds after taking the strip out of the urine.
- If the tape indicates 0.5% or higher, wait an additional 60 seconds to make the final color comparison.
- Record the results.

### Precautions

- Keep the test strip container tightly closed to prevent deterioration of strips by exposure to light or moisture.
- Store the container in a cool place (under 86° F [30° C]) to avoid heat degradation.

DO'S & DON'TS

 Don't use discolored or darkened Clinistix or Diastix or dark yellow or yellow-brown Tes-Tape.

## Ketones

In the ketone test—a routine, semiquantitative screening test—a commercially prepared product is used to measure the urine level of ketone bodies. Ketone bodies are the by-products of fat metabolism; they include acetoacetic acid, acetone, and beta-hydroxybutyric acid. Excessive amounts may appear in the patient with carbohydrate dehydration, which may occur in starvation or diabetic ketoacidosis (DKA).

Commercially available tests include the Acetest tablet, Chemstrip K, Ketostix, or Keto-Diastix. Each product measures a specific ketone body. For example, Acetest measures acetone, and Ketostix measures acetoacetic acid.

## Normal results
- No ketones are present in urine.

## Abnormal results
- Ketonuria may occur in uncontrolled diabetes mellitus or starvation or as a metabolic complication of total parenteral nutrition.

## Purpose
- To screen for ketonuria
- To identify DKA and carbohydrate deprivation
- To distinguish between a diabetic and a nondiabetic coma
- To monitor control of diabetes mellitus, ketogenic weight reduction, and treatment of DKA

## Patient preparation
- Explain that the ketone test evaluates fat metabolism.
- If the patient is newly diagnosed with diabetes, tell him how to perform the test.

**DRUG CHALLENGE**

Levodopa, phenazopyridine, or sulfobromophthalein (inaccurate results with reagent strips)

## Procedure and posttest care
- Confirm the patient's identity using two patient identifiers according to facility policy.
- Instruct the patient to void and then to drink a glass of water.
- Collect a second-voided midstream specimen about 30 minutes later.

### Acetest
- If the patient is taking levodopa or phenazopyridine or has recently received sulfobromophthalein, use Acetest tablets because reagent strips may produce inaccurate results.

- Lay the tablet on a piece of white paper and place one drop of urine on the tablet.
- Compare the tablet color (white, lavender, or purple) with the color chart after 30 seconds.

### Ketostix
- Dip the reagent stick into the specimen and remove it immediately.
- Compare the stick color (buff or purple) with the color chart after 15 seconds.
- Record the results as negative, small, moderate, or large amounts of ketones.

### Keto-Diastix
- Dip the reagent strip into the specimen and remove it immediately.
- Tap the edge of the strip against the container or a clean, dry surface to remove excess urine.
- Hold the strip horizontally to prevent mixing the chemicals from the two areas.
- Interpret each area of the strip separately. Compare the color of the ketone section (buff or purple) with the appropriate color chart after exactly 15 seconds; compare the color of the glucose section after 30 seconds.
- Ignore color changes that occur after the specified waiting periods.
- Record the results as negative or positive for small, moderate, or large amounts of ketones.

## Precautions
- Test the specimen within 60 minutes after it's obtained; otherwise, you must refrigerate it.
- Allow refrigerated specimens to return to room temperature before testing.
- Don't use tablets or strips that have become discolored or darkened.

# Urine vitamins and minerals

## Vitamin assays

### Tryptophan challenge

This test measures urine xanthurenic acid after a challenge dose of tryptophan to confirm vitamin $B_6$ deficiency long before symptoms appear.

Although vitamin $B_6$ isn't directly involved in energy metabolism, it's essential for reactions that occur in protein metabolism and for amino acid synthesis. Vitamin $B_6$ deficiency can cause hypochromic microcytic anemia without iron deficiency and central nervous system disturbances. When normal magnesium levels accompany a vitamin $B_6$ deficiency, urinary citrate and oxalate solubility may decrease, causing urinary calculi formation.

#### Reference values
▪ Urine level of xanthurenic acid after a tryptophan challenge dose is less than 50 mg/24 hours.

#### Abnormal results
▪ Urine levels of xanthurenic acid exceeding 100 mg/24 hours indicate vitamin $B_6$ deficiency, a rare disorder caused by malnutrition, malignancy, pregnancy, familial xanthurenic aciduria, or the use of hormonal contraceptives, hydralazine, D-penicillamine, or isoniazid.

DRUG CHALLENGE

Hormonal contraceptives, hydralazine, and isoniazid (decrease)

#### Purpose
▪ To detect vitamin $B_6$ deficiency

#### Patient preparation
▪ Explain that the tryptophan challenge test determines the body's stores of vitamin $B_6$.
▪ Tell the patient that he'll receive an oral dose of medication.
▪ Explain that this test requires urine collection over a 24-hour period.
▪ Notify the laboratory and practitioner of medications the patient is taking that may affect test results; the medications may need to be restricted.

#### Procedure and posttest care
▪ Confirm the patient's identity using two patient identifiers according to facility policy.
▪ Give L-tryptophan by mouth (usually, 50 mg/kg for children and up to 2 g/kg for adults).

- Have the patient void and discard the urine. Immediately begin collection of a 24-hour urine specimen.

- Inform the patient with vitamin $B_6$ deficiency that yeast, wheat, corn, liver, and kidneys are good sources of pyridoxine.
- Tell the patient to resume his medications, as ordered.

### Precautions
- Make sure the specimen bottle contains a crystal of thymol, a preservative.

# Vitamin $B_1$, urine

The vitamin $B_1$ test is used to detect a deficiency of vitamin $B_1$ (thiamine), a condition called beriberi. This water-soluble vitamin, which requires folic acid (folate) for effective uptake, is absorbed in the duodenum and excreted in the urine. Urine levels of vitamin $B_1$ reflect dietary intake and metabolic storage of thiamine. A coenzyme in decarboxylase reactions with citric acids, vitamin $B_1$ helps metabolize carbohydrates, fats, and proteins.

Rare in the United States, vitamin $B_1$ deficiency is most common in Asians because of their subsistence on polished rice. Vitamin $B_1$ deficiency may result from inadequate dietary intake (usually associated with alcoholism), impaired absorption (malabsorption syndrome), impaired utilization (hepatic disease), or conditions that increase metabolic demand (pregnancy, lactation, fever, exercise, hyperthyroidism, surgery, and high carbohydrate intake). High dietary intake of fats and proteins spares the vitamin $B_1$ necessary for tissue respiration.

The clinical effects of vitamin $B_1$ deficiency vary. Early deficiency produces nonspecific symptoms that may include fatigue, irritability, sleep disturbances, and abdominal and precordial discomfort. Severe deficiency states vary in several distinct patterns: Infantile beriberi produces abdominal pain, edema, irritability, vomiting, pallor and, possibly, seizures; wet, or edematous, beriberi (a complication of chronic alcoholism) produces severe neurologic symptoms—which may lead to Wernicke-Korsakoff's syndrome and Korsakoff's psychosis—emaciation, and edema that rises from the legs. Beriberi also causes arrhythmias, cardiomegaly, and circulatory collapse.

### Reference values
- Normal urinary excretion ranges from 100 to 200 mcg/24 hours.

### Abnormal results
- Deficient urine levels of vitamin $B_1$ can result from inadequate dietary intake, hyperthyroidism, alcoholism, severe hepatic disease, chronic diarrhea, or prolonged diuretic therapy.
- Negative results indicate neuritis unrelated to deficiency.

### Purpose
- To help confirm vitamin $B_1$ deficiency (beriberi) and to distinguish it from other causes of polyneuritis

### Patient preparation
- Explain to the patient that this test evaluates the body's stores of vitamin $B_1$.
- Tell the patient that the test requires a 24-hour urine specimen. If the patient is to collect the specimen, teach him the proper technique.

- Check the patient's diet history to rule out a deficiency due to inadequate intake.

### Procedure and posttest care
- Confirm the patient's identity using two patient identifiers according to facility policy.
- Collect a 24-hour urine specimen.

 Refrigerate the specimen or place it on ice during the collection period.

- Educate the patient who's deficient in vitamin $B_1$ about good dietary sources of this vitamin: beef, pork, organ meats, fresh vegetables (especially peas and beans), and wheat and other whole grains.

### Precautions
- Tell the patient to save all urine voided in a 24-hour period and not to contaminate the urine specimen with toilet tissue or stool. If any urine is lost, discard the entire specimen and restart collecting with the next void.

# Mineral assays

## Calcium and phosphates, urine

The calcium and phosphates test measures the urine levels of calcium and phosphates, elements essential for bone formation and resorption. Urine calcium and phosphate levels generally parallel serum levels.

Normally absorbed in the upper intestine and excreted in stool and urine, calcium and phosphates help maintain tissue and fluid pH, electrolyte balance in cells and extracellular fluids, and permeability of cell membranes. Calcium promotes enzymatic processes, aids blood coagulation, and lowers neuromuscular irritability; phosphates aid carbohydrate metabolism.

### Reference values
- Normal values depend on dietary intake.
- In a normal diet, urine calcium levels range from 100 to 300 mg/24 hours (SI, 2.5 to 7.5 mmol/d).
- Excretion of phosphate is less than 1,000 mg/24 hours.

### Abnormal results
- Many disorders may affect calcium and phosphorus levels. (See *Disorders that affect urine calcium and urine phosphorus levels,* page 284.)

 Parathyroid hormones (increases phosphate excretion and decrease calcium excretion); thiazide diuretics (decreases calcium excretion); prolonged inactivity and ingestion of corticosteroids, sodium phosphate, calcitonin (increases calcium excretion); vitamin D (increases phosphate absorption and excretion)

### Purpose
- To evaluate calcium and phosphate metabolism and excretion
- To monitor treatment of calcium or phosphate deficiency

### Patient preparation
- Explain that the urine calcium and phosphates test measures the amount of calcium and phosphates in the urine.
- Encourage the patient to be as active as possible before the test.
- Tell the patient that the test requires urine collection over a 24-hour period.

## Disorders that affect urine calcium and urine phosphorus levels

| Disorder | Urine calcium level | Urine phosphate level |
| --- | --- | --- |
| Hyperparathyroidism | High | High |
| Vitamin D intoxication | High | Low |
| Metastatic carcinoma | High | Normal |
| Sarcoidosis | High | Low |
| Renal tubular acidosis | High | High |
| Multiple myeloma | High or normal | High or normal |
| Paget's disease | Normal | Normal |
| Milk-alkali syndrome | Low or normal | Low or normal |
| Hypoparathyroidism | Low | Low |
| Acute nephrosis | Low | Low or normal |
| Chronic nephrosis | Low | Low |
| Acute nephritis | Low | Low |
| Renal insufficiency | Low | Low |
| Osteomalacia | Low | Low |
| Steatorrhea | Low | Low |

If the patient is to collect the specimen, teach him the proper technique.
- Provide a diet that contains about 130 mg of calcium/24 hours for 3 days before the test, or give the patient a copy of the diet to follow at home.
- Notify the laboratory and practitioner of medications the patient is taking that may affect test results; the medications may need to be restricted.

### Procedure and posttest care
- Confirm the patient's identity using two patient identifiers according to facility policy.
- Collect the patient's urine over a 24-hour period, discarding the first specimen and retaining the last.

ALERT

Observe the patient with low urine calcium levels for tetany.

■ Tell the patient to resume his usual diet, activities, and medications, as ordered.

# Magnesium, urine

Measurement of urine magnesium is especially useful because magnesium deficiency is detectable in urine before it's detectable in serum. This test may be used to rule out magnesium deficiency as the cause of neurologic symptoms and to help evaluate glomerular function in suspected renal disease.

Magnesium is a cation found primarily in the bones and in intracellular fluid; a small amount is present in extracellular fluid. This element activates many enzyme systems, helps transport sodium and potassium across cell membranes, affects nucleic acid and protein metabolism, and influences intracellular calcium levels through its effect on parathyroid hormone secretion.

### Reference values
■ Urine magnesium levels are 6 to 10 mEq/24 hours (SI, 3 to 5 mmol/d).

### Abnormal results
■ Low urine magnesium levels may result from malabsorption, decreased dietary intake of magnesium, acute or chronic diarrhea, diabetic ketoacidosis, dehydration, pancreatitis, advanced renal failure, and primary aldosteronism.
■ High urine magnesium levels may result from early chronic renal disease, adrenocortical insufficiency (Addison's disease), chronic alcoholism, or chronic ingestion of magnesium-containing antacids.

### DRUG CHALLENGE

Spirolactone (decrease); increased calcium intake (decrease); magnesium-containing antacids, ethacrynic acid, thiazide diuretics, and aldosterone (possible increase)

### Purpose
■ To rule out magnesium deficiency in the patient with symptoms of central nervous system irritation
■ To detect excessive urinary excretion of magnesium
■ To help evaluate glomerular function in renal disease

### Patient preparation
■ Explain that the urine magnesium test determines urine magnesium levels.
■ Tell the patient that this test requires urine collection over a 24-hour period.
■ Notify the laboratory and practitioner of medications the patient is taking that may affect test results; the medications may need to be restricted.
■ Tell the patient to avoid strenuous exercise during the collection period.

### Procedure and posttest care
■ Confirm the patient's identity using two patient identifiers according to facility policy.
■ Collect the patient's urine over a 24-hour period, discarding the first specimen and retaining the last.
■ Tell the patient to resume his medications, as ordered.

# Oxalate

Oxalate, a salt of oxalic acid, is an end product of metabolism and is excreted almost exclusively in the urine. Measuring urine levels of oxalate detects hyperoxaluria, a disorder in which oxalate accumulates in the soft and connective tissue, especially in the kidneys and bladder, causing chronic inflammation and fibrosis. Calcium oxalate deposits are the most common cause of renal calculi, which can damage the kidney.

## Reference values
- Urine oxalate levels are less than or equal to 40 mg/24 hours (SI, ≤ 456 µmol/d).

## Abnormal results
- High urine oxalate levels (hyperoxaluria) up to 400 mg/24 hours (SI, 4,560 µmol/d) may result from excessive metabolic production of oxalate or increased oxalate intake.
- Primary hyperoxaluria, a rare inborn metabolic disorder, causes excessive production and urinary excretion of oxalate. In this type of hyperoxaluria, levels in urine become elevated before those in serum.
- Secondary hyperoxaluria can result from pancreatic insufficiency, diabetes mellitus, cirrhosis, pyridoxine deficiency, Crohn's disease, ileal resection, or ingestion of antifreeze (ethylene glycol) or stain remover; it may also occur as a reaction to a methoxyflurane anesthetic.

### DRUG CHALLENGE

 Vitamin C (increase in oxalate excretion, which may be a risk for calcium oxalate nephrolithiasis in individuals consuming megadoses of this vitamin)

## Purpose
- To detect primary hyperoxaluria in infants
- To rule out hyperoxaluria in renal insufficiency
- To evaluate patients with malabsorption syndrome

## Patient preparation
- Explain to the patient (or to the parents if the patient is a child) that the urine oxalate test determines if the urine contains excess oxalate.
- Tell the patient or parents that the test requires urine collection over a 24-hour period.
- Tell the patient to avoid foods high in oxalate—such as tomatoes, strawberries, rhubarb, and spinach—for 1 week before the test.

## Procedure and posttest care
- Confirm the patient's identity using two patient identifiers according to facility policy.
- Collect the patient's urine over a 24-hour period, discarding the first specimen and retaining the last. Use a light-protected container with 30 ml of 6 N hydrochloric acid.
- Inform the patient to resume his usual diet.

## Precautions
- Ingestion of tomatoes, strawberries, rhubarb, and spinach may cause a possible false increase.

# Potassium, urine

The urine potassium test is a quantitative test that measures urine levels of potassium, a major intracellular cation that helps regulate acid-base balance and neuromuscular function. Potassium imbalance may cause such signs and symptoms as muscle weakness, nausea, diarrhea, confusion, hypotension, and electrocardiogram changes; severe imbalance may lead to cardiac arrest.

Most commonly, a serum potassium test is performed to detect hyperkalemia (abnormally high levels) or hypokalemia (abnormally low levels). A urine potassium test may be performed to evaluate hypokalemia when a history and physical examination fail to uncover the cause. If results suggest a renal disorder, additional renal function tests may be ordered.

## Reference values
- In adults, potassium excretion is 25 to 125 mmol/24 hours (SI, 25 to 125 mmol/d) but varies with diet.
- In children, potassium excretion is 22 to 57 mmol/24 hours (SI, 22 to 57 mmol/d).

## Abnormal results
- In a patient with hypokalemia, potassium excretion less than 10 mmol/24 hours (SI, < 10 mmol/d) suggests normal renal function, indicating that potassium loss is most likely the result of a GI disorder such as malabsorption syndrome.
- In a patient with hypokalemia lasting more than 3 days, urine potassium level above 10 mmol/24 hours (SI, > 10 mmol/d) indicates renal loss of potassium, resulting from aldosteronism, renal tubular acidosis, or chronic renal failure.
- Extrarenal disorders, such as dehydration, starvation, Cushing's disease, or salicylate intoxication, may elevate urine potassium levels.

### Drug challenge

Potassium-wasting medications, such as ammonium chloride, thiazide diuretics, and acetazolamide (increase)

## Purpose
- To determine whether hypokalemia is caused by renal or extrarenal disorders

## Patient preparation
- Explain that the urine potassium test evaluates his kidney function.
- Tell the patient that he doesn't have to restrict food or fluids.
- Tell him that the test requires urine collection over a 24-hour period.
- If the specimen is to be collected at home, teach the patient the correct collection technique.

- Notify the laboratory and practitioner of medications the patient is taking that may affect test results; the medications may need to be restricted.

## Procedure and posttest care
- Confirm the patient's identity using two patient identifiers according to facility policy.
- Collect the patient's urine over a 24-hour period, discarding the first specimen and retaining the last.

### Do's & don'ts

Refrigerate the specimen or place it on ice during the collection period.

- Give potassium supplements and monitor serum levels as appropriate.
- Provide dietary supplements and nutritional counseling as necessary.
- Replace fluid volume loss with I.V. or oral fluids as necessary.
- Tell the patient to resume his medications, as ordered.
- Don't use a metallic bedpan for collection.

## Precautions
- Excessive vomiting or stomach suctioning may cause decreased potassium levels.

# ▌Sodium and chloride, urine

The sodium and chloride test determines urine levels of sodium, the major extracellular cation, and of chloride, the major extracellular anion. Less significant than serum levels and, consequently, performed less frequently, the measurement of urine sodium and chloride levels is used to evaluate renal conservation of these two electrolytes and to confirm serum sodium and chloride values.

Normal ranges of sodium and chloride in the urine vary greatly with dietary salt intake and perspiration.

## Reference values

- Urine sodium excretion in adults ranges from 40 to 220 mEq/L/24 hours (SI, 40 to 220 mmol/d); in infants and children, from 41 to 115 mEq/L/24 hours (SI, 41 to 115 mmol/d).
- Urine chloride excretion in adults ranges from 110 to 250 nmol/24 hours (SI, 110 to 250 mmol/d); in children, from 15 to 40 nmol/24 hours (SI, 15 to 40 mmol/d); and in infants, from 2 to 10 mmol/24 hours (SI, 2 to 10 mmol/d).

## Abnormal results

- High urine sodium levels may reflect increased salt intake, adrenal failure, salicylate toxicity, diabetic acidosis, salt-losing nephritis, and water-deficient dehydration.
- Low urine sodium levels suggest decreased salt intake, primary aldosteronism, acute renal failure, and heart failure.
- High urine chloride levels may result from water-deficient dehydration, salicylate toxicity, diabetic ketoacidosis, adrenocortical insufficiency (Addison's disease), or salt-losing renal disease.
- Low urine chloride levels may result from excessive diaphoresis, heart failure, hypochloremic metabolic alkalosis, or prolonged vomiting or gastric suctioning.
- Most commonly, urine sodium and urine chloride levels are parallel, rising and falling in tandem. Abnormal levels of both minerals may indicate the need for more specific testing. To evaluate fluid-electrolyte imbalance, results must be correlated with findings of serum electrolyte studies.

**DRUG CHALLENGE**

 Sodium bicarbonate and thiazide diuretics (increase in sodium); steroids (decrease in sodium); ammonium chloride and potassium chloride (increase in chloride)

## Purpose

- To help evaluate fluid and electrolyte imbalance
- To help evaluate acid-base imbalance
- To monitor the effects of a low-salt diet
- To help evaluate renal and adrenal disorders

## Patient preparation

- Explain that the urine sodium and chloride test helps determine the balance of salt and water in the body.
- Tell the patient that he doesn't need to restrict food or fluids.
- Tell him that the test requires urine collection over a 24-hour period.
- If the specimen is to be collected at home, instruct the patient on proper collection technique.
- Notify the laboratory and practitioner of medications the patient is taking that may affect test results; the medications may need to be restricted.

## Procedure and posttest care

- Confirm the patient's identity using two patient identifiers according to facility policy.
- Collect the patient's urine over a 24-hour period, discarding the first specimen and retaining the last.

**DO'S & DON'TS**

 Keep a 24-hour urine specimen on ice or in the refrigerator.

- Tell the patient to resume his medications, as ordered.

# III

# Histologic and microbiologic tests

# Histology

## Gland biopsies

### 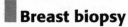 Breast biopsy

Breast biopsy is performed to confirm or rule out breast cancer after examination, mammography, or thermography has identified a mass. *Fine-needle* or *needle biopsy* is usually done on a mass that has been identified by ultrasonography as being fluid-filled. Both methods have limited diagnostic value because of the small and perhaps unrepresentative specimens they provide. *Open, or incisional, biopsy* provides larger specimens, which can be sectioned to allow more accurate evaluation. Local anesthesia can usually be given to outpatients for these three techniques. *Stereotactic breast biopsy* immobilizes the breast and allows the computer to calculate the exact location of the mass based on X-rays from two angles.

An *excisional biopsy* may be done under general anesthesia. If sufficient tissue is obtained and the mass is found to be a malignant tumor, specimens are sent for estrogen and progesterone receptor assays to assist in determining future therapy and the prognosis.

Because breast cancer remains the most prevalent cancer in women, genetic researchers are continually working to identify women at risk. (See *BRCA testing*.)

### Normal results

- Breast tissue consists of cellular and noncellular connective tissue, fat lobules, and various lactiferous ducts.
- Breast tissue is pink, more fatty than fibrous, and shows no abnormal development of cells or tissue elements.

### Abnormal results

- Benign tumors include fibrocystic disease, adenofibroma, intraductal papilloma, mammary fat necrosis, and plasma cell mastitis (mammary duct ectasia).
- Malignant tumors include adenocarcinoma, cystosarcoma, intraductal carcinoma, infiltrating carcinoma, inflammatory carcinoma, medullary or circumscribed carcinoma, colloid carcinoma, lobular carcinoma, sarcoma, and Paget's disease.

### Purpose

- To differentiate between benign and malignant breast tumors

### Patient preparation

- Describe the procedure to the patient and explain that this test permits microscopic examination of a breast tissue specimen. Offer her emotional support and assure her that breast masses don't always indicate cancer.
- Explain that pretest studies, such as blood tests, urine tests, and chest X-rays, may be required.

- Tell the patient who will perform the biopsy and where it will be done.
- Make sure she has signed an informed consent form.
- Check her history for hypersensitivity to anesthetics.
- If the patient is to receive a local anesthetic, tell her that she doesn't need to restrict food, fluids, or medication.
- If the patient is to receive a general anesthetic, tell her to fast from midnight before the test until after the biopsy.

### Procedure and posttest care

- Confirm the patient's identity using two patient identifiers according to facility policy.
- Double-check with the patient and the other members of team performing the procedure the side of the body the procedure is being done on.

#### Needle biopsy

- Instruct the patient to undress to the waist and guide her to a sitting or recumbent position with her hands at her sides, reminding her to remain still.
- The biopsy site is prepared, a local anesthetic is administered and the syringe (Luer-lock syringe for aspiration, Vim-Silverman needle for tissue specimen) is introduced into the lesion.
- Fluid aspirated from the breast is expelled into a properly labeled, heparinized tub; the tissue specimen is placed in a labeled specimen bottle containing normal saline solution or formalin.
- With fine-needle aspiration, a slide is made for cytology and viewed immediately under a microscope.
- Pressure is exerted on the biopsy site and, after bleeding stops, an adhesive bandage is applied. Because breast fluid aspiration isn't considered diagnostically accurate, some physicians aspirate fluid only from cysts. If such fluid is clear yellow and the mass disappears, the aspiration procedure is diagnostic and thera-

## BRCA testing

Genetic researchers have located two genes, BRCA1 and BRCA2, that have been linked to certain forms of breast cancer. BRCA testing can detect the presence of BRCA gene mutations, which may increase an individual's susceptibility to some breast cancers.

The test, performed on a blood sample, is available for women with a family history of breast cancer. Controversy continues over whether BRCA testing should be made available to the general public.

peutic, and the aspirate is discarded. If aspiration yields no fluid or if the lesion recurs two or three times, an open biopsy is then considered appropriate.

#### Open biopsy

- After the patient receives a general or local anesthetic, an incision is made in the breast to expose the mass.
- The examiner may then incise a portion of tissue or excise the entire mass. If the mass is smaller than 2 cm in diameter and appears benign, it's usually excised; if it's larger or appears malignant, a specimen is usually incised before the mass is excised.
- The specimen is placed in a properly labeled specimen bottle containing 10% formalin solution. Tissue that appears malignant is sent for frozen section and receptor assays. Receptor assay specimens must not be placed in the formalin solution.
- The wound is sutured and an adhesive bandage applied.

#### All procedures

- If the patient has received a general or local anesthetic, check her vital signs, and provide medication for pain. If she has received a general anesthetic, check her vital signs every 15 minutes for 1 hour, every 30 minutes for 2 hours, every hour for the next 4 hours, and then every 4 hours.

■ Give an analgesic, as ordered. An ice bag may provide comfort. Instruct the patient to wear a support bra at all times until healing is complete.

■ Watch for and report bleeding, tenderness, and redness at the biopsy site.

■ Provide emotional support to the patient who's awaiting diagnosis.

### Precautions

■ Open breast biopsy is contraindicated in the patient with a condition that precludes surgery, such as coagulopathies, late-stage pregnancy, and severe cardiac or respiratory disease.

### Complications

■ Bleeding

■ Infections

## Lymph node biopsy

Lymph node biopsy is the surgical excision of an active lymph node or the needle aspiration of a nodal specimen for histologic examination.

### Normal results

■ The lymph node is encapsulated by collagenous connective tissue and divided into smaller lobes by tissue strands called trabeculae.

■ The lymph node has an outer cortex, composed of lymphoid cells and nodules or follicles containing lymphocytes, and an inner medulla, composed of reticular phagocytic cells that collect and drain fluid.

### Abnormal results

■ Histologic examination of the tissue specimen distinguishes between malignant and nonmalignant causes of lymph node enlargement.

■ When histologic results aren't clear or nodular material isn't involved, mediastinoscopy or laparotomy can provide another nodal specimen.

■ Lymph node cancer may also result from metastatic cancer.

### Purpose

■ To determine the cause of lymph node enlargement

■ To distinguish between benign and malignant lymph node processes

■ To stage metastatic cancer

### Patient preparation

■ Explain that this test allows microscopic study of lymph node tissue.

■ Describe the procedure to the patient and answer his questions.

■ For excisional biopsy, instruct the patient to restrict food after midnight and to drink only clear liquids on the morning of the test (if general anesthesia is needed for deeper nodes, he must also restrict fluids).

■ For needle biopsy, inform the patient that he doesn't need to restrict food and fluids. Tell him who will perform the biopsy and where it will be done.

■ Make sure the patient has signed an informed consent form.

■ Check the patient's history for hypersensitivity to the anesthetic.

■ If the patient is to receive a local anesthetic, explain that he may experience slight discomfort during the injection.

■ Record the patient's baseline vital signs just before the biopsy.

### Procedure and posttest care

■ Confirm the patient's identity using two patient identifiers according to facility policy.

■ Double-check with the patient and the other members of the team performing the procedure the site of the biopsy.

### Excisional biopsy

- After the skin over the biopsy site is prepared and draped, the local anesthetic is given.
- The physician makes an incision, removes an entire node, and places it in a properly labeled bottle containing normal saline solution.
- The wound is sutured and a sterile dressing is applied.

### Needle biopsy

- After preparing the biopsy site and giving a local anesthetic, the physician grasps the node between his thumb and forefinger, inserts the needle directly into the node, and obtains a small core specimen.
- The needle is removed and the specimen placed in a properly labeled bottle containing normal saline solution.
- Pressure is exerted at the biopsy site to control bleeding and an adhesive bandage is applied.

### Both procedures

- Check the patient's vital signs and watch for bleeding, tenderness, and redness at the biopsy site.
- Inform the patient that he may resume his usual diet.
- Provide emotional support to the patient.

## Precautions

- Storing the tissue specimen in normal saline solution instead of 10% formalin solution allows part of the specimen to be used for cytologic impression smears, which are studied along with the biopsy specimen.

## Complications

- Bleeding
- Infection

# ▋ Prostate gland biopsy

Prostate gland biopsy is the needle excision of a prostate tissue specimen for histologic examination. Indications include potentially malignant prostatic hypertrophy and prostatic nodules. A perineal, transrectal, or transurethral approach may be used—the transrectal approach is used for high prostatic lesions.

## Normal results

- A thin, fibrous capsule surrounds the stroma, which is made up of elastic and connective tissues and smooth-muscle fibers.
- The epithelial glands found in these tissues and muscle fibers drain into the chief excreting ducts.
- No cancer cells are found.

## Abnormal results

- Histologic examination can confirm prostate cancer and can detect benign prostatic hyperplasia, prostatitis, tuberculosis, lymphomas, and rectal or bladder cancer.
- Acid phosphatase levels tend to be low in cancer that's confined to the prostatic capsule and usually rise in metastatic prostate cancer.

## Purpose

- To confirm prostate cancer
- To determine the cause of prostatic hyperplasia

## Patient preparation

- Describe the procedure to the patient, answer his questions, and tell him that the test provides a tissue specimen for microscopic study.
- Tell the patient who will perform the biopsy, where it will be done, and that he'll receive a local anesthetic.
- Make sure the patient has signed an informed consent form.

- Check the patient's history for hypersensitivity to the anesthetic or other drugs.
- For a transrectal approach, give the patient enemas until the return is clear and give him an antibacterial to minimize the risk of infection. This approach may be performed on an outpatient without an anesthetic.
- Just before the biopsy, check the patient's vital signs and give him a sedative.
- Give a prophylactic antibiotic, as ordered.
- Instruct the patient to remain still during the procedure and to follow instructions.

## Procedure and posttest care

- Confirm the patient's identity using two patient identifiers according to facility policy.

### Perineal approach

- Place the patient in the proper position (left lateral, knee-chest, or lithotomy) and clean the perineal skin.
- After the local anesthetic is administered, a 2-mm incision may be made into the perineum.
- The examiner immobilizes the prostate by inserting a finger into the rectum and introduces the biopsy needle into a prostate lobe. The needle is rotated gently, pulled out about 5 mm, and reinserted at another angle. The procedure is repeated at several areas.
- Pressure is exerted on the puncture site, which is then bandaged.

### Transrectal approach

- Place the patient in the left lateral position.
- A digital rectal examination is performed before an ultrasound probe is inserted. A curved needle guide is attached to the finger palpating the rectum. The biopsy needle is pushed along the guide into the prostate that was localized by ultrasonography.
- As the needle enters the prostate, the patient may experience pain. The needle is rotated to cut off the tissue and is then withdrawn.
- An alternative method of transrectal detection is the automated cone biopsy, in which the physician uses a spring-powered device with an inner trocar needle to cut through prostatic tissue. This technique is quick and reportedly painless.

### Transurethral approach

- An endoscopic instrument is passed through the urethra, permitting direct viewing of the prostate and passage of a cutting loop.
- The loop is rotated to obtain tissue and then withdrawn.

### All approaches

- The specimen is placed immediately in a labeled specimen bottle containing 10% formalin solution and sent to the laboratory for analysis.
- Check the patient's vital signs immediately after the procedure, every 2 hours for 4 hours, and then every 4 hours.
- Observe the biopsy site for hematoma and for signs and symptoms of infection, such as redness, swelling, and pain. Watch for urine retention, urinary frequency, and hematuria.

## Complications

- Bleeding into the prostatic urethra and bladder
- Infection
- Urinary retention

# Thyroid biopsy

Thyroid biopsy is the excision of a thyroid tissue specimen for histologic examination. This procedure is indicated in patients with thyroid enlargement or nodules (even if serum triiodothyronine [$T_3$] and thyroxine [$T_4$] levels are normal), breathing and swallowing difficulties, vocal cord paralysis, weight loss, hemoptysis, and a sensation of fullness in the neck. It's commonly performed when noninvasive tests, such as thyroid ultrasonography and scans, are abnormal or inconclusive. Coagulation studies should always precede thyroid biopsy.

Thyroid tissue may be obtained with a hollow needle under local anesthesia or during open (surgical) biopsy under general anesthesia. Fine-needle aspiration with a cytologic smear examination can aid in diagnosis and replace an open biopsy. Open biopsy, performed in the operating room, provides more information than needle biopsy; it also permits direct examination and immediate excision of suspicious tissue.

## Normal results

- Fibrous networks divide the gland into pseudolobules that are made up of follicles and capillaries.
- Cuboidal epithelium lines the follicle walls and contains the protein thyroglobulin, which stores $T_4$ and $T_3$.

## Abnormal results

- Malignant tumors appear as well-encapsulated, solitary nodules of uniform but abnormal structure.
- Benign tumors, such as nontoxic nodular goiter, demonstrate hypertrophy, hyperplasia, and hypervascularity.
- Distinct histologic patterns characterize subacute granulomatous thyroiditis, Hashimoto's thyroiditis, and hyperthyroidism.

## Purpose

- To differentiate between benign and malignant thyroid disease
- To help diagnose Hashimoto's disease, hyperthyroidism, and nontoxic nodular goiter

## Patient preparation

- Describe the procedure to the patient and answer his questions.
- Explain that this test permits microscopic examination of a thyroid tissue specimen.
- Inform the patient that he doesn't need to restrict food and fluids (unless he'll receive a general anesthetic).
- Tell the patient who will perform the biopsy and where it will be done.
- Make sure the patient or a responsible family member has signed an informed consent form.
- Check the patient's history for hypersensitivity to anesthetics or analgesics.
- Tell the patient that he'll receive a local anesthetic to minimize pain during the procedure but may experience some pressure when the tissue specimen is procured.
- Check the results of the patient's coagulation studies and make sure they're in his chart.
- Advise the patient that he may have a sore throat the day after the test.
- Give the patient a sedative 15 minutes before biopsy.

## Procedure and posttest care

- Confirm the patient's identity using two patient identifiers according to facility policy.
- For needle biopsy, place the patient in the supine position with a pillow under his shoulder blades. (This position pushes the trachea and thyroid forward and allows the neck veins to fall backward.)
- Prepare the skin over the biopsy site.
- As the physician prepares to inject the local anesthetic, warn the patient not to swallow.
- After the anesthetic is injected, the carotid artery is palpated and the biopsy needle is inserted parallel to the thyroid cartilage to prevent damage to the deep structures and the larynx.

■ When the specimen is obtained, the needle is removed and the specimen is placed in formalin immediately.

■ Apply pressure to the biopsy site to stop bleeding. If bleeding continues for more than a few minutes, press on the site for up to an additional 15 minutes. Apply an adhesive bandage. (Bleeding may persist in a patient with a prolonged prothrombin time [PT] or partial thromboplastin time [PTT] or in a patient with a large, vascular thyroid with distended veins.)

■ To make the patient more comfortable, place him in the semi-Fowler position; tell him to avoid straining the biopsy site by putting both hands behind his neck when he sits up.

■ Watch for tenderness or redness and report signs of bleeding at the biopsy site immediately. Check the back of the patient's neck and his pillow for bleeding every hour for 8 hours. Observe for difficult breathing due to edema or hematoma, with resultant tracheal collapse.

■ Keep the biopsy site clean and dry.

### Precautions
■ Thyroid biopsy should be used cautiously in the patient with coagulation defects, as indicated by a prolonged PT or PTT.

### Complications
■ Bleeding
■ Infection
■ Respiratory compromise

# Organ biopsies

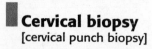

## Cervical biopsy
[cervical punch biopsy]

Cervical biopsy is the excision by sharp forceps of a tissue specimen from the cervix for histologic examination. Generally, multiple biopsies are done to obtain specimens from all areas with abnormal tissue or from the squamocolumnar junction and other sites around the cervical circumference. The biopsy site is selected by direct visualization of the cervix with a colposcope or by Schiller's test, which stains normal squamous epithelium a dark mahogany, but fails to color abnormal tissue. Other biopsies are done to detect other gynecological disorders. (See *Endometrial and ovarian biopsies.*) The biopsy is performed when the cervix is least vascular, usually 1 week after menses.

### Normal results
■ Normal cervical tissue is composed of columnar and squamous epithelial cells, loose connective tissue, and smooth-muscle fibers.

■ No dysplasia or abnormal cell growth are present.

### Abnormal results
■ Dysplasia or abnormal cell growth on histologic examination of a cervical tissue specimen may suggest intraepithelial neoplasia or invasive cancer.

### Purpose
■ To evaluate suspicious cervical lesions
■ To diagnose cervical cancer

### Patient preparation
■ Describe the procedure to the patient and explain that it provides a cervical tissue specimen for microscopic study.

■ Tell the patient who will perform the biopsy and where it will be done.

■ Tell the patient that she may experience mild discomfort during and after the biopsy.

■ Advise the outpatient to have someone accompany her home after the biopsy.

■ Make sure the patient has signed an informed consent form.

# Endometrial and ovarian biopsies

This table shows purposes and special considerations involved in endometrial and ovarian biopsies.

| Method | Purpose | Special considerations |
|---|---|---|
| **Endometrial biopsy** | | |
| ▪ Dilatation and curettage (D&C) <br> ▪ Endometrial washing (by jet irrigation, aspiration, or brushing) | ▪ To evaluate uterine bleeding <br> ▪ To diagnose suspected endometrial cancer | ▪ Time of menstrual cycle affects the accuracy of biopsy results. <br> ▪ The type of specimen obtained depends on the patient's age and the disorder. <br> ▪ D&C by endometrial washing may follow a negative biopsy. <br> ▪ Specimens obtained by D&C may be processed as frozen sections. |
| **Ovarian biopsy** | | |
| ▪ Transrectal or transvaginal fine-needle biopsy <br> ▪ Aspiration biopsy during laparoscopy | ▪ To diagnose a missed abortion <br> ▪ To detect an ovarian tumor <br> ▪ To determine the spread of cancer | ▪ Fine-needle biopsy may follow palpation, laparoscopy, or computed tomography that detects an abnormal ovary. <br> ▪ Aspiration during laparoscopy is particularly useful for young women who are infertile or who have lesions that appear benign. |

▪ Ask the patient to void just before the biopsy.

## Procedure and posttest care
▪ Confirm the patient's identity using two patient identifiers according to facility policy.
▪ Place the patient in the lithotomy position and tell her to relax as the unlubricated speculum is inserted.
▪ For direct visualization, the colposcope is inserted through the speculum, the biopsy site is located, and the cervix is cleaned with a swab soaked in 3% acetic acid solution. The biopsy forceps are then inserted through the speculum or the colposcope and tissue is removed from any lesion or from selected sites, starting from the posterior lip to avoid obscuring other sites with blood. Each specimen is immediately put in 10% formalin solution in a labeled bottle. To control bleeding after biopsy, the cervix is swabbed with 5% silver nitrate solution (cautery or sutures may be used instead). If bleeding persists, the physician may insert a tampon.
▪ For Schiller's test, an applicator stick saturated with iodine solution is insert-

ed through the speculum. This stains the cervix to identify lesions for biopsy.

■ Record the patient's and physician's names and the biopsy sites on the laboratory request.

■ Instruct the patient to avoid strenuous exercise for 24 hours after the biopsy. Encourage the outpatient to rest briefly before leaving the office.

■ If a tampon was inserted after the biopsy, tell the patient to leave it in place for 8 to 24 hours. Inform her that some bleeding may occur, but she should report heavy bleeding (heavier than menses). Warn the patient to avoid using tampons, except for the tampon placed after the biopsy, because they can irritate the cervix and provoke bleeding.

■ Tell the patient to avoid douching and intercourse for 2 weeks, or as directed, if she has undergone cryotherapy or laser treatment during the procedure.

■ Tell the patient that a foul-smelling, gray-green vaginal discharge is normal for several days after the biopsy and may persist for 3 weeks.

## Complications
■ Bleeding
■ Infection

# Lung biopsy

In lung biopsy, a specimen of pulmonary tissue is excised by closed or open technique for histologic examination. *Needle biopsy* is appropriate when the lesion is readily accessible, originates in the lung parenchyma and is confined to it, or is affixed to the chest wall; it provides a much smaller specimen than the open technique. *Transbronchial biopsy,* the removal of multiple tissue specimens through a fiber-optic bronchoscope, may be used in patients with diffuse infiltrative pulmonary disease or tumors or when severe debilitation contraindicates open biopsy.

Open biopsy is appropriate for the study of a well-circumscribed lesion that may require resection.

## Normal results
■ Pulmonary tissue shows uniform texture of the alveolar ducts, alveolar walls, bronchioles, and small vessels.

## Abnormal results
■ Histologic examination of a pulmonary tissue specimen can reveal squamous cell or oat cell carcinoma and adenocarcinoma.

## Purpose
■ To confirm a diagnosis of diffuse parenchymal pulmonary disease and pulmonary lesions

## Patient preparation
■ Explain to the patient that this test is used to confirm or rule out a diagnostic finding in the lung.

■ Describe the procedure to the patient and answer his questions.

■ Tell the patient that a chest X-ray and blood studies (prothrombin time, partial thromboplastin time, and platelet count) will be performed before the biopsy.

■ Tell the patient who will perform the biopsy and where it will be done.

■ Instruct the patient to fast for 8 hours before the procedure. (Sometimes the patient is permitted to have clear liquids the morning of the test.)

■ Make sure the patient or a responsible family member has signed an informed consent form.

■ Check the patient's history for hypersensitivity to the local anesthetic.

■ Administer a mild sedative, as ordered, 30 minutes before the biopsy to help the patient relax. Tell him that he'll receive a local anesthetic, but he may experience a sharp, transient pain when the biopsy needle touches the lung.

- Reinforce that the patient needs to lie still during the procedure because any movement or coughing can result in laceration of lung tissue by the biopsy needle.

## Procedure and posttest care

- Confirm the patient's identity using two patient identifiers according to facility policy.
- Double-check with the patient and the other members of the team the correct side of the body for the procedure to be done.
- After the biopsy site is selected but before the start of the procedure, lead markers are placed on the patient's skin and X-rays are ordered to verify their correct placement.
- Position the patient in a sitting position with his arms folded on a table in front of him; instruct him to maintain this position, remaining as still as possible, and to refrain from coughing.
- Prepare the skin over the biopsy site with povidone-iodine or chlorhexidine and drape the appropriate area.
- With a 25G needle, the local anesthetic is injected just above the rib below the selected site to prevent damage to the intercostal nerves and vessels.
- Using a 22G needle, the physician anesthetizes the intercostal muscles and parietal pleura, makes a small incision (2 to 3 mm) with a scalpel, and introduces the biopsy needle through the incision, chest wall, and pleura into the tumor or pulmonary tissue.
- If the intercostal space at the incision site is wide, the needle is inserted at a 90-degree angle; if the ribs overlap and the intercostal space is narrow, the needle is inserted at a 45-degree angle. When the needle is in the tumor or pulmonary tissue, the specimen is obtained and the needle withdrawn.
- The specimen is divided immediately. The tissue for histology is placed in a properly labeled bottle containing 10% neutral buffered formalin solution; the tissue for microbiology is placed in a sterile container.
- Immediately after the procedure, apply pressure on the biopsy site to stop bleeding and apply a small bandage.

 Check the patient's vital signs every 15 minutes for 1 hour, every 30 minutes for 2 hours, every hour for 4 hours, and then every 4 hours. Watch for bleeding, dyspnea, elevated pulse rate, diminished breath sounds on the biopsy side and, eventually, cyanosis. Complications include pneumothorax and bleeding. Make sure the chest X-ray is repeated as soon as the biopsy has been completed.

- Tell the patient to resume his usual diet.

## Precautions

- Needle biopsy is contraindicated in the patient with a lesion that's separated from the chest wall or accompanied by emphysematous bullae, cysts, or gross emphysema and in the patient with coagulopathy, hypoxia, pulmonary hypertension, or cardiac disease with cor pulmonale.

ACTION STAT!

 During biopsy, observe for signs of respiratory distress, such as shortness of breath, elevated pulse rate, and cyanosis (late sign). If such signs develop, report them immediately.

- Because coughing and movement during biopsy can cause lung tearing by the biopsy needle, keep the patient calm and still.

# Percutaneous liver biopsy

Percutaneous biopsy of the liver is the needle aspiration of a core of liver tissue for histologic analysis. This procedure is performed under local or general anesthesia using a special needle. (See *Using a Menghini needle*.) Findings may help to identify hepatic disorders after ultrasonography, computed tomography scan, and radionuclide studies have failed to detect them. Because many patients with hepatic disorders have clotting defects, they should be tested for hemostasis before liver biopsy.

## Normal results

- The liver consists of sheets of hepatocytes supported by a reticulin framework.

## Abnormal results

- The hepatic tissue may reveal diffuse hepatic disease, such as cirrhosis or hepatitis, or granulomatous infections such as tuberculosis.
- Primary malignant tumors include hepatocellular carcinoma, cholangiocellular carcinoma, and angiosarcoma, but hepatic metastasis is more common.
- Nonmalignant findings with a known focal lesion require further studies, such as laparotomy or laparoscopy with biopsy.

## Purpose

- To diagnose hepatic parenchymal disease, malignant tumors, and granulomatous infections

## Patient preparation

- Explain that this test is used to diagnose liver disorders.
- Describe the procedure to the patient and answer his questions.
- Instruct the patient to restrict food and fluids for 4 to 8 hours before the test.
- Tell the patient who will perform the biopsy and where it will be done.
- Make sure the patient has signed an informed consent form.
- Check the patient's history for hypersensitivity to the local anesthetic.
- Make sure coagulation studies (prothrombin time [PT], partial thromboplastin time, and platelet counts) have been performed and that the results are recorded on the patient's chart.
- A blood sample is usually drawn for baseline hematocrit assessment.
- Just before the biopsy, tell the patient to void and then record his vital signs.
- Inform the patient that he'll receive a local anesthetic but may experience pain similar to that of a punch in his right shoulder as the biopsy needle passes the phrenic nerve.

## Procedure and posttest care

- Confirm the patient's identity using two patient identifiers according to facility policy.
- For aspiration biopsy using the Menghini needle, place the patient in a supine position with his right hand under his head. Instruct him to maintain this position and remain as still as possible during the procedure.
- The liver is palpated, the biopsy site is selected and marked, and the local anesthetic is then injected.
- The needle flange is set to control the depth of penetration and 2 ml of sterile normal saline solution are drawn into the syringe.
- The syringe is attached to the biopsy needle and the needle is introduced into the subcutaneous tissue through the right eighth or ninth intercostal space at the midaxillary line and advanced up to the pleura.
- Next, 1 ml of normal saline solution is injected to clear the needle and the plunger, and then the plunger is drawn

## Using a Menghini needle

In percutaneous liver biopsy, a Menghini needle attached to a 5-ml syringe containing normal saline solution is introduced through the chest wall and intercostal space (1). Negative pressure is created in the syringe. Then the needle is pushed rapidly into the liver (2) and pulled out of the body entirely (3) to obtain a tissue specimen.

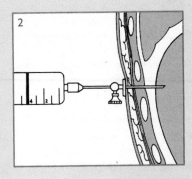

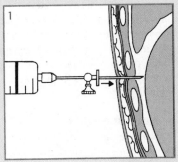

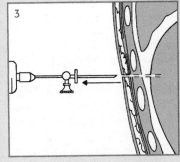

back to the 4-ml mark to create negative pressure.

■ At this point in the procedure, ask the patient to take a deep breath, exhale, and hold his breath at the end of expiration to prevent movement of the chest wall.

■ As the patient holds his breath, the biopsy needle is quickly inserted into the liver and withdrawn in 1 second.

■ For the patient who can't hold his breath, the biopsy needle is quickly inserted and withdrawn at the end of expiration.

■ After the needle is withdrawn, tell the patient to resume normal respirations.

■ The tissue specimen is then placed in a properly labeled specimen cup containing 10% formalin solution. This is done by releasing negative pressure while the point of the needle is in the formalin so-

lution. Send the specimen to the laboratory immediately.

■ Again, 1 ml of normal saline solution is injected to clear the needle of the tissue specimen.

■ Apply pressure to the biopsy site to stop bleeding.

■ Position the patient on his right side for 2 to 4 hours with a small pillow or sandbag under the costal margin to provide extra pressure. Advise bed rest for at least 24 hours.

■ Check the patient's vital signs every 15 minutes for 1 hour, every 30 minutes for 4 hours, and every 4 hours thereafter for 24 hours. Throughout, observe him carefully for signs of shock.

**ALERT**

 Immediately report bleeding or signs of bile peritonitis, such as tenderness and rigidity around the biopsy site. Be alert for symptoms of pneumothorax, such as rising respiratory rate, depressed breath sounds, dyspnea, persistent shoulder pain, and pleuritic chest pain. Report such complications promptly.

- If the patient experiences pain, which may persist for several hours after the test, give him an analgesic.
- Tell the patient to resume his usual diet, as ordered.

### Precautions

- Percutaneous liver biopsy is contraindicated in a patient with a platelet count below 100,000/µl; PT time longer than 15 seconds; empyema of the lungs, pleurae, peritoneum, biliary tract, or liver; vascular tumor; hepatic angiomas; hydatid cyst; or tense ascites. If extrahepatic obstruction is suspected, ultrasonography or subcutaneous transhepatic cholangiography should rule out this condition before the biopsy is considered.
- Pain in the abdomen or dyspnea after the biopsy may indicate perforation of an abdominal organ or pneumothorax, respectively. In such cases, complete a thorough assessment and notify the practitioner at once.
- Instruct the patient to hold his breath while the needle is in place.

### Complications

- Peritonitis
- Pneumothorax
- Bleeding
- Infection

# Percutaneous renal biopsy

Percutaneous renal biopsy is the needle excision of a core of kidney tissue for histologic examination. This biopsy may help assess histologic changes caused by acute or chronic glomerulonephritis, pyelonephritis, renal vein thrombosis, amyloid infiltration, and systemic lupus erythematosus. In the case of a mass, results can differentiate a primary renal cancer from a metastatic lesion.

This procedure is safer than open biopsy, which is the preferred method for sampling a solid lesion, but noninvasive procedures, especially renal ultrasonography and computed tomography, have replaced percutaneous renal biopsy in many facilities. (See *Urinary tract brush biopsy.*)

### Normal results

- Normal results should reveal Bowman's capsule—the area between two layers of flat epithelial cells—the glomerular tuft, and the capillary lumen.
- The proximal tubule is one layer of epithelial cells with microvilli that form a brush border.
- The descending loop of Henle has flat squamous epithelial cells.
- The ascending loop is convoluted distally and collecting tubules are lined with squamous epithelial cells.

### Abnormal results

- Cancer (Wilms' tumor) or renal disease (disseminated lupus erythematosus, amyloid infiltration, acute or chronic glomerulonephritis, renal vein thrombosis, or pyelonephritis) is present.

### Purpose

- To help diagnose renal parenchymal disease

# Urinary tract brush biopsy

Retrograde brush biopsy of the urinary tract may be used to obtain a renal tissue specimen when X-rays show a lesion in the renal pelvis or calyx. It can also be used to obtain specimens from other areas of the urinary tract. Retrograde brush biopsy is contraindicated in the patient with an acute urinary tract infection or an obstruction at or below the biopsy site.

### Patient preparation

To prepare the patient for brush biopsy, describe the procedure and tell him that he may experience some discomfort. Inform him who will perform the biopsy and when. Tell the patient that the procedure will take 30 to 60 minutes.

Make sure the patient has signed an informed consent form. Because this procedure requires the use of a contrast medium and a general, local, or spinal anesthetic, check the patient's history for hypersensitivity to anesthetics, contrast media, or iodine-containing foods such as shellfish. Just before the biopsy procedure, administer a sedative to the patient.

### Obtaining the biopsy

After the patient has received a sedative and an anesthetic, place him in the lithotomy position. Using a cystoscope, a guide wire is passed up the ureter and a urethral catheter is passed over the guide wire. Contrast medium is instilled through the catheter, which is positioned next to the lesion under fluoroscopic guidance. The contrast medium is washed out with normal saline solution to prevent cell distortions from the dye. A nylon or steel brush is passed up the catheter and the lesion is brushed. This procedure is repeated at least six times, using a new brush each time.

As each brush is removed from the catheter, a smear is made for Papanicolaou staining and the brush tip is cut off and placed in formalin solution for 1 hour. The biopsy material is then removed from the brush tip for histologic examination. When the last brush is withdrawn, the catheter is irrigated with normal saline solution to remove additional cells. These cells are also sent for histologic examination.

Results differentiate between malignant and benign lesions, which may appear the same on X-rays.

### Posttest care

Because brush biopsy may cause complications, such as perforation, hemorrhage, sepsis, and contrast medium extravasation, carefully monitor the patient's vital signs. Be sure to record the time, color, and amount of voiding, being alert for hematuria and abdominal or flank pain. Report abnormal findings immediately and administer analgesics and antibiotics, as ordered.

■ To monitor the progression of renal disease and assess the effectiveness of therapy

### Patient preparation

■ Explain that this test is used to diagnose kidney disorders.
■ Describe the procedure to the patient and answer his questions.
■ Instruct the patient to restrict food and fluids for 8 hours before the test.
■ Tell the patient who will perform the biopsy and where it will be done.
■ Ensure that blood samples and urine specimens are collected and tested before the biopsy and that results of other tests to determine the biopsy site, such as excretory urography, ultrasonography,

and an erect film of the abdomen, are available.

■ Make sure the patient has signed an informed consent form.

■ Check the patient's history for hemorrhagic tendencies and hypersensitivity to the local anesthetic.

■ Give a mild sedative 30 minutes to 1 hour before the biopsy to help the patient relax, as ordered.

■ Inform the patient that he'll receive a local anesthetic but may experience a pinching pain when the needle is inserted through the back into the kidney.

■ Check the patient's vital signs and tell him to void just before the test.

## Procedure and posttest care

■ Confirm the patient's identity using two patient identifiers according to facility policy.

■ Double-check with the patient and other team members to verify the correct side for the procedure.

■ Place the patient in a prone position on a firm surface with a sandbag beneath his abdomen.

■ Tell him to take a deep breath while his kidney is being palpated.

■ A 7″ 20G needle is used to inject the local anesthetic into the skin at the biopsy site. Instruct the patient to hold his breath and remain still as the needle is inserted through the back muscles, the deep lumbar fascia, the perinephric fat, and the kidney capsule. After the needle is inserted, tell the patient to take several deep breaths. If the needle swings smoothly during deep breathing, it has penetrated the kidney capsule. After the penetration depth is marked on the needle shaft, instruct the patient to hold his breath and remain as still as possible while the needle is withdrawn.

■ After a small incision is made in the anesthetized skin, instruct the patient to hold his breath and remain still while the Vim-Silverman needle with stylet is inserted to the measured depth.

■ Tell the patient to breathe deeply and to remain still while the tissue specimen is obtained.

■ The tissue is examined immediately under a hand lens to ensure that the specimen contains tissue from the cortex and medulla. Then it's placed on a saline-soaked gauze pad and placed in a properly labeled container.

■ If an adequate tissue specimen hasn't been obtained, the procedure is repeated immediately.

■ After an adequate specimen is secured, apply pressure to the biopsy site for 3 to 5 minutes to stop superficial bleeding. Then apply a pressure dressing.

■ Instruct the patient to lie flat on his back without moving for at least 12 hours to prevent bleeding. Check his vital signs every 15 minutes for 4 hours, every 30 minutes for 4 hours, every hour for 4 hours and, finally, every 4 hours. Report any changes.

■ Examine the patient's urine for blood; small amounts may be present after the biopsy but should disappear within 8 hours. Hematocrit may be monitored after the procedure to screen for internal bleeding.

■ Encourage fluid ingestion to minimize colic and obstruction from blood clotting within the renal pelvis.

■ Tell the patient to resume his usual diet.

■ Tell him to avoid strenuous activities for several days after the procedure to prevent possible bleeding.

## Precautions

■ Percutaneous renal biopsy is contraindicated in a patient with a severe bleeding disorder, markedly reduced plasma or blood volume, severe hypertension, hydronephrosis, perinephric abscess, advanced renal failure with uremia, or only one kidney.

- Instruct the patient to hold his breath and remain still whenever the needle or prongs are advanced into or retracted from the kidney.

### Complications
- Bleeding
- Infection

# Pleural biopsy

Pleural tissue biopsy is the removal of pleural tissue by needle biopsy or open biopsy for histologic examination. *Needle pleural biopsy* is performed under local anesthesia. It's usually done in conjunction with or after thoracentesis (aspiration of pleural fluid), which is performed when the cause of an effusion is unknown, but it can also be performed separately.

*Open pleural biopsy*, performed in the absence of pleural effusion, permits direct visualization of the pleura and the underlying lung. It's performed in the operating room.

### Normal results
- Mesothelial cells that are flattened in a uniform layer.
- Layers of areolar connective tissue that contain blood vessels, nerves, and lymphatics lie below.

### Abnormal results
- Malignant disease, tuberculosis, and viral, fungal, parasitic, or collagen vascular disease are present.
- Primary neoplasms of the pleura are generally fibrous and epithelial.

### Purpose
- To differentiate between nonmalignant and malignant disease
- To diagnose viral, fungal, or parasitic disease and collagen vascular disease of the pleura

### Patient preparation
- Explain that this test permits microscopic examination of pleural tissue.
- Describe the procedure to the patient and answer his questions.
- Tell the patient who will perform the biopsy, where it will be done, and that no fasting is required.
- Explain that blood studies will precede the biopsy and chest X-rays will be taken before and after the biopsy.
- Make sure the patient has signed an informed consent form.
- Check the patient's history for hypersensitivity to the local anesthetic.
- Tell the patient that he'll receive a local anesthetic to help reduce his pain.
- Record the patient's vital signs just before the procedure.

### Procedure and posttest care
- Confirm the patient's identity using two patient identifiers according to facility policy.
- Double-check with the patient and other team members to verify the correct side for the procedure.
- Seat the patient on the side of the bed, with his feet resting on a stool and his arms on the overbed table or supported by his upper body. Tell him to hold this position and remain still during the procedure.
- Prepare the skin and drape the area.
- The local anesthetic is given.
- In a Vim-Silverman needle biopsy, a needle is inserted through the appropriate intercostal space into the biopsy site with the outer tip distal to the pleura and the central portion pushed in deeper and held in place. The outer case is inserted about ⅜″ (1 cm), the entire assembly is rotated 360 degrees, and the needle and tissue specimen are withdrawn. In Cope's needle biopsy, a trocar is introduced through the appropriate intercostal space into the biopsy site. To obtain the specimen, a hooked stylet is

# Using Cope's needle

Cope's needle, which is used to obtain a pleural biopsy specimen, consists of three parts: a sharp obturator (A) and a cannula (B), which when fitted together are called a trocar, and a blunt-ended, hooked stylet (C). The trocar is used to gain access to the pleural cavity. Then the obturator is removed, leaving the cannula in place. The stylet is passed through the cannula to excise a tissue specimen, as shown below.

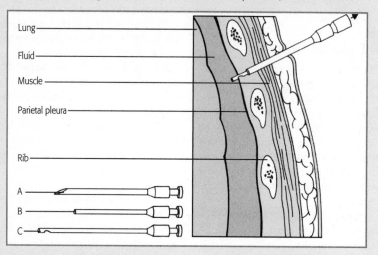

inserted through the trocar. While the outer tube is held stationary, the inner tube is twisted to cut off the tissue specimen, and the assembly is withdrawn. (See *Using Cope's needle.*)

■ After the specimens are obtained, additional parietal fluid may be removed to treat the effusion.

■ Put the specimen immediately into a 10% neutral buffered formalin solution in a labeled specimen bottle and send it to the laboratory immediately.

■ Clean the skin around the biopsy site and apply an adhesive bandage.

■ Make sure the chest X-ray is repeated immediately after the biopsy.

■ Check the patient's vital signs every 15 minutes for 1 hour and then every hour for 4 hours or until stable.

**ALERT**

 Watch for signs of respiratory distress (dyspnea), shoulder pain, and such complications as pneumothorax (immediate), pneumonia (delayed), and hemorrhage.

■ Instruct the patient to lie on his unaffected side to promote healing of the biopsy site, as indicated.

### Precautions

■ Pleural biopsy is contraindicated in the patient with a severe bleeding disorder.

### Complications

■ Pneumothorax
■ Bleeding
■ Infection

# Skin biopsy

Skin biopsy is the removal of a small piece of tissue under local anesthesia from a lesion suspected of being malignant or from other dermatoses. One of three techniques may be used: shave biopsy, punch biopsy, or excisional biopsy. *Shave biopsy* uses a scalpel to slice a superficial specimen from the site. *Punch biopsy* removes an oval core from the center of a lesion down to the dermis or subcutaneous tissue. *Excisional biopsy* removes the entire lesion with a small border of normal skin.

Lesions suspected of being malignant usually have changed color, size, or appearance or have failed to heal properly after injury. Fully developed lesions should be selected for biopsy whenever possible because they provide more diagnostic information than lesions that are resolving or in early developing stages.

## Normal results

- Skin consists of squamous epithelium (epidermis) and fibrous connective tissue (dermis).

## Abnormal results

- Histologic examination of the tissue specimen may reveal a benign or malignant lesion.
- Benign growths include cysts, seborrheic keratoses, warts, pigmented nevi (moles), keloids, dermatofibromas, and multiple neurofibromas.
- Malignant tumors include basal cell carcinoma, squamous cell carcinoma, and malignant melanoma. Basal cell carcinoma occurs on hair-bearing skin; the most common location is the face, including the nose and its folds. Squamous cell carcinoma most commonly appears on the lips, mouth, and genitalia.

## Purpose

- To provide differential diagnosis among basal cell carcinoma, squamous cell carcinoma, malignant melanoma, and benign growths
- To diagnose chronic bacterial or fungal skin infections

## Patient preparation

- Explain that the biopsy provides a specimen for microscopic study.
- Describe the procedure to the patient and answer his questions.
- Inform the patient that he doesn't need to restrict food and fluids.
- Tell the patient who will perform the procedure and where it will be done.
- Tell the patient that he'll receive a local anesthetic to minimize pain during the procedure.
- Make sure the patient has signed an informed consent form.
- Check the patient's history for hypersensitivity to the local anesthetic.

## Procedure and posttest care

- Confirm the patient's identity using two patient identifiers according to facility policy.
- Double-check with the patient and other team members to verify the correct site for the procedure.
- Position the patient comfortably and clean the biopsy site before the local anesthetic is given.

### Shave biopsy

- The protruding growth is cut off at the skin line with a #15 scalpel and the tissue is placed immediately in a properly labeled specimen bottle containing 10% formalin solution.
- Apply pressure to the area to stop the bleeding.

### Punch biopsy

- The skin surrounding the lesion is pulled taut and the punch is firmly introduced into the lesion and rotated to obtain a tissue specimen. The plug is lifted with forceps or a needle and severed as deeply into the fat layer as possible.
- The specimen is placed in a properly labeled specimen bottle containing 10% formalin solution or in a sterile container, if indicated.
- Closing the wound depends on the size of the punch. A 3-mm punch requires only an adhesive bandage, a 4-mm punch requires one suture, and a 6-mm punch requires two sutures.

### Excisional biopsy

- A #15 scalpel is used to excise the entire lesion; the elliptical incision is made as wide and as deep as necessary.
- The tissue specimen is removed and placed immediately in a properly labeled specimen bottle containing 10% formalin solution.
- Apply pressure to the site to stop bleeding.
- The wound is closed using 4-0 suture. If the incision is large, skin grafting may be required.

### All procedures

- Check the biopsy site for bleeding.
- If the patient experiences pain, give an analgesic, as ordered.
- Advise the patient with sutures to keep the area as clean and dry as possible. Facial sutures are removed in 3 to 5 days; trunk sutures, in 7 to 14 days. Tell the patient with adhesive strips to leave them in place for 14 to 21 days or until they fall off.

## Complications

- Bleeding
- Infection

# Skeletal biopsies

## ▮ Bone biopsy

Bone biopsy is the removal of a piece or a core of bone for histologic examination. It's performed either by using a special drill needle under local anesthesia or by surgical excision under general anesthesia.

Bone biopsy is indicated in patients with bone pain and tenderness after bone scan, computed tomography scan, X-ray, or arteriography reveals a mass or deformity. Excision provides a larger specimen than drill biopsy and permits immediate surgical treatment if quick histologic analysis of the specimen reveals cancer.

### Normal results

- Bone tissue consists of fibers of collagen, osteocytes, and osteoblasts.
- Compact bone has dense, concentric layers of mineral deposits, or lamellae.
- Cancellous bone has widely spaced lamellae, with osteocytes and red and yellow marrow between them.

### Abnormal results

- Benign tumors, generally well circumscribed and nonmetastasizing, include osteoid osteoma, osteoblastoma, osteochondroma, unicameral bone cyst, benign giant-cell tumor, and fibroma.
- Malignant tumors, which spread irregularly and rapidly, most commonly include multiple myeloma and osteosarcoma; the most lethal is Ewing's sarcoma.

### Purpose

- To distinguish between benign and malignant bone tumors

### Patient preparation

- Explain that this test permits microscopic examination of a bone specimen.

- Describe the procedure to the patient and answer his questions.
- If the patient will have a drill biopsy, he doesn't need to restrict food and fluids; if he will have open biopsy, he must fast overnight before the test.
- Tell the patient who will perform the biopsy and where it will be done.
- Tell the patient that he'll receive a local anesthetic but will still experience discomfort and pressure when the biopsy needle enters the bone.
- Explain that a special drill forces the needle into the bone; if possible, show him a photograph of the bone drill. Stress the importance of his cooperation during the biopsy.
- Make sure the patient or a responsible family member has signed an informed consent form.
- Check the patient's history for hypersensitivity to the local anesthetic.

### Procedure and posttest care
- Confirm the patient's identity using two patient identifiers according to facility policy.
- Double-check with the patient and other team members to verify the correct site for the procedure.

#### *Drill biopsy*
- The patient is properly positioned and the biopsy site is shaved and prepared.
- After the local anesthetic is injected, a small incision (usually about 3 mm) is made and the biopsy needle is pushed with a pointed trocar into the bone, then it's rotated about 180 degrees.
- When the bone core is obtained, the trocar is withdrawn and the specimen is placed in a properly labeled bottle containing 10% formalin solution. Then pressure is applied to the site with a sterile gauze pad.
- When bleeding stops, apply a topical antiseptic (povidone-iodine ointment) and an adhesive bandage or other sterile

covering to close the wound and prevent infection.

#### *Open biopsy*
- The patient is anesthetized and the biopsy site is clipped, cleaned with surgical soap, and disinfected with an iodine wash and alcohol.
- An incision is made and a piece of bone is removed and sent to the histology laboratory immediately for analysis. Further surgery can then be performed, depending on findings.

#### *Both procedures*
- Check the patient's vital signs and the dressing at the biopsy site. Determine how much drainage is expected and report excessive drainage to the practitioner.
- If the patient experiences pain, give an analgesic.

 ALERT  For several days after the biopsy, watch for indications of bone infection, such as fever, headache, pain on movement, and redness or abscess near the biopsy site. Notify the practitioner if these symptoms develop.

- Tell the patient to resume his usual diet.

### Precautions
- Bone biopsy should be performed cautiously in the patient with coagulopathy.

### Complications
- Bone fracture
- Infection (osteomyelitis)

# ▌Bone marrow aspiration and biopsy

Bone marrow, the soft tissue contained in the medullary canals of the long bone

## Common sites of bone marrow aspiration and biopsy

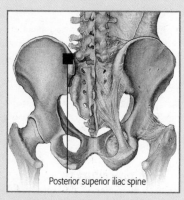

Posterior superior iliac spine

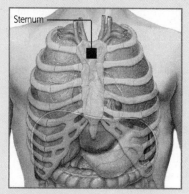

Sternum

The *posterior superior iliac spine* is usually the preferred site for bone marrow aspiration and biopsy because no vital organs or vessels are located nearby. With the patient in a lateral position with one leg flexed, the practitioner inserts the needle several centimeters lateral to the iliosacral junction, entering the bone plane crest with the needle directed downward and toward the anterior inferior spine, or entering a few centimeters below the crest at a right angle to the surface of the bone.

The *sternum* involves the greatest risk but is commonly used for marrow aspiration because it's near the surface, the cortical bone is thin, and the marrow cavity contains numerous cells and relatively little fat or supporting bone. For this procedure, the patient is in a supine position on a firm bed or examining table with a small pillow beneath the shoulders to elevate the chest and lower the head. The practitioner secures the needle guard 3 to 4 mm from the tip of the needle to avoid accidental puncture of the heart or a major vessel. Then he inserts the needle at the midline of the sternum at the second intercostal space.

and in the interstices of cancellous bone, may be removed by aspiration or needle biopsy under local anesthesia. The histologic and hematologic examination of bone marrow provides reliable diagnostic information about blood disorders. In *aspiration biopsy,* a fluid specimen in which pustulae of marrow are suspended is removed from the bone marrow. In *needle biopsy,* a core of marrow cells (not fluid) is removed. These methods are typically used concurrently to obtain the best possible marrow specimens. (See *Common sites of bone marrow aspiration and biopsy.*)

### Normal results

- Yellow marrow contains fat cells and connective tissue.
- Red marrow contains hematopoietic cells, fat cells, and connective tissue.
- The iron stain, which is used to measure hemosiderin (storage iron), has a +2 level.
- The result of the Sudan black B (SBB) fat stain, which shows granulocytes, is negative.
- The result of the periodic acid–Schiff (PAS) stain, which detects glycogen reactions, is negative.

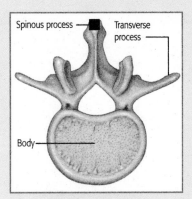

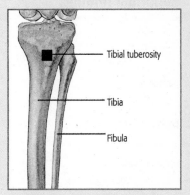

The *spinous process* is the preferred site if multiple punctures are necessary, marrow is absent at other sites, or the patient objects to sternal puncture. For this procedure, the patient sits on the edge of the bed, leaning over the bedside stand or, if he's uncooperative, he may be placed in the prone position with restraints. The practitioner selects the spinous process of the third or fourth lumbar vertebra and inserts the needle at the crest or slightly to one side, advancing the needle in the direction of the bone plane.

The *tibia* is the site of choice for infants under age 1. The infant is placed in a prone position on a bed or examining table with a sandbag beneath the leg. The foot is taped to the surface of the table, or an assistant holds the leg stationary by placing a hand under it. The practitioner inserts the needle about ⅜" (1 cm) below the tibial tuberosity and slightly toward the medial side, being careful to angle the needle point toward the foot to avoid epiphyseal injury.

Illustrations from Anatomical Chart Company. *Atlas of Human Anatomy.* Springhouse, Pa.: Springhouse Corp., 2001.

## Abnormal results

- Histologic examination of a bone marrow specimen can detect myelofibrosis, granulomas, lymphoma, and cancer.
- Hematologic analysis, including the differential count and myeloid-erythroid ratio, can implicate a wide range of disorders. (See *Bone marrow: Normal values and implications of abnormal findings,* pages 312 and 313.)
- Low hemosiderin levels may indicate a true iron deficiency.

- High hemosiderin levels may accompany other types of anemias and blood disorders.
- A positive SBB stain can differentiate acute granulocytic leukemia from acute lymphocytic leukemia (SBB-negative) or may indicate granulation in myeloblasts.
- A positive PAS stain may indicate acute or chronic lymphocytic leukemia, amyloidosis, thalassemia, lymphomas, infectious mononucleosis, iron deficiency anemia, or sideroblastic anemia.

*(Text continues on page 314.)*

# Bone marrow: Normal values and implications of abnormal findings

| Cell types | Normal mean values | | |
|---|---|---|---|
| | *Adults* | *Children* | *Infants* |
| **Basophils** | 0.01% | 0.06% | 0.07% |
| **Eosinophils** | 3.1% | 3.6% | 2.6% |
| **Lymphocytes** | 16.2% | 16% | 49% |
| **Megakaryocytes** | 0.1% | 0.1% | 0.05% |
| **Myeloid:erythroid ratio** | 2:1 to 4:1 | 2.9:1 | 4.4:1 |
| **Neutrophils, total** | 56.5% | 57.1% | 32.4% |
| Myeloblasts | 0.2% to 1.5% | 1.2% | 0.62% |
| Promyelocytes | 2.1% to 4.1% | 1.4% | 0.76% |
| Myelocytes | 8.2% to 15.7% | 18.3% | 2.5% |
| Metamyelocytes | 9.6% to 24.6% | 23.3% | 11.3% |
| Bands | 9.5% to 15.3% | 0 | 14.1% |
| Segmented | 6% to 12% | 12.9% | 3.6% |
| **Normoblasts, total** | 25.6% | 23.1% | 8% |
| Pronormoblasts | 0.2% to 1.3% | 0.5% | 0.1% |
| Basophilic | 0.5% to 2.4% | 1.7% | 0.34% |
| Polychromatic | 17.9% to 29.2% | 18.2% | 6.9% |
| Orthochromatic | 0.4% to 4.6% | 2.7% | 0.54% |
| **Plasma cells** | 1.3% | 0.4% | 0.02% |

## Clinical implications

*High values:* no relation between basophil count and symptoms
*Low values:* no relation between basophil count and symptoms

*High values:* bone marrow carcinoma, lymphadenoma, myeloid leukemia, eosinophilic leukemia, pernicious anemia (in relapse)

*High values:* B- and T-cell chronic lymphocytic leukemia, other lymphatic leukemias, lymphoma, mononucleosis, aplastic anemia, macroglobulinemia

*High values:* advanced age, chronic myeloid leukemia, polycythemia vera, megakaryocytic myelosis, infection, idiopathic thrombocytopenic purpura, thrombocytopenia
*Low values:* pernicious anemia

*High values:* myeloid leukemia, infection, leukemoid reactions, depressed hematopoiesis
*Low values:* agranulocytosis, hematopoiesis after hemorrhage or hemolysis, iron deficiency anemia, polycythemia vera

*High values:* acute myeloblastic or chronic myeloid leukemia
*Low values:* lymphoblastic, lymphatic, or monocytic leukemia; aplastic anemia

*High values:* polycythemia vera
*Low values:* vitamin $B_{12}$ or folic acid deficiency; hypoplastic or aplastic anemia

*High values:* myeloma, collagen disease, infection, antigen sensitivity, malignancy

## Preparing a child for bone marrow biopsy

To prepare a child for a bone marrow biopsy, give him his own biopsy kit: a syringe without a needle, cotton balls, and adhesive bandages. Act out the procedure by using a doll or a stuffed animal as a model. This will help you gain the child's confidence and answer any questions he may have. Be sure to prepare him by describing the kinds of pressure and discomfort he will feel during the procedure.

Before the biopsy, explain the equipment on the tray to the child. Encourage the parents to get involved by helping you hold the child still and reassuring him. Tell the child that he'll feel some pain when the physician aspirates the bone marrow and that it's okay to cry or yell if he wants to, but the pain will go away quickly.

### Purpose

- To diagnose thrombocytopenia, leukemias, and granulomas as well as aplastic, hypoplastic, and pernicious anemias
- To diagnose primary and metastatic tumors
- To determine the cause of infection
- To help stage diseases such as Hodgkin's disease
- To evaluate the effectiveness of chemotherapy and monitor myelosuppression

### Patient preparation

- Explain that the test permits microscopic examination of a bone marrow specimen.
- Describe the procedure to the patient and answer his questions.
- Inform the patient that he doesn't need to restrict food and fluids.
- Tell him who will perform the biopsy and where it will be done.
- Inform the patient that more than one bone marrow specimen may be required and that a blood sample will be collected before biopsy for laboratory testing.
- Make sure the patient has signed an informed consent form.
- Check the patient's history for hypersensitivity to the local anesthetic.
- Tell the patient which bone—the sternum, anterior or posterior iliac crest, vertebral spinous process, rib, or tibia—will be the biopsy site.
- Inform the patient that he'll receive a local anesthetic but will feel pressure on insertion of the biopsy needle and a brief, pulling pain on removal of the marrow. Give a mild sedative 1 hour before the test, as ordered.
- Preparation for children requires additional steps. (See *Preparing a child for bone marrow biopsy*.)

### Procedure and posttest care

- Confirm the patient's identity using two patient identifiers according to facility policy.
- Double-check with the patient and other team members to verify the correct site for the procedure.
- After positioning the patient, instruct him to remain as still as possible.
- Offer emotional support during the biopsy by talking quietly to the patient, describing what's being done and answering questions.

#### Aspiration biopsy

- After the skin over the biopsy site is prepared and the area draped, the local anesthetic is injected. With a twisting motion, the marrow aspiration needle is inserted through the skin, the subcutaneous tissue, and the cortex of the bone.
- The stylet is removed from the needle and a 10- to 20-ml syringe is attached.

The physician aspirates 0.2 to 0.5 ml of marrow and then withdraws the needle.
- Apply pressure to the site for 5 minutes, while the marrow slides are being prepared. (If the patient has thrombocytopenia, apply pressure to the site for 10 to 15 minutes.)
- The biopsy site is cleaned again and a sterile adhesive bandage is applied.
- If an adequate marrow specimen isn't obtained on the first attempt, the needle may be repositioned within the marrow cavity or removed and reinserted in another site within the anesthetized area. If the second attempt fails, a needle biopsy may be needed.

### Needle biopsy
- After preparing the biopsy site and draping the area, the physician marks the skin at the site with an indelible pencil or marking pen.
- A local anesthetic is then injected intradermally, subcutaneously, and at the bone's surface.
- The biopsy needle is inserted into the periosteum and the needle guard is set as indicated. The needle is advanced with a steady boring motion until the outer needle passes through the bone's cortex.
- The inner needle with trephine tip is inserted into the outer needle. By rotating the inner needle alternately clockwise and counterclockwise, the examiner directs the needle into the marrow cavity and then removes a tissue plug.
- The needle assembly is withdrawn and the marrow is expelled into a labeled bottle containing Zenker's acetic acid solution.
- After the biopsy site is cleaned, a sterile adhesive bandage or a pressure dressing is applied.

### Both procedures
- Check the biopsy site for bleeding and inflammation.
- Observe the patient for signs of hemorrhage and infection, such as rapid pulse rate, low blood pressure, and fever.

## Precautions
- Bone marrow biopsy is contraindicated in the patient with a severe bleeding disorder.

## Complications
- Hemorrhage
- Infection
- Puncture of the mediastinum

# 19
# Microbes and parasites

## Cultures for bacteria and viruses

### Bioterrorism infectious agents testing

Numerous agents can be used to treat the effects of bioterrorism. The most common infections associated with bioterrorism include botulism, anthrax, hemorrhagic and yellow fever (including Hantaan virus and Ebola virus), plague, smallpox, and tularemia. Various specimen collection methods may be used to diagnose an infection with a bioterrorist agent depending on the causative agent and site of entry. (See *Understanding bioterrorism infectious agents.*) These methods include cultures of blood, sputum, urine, emesis or gastric aspirate, stool, lymph node aspirate, or scrapings from lesions. Regardless of the method used, suspected cases of infection must be reported to local, state, and federal health departments.

#### Normal results
- Cultures are negative for the suspected organism.

- If an electromyogram was done for a patient suspected of botulism, the response to repetitive nerve stimulation reveals no increase.

#### Abnormal results
- Evidence of growth of the causative organism indicates infection.
- For smallpox, Guarnieri's bodies are present in the lesion scrapings, and brick-shaped virions are noted when the specimen is viewed by an electron microscope.

#### Purpose
- To isolate and identify the causative organism

#### Patient preparation
- Explain to the patient that this test helps identify the organism causing his symptoms.
- Describe the method and procedure to be used to obtain the specimen, such as blood, stool, or sputum.
- Tell the patient when the specimen will be collected, who will be collecting it, and how many samples will be needed.
- Tell him that he doesn't need to restrict food or fluids.

# Understanding bioterrorism infectious agents

| Infectious agent | Mode of transmission | Mode of entry | Specimen for testing |
|---|---|---|---|
| *Bacillus anthracis* (spore-forming, gram-positive bacillus causing anthrax) | ■ Undercooked meat from infected animals<br>■ Inhalation of animal products such as the animal's wool<br>■ Intentional release of spores | ■ Skin<br>■ Inhalation<br>■ GI tract | ■ Blood, sputum, or stool<br>■ Fluid from lesion |
| *Clostridium botulinum* (spore-forming obligate anaerobe causing botulism) | ■ Soil<br>■ Undercooked food not kept warm | ■ Mucosal surface (GI tract, lung)<br>■ Wound | ■ Blood, stool, gastric aspirate, emesis<br>■ Suspected contaminated food substance |
| *Francisella tularensis* (intracellular parasite causing tularemia) | ■ Infected animals, such as mice, squirrels, or rabbits<br>■ Contaminated water, soil, or vegetation | ■ Skin, mucous membranes<br>■ Lungs<br>■ GI tract | ■ Respiratory secretions and blood<br>■ Lymph node biopsy<br>■ Lesion scrapings |
| Variola virus (causing smallpox) | ■ Airborne via coughing<br>■ Direct contact<br>■ Contaminated clothing or bedding | ■ Lungs | ■ Fluid from lesion |
| Viruses for hemorrhagic fever and yellow fever (including Hantaan virus, Ebola virus) | ■ Bite of infected animal, rodent, or insect | ■ Skin | ■ Blood, sputum, tissue, or urine |
| *Yersinia pestis* (causing plague) | ■ Infected flea bite | ■ Skin | ■ Blood, sputum, or lymph node aspirate |

■ If botulism is suspected, inform the patient that an electromyogram may be done to identify the cause of acute flaccid paralysis.

### Procedure and posttest care
■ Confirm the patient's identity using two patient identifiers according to facility policy.

■ Obtain the specimens as ordered based on the suspicion of infectious agent.

### DO'S & DON'TS

Place blood samples on ice; refrigerate all specimens for botulinum toxin testing.

ALERT

 If stool is being cultured for botulism testing and the patient is constipated, give him an enema using sterile water as the solution to make sure that an adequate sample is obtained.

- Send the specimen to the laboratory for a "mouse" assay to evaluate for botulinum toxin.
- Collect vesicular fluid from a previously unopened lesion on at least one culture swab when testing for cutaneous anthrax and smallpox.
- Obtain three blood cultures along with specimens of gastric aspirate, stool, or food if GI anthrax is suspected.
- When obtaining specimens for tularemia, have the patient provide a forced deep cough for a sputum specimen; obtain a lesional specimen from the leading edge of the lesion.
- Send any food that's being tested (for botulism) in its original container.
- Send all specimens to the laboratory immediately.

### Precautions
- Adhere to standard precautions during collection of all specimens.
- Use of anticholinergic agents by a patient being tested for botulism may alter the results.
- Institute airborne precautions and use negative pressure rooms for patients with suspected infection of hemorrhagic fever, Hantaan virus, Ebola virus, and yellow fever.
- Clean contaminated surfaces and spills with appropriate solution such as a hypochlorite bleach solution.
- Make sure that examinations of specimens for smallpox are performed in a Biosafety laboratory (level 4); examinations of specimens for other infections are performed in a Biosafety laboratory (level 2).

# Blood culture

A blood culture is performed to isolate and aid in the identification of the pathogens in bacteremia (bacterial invasion of the bloodstream) and septicemia (systemic spread of such infection). It requires inoculating a culture medium with a blood sample and incubating it.

Blood culture can identify about 67% of pathogens within 24 hours and up to 90% within 72 hours.

The timing of specimen collection for blood cultures varies; it usually depends on the type of bacteremia (intermittent or continuous) suspected and on whether drug therapy needs to be started regardless of test results.

### Normal results
- Blood cultures are negative for pathogens.

### Abnormal results
- Positive blood cultures don't necessarily confirm pathologic septicemia.
- Mild, transient bacteremia may occur during the course of many infectious diseases or may complicate other disorders.
- Persistent, continuous, or recurrent bacteremia reliably confirms the presence of serious infection. To detect most causative agents, blood cultures are ideally drawn on 2 consecutive days.
- Isolation of most organisms takes about 72 hours; negative cultures are held for 1 or more weeks before being reported negative.
- Common blood pathogens include *Streptococcus pneumoniae* and other Streptococcus species, *Haemophilus influenzae, Staphylococcus aureus, Pseudomonas aeruginosa, Bacteroides, Brucella, Enterobacteriaceae,* coliform bacilli, and *Candida albicans.*
- Although 2% to 3% of cultured blood samples are contaminated by skin bacte-

ria, such as *Staphylococcus epidermidis,* diphtheroids, and Propionibacterium, these organisms may be clinically significant when isolated from multiple cultures or from immunocompromised patients.

■ Debilitated or immunocompromised patients may have isolates of *C. albicans.* In patients with human immunodeficiency virus infection, *Mycobacterium tuberculosis* and *M. avium* complex may be isolated as well as other Mycobacterium species on a less frequent basis.

### DRUG CHALLENGE

 Previous or current antimicrobial therapy on the laboratory request (possible false-negative)

### Purpose

■ To confirm bacteremia
■ To identify the causative organism in bacteremia and septicemia

### Patient preparation

■ Explain that this procedure helps identify the organism causing his symptoms.
■ Inform the patient that he need not restrict food and fluids.
■ Tell the patient how many samples the test will require and who will perform the venipunctures and when.
■ Inform the patient that he may experience slight discomfort from the needle punctures and the tourniquet.

### Procedure and posttest care

■ Confirm the patient's identity using two patient identifiers according to facility policy.
■ Put on gloves.
■ Clean the venipuncture site with an alcohol swab and then with an iodine swab, working in a circular motion from the site outward.

■ Wait at least 1 minute for the skin to dry, and remove the residual iodine with an alcohol swab, or remove the iodine after venipuncture.
■ Apply the tourniquet.
■ Perform a venipuncture; draw 10 to 20 ml of blood for an adult or 2 to 6 ml for a child.

### DO'S & DON'TS

 Don't draw blood from an existing I.V. catheter. Use a vein below an I.V. catheter or in the opposite arm.

■ Clean the diaphragm tops of the culture bottles with alcohol or iodine, and change the needle on the syringe.
■ If broth is used, add blood to each bottle until a 1:5 or 1:10 dilution is obtained. For example, add 10 ml of blood to a 100-ml bottle. (The size of the bottle varies, depending on facility procedure.)
■ If a special resin is used, add blood to the resin in the bottles, and invert them gently to mix.
■ If you're using the lysis-centrifugation technique (Isolator), draw the blood directly into a special collection and processing tube.
■ Indicate the tentative diagnosis on the laboratory request, and note current or recent antimicrobial therapy.
■ Apply direct pressure to the venipuncture site until bleeding stops.
■ If a hematoma develops at the venipuncture site, apply warm soaks.

### Precautions

■ Removing the culture bottle caps or use of the incorrect media or bottle may prevent proper growth.
■ Whenever possible, blood cultures should be collected before administering antimicrobial agents.

# Culture for chlamydia

The most common sexually transmitted disease in the United States, chlamydia is caused by the organism *Chlamydia trachomatis*. Identification of this parasite requires cultivation in the laboratory. After incubation, Chlamydia-infected cells can be detected by fluorescein isothiocyanate-conjugated monoclonal antibodies or by iodine stain. Detection in cell cultures of *C. psittaci* and *C. pneumoniae* requires specific technical manipulations and reagents; deoxyribonucleic acid detection may also be performed in women who may be susceptible to the infections, whether they have symptoms or not.

Culture is the detection method of choice, but rapid noncultural (antigen detection) procedures are also available.

## Normal results

- No *C. trachomatis* appears in the culture.

## Abnormal results

- A positive culture confirms *C. trachomatis* infection.

**DRUG CHALLENGE**

Using an antimicrobial drug within a few days before specimen collection (possible inability to recover *C. trachomatis*)

## Purpose

- To confirm infections caused by *C. trachomatis*

## Patient preparation

- Explain the purpose of the test to the patient.
- Describe the procedure for collecting a specimen for culture.
- If the specimen will be collected from the patient's genital tract, instruct him

not to urinate for 3 to 4 hours before the specimen is taken.
- If the patient is a woman, tell her not to douche for 24 hours before the test.
- If the patient is a man, tell him that he may experience some burning and pressure as the culture is taken but that the discomfort will subside after a few minutes.

## Procedure and posttest care

- Confirm the patient's identity using two patient identifiers according to facility policy.
- Obtain a specimen of the epithelial cells from the infected site. In adults, these sites may include the eye, urethra (rather than from the purulent exudate that may be present), endocervix, and rectum.
- Obtain a urethral specimen by inserting a cotton-tipped applicator ¾" to 2" (2 to 5 cm) into the urethra.
- To collect a specimen from the endocervix, use a microbiologic transport swab or cytobrush.
- Extract the specimen into 2SP transport medium.
- Specimens collected from the throat, eye, or nasopharynx and aspirates from infants should also be extracted into 2SP transport medium. These specimens are sent to the laboratory at 39.2° F (4° C).
- If the anticipated time between specimen collection and inoculation into cell culture is more than 24 hours, freeze the 2SP transport medium, and send it to the laboratory with dry ice.

**ALERT**

In the patient suspected of being sexually abused, be sure to process the specimen by culture rather than by antigen detection methods.

- Advise the patient to avoid all sexual contact until after test results are available.
- If the culture confirms infection, provide counseling for the patient about treatment of sexual partners.
- Tell the patient that positive culture findings must be reported to the local health department.

### Precautions
- Place the male patient in the supine position to prevent him from falling if vasovagal syncope occurs when the cotton swab or wire loop is introduced into the urethra. Observe for profound hypotension, bradycardia, pallor, and sweating.
- Collect a urethral specimen at least 1 hour after the patient has voided to prevent loss of urethral secretions.
- After collecting the specimens, carefully dispose of gloves, swabs, and speculum to prevent staff exposure.

## Culture for gonorrhea

Gonorrhea almost always results from sexual transmission of *Neisseria gonorrhoeae*. A stained smear of genital exudate can confirm gonorrhea in 90% of males with characteristic symptoms, but a culture is usually necessary, especially in asymptomatic women. Possible culture sites include the urethra (usual site in men), endocervix (usual site in women), anal canal, and throat.

### Normal results
- No *N. gonorrhoeae* appears in the culture.

### Abnormal results
- A positive culture confirms gonorrhea.

### Purpose
- To confirm gonorrhea

### Patient preparation
- Describe the procedure to the patient. Explain that this test is used to confirm gonorrhea.
- Inform the patient who will perform the test and when.
- If the patient is a woman, tell her not to douche for 24 hours before the test.
- If the patient is a man, tell him not to void during the hour preceding the test. Warn him that men sometimes experience nausea, sweating, weakness, and fainting due to stress or discomfort when the cotton swab or wire loop is introduced into the urethra.

### Procedure and posttest care
- Confirm the patient's identity using two patient identifiers according to facility policy.

#### Endocervical culture
- Place the patient in the lithotomy position, drape her appropriately, and instruct her to take deep breaths.
- Using gloved hands, insert a vaginal speculum that has been lubricated only with warm water. Clean mucus from the cervix, using cotton balls in ring forceps.
- Insert a dry, sterile cotton swab into the endocervical canal, and rotate it from side to side. Leave the swab in place for several seconds for optimum absorption of organisms.
- In cases of deep pelvic inflammatory disease, cultures of the endometrium or aspirations by laparoscopy or culdoscopy may be necessary. Endometrial specimens are obtained by inserting stents through a narrow-bore catheter introduced into the cervical canal.

#### Urethral culture
- Place the patient in a supine position, and drape him appropriately.
- Clean the urethral meatus with sterile gauze or a cotton swab, and then insert a thin urogenital alginate swab or a wire

# Culturing for *Neisseria gonorrhoeae*

Culturing for *Neisseria gonorrhoeae* requires use of a modified Thayer-Martin (MTM) medium. If a laboratory isn't readily available, you may use Transgrow medium.

## Modified Thayer-Martin medium

MTM medium is a combination of hemoglobin, gonococcal growth-enhancing chemicals, and antimicrobial agents for culturing endocervical, urethral, and rectal specimens. To inoculate a culture plate treated with MTM medium and to spread organisms out of their associated mucus, take these steps:

■ Roll the swab in a Z pattern (illustration 1)

■ Using the swab or a sterile wire loop, immediately cross-streak the plate (illustration 2).

Incubate within 15 minutes of streaking.

Two-step method of streaking Thayer-Martin medium

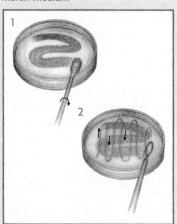

## Transgrow medium

A modification of MTM medium, Transgrow is available in a screwcap bottle containing air and carbon dioxide. Transgrow bottles are used to transport suspect cultures when laboratory facilities aren't available at the site of specimen collection. Use this procedure:

■ To prevent loss of carbon dioxide, inoculate the specimen bottle while it's upright.

■ After uncapping the bottle, immediately insert the swab, and soak up all excess moisture.

■ Starting at the bottom of the bottle, roll the swab from side to side across the medium.

■ Recap the bottle, and send it to the laboratory immediately. Subculturing should begin within 24 to 48 hours.

One-step method of streaking Transgrow medium

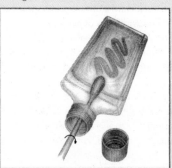

bacteriologic loop ⅜" to ¾" (1 to 2 cm) into the urethra, and rotate the swab or loop from side to side. Leave it in place for several seconds for optimum absorption of organisms. If permitted, the patient may milk the urethra, bringing urethral secretions to the meatus for collection on a cotton swab.

### *Rectal culture*

■ After obtaining an endocervical or a urethral specimen (while the patient is still on the examination table), insert a

sterile cotton swab into the anal canal about 1″ (2.5 cm), move the swab from side to side, and leave it in place for several seconds for optimum absorption.
- If the swab is contaminated with stool, discard it, and repeat the procedure with a clean swab.

### Throat culture
- Position the patient with his head tilted back.
- Check his throat for inflamed areas using a tongue blade. Rub a sterile swab from side to side over the tonsillar areas, including inflamed or purulent sites. Be careful not to touch the teeth, cheeks, or tongue with the swab.

### After specimen collection
- Roll the swab in a Z pattern in a plate containing modified Thayer-Martin medium. Then cross-streak the medium with a sterile wire loop or the tip of the swab, and cover the plate. (See *Culturing for* Neisseria gonorrhoeae.)
- Label the specimen with the patient's name and room number (if applicable), the practitioner's name, and the date and time of collection.
- Direct smears of obtained material should be made immediately to prepare the Gram stain. Remaining material must be quickly inoculated into selective culture media or into a transport system. A culturette transport tube or a swab transport medium containing charcoal can be used. Charcoal helps neutralize toxic materials in the specimen.
- If laboratory facilities aren't readily available, do the following: Uncap the Transgrow medium specimen bottle just before inserting the swab of test material into the bottle. Keep the bottle upright to minimize loss of carbon dioxide. With the swab, absorb the excess moisture within the bottle, and then roll the swab across the Transgrow medium.

Discard the swab. Place the lid on the bottle, and label it appropriately.
- Advise the patient to avoid all sexual contact until test results are available.
- Explain that treatment usually begins after confirming a positive culture, except in a person who has symptoms of gonorrhea or who has had intercourse with someone with gonorrhea.
- Advise the patient that a repeat culture is required 1 week after completion of treatment to evaluate the effectiveness of therapy.
- Tell the patient that positive culture findings must be reported to the local health department and that all recent sexual partners must also be informed and treated.

## Precautions
- If the patient is a man, place him in the supine position to prevent him from falling if vasovagal syncope occurs when the cotton swab or wire loop is introduced into the urethra. Observe for profound hypotension, bradycardia, pallor, and sweating.
- Collect a urethral specimen at least 1 hour after the patient has voided to prevent loss of urethral secretions.
- After collecting the specimens, carefully dispose of gloves, swabs, and speculum to prevent staff exposure.

## ▌Culture for herpes simplex virus
Herpes simplex virus (HSV) produces a wide spectrum of clinical signs and symptoms, including keratitis, gingivostomatitis, and encephalitis. In the immunocompromised individual, it may lead to disseminated illness. The herpesvirus group includes Epstein-Barr virus, cytomegalovirus (CMV), varicella-zoster virus (VZV), human herpesvirus-6, herpesvirus-7, herpesvirus-8, and the two closely related serotypes of HSV—

type 1 and type 2. Only CMV, VZV, and HSV replicate in the standard cell cultures used in diagnostic laboratories.

About 50% of HSV strains can be detected by characteristic cytopathic effects (CPE) within 24 hours after the laboratory receives the specimen; 5 to 7 days are required to detect the remaining HSV strains.

Alternatively, early HSV antigens can be detected by monoclonal antibodies in shell vial cell cultures within 16 hours after receipt of the specimen with the same sensitivity and specificity as standard tube cell cultures.

## Normal results
▪ HSV is seldom recovered from an immunocompetent patient who shows no overt signs of disease.

## Abnormal results
▪ HSV detected in specimens taken from dermal lesions, the eye, or cerebrospinal fluid is highly significant.
▪ Specimens from the upper respiratory tract may be associated with intermittent shedding of the virus, particularly in an immunocompromised patient.
▪ Like other herpesviruses, HSV can be shed from the immunocompromised patient intermittently in the absence of apparent disease.
▪ For epidemiologic purposes, HSV detected by CPE in standard tube cell cultures is confirmed and identified as type 1 or 2.

DRUG CHALLENGE

Administration of antiviral drugs before specimen collection

## Purpose
▪ To confirm diagnosis of HSV infection by culturing the virus from specimens

## Patient preparation
▪ Explain that this test detects HSV infection.
▪ Tell the patient that specimens will be collected from suspected lesions during the prodromal and acute stages of clinical infection.

## Procedure and posttest care
▪ Confirm the patient's identity using two patient identifiers according to facility policy.
▪ Collect a specimen for culture in the appropriate collection device. Vesicle fluid can be obtained with a 27G needle or a tuberculin syringe. If the fluid is scant, the base of the ulcer can be scraped with a swab to remove cells.
▪ For the throat, skin, eye, or genital area, use a microbiologic transport swab.
▪ For body fluids or other respiratory specimens (washings, lavage), use a sterile screw-capped jar.
▪ Transport the specimen to the laboratory as soon as possible after collection. If the anticipated time between collection and inoculation of cell cultures is more than 3 hours, the specimen should be stored and transported at 39.2° F (4° C).

## Precautions
▪ Don't allow the specimen to dry up.

# ▌Nasopharyngeal culture

A nasopharyngeal culture evaluates nasopharyngeal secretions for the presence of pathogenic organisms. It requires direct microscopic examination of a Gram-stained smear of the specimen. Preliminary identification of organisms may be used to guide clinical management and determine the need for additional testing. Cultured pathogens may then require susceptibility testing to determine appropriate antimicrobial therapy.

## Normal results
■ Nonhemolytic streptococci, alpha-hemolytic streptococci, *Neisseria* species (except *N. meningitidis* and *N. gonorrhoeae*), coagulase-negative staphylococci such as *Staphylococcus epidermidis* and, occasionally, the coagulase-positive *S. aureus* are present.

## Abnormal results
■ Group A beta-hemolytic streptococci; occasionally groups B, C, and G beta-hemolytic streptococci; *B. pertussis, C. diphtheriae,* and *S. aureus;* large numbers of pneumococci; *Haemophilus influenzae; Myxovirus influenzae;* paramyxoviruses; *Candida albicans;* mycoplasma species; and *Mycobacterium tuberculosis* may be present.

### DRUG CHALLENGE

Recent antimicrobial therapy (decrease in bacterial growth)

## Purpose
■ To identify pathogens causing upper respiratory tract symptoms
■ To identify proliferation of normal nasopharyngeal flora, which may be pathogenic in debilitated and other immuno-compromised patients
■ To identify *B. pertussis* and *N. meningitidis,* especially in very young, elderly, or debilitated patients and asymptomatic carriers
■ To isolate viruses (infrequently), especially to identify carriers of influenza virus A and B

## Patient preparation
■ Explain that this test isolates the cause of nasopharyngeal infection.

■ Describe the procedure to the patient; tell him that secretions will be obtained from the back of the nose and the throat, using a cotton-tipped swab, and who will collect the specimen.
■ Warn the patient that he may experience slight discomfort and gagging, but reassure him that obtaining the specimen takes less than 15 seconds.

## Procedure and posttest care
■ Confirm the patient's identity using two patient identifiers according to facility policy.
■ Put on gloves.
■ Moisten the swab with sterile water or saline.
■ Ask the patient to cough before you begin collecting the specimen.
■ Position the patient with his head tilted back.
■ Using a penlight and a tongue blade, inspect the nasopharyngeal area.
■ Gently pass the swab through the nostril and into the nasopharynx, keeping the swab near the septum and floor of the nose. Rotate the swab quickly and remove it.
■ Alternatively, place the glass tube in the patient's nostril, and carefully pass the swab through the tube into the nasopharynx. (See *Obtaining a nasopharyngeal specimen,* page 326.) Rotate the swab for 5 seconds, and place it in the culture tube with the transport medium. Remove the glass tube.
■ Label the specimen with the patient's name, the practitioner's name, the date and time of collection, the origin of the material, and the suspected organism.
■ Ideally, specimens for *B. pertussis* should be inoculated to fresh culture medium at the patient's bedside because of the organism's susceptibility to environmental changes.
■ If the purpose of specimen collection is to isolate a virus, follow the laboratory's recommended collection technique.

# Obtaining a nasopharyngeal specimen

When the swab passes into the nasopharynx, gently but quickly rotate it to collect a specimen. Then remove the swab, taking care not to injure the nasal mucous membrane.

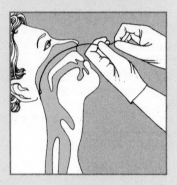

## Precautions

- Don't let the swab touch the sides of the patient's nostril or his tongue to prevent specimen contamination.
- Note antimicrobial therapy or chemotherapy on the laboratory request.
- Keep the container upright.
- Tell the laboratory if the suspected organism is *Corynebacterium diphtheriae* or *B. pertussis* because these need special growth media.
- Refrigerate a viral specimen according to your laboratory's procedure.
- If *B. pertussis* is suspected, Dacron or calcium alginate mini-tipped swabs should be used for collection.
- When specimens can't be directly placed onto growth media, the best media-based transport is one supplemented with antibiotics to reduce the growth of normal flora.

## Complications

 Laryngospasm may occur after the culture is obtained if the patient has epiglottiditis or diphtheria. Keep resuscitation equipment nearby.

# ■ SARS viral testing

Severe acute respiratory syndrome (SARS) viral testing involves the use of one of three different tests to identify infection with the SARS virus. The SARS virus is a coronavirus (CoV) that causes a pneumonia-like infection. The incubation period is about 8 to 10 days. Typically, the person has traveled to an area or lives in an area in which the infection has been identified. Usually SARS testing is performed only if there's a high index of suspicion—that is, in patients for whom infection from other causes has been ruled out.

The three tests used for SARS testing are:
- Enzyme-linked immunosorbent assay (ELISA)—identifies antibodies to the SARS virus, usually about 20 days after the onset of symptoms
- Immunofluorescence assay—identifies antibodies to the SARS virus possibly as early as 10 days after infection but can be time consuming because it involves growing the virus in the laboratory
- Reverse transcriptase-polymerase chain reaction (RT-PCR)—identifies the infection early on, with results available in as few as 2 days; identifies genetic information of the virus's RNA.

Specimens for SARS testing may be obtained from the nasopharyngeal, oropharyngeal, or bronchoalveolar area; trachea; pleural fluid; sputum; or postmortem tissue. Testing with RT-PCR usually involves serum and blood specimens.

## Normal results
- No antibodies to the SARS virus are found.

## Abnormal results
- The specimen tests positive for the SARS virus, indicating infection with SARS.
- SARS is diagnosed when positive test results occur:
  - in a single specimen, which is tested at two distinct times
  - in two specimens from two different areas
  - in two specimens from the same area but tested on different days.

## Purpose
- To identify the SARS CoV as the cause of the infection

## Patient preparation
- Explain that the SARS viral test identifies the organism causing respiratory tract infection.
- Tell the patient about the types of specimens that will be collected. Explain when the specimens will be collected and how.
- If the specimen will be collected by expectoration, encourage fluid intake the night before collection to help sputum production, unless contraindicated by a fluid restriction. Teach the patient how to expectorate by taking three deep breaths and forcing a deep cough; emphasize that sputum isn't the same as saliva, which is unacceptable for culturing. Tell him to brush his teeth and gargle with water before the specimen collection to reduce contaminating oropharyngeal bacteria.
- If the specimen will be collected by swabbing the area, warn the patient that he may feel a slight itching sensation.
- If the specimen will be collected by tracheal suctioning, tell the patient that

he'll experience discomfort as the catheter passes into the trachea.
- If the specimen will be collected by bronchoscopy, instruct the patient to fast for 6 hours before the procedure.
- Make sure the patient or a responsible family member has signed an informed consent form.

## Procedure and posttest care
- Confirm the patient's identity using two patient identifiers according to facility policy.
- Put on gloves.

### Washing or aspirating the nasopharyngeal area
- Have the patient sit with his head tilted slightly back.
- Insert a syringe filled with 1 to 1.5 ml of saline (nonbacteriostatic) into one nostril and instill the saline.
- Attach a small plastic catheter or tubing to the syringe and flush it with 2 to 3 ml of saline.
- Insert the tubing into the nostril, and aspirate the secretions; then repeat in the other nostril.

### Swabbing the nasopharyngeal or oropharyngeal area
- Obtain sterile swabs that have plastic sticks and Dacron or rayon tips.

ALERT

Never use cotton-tipped applicators or swabs with wooden sticks. Some viruses can become inactivated by the substances contained in these swabs, thereby interfering with RT-PCR testing.

- Insert the swab into the nostril, and let it remain there for several seconds to absorb the secretions; if swabbing the oropharyngeal area, run the swab along the posterior pharynx and tonsils. Avoid touching the tongue.

### Expectorating sputum

- Have the patient rinse his mouth with water.
- Instruct the patient to cough deeply and expectorate into the sterile dry container.

### Collecting blood and plasma specimens

- Perform a venipuncture, and collect 5 to 10 ml of whole blood in a serum separator tube (for serum RT-PCR or ELISA antibody testing) or an EDTA tube (for plasma testing).

### Collecting other specimens

- Assist with tracheal suctioning, bronchoscopy, or thoracentesis as appropriate.

### All tests

- Make sure that all specimens are placed in the appropriate sterile container for transport.
- Dispose of equipment properly; seal the container in a biohazard bag before sending it to the laboratory.
- Label the container with the patient's name and the practitioner's name. Include on the test request form the nature and origin of the specimen, the date and time of collection, the initial diagnosis, and any current antimicrobial therapy.
- Provide mouth care as indicated.

## Precautions

- Be sure to wear gloves when performing the procedure and handling specimens; adhere to your facility's infection control policies at all times.
- Because the patient may cough violently during suctioning, wear gloves, a mask and, if necessary, a gown to avoid exposure to pathogens.

## ▌Sputum culture
[sputum C&S]

Bacteriologic examination of sputum (material raised from the lungs and bronchi) is an important aid to the management of lung disease.

The usual method of specimen collection is expectoration (which may require ultrasonic nebulization, hydration, physiotherapy, or postural drainage); other methods include tracheal suctioning and bronchoscopy. (See *Using an in-line trap.*)

A Gram stain of expectorated sputum must be examined to make sure that it's a representative specimen of secretions from the lower respiratory tract (many white blood cells [WBCs], few epithelial cells) rather than one contaminated by oral flora (few WBCs, many epithelial cells). Careful examination of an acid-fast smear of sputum may provide presumptive evidence of a mycobacterial infection such as tuberculosis.

### Normal results

- Flora commonly found in the respiratory tract include alpha-hemolytic streptococci, *Neisseria* species, and diphtheroids.
- The presence of normal flora doesn't rule out infection.

### Abnormal results

- Because sputum is invariably contaminated with normal oropharyngeal flora, a culture isolate must be interpreted in light of the patient's overall clinical condition.
- Isolation of *M. tuberculosis* is always a significant finding.
- Isolation of pathogenic organisms most often includes *Streptococcus pneumoniae*, *M. tuberculosis*, *Klebsiella pneumoniae* (and other *Enterobacteriaceae*),

*Haemophilus influenzae, Staphylococcus aureus,* and *Pseudomonas aeruginosa.*

### Purpose
■ To isolate and identify the cause of pulmonary infection, helping to diagnose respiratory diseases (most commonly bronchitis, tuberculosis, lung abscess, and pneumonia)

### Patient preparation
■ Explain that this test identifies the organism causing a respiratory tract infection.
■ Tell the patient the test requires a sputum specimen. Explain who will collect the specimen and when it will be done.
■ If the suspected organism is *M. tuberculosis,* tell the patient that as many as three consecutive morning specimens may be required; diagnosis of this disorder usually depends on the symptoms, a smear for acid-fast bacilli, a chest X-ray, and response to a purified protein derivative skin test.
■ If the specimen will be collected by expectoration, encourage fluid intake the night before collection to help sputum production, unless contraindicated by a fluid restriction. Teach the patient how to expectorate by taking three deep breaths and forcing a deep cough; emphasize that sputum isn't the same as saliva, which is unacceptable for culturing. Tell him to brush his teeth and gargle with water before the specimen collection to reduce contaminating oropharyngeal bacteria.
■ If the specimen will be collected by tracheal suctioning, tell the patient that he'll experience discomfort as the catheter passes into the trachea.
■ If the specimen will be collected by bronchoscopy, instruct the patient to fast for 6 hours before the procedure. Also make sure that the patient or a responsible family member has signed an inform consent form.

## Using an in-line trap

Push the suction tubing onto the male adapter of the in-line trap.

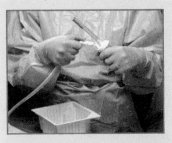

Put on sterile gloves; with one hand, insert the suction catheter into the rubber tubing of the trap. Then suction the patient.

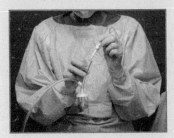

After suctioning, disconnect the in-line trap from the suction tubing and catheter. To seal the container, connect the rubber tubing to the female adapter of the trap.

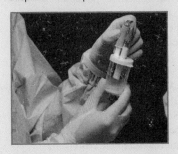

■ Tell the patient that he'll receive a local anesthetic just before the test to minimize discomfort during passage of the tube.

## Procedure and posttest care

- Confirm the patient's identity using two patient identifiers according to facility policy.

### *Expectoration*

- Put on gloves.
- Instruct the patient to cough deeply and expectorate into the container. If the cough is nonproductive, use chest physiotherapy or a heated aerosol spray (nebulization) to induce sputum. Using sterile technique, close the container securely.
- Dispose of equipment properly; seal the container in a leakproof bag before sending it to the laboratory.

### *Tracheal suctioning*

- Give the patient oxygen before and after the procedure if necessary.
- Attach the sputum trap to the suction catheter. Using sterile gloves, lubricate the catheter with normal saline solution, and pass it through the patient's nostril without suction. (He'll cough when the catheter passes through the larynx.) Advance the catheter into the trachea. Apply suction for no longer than 15 seconds to obtain the specimen.
- Stop suction and gently remove the catheter. Discard the catheter and gloves in the proper receptacle. Then detach the in-line sputum trap from the suction apparatus, and cap the opening.

### *Bronchoscopy*

- After a local anesthetic is sprayed into the patient's throat or after he gargles with a local anesthetic, the bronchoscope is inserted through the pharynx and trachea into the bronchus.
- Secretions are then collected with a bronchial brush or aspirated through the inner channel of the scope using an irrigating solution, such as normal saline solution, if necessary.

- After the specimen is obtained, the bronchoscope is removed.

### *All collection methods*

- Provide good mouth care.
- Label the container with the patient's name and the practitioner's name. Include on the test request form the nature and origin of the specimen, the date and time of collection, the initial diagnosis, and any current antimicrobial therapy.

## Precautions

- Tracheal suctioning is contraindicated in the patient with esophageal varices.

ALERT

 In a patient with asthma or chronic bronchitis, watch for aggravated bronchospasms when using normal saline solution or acetylcysteine in an aerosol.

- During tracheal suctioning, suction for only 5 to 10 seconds at a time. Never suction longer than 15 seconds. If the patient becomes hypoxic or cyanotic, remove the catheter immediately and administer oxygen.
- Because the patient may cough violently during suctioning, wear gloves, a mask and, if necessary, a gown to avoid exposure to pathogens.
- Don't use more than 20% propylene glycol with water as an inducer for a specimen scheduled for tuberculosis culturing because higher concentrations inhibit the growth of *M. tuberculosis*. (If propylene glycol isn't available, use 10% to 20% acetylcysteine with water or saline solution.)

## Complications

ALERT

 During and after bronchoscopy, observe the patient carefully for signs of hypoxemia (change in mental status), laryngospasm (laryngeal stridor), bronchospasm (paroxysms of coughing or wheezing), pneumothorax (dyspnea, cyanosis, pleural pain, tachycardia), perforation of the trachea or bronchus (subcutaneous crepitus), and trauma to respiratory structures (blood-tinged sputum, coughing up blood). Also, check for difficulty in breathing or swallowing. Don't give liquids until the gag reflex returns.

- Cardiac arrhythmias
- Bleeding

# Throat culture

A throat culture is used primarily to isolate and identify pathogens, thus allowing early treatment of pharyngitis and prevention of sequelae, such as rheumatic heart disease and glomerulonephritis.

A throat culture requires swabbing the throat, streaking a culture plate, and allowing the organisms to grow for isolation and identification of pathogens. A Gram-stained smear may provide preliminary identification, which may guide clinical management and determine the need for further tests. Culture results are considered in relation to the patient's clinical status, recent antimicrobial therapy, and amount of normal flora.

## Normal results
- Normal flora include nonhemolytic and alpha-hemolytic streptococci, *Neisseria* species, staphylococci, diphtheroids, some *Haemophilus* species, *pneumococci*, yeasts, enteric gram-negative rods, spirochetes, *Veillonella* species, and *Micrococcus* species.

## Abnormal results
- Group A beta-hemolytic streptococci (*Streptococcus pyogenes*), which can cause scarlet fever and pharyngitis, is detected.

- *Candida albicans*, which can cause thrush, is present.
- *Corynebacterium diphtheriae*, which can cause diphtheria, is present.
- *B. pertussis*, which can cause whooping cough, is detected.
- *Legionella* species and *Mycoplasma pneumoniae* suggest bacterial pneumonia.
- *Histoplasma capsulatum*, *Coccidioides immitis*, and *Blastomyces dermatitidis* suggest fungal infections.
- Adenovirus, enterovirus, herpesvirus, rhinovirus, influenza virus, and parainfluenza virus suggest viral infections.

## Purpose
- To isolate and identify group A beta-hemolytic streptococci
- To screen asymptomatic carriers of pathogens, especially *N. meningitidis*

## Patient preparation
- Explain to the patient that this test identifies microorganisms that may be causing his symptoms or screens for asymptomatic carriers.
- Inform the patient that he need not restrict food and fluids.
- Tell the patient that a specimen will be collected from his throat, who will collect the specimen, and when.
- Describe the procedure, and warn the patient that he may gag during the swabbing.
- Check the patient's history for recent antimicrobial therapy. Determine immunization history if it's pertinent to the preliminary diagnosis.

## Procedure and posttest care
- Confirm the patient's identity using two patient identifiers according to facility policy.
- Tell the patient to tilt his head back and close his eyes.

- With the throat well illuminated, check for inflamed areas using a tongue blade.
- Swab the tonsillar areas from side to side; include inflamed or purulent sites.

### Do's & don'ts

Don't touch the tongue, cheeks, or teeth with the swab.

- Immediately place the swab in the culture tube.
- If a commercial sterile collection and transport system is used, crush the ampule, and force the swab into the medium to keep the swab moist.
- Note recent antimicrobial therapy on the laboratory request; label the specimen with the patient's name, the practitioner's name, the date and time of collection, and the origin of the specimen; indicate the suspected organism, especially *C. diphtheriae* (requires two swabs and a special growth medium), *B. pertussis* (requires a nasopharyngeal culture and a special growth medium), and *N. meningitidis* (requires enriched selective media).
- Nonculture antigen testing methods can be used to detect group A streptococcal antigen in as few as 5 minutes. Cultures are then performed on negative specimens.

### Precautions

- Procure the throat specimen before beginning antimicrobial therapy.
- Send the specimen to the laboratory immediately. Unless a commercial sterile collection and transport system is used, keep the container upright during transport.

## Complications

Laryngospasm may occur after the culture is obtained if the patient has epiglottiditis or diphtheria. Keep resuscitation equipment nearby.

# Urine culture
## [urine C&S]

Laboratory examination and culture of urine evaluates urinary tract infections (UTIs), especially bladder infections. Urine in the kidneys and bladder is normally sterile, but a urine specimen may contain various organisms due to bacteria in the urethra and on external genitalia. Bacteriuria generally results from one prevalent bacteria type; the presence of more than two bacterial species in a specimen strongly suggests contamination during collection. A single negative culture doesn't always rule out infection; a quantitative examination of urine culture is needed.

Significant results of urine culture are possibly only after quantitative examination. To distinguish between true bacteriuria and contamination, it's necessary to know the number or organisms in a milliliter of urine, estimated by a culture technique known as "colony count." In addition, a quick centrifugation test can determine where a UTI originates. (See *Quick centrifugation test.*)

Clean-voided midstream collection, rather than suprapubic aspiration of catheterization, is now the method of choice for obtaining a urine specimen.

### Normal results

- The urine is sterile with no bacterial growth.

## Quick centrifugation test

The quick centrifugation test can determine whether the source of a urinary tract infection is in the lower tract (bladder) or the upper tract (kidneys). The test involves centrifugation of urine in a test tube, followed by staining of the sediment with fluorescein. If one-quarter of the bacteria fluoresce when viewed under a fluorescent microscope, an upper tract infection is present; if bacteria don't fluoresce, a lower tract infection is present.

### Abnormal results

- Bacterial counts of 100,000/ml or more of a single microbe species indicate a probable UTI. Counts under 100,000/ml may be significant, depending on the patient's age, sex, history, and other individual factors.
- Counts under 10,000/ml usually suggest that the organisms are contaminants, except in symptomatic patients, those with urologic disorders, and those whose urine specimens were collected by suprapubic aspiration.
- A special test for acid-fast bacteria isolates *Mycobacterium tuberculosis,* thus indicating tuberculosis of the urinary tract.
- *Escherichia coli* causes the majority of lower UTI infections.
- Isolation of more than two species of organisms or of vaginal or skin organisms usually suggests contamination and requires a repeat culture. Prolonged catheterization or urinary diversion may cause polymicrobial infection.

DRUG CHALLENGE

 Fluid- or drug-induced diuresis and antimicrobial therapy (possible decrease)

### Purpose

- To diagnose UTI
- To monitor microorganism colonization after urinary catheter insertion

### Patient preparation

- Explain that this test detects UTIs.
- Inform the patient that the test requires a urine specimen and that no restriction of food and fluids is necessary.
- Instruct him how to collect a clean-voided midstream specimen; emphasize that external genitalia must be cleaned thoroughly.
- If appropriate, explain catheterization or suprapubic aspiration to the patient, and inform him that he may experience some discomfort during specimen collection.
- For the patient with suspected tuberculosis, specimen collection may be required on three consecutive mornings.
- Check the patient's history for current antimicrobial therapy.

### Procedure and posttest care

- Confirm the patient's identity using two patient identifiers according to facility policy.
- Collect a urine specimen as ordered.
- When obtaining a specimen from an indwelling urinary catheter, clamp the tubing below the collection port to collect a specimen in the tubing. Then use an alcohol pad to clean the port. Next, using a sterile needle and syringe, aspirate a 4-ml specimen from the port, and transfer it into a sterile specimen cup.
- Seal the cup with a sterile lid, and send it to the laboratory immediately. If transport is delayed longer than 30 minutes, store the specimen at 39.2° F (4° C) or place it on ice, unless a urine

transport tube containing preservative is used.

- When collecting a clean-voided urine specimen, instruct the patient to wash his hands and then clean the urethral area with antiseptic towelettes. Tell the patient to begin urinating in the toilet and then stop and continue to urinate into the sterile cup, without touching the inside of the cup.
- Record on the laboratory request the suspected diagnosis, the collection time and method, current antimicrobial therapy, and fluid- or drug-induced diuresis.

### Precautions
- Collect at least 3 ml of urine, but don't fill the specimen cup more than halfway.

### Complications
- Possible infection when specimens are obtained by catheterization

# Wound culture
## [wound C&S]

Performed to confirm infection, a wound culture is a microscopic analysis of a specimen from a lesion. Wound cultures may be aerobic, for detection of organisms that usually appear in a superficial wound, or anaerobic, for organisms that need little or no oxygen and appear in areas of poor tissue perfusion, such as postoperative wounds, ulcers, and compound fractures. Indications for wound culture include fever as well as inflammation and drainage in damaged tissue.

### Normal results
- No pathogenic organisms are present.

### Abnormal results
- *Staphylococcus aureus*, group A beta-hemolytic streptococci, *Proteus*, *Escherichia coli* and other *Enterobacteriaceae*,

and some *Pseudomonas* species may be detected.
- The most common anaerobic pathogens include some *Clostridium*, *Peptococcus*, *Bacteroides*, and *Streptococcus* species.

### Purpose
- To identify an infectious microbe in a wound

### Patient preparation
- Explain that this test identifies infectious microbes.
- Describe the procedure, informing the patient that a drainage specimen from the wound is withdrawn by a syringe or removed on sterile cotton swabs.
- Tell the patient who will collect the specimen and when it will be done.

### Procedure and posttest care
- Confirm the patient's identity using two patient identifiers according to facility policy.
- Put on gloves, prepare a sterile field, and clean the area around the wound with antiseptic solution.
- For an aerobic culture, express the wound, and swab as much exudate as possible, or insert the swab deeply into the wound, and gently rotate. Immediately place the swab in the aerobic culture tube.
- For an anaerobic culture, insert the swab deeply into the wound, gently rotate, and immediately place the swab in the anaerobic culture tube. (See *Anaerobic specimen collector.*) Or, insert the needle into the wound, aspirate 1 to 5 ml of exudate into the syringe, and immediately inject the exudate into the anaerobic culture tube. If the needle is covered with a rubber stopper, the aspirate may be sent to the laboratory in the syringe.
- Obtain exudate from the entire wound, using more than one swab if necessary.

# Anaerobic specimen collector

Some anaerobes die when exposed to oxygen. To facilitate anaerobic collection and culturing, tubes filled with carbon dioxide ($CO_2$) or nitrogen are used for oxygen-free transport.

The anaerobic specimen collector shown here consists of a rubber-stopper tube filled with $CO_2$, a small inner tube, and a swab attached to a plastic plunger. The drawing (near right) shows the tube before specimen collection. The small inner tube containing the swab is held in place by the rubber stopper.

After specimen collection (far right), the swab is quickly replaced in the inner tube, and the plunger is depressed. This separates the inner tube from the stopper, forcing it into the larger tube and exposing the specimen to the $CO_2$-rich environment.

The tube should be kept upright.

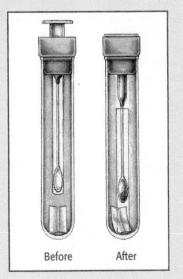

Before          After

■ Record on the laboratory request recent antimicrobial therapy, the source of the specimen, and the suspected organism. Label the specimen container with the patient's name, the practitioner's name, the facility number, the wound site, and the time of collection.
■ Dress the wound.

## Precautions

■ Clean the area around the wound thoroughly to limit contamination of the culture by normal skin flora, such as diphtheroids, *Staphylococcus epidermidis*, and alpha-hemolytic streptococci. Don't clean the area around a perineal wound.

DO'S & DON'TS

Make sure no antiseptic enters the wound.

■ Because some anaerobes die in the presence of even a small amount of oxygen, place the specimen in the culture tube quickly, take care that no air enters the tube, and check that double stoppers are secure.
■ Keep the specimen container upright, and send it to the laboratory within 15 minutes to prevent growth or deterioration of microbes.

## Complications
■ Spread of existing infection

# IV

# Organ tests

# 20 Thyroid

## Scanning

### Radionuclide thyroid imaging

In radionuclide thyroid imaging, the thyroid is studied by gamma camera after the patient receives a radioisotope (iodine-123 [$^{123}$I], technetium [$^{99m}$Tc] pertechnetate, or iodine-131 [$^{131}$I]). Thyroid imaging typically follows discovery of a palpable mass, an enlarged gland, or an asymmetrical goiter and is performed concurrently with thyroid uptake tests and measurements of serum triiodothyronine ($T_3$) and serum thyroxine ($T_4$) levels.

### Normal results
- The thyroid gland is about 2″ (5 cm) long and 1″ (2.5 cm) wide, with a uniform uptake of the radioisotope and without tumors.
- The gland is butterfly-shaped, with the isthmus located at the midline. Occasionally, a third lobe called the pyramidal lobe may be present; this is a normal variant.

### Abnormal results
- Hyperfunctioning nodules (areas of excessive iodine uptake) appear as black regions called *hot spots*. The presence of hot spots requires a follow-up $T_3$ thy-

roid suppression test to determine if the hyperfunctioning areas are autonomous.
- Hypofunctioning nodules (areas of little or no iodine uptake) appear as white or light gray regions called *cold spots*. If a cold spot appears, thyroid ultrasonography may be performed to rule out cysts, and fine-needle aspiration and biopsy of the nodules may be performed to rule out malignancy. (See *Results of thyroid imaging in thyroid disorders*.)

### DRUG CHALLENGE

 An iodine-deficient diet and phenothiazines (increase); ingestion of iodized salt, iodine preparations, iodinated salt substitutes, or seafood; thyroid hormones, thyroid hormone antagonists, aminosalicylic acid, corticosteroids, multivitamins, or cough syrups containing inorganic iodine (decrease)

### Purpose
- To assess the size, structure, and position of the thyroid gland
- To evaluate thyroid function (in conjunction with other thyroid tests)

### Patient preparation
- Explain that this procedure helps determine the cause of thyroid dysfunction.
- If $^{123}$I or $^{131}$I will be used, tell the patient to fast after midnight the night be-

# Results of thyroid imaging in thyroid disorders

This table shows the characteristic findings in radionuclide imaging tests that are associated with various thyroid disorders as well as the possible causes of those disorders.

| Condition | Findings | Causes |
|---|---|---|
| Hypothyroidism | - Glandular damage or absent gland | - Surgical removal of gland<br>- Inflammation<br>- Radiation<br>- Neoplasm (rare) |
| Hypothyroid goiter | - Enlarged gland<br>- Decreased uptake (of radioactive iodine) if glandular destruction is present<br>- Increased uptake possible from congenital error in thyroxine synthesis | - Insufficient iodine intake<br>- Hypersecretion of thyroid-stimulating hormone (TSH) caused by thyroid hormone deficiency |
| Myxedema (cretinism in children) | - Normal or slightly reduced gland size<br>- Uniform pattern<br>- Decreased uptake | - Defective embryonic development, resulting in congenital absence or underdevelopment of thyroid gland<br>- Maternal iodine deficiency |
| Hyperthyroidism (Graves' disease) | - Enlarged gland<br>- Uniform pattern<br>- Increased uptake | - Unknown, but may be hereditary<br>- Production of thyroid-stimulating immunoglobulins |
| Toxic nodular goiter | - Multiple hot spots | - Long-standing simple goiter |
| Hyperfunctioning adenomas | - Solitary hot spot | - Adenomatous production of triiodothyronine and thyroxine, suppressing TSH secretion and producing atrophy of other thyroid tissue |
| Hypofunctioning adenomas | - Solitary cold spot | - Cyst or nonfunctioning nodule |
| Benign multinodular goiter | - Multiple nodules with variable or no function | - Local inflammation<br>- Degeneration |
| Thyroid carcinoma | - Usually a solitary cold spot with occasional or no function | - Neoplasm |

fore the test. Fasting isn't required if an I.V. injection of $^{99m}$Tc pertechnetate is used.

- Explain to the patient that after he receives the radiopharmaceutical, a gamma camera will be used to produce an image of his thyroid. Tell him that the imaging procedure will take about 30 minutes, and assure him that his exposure to radiation is minimal.

- Ask the patient if he has undergone tests that used radiographic contrast media within the past 60 days. Note previous radiographic contrast media exposure on the X-ray request.

- Check the patient's diet and medication history. Medications such as thyroid hormones, thyroid hormone antagonists, and iodine preparations (Lugol's solution, some multivitamins, and cough syrups) should be stopped 2 to 3 weeks before the test as ordered. Phenothiazines, corticosteroids, salicylates, anticoagulants, and antihistamines should be stopped 1 week before the test as ordered. Instruct the patient to stop consuming iodized salt, iodinated salt substitutes, and seafood for 14 to 21 days as ordered. Liothyronine, propylthiouracil, and methimazole should be stopped 3 days before the test, and $T_4$ should be stopped 10 days before the test as ordered.

- Just before the test, tell the patient to remove dentures, jewelry, and other materials that may interfere with the imaging process.

- Make sure the patient or a responsible family member has signed an informed consent form, if required.

- The patient receives $^{123}$I or $^{131}$I (oral) or $^{99m}$Tc pertechnetate (I.V.). Record the date and the time of administration.

- The patient receiving an oral radioisotope should fast for another 2 hours after administration.

## Procedure and posttest care

- Confirm the patient's identity using two patient identifiers according to facility policy.

- The test is performed 24 hours after oral administration of $^{123}$I or $^{131}$I or 20 to 30 minutes after I.V. injection of $^{99m}$Tc pertechnetate. Just before the test, tell the patient to remove his dentures and any jewelry that could interfere with visualization of the thyroid.

- The patient is placed in a supine position with his neck extended; the thyroid gland is palpated. The gamma camera is positioned above the anterior portion of his neck.

- Images of the patient's thyroid gland are projected on a monitor and are recorded on X-ray film. Three views of the thyroid are obtained: a straight-on anterior view and two bilateral oblique views.

- Tell the patient that he may resume his usual diet and medications as ordered.

### Precautions

- Radionuclide thyroid imaging is contraindicated during pregnancy and lactation and in the patient with a previous allergy to iodine, shellfish, or radioactive tracers.

- Severe diarrhea and vomiting, impairing GI absorption of radioiodine, may decrease results.

### Complications

- Adverse reaction to the isotope

# Ultrasonography

## Thyroid ultrasonography

In thyroid ultrasonography, high-frequency sound waves emitted from a transducer are directed at the thyroid gland and reflected back to produce structural images on a monitor.

When a mass is located by palpation or by thyroid imaging, thyroid ultrasonography can differentiate between a cyst and a tumor larger than 1 cm with a high degree of accuracy. This test is also used to evaluate thyroid nodules during pregnancy because it doesn't require use of radioactive iodine.

### Normal results

- A uniform echo pattern is evident throughout the gland.

### Abnormal results

- Cysts appear as smooth-bordered, echo-free areas with enhanced sound transmission.
- Adenomas and carcinomas appear either solid and well demarcated with identical echo patterns or, less commonly, solid with cystic areas. Carcinoma infiltrating the gland may not be well demarcated.
- Identification of a tumor is generally followed up by fine-needle aspiration or an excisional biopsy to determine malignancy.

### Purpose

- To evaluate thyroid structure
- To differentiate between a cyst and a solid tumor
- To monitor the size of the thyroid gland during suppressive therapy

### Patient preparation

- Describe the procedure to the patient, and explain that this test defines the size and shape of the thyroid gland.
- Tell the patient that he doesn't need to restrict food and fluids.
- Tell him who will perform the procedure, where it will be done, and that it's painless and safe.

### Procedure and posttest care

- Confirm the patient's identity using two patient identifiers according to facility policy.
- The patient is placed in a supine position with a pillow under his shoulder blades to hyperextend his neck.
- His neck is coated with water-soluble conductive gel.
- The transducer then scans the thyroid, projecting its echographic image on the oscilloscope screen.
- The image on the monitor is photographed for subsequent examination.
- Accurate visualization of the anterior portion of the thyroid requires use of a short-focused transducer.
- Thoroughly clean the patient's neck to remove the conductive gel.

# 21
# Eye

## Subjective tests

### Color vision

The human eye perceives color through the cones of the retina, which are also responsible for central visual acuity. The most widely accepted theories of color vision propose that these retinal cones contain three different photosensitive pigments, each of which absorbs light of different wavelengths. Specifically, these pigments are sensitive to red, green, and blue—the primary colors of light. Mixtures of these three pigments allow perception of other colors.

Color vision tests assess the ability to recognize differences in color. They're commonly used to evaluate patients with suspected retinal disease or with a family history of color vision deficiency. These tests are also used to screen applicants for jobs in which accurate color perception is vital, as in the military and electronics fields.

The most common color vision tests use pseudoisochromatic plates made up of dot patterns of the primary colors superimposed on backgrounds of randomly mixed colors. A patient with normal color vision can identify the dot pattern; a patient with a color vision deficiency can't distinguish between the pattern and the background. Basic color vision tests merely indicate the presence of a deficiency; more sophisticated tests can determine the degree of deficiency.

### Normal results
- A person with normal color vision—a *trichromat*—can identify all the patterns or symbols.

### Abnormal results
- A patient with deficit color vision—an *anomalous trichromat*—can't identify all the patterns or symbols. The deficit is diagnosed more precisely by noting the combinations of colors that elicit incorrect responses.
- A patient with *protanopia,* a deficiency of the retinal pigment sensitive to red, can't distinguish between red-green and blue-green.
- A patient with *deuteranopia*, a deficiency of the retinal pigment sensitive to green, can't distinguish between green-purple and red-purple.
- A patient with *tritanopia*, a deficiency of the retinal pigment sensitive to blue, can't distinguish between blue-green and yellow-green.
- *Achromatopsia*—true color blindness—is a rare disease inherited as a Mendelian autosomal dominant or autosomal recessive trait. Patients with achromatopsia, called *monochromats*, see all colors as shades of gray. These patients may also have impaired visual acuity, nystagmus, and photophobia from reduced or absent cone function.

- Inherited color deficiency affects both eyes; acquired deficiency may affect only one eye. The patient with an acquired deficiency may complain of an inability to recognize colors that were formerly recognizable.
- Abnormalities of the ocular media, retina, or optic nerve can cause deficient color vision. For this reason, a patient with an acquired or inherited color vision deficiency accompanied by a loss of visual acuity should be referred for a complete ophthalmologic examination to determine the source of the deficiency.

### Purpose
- To detect color vision deficiency

### Patient preparation
- Explain that this test evaluates color perception, takes only a few minutes, and causes no pain.
- If the patient normally wears glasses or contact lenses, tell him to wear them during the test.

### Procedure and posttest care
- Confirm the patient's identity using two patient identifiers according to facility policy.
- After seating the patient comfortably, occlude one of his eyes.
- Hold the test book about 14" (35.5 cm) in front of his unoccluded eye, and give him the pointer.
- Explain to the patient what patterns or symbols he may see. Show him the sample plates—which can be deciphered in most cases—and tell him you'll ask him to identify the symbols and then to trace them with the pointer. Inform him that some symbols are more difficult to see than others.
- Conduct the test, eliciting immediate responses from the patient.
- Record the responses according to the instructions included with the test kit.

- When testing the other eye (or repeating the test, if necessary), rotate the plates 90 to 180 degrees to minimize recall.

### Precautions
- To prevent discoloration of the plates, keep the test book closed when it isn't being used, and turn the pages by their edges.
- Don't allow too much time for a response, as that may alter the test results.

## Refraction

Refraction—the bending of light rays by the cornea, aqueous humor, lens, and vitreous humor in the eye—enables images to focus on the retina and directly affects visual acuity. The refraction test, done routinely during a complete eye examination or whenever a patient complains of a change in vision, defines the refractive error and determines the degree of correction required to improve visual acuity with corrective lenses. The ophthalmologist generally performs a refraction objectively, by using a retinoscope, and subjectively, by asking the patient about his visual acuity while placing trial lenses before his eyes.

### Normal results
- Refractive power, measured in diopters, is greatest at the cornea (about 44 diopters) because of its curvature. The aqueous humor has the same refractive power as the cornea and is considered to be the same medium.
- The lens, normally a convex structure, has a refractive power of about 10 to 14 diopters but can alter this power by changing its shape. This phenomenon is known as *accommodation* and occurs when the eye views objects closer than 20' (6.1 m).

- The vitreous humor, a gelatinous medium, has little refractive power and mainly transmits light.
- In the absence of accommodation, the average refractive power of the human eye is 58 diopters.
- Ideally, the eyes have no refractive error (*emmetropia*). Parallel light rays emanating from a point source can be focused directly on the retina to produce a clear image.

## Abnormal results

- Most patients show some degree of refractive error (*ametropia*). *Hyperopia*, or farsightedness, occurs when the eyeball is too short and parallel light rays focus behind the retina. Retinoscopic examination shows a red reflex moving in the same direction as the retinoscope's light. A patient with hyperopia sees clearly at a distance but experiences blurring of near objects.
- *Myopia*, or nearsightedness, occurs when the eyeball is too long and parallel light rays focus in front of the retina. Retinoscopic examination shows a reflex motion opposite to the movement of the retinoscope's light. A patient with myopia sees near objects clearly but experiences blurring of distant images. (See *Normal and abnormal refraction*.)
- When light rays entering the eye aren't refracted uniformly and a clear focal point on the retina isn't attained, the patient has astigmatism. This disorder is usually caused by unequal curvature of the cornea and is typically associated with some degree of hyperopia or myopia.

## Purpose

- To diagnose refractive error and prescribe corrective lenses, if necessary

## Patient preparation

- Explain that the test helps determine whether the patient needs corrective lenses.
- Tell the patient that eyedrops may be instilled to dilate his pupils and that the test takes 10 to 20 minutes.
- Reassure him that the test is painless and safe.
- Don't give dilating eyedrops to a patient who has angle-closure glaucoma or a history of hypersensitivity reactions to these drops.

## Procedure and posttest care

- Confirm the patient's identity using two patient identifiers according to facility policy.
- After short-acting mydriatic eyedrops are given, if ordered, the ophthalmologist directs the light of the retinoscope at the pupillary opening.
- Through the aperture at the top of the instrument, the ophthalmologist looks for an orange glow—the retinoscopic, or red, reflex, which represents the reflection of light from the retinoscope—and notes its brightness, clarity, and uniformity.
- Moving the retinoscope's light across the pupil, the ophthalmologist observes the reflex for any movement.
- The ophthalmologist then places trial lenses before the patient's eyes and adjusts the lens power to make the reflex clear, bright, and uniform and to neutralize its motion. The lens power necessary to make this adjustment is recorded.
- Objective findings can be refined by altering the trial lenses and having the patient read lines on a standardized visual chart. This helps determine which lens or combination of lenses provides the best correction of his visual acuity.
- If corrective lenses are prescribed, the patient is advised that images may appear blurred the first time he wears the

# Normal and abnormal refraction

### Emmetropia

The eye is considered emmetropic when parallel light rays focus directly on the retina.

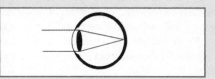

### Hyperopia

In hyperopia, parallel light rays focus behind the retina (left). This defect is corrected by placing a convex lens in front of the eye, which causes the rays to converge so they focus on the retina (right).

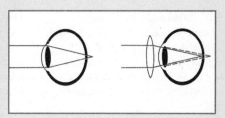

### Myopia

In myopia, parallel light rays focus in front of the retina (left). A concave lens placed in front of the eye can correct this defect by diverging the rays so they focus on the retina (right).

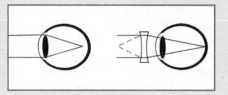

lenses; eventually his eyes will adjust to the prescription.

- If the patient has worn glasses or contact lenses previously, the patient should wear only his new prescription lenses because changing back and forth from the old prescription to the new one will prevent his eyes from making the required adjustment to the new lenses.
- Laser-assisted in situ keratomileusis (LASIK) or optic laser surgery also may be used to correct refractive errors.

## Precautions

### DO'S & DON'TS

 Don't give dilating eyedrops to a patient who has angle-closure glaucoma or to one who has had a hypersensitivity reaction to such drops. Instruct the patient to report ocular discomfort or redness immediately.

## Complications

- Hypersensitivity reaction or ocular discomfort from the eyedrops

# Visual acuity

The visual acuity test evaluates the patient's ability to distinguish the form and detail of an object. The patient is asked to read letters on a standardized visual chart, commonly called the *Snellen chart*, from a distance of 20' (6.1 m). A chart showing the letter "E" in various positions and sizes—the *Lea symbol chart*—are used for young children and other people who can't read. The smaller the symbol the patient can identify, the sharper his visual acuity. A patient's near (reading) vision may be tested as well, using a standardized chart such as the *Jaeger card* (a card with print in graded sizes).

The Snellen chart test should be performed on all patients with eye complaints. The near-vision test is routine for those complaining of eyestrain or reading difficulty and for everyone over age 40. Results serve as a baseline for treatments, follow-up examinations, and referrals.

### Normal results

- Distance visual acuity is 20/20, which means that the smallest symbol the patient can identify at 20' (6.1 m) is the same symbol a patient with normal vision can identify from the same distance.
- Normal near visual acuity is usually recorded as 14/14 because standard testing charts, such as the Jaeger card, are generally held 14" (35.6 cm) from the patient's eyes.
- Normal or better-than-normal visual acuity doesn't necessarily indicate normal vision. For example, a visual field defect may be present if the patient consistently misses the letters on one side of all the lines.

### Abnormal results

- If the denominator is more than 20 (for example, 40), the patient's visual acuity is less than normal. In this case, it means he reads at 20' what a person with normal vision can read at 40' (12.2 m). A person with visual acuity of 20/200 in the better corrected eye is considered legally blind.
- Similarly, if the denominator is less than 20, the patient's distance visual acuity is better than normal. For example, 20/15 vision means that the patient can read at 20' what a person with normal visual acuity can see at 15' (4.6 m).
- Decreased near visual acuity is indicated by a larger denominator. For example, 14/20 near vision means that the patient can read at 14" what a person

with normal vision can read at 20" (50.8 cm).

- A field defect is present if the patient states that one or more of the letters disappear or become illegible when he's looking at a nearby letter. Such findings indicate the need for further visual field testing, such as Amsler's grid test or the tangent screen examination.
- Patients with less-than-normal visual acuity require further testing, including refraction and complete ophthalmologic examination, to determine whether visual loss is due to injury, disease, or a need for corrective lenses.

### Purpose

- To test distance and near visual acuity
- To identify refractive errors in vision

### Patient preparation

- Explain that the tests evaluate distant and near vision.
- Tell the patient that the tests take only a few minutes. If he wears glasses, tell him to bring them to the examination.

### Procedure and posttest care
#### *Distance visual acuity*

- Have the patient sit 20' (6.1 m) away from the eye chart. If he's wearing glasses, tell him to remove them so his uncorrected vision can be tested first.
- Begin with the right eye, unless vision in the left eye is known to be more acute. Have the patient occlude the left eye; then ask him to read the smallest line of letters he can see on the chart. Encourage him to try to read lines he can't see clearly because intelligent guesses usually indicate that the patient can recognize some of the symbols' details.
- Instruct the patient not to place pressure on the occluded eye to avoid blurry vision during the examination.
- Record the number of the smallest line the patient can read. This number is ex-

pressed as a fraction. The numerator is the distance between the patient and the chart; the denominator is the distance from which a patient with normal vision can read the line. The greater the denominator, the poorer the vision.

■ If the patient makes an error on a line, record the results with a minus number. For example, if the patient reads the 20/40 line but makes one error, record his vision as 20/40 −1. If the patient reads the 20/40 line and one symbol on the next line, record his vision as 20/40 +1.

■ Have the patient occlude the right eye; then repeat the test for the left eye. To minimize recall, use a different set of symbols, or have the patient read the lines backward.

■ If the patient can't read the largest letter on the chart, further testing is necessary. (See *Special procedures for testing vision.*)

■ In recording the patient's responses, indicate which eye was tested and

## Special procedures for testing vision

These tests may be performed if the patient can't identify the largest letter on the Snellen chart.

### Pinhole test

The pinhole test can determine whether the cause of the patent's vision problem is refractive error or organic disease. In this test, the patient is asked to look at the visual acuity chart through a pinhole in the center of a disk. Looking through the tiny opening eliminates peripheral light rays and improves the patient's vision if impairment is related to refractive error. If impairment results from organic disease, vision fails to improve.

### Changing the distance

If the patient can't identify the largest letter or symbol on the chart (line 20/200), tell him to walk toward the chart until he can correctly identify it. Record the distance at which the patient can identify the symbol as the numerator. For example, 2/200 means the patient can identify a symbol at 2′ (0.6 m) that a person with normal vision can identify at 200′ (61 m).

### Counting fingers

If the patient can't identify the largest symbol at any distance, hold up your fingers at various distances in front of his

eyes. When the patient correctly identifies the number of fingers in front of him, note the distance—for example, 4′/CF.

### Hand motion

If the patient can't identify the number of fingers at any distance, wave your hand in front of his eyes at various distances. If he can detect hand movement, note the distance—for example, 2′/HM.

### Light projection

If the patient can't identify hand motion at any distance, darken the room, and tell him to look straight ahead. Shine a penlight in each quadrant—nasal, temporal, superior, and inferior—of each eye. Note in which quadrants the patient can perceive light—for example, light projection/superior and nasal quadrants.

### Light perception

If the patient can't perceive light projection at all, ask if he can tell whether the light is on or off. If the patient has no light perception, note NLP; otherwise, note that light perception exists.

whether it was tested with or without corrective lenses.

- If the patient wears glasses, test his corrected vision using the same procedure. If he normally wears glasses but doesn't have them with him, note this on the test results.
- Use the Lea symbol chart when testing preschool children or others who can't read.

### Near visual acuity

- Have the patient remove his glasses and occlude the left eye. Ask him to read the Jaeger card at his customary reading distance. Both eyes are tested with and without corrective lenses.
- In reporting near visual acuity, specify the size of the smallest print legible to the patient and the nearest distance at which reading is possible.

## Objective tests

### Exophthalmometry

Exophthalmometry determines the relative forward protrusion of the eye from its orbit by using an exophthalmometer to measure the distance from the apex of the cornea to the lateral orbital margin. The exophthalmometer is a horizontal calibrated bar with movable carriers on both sides. These carriers hold mirrors inclined at a 45-degree angle that reflect the scale readings and the corneal apex in profile.

This test provides information that's useful in detecting and evaluating thyroid disease, eye tumors, and any condition that displaces the eye in the orbit.

#### Normal results

- Readings range from 12 to 20 mm.

- Measurements for each eye are similar, usually differing by 1.5 mm or less and rarely by more than 3 mm.

#### Abnormal results

- A difference between the eyes of more than 3 mm may indicate *exophthalmos* (outward displacement) or *enophthalmos* (inward displacement).
- Readings under 12 mm may indicate enophthalmos.
- A single reading that exceeds 20 mm may indicate exophthalmos.
- Bilateral exophthalmos suggests a possible systemic disorder such as thyroid disease as well as xanthomatosis or a blood dyscrasia.

#### Purpose

- To measure the amount of forward eye protrusion
- To evaluate the progression or regression of exophthalmos

#### Patient preparation

- Explain that this test determines the degree of eye protrusion.

#### Procedure and posttest care

- Confirm the patient's identity using two patient identifiers according to facility policy.
- Ask the patient to sit upright facing you with his eyes on the same level as yours.
- Hold the horizontal bar of the exophthalmometer in front of the patient's eyes, parallel to the floor.
- Move the device's two small concave carriers against the lateral orbital margins, and carefully record the calibrated bar reading. The baseline reading should be used during follow-up examinations.
- If the patient has already been measured with an exophthalmometer, set the calibrated bar at the baseline reading. Tighten the locking screws on the mirrors to keep them properly positioned.

- Measure each eye separately.
- First, instruct the patient to fixate his right eye on your left eye. Using the inclined mirrors, superimpose the apex of the right cornea on the millimeter scale, and record the reading, which represents the eye's relative forward displacement from its orbit.
- Then instruct the patient to fixate his left eye on your right eye, and repeat the procedure.
- Refer the patient to an appropriate specialist as needed.

### Precautions
- For follow-up examinations, set the calibrated bar at the baseline reading.

# Fluorescein angiography

In fluorescein angiography, a special camera takes rapid-sequence photographs of the fundus following I.V. injection of sodium fluorescein (a contrast medium), thereby recording the appearance of blood vessels within the eye. This technique provides enhanced visibility of the microvascular structures of the retina and choroid, which permits the evaluation of the entire retinal vascular bed, including retinal circulation.

### Normal results
- After rapid injection into the antecubital vein, sodium fluorescein reaches the retina in 12 to 15 seconds (filling phase).
- As the choroidal vessels and choriocapillaries fill, the background of the retina fluoresces, taking on an evenly mottled appearance known as the *choroidal flush*.
- The dye fills the arteries (arterial phase).
- There is no leakage from the retinal vessels.

### Abnormal results
- Abnormalities detected in the early filling phase may include microaneurysms, AV shunts, and neovascularization.
- The test may identify arterial occlusion by showing delayed or absent flow of the dye through the arteries, stenosis, and prolonged venous drainage.
- Venous occlusion may be associated with vessel dilation and fluorescein leakage.
- Chronic obstruction may produce recanalization and collateral circulation.
- In hypertensive retinopathy, abnormalities may include areas of increased vascular tortuosity, microaneurysms around zones of capillary nonperfusion, and generalized suffusion of the dye in the retina.
- Aneurysms and capillary hemangiomas may leak fluorescein and are typically surrounded by hard yellow exudate.
- Tumors exhibit variable fluorescein patterns, depending on the histologic type.
- Retinal edema or inflammation and fibrous tissue may show variable degrees of fluorescence.
- Papilledema produces vascular leakage in the disk area.

### Purpose
- To document retinal circulation when evaluating intraocular abnormalities, such as retinopathy, tumors, and circulatory or inflammatory disorders

### Patient preparation
- Explain that the test evaluates the small blood vessels in the eyes and takes about 30 minutes.
- Make sure the patient or a responsible family member has signed an informed consent form.
- Check the patient's history for glaucoma and hypersensitivity reactions or allergies, especially to contrast media and

dilating eyedrops. If necessary, tell a patient with glaucoma not to use miotic eyedrops on the day of the test.

- Explain that eyedrops will be instilled to dilate his pupils and that a dye will be injected into his arm. Tell him that his eyes will be photographed with a special camera before and after the injection. Stress that these are photographs, not X-rays.
- Warn the patient that his skin may be discolored and his urine may appear orange for 24 to 48 hours after the procedure.
- Have the patient arrange for transportation after the test as his vision may be blurred for up to 12 hours.

## Procedure and posttest care

- Confirm the patient's identity using two patient identifiers according to facility policy.
- Give mydriatic eyedrops. Usually, two instillations are necessary to achieve maximum mydriasis within 15 to 40 minutes.
- After mydriasis, seat the patient comfortably in the examining chair facing the camera.
- Have the patient loosen or remove any restrictive clothing around his neck.
- Tell the patient to place his chin in the chin rest and his forehead against the bar. Have him open his eyes wide and stare straight ahead, while keeping his teeth together and maintaining normal breathing and blinking.
- The antecubital vein is prepared and punctured; however, dye isn't injected yet. At this time, a few photographs may be taken. Make sure the patient keeps his arm extended; if necessary, use an arm board.
- Warn the patient that the dye will be injected rapidly. Remind him to maintain his position and to continue to stare straight ahead, and then inject the dye.

- The patient may experience nausea and a feeling of warmth. Provide reassurance and observe him for hypersensitivity reactions, such as vomiting, dry mouth, metallic taste, suddenly increased salivation, sneezing, light-headedness, fainting, or hives. In rare instances, anaphylactic shock may occur.
- As the dye is injected, 25 to 30 photographs are taken in rapid sequence. Each photograph is taken 1 second after the other.
- The needle and syringe are removed carefully; pressure and a dressing are applied to the injection site.
- If late-phase photographs are needed, tell the patient to sit and relax for 20 minutes, and then reposition him for 5 to 10 photographs. If necessary, photographs may be taken up to 1 hour after the injection.
- Remind the patient that his skin and urine will be slightly discolored for 24 to 48 hours after the test. Encourage the patient to drink increased amounts of fluids to help excrete the dye.
- Explain to the patient that his near vision will be blurred for up to 12 hours and that he should avoid direct sunlight and refrain from driving during this time.

## Precautions

- Don't leave the patient unattended because he may experience mild adverse reactions, such as nausea, vomiting, sneezing, paresthesia of the tongue, and dizziness.

### ACTION STAT!

 Have emergency resuscitation equipment at hand. Serious adverse effects (laryngeal edema, bronchospasm, and respiratory arrest) are possible. If a reaction occurs, note it on the patient's allergy history.

## Complications

- Extravasation of the dye, which is painful and toxic to the tissues

# Ophthalmoscopy

Ophthalmoscopy allows magnified examination of the vascular and nerve tissue of the fundus, including the optic disk, retinal vessels, macula, and retina. This test is conducted with either a direct or an indirect ophthalmoscope—one of the most important diagnostic tools in ophthalmology. Generally, examiners use the direct ophthalmoscope, a small, handheld instrument consisting of a light source, a viewing device, a reflecting device to channel light into the patient's eyes, and spherical lenses to correct refractive error of the patient or examiner. The practitioner may also use the ophthalmoscope to examine the patient's cornea, iris, and lens.

If an abnormality of the retina is suspected, further testing, such as fluorescein angiography, may be necessary.

### Normal results

- The red reflex should be visible through the aperture.
- The slightly oval optic disk lies to the nasal side of the fundus center. Although its color varies widely, it's usually pink with darker edges at its nasal border.
- The physiologic cup, a pale depression in the center of the optic disk, varies widely in size; it tends to be larger in the patient with myopia and smaller in one with hyperopia.
- The semitransparent retina surrounds the optic disk.
- Branching out from the disk are the retinal vessels, including the venules and the slightly smaller arterioles.
- Vessel diameter progressively decreases with distance from the optic disk.

- Retinal arterioles generally have a medium red color; venules appear dark red or blue.
- The macula is the most darkly pigmented area of the retina. In its center lies a small, even darker spot—the fovea.
- A tiny light reflex can be seen at the center of the fovea, caused by reflection of the ophthalmoscopic light from the concave inner surface of the area.

### Abnormal results

- An absent or a diminished red reflex may be due to gross corneal lesions, dense opacities of the aqueous or vitreous (such as from blood after hemorrhage), cataracts, or a detached retina.
- A cloudy vitreous that obscures the fundus may be caused by inflammatory disease of the optic disk, retina, or uvea. Fundal lesions should be sketched or photographed for further study.
- Optic neuritis causes the optic disk to become elevated and more vascular; small hemorrhages may also occur. Optic nerve atrophy causes the disk to appear white.
- Papilledema, which may result from increased intracranial pressure, causes an abnormal elevation of the disk, blurring of disk margins, engorged vessels, and hemorrhages.
- In glaucoma, the physiologic cup may appear enlarged and gray with white edges.
- A milky white retina characterizes the acute phase of a central retinal artery occlusion; the fovea, in contrast to the ischemic macula, appears as a bright red spot.
- Central retinal vein occlusion is marked by widespread retinal hemorrhaging, patches of white exudate, and disk elevation.
- Retinal detachments appear as gray elevated areas, possibly with areas of red

vascular choroid exposed by retinal tears.

▪ A choroidal tumor appears as a dark lesion.

### Purpose

▪ To detect and evaluate eye disorders as well as ocular manifestations of systemic disease

### Patient preparation

▪ Explain that this test permits examination of the back of the eye.

▪ Describe the test, including who will perform it, where it will take place, and how long it will last.

▪ Advise the patient that eyedrops may be used to dilate the pupils for a clearer examination, but reassure him that he'll experience no discomfort during the test.

▪ Don't give dilating eyedrops to a patient who has angle-closure glaucoma or a history of hypersensitivity reactions to these drops.

### Procedure and posttest care

▪ Confirm the patient's identity using two patient identifiers according to facility policy.

▪ Routine examination of the ocular media and fundus is usually conducted without dilating the pupil if there's sufficient light in the ophthalmoscope and room lighting is subdued. If indicated, two instillations of mydriatic eyedrops are usually necessary to achieve maximum dilation.

▪ The patient sits upright in the examination chair, and the room lights are dimmed to keep irregular reflections from interfering with the examination.

▪ The practitioner sits about 2′ (0.6 m) away from the patient and slightly to his right. The examination begins with the patient's right eye. The ophthalmoscope is held in the right hand in front of the practitioner's right eye. A small adjustment near the forefinger allows him to select different lenses quickly.

▪ The illuminated dial should be set to zero and the patient told to look straight ahead at a specific object 20′ (6.1 m) away—for example, a large symbol on a standardized vision chart—for the duration of the examination.

▪ Remaining on the patient's right side, the practitioner moves forward until he's within 6″ (15 cm) of the patient. At this point, he directs the light beam into the pupil and looks for the red reflex (red reflection from the fundus), which is visible without magnification. Then he focuses on the optic disk, noting its size, shape, and color.

▪ Next, the practitioner looks for a white central depression in the optic disk—the physiologic cup—and observes the retinal vessels that emerge from the disk.

▪ Finally, the practitioner focuses on the macula—a yellowish depression slightly below the center of the optic disk—and its center, the fovea. The examiner tells the patient to look up, down, and to each side to examine the extreme periphery. The superior, inferior, temporal, and nasal portions of the retina are examined respectively.

▪ This procedure is then repeated for the left eye, with the practitioner moving slightly to the patient's left side and holding the ophthalmoscope in the left hand and in front the examiner's left eye.

### Precautions

▪ Don't give dilating eyedrops to a patient who has angle-closure glaucoma or a history of hypersensitivity reactions to these drops.

▪ Make sure the patient maintains fixation throughout the procedure.

### Complications

▪ If mydriatics are used, photophobia and increased intraocular pressure possible

# Schirmer's test

Schirmer's test assesses the function of the major lacrimal glands, which are responsible for reflex tearing in response to stressful situations such as the presence of a foreign body. Reflex tearing is stimulated by inserting a strip of filter paper into the lower conjunctival sac, followed by measuring the amount of moisture absorbed by the paper. (See *Proper filter placement in Schirmer's test.*) Both eyes are tested simultaneously.

A variation of this test evaluates the function of the accessory lacrimal glands of Krause and Wolfring by instilling a topical anesthetic before inserting the filter papers. The anesthetic inhibits reflex tearing by the major lacrimal glands, ensuring measurement of only the basic tear film normally produced by the accessory glands. This tear film usually maintains adequate corneal moisture under normal circumstances.

### Normal results

- The test strip shows at least 15 mm of moisture after 5 minutes. Both eyes usually secrete the same amount of tears.
- Because tear production decreases with age, normal test results in a patient over age 40 may range from 10 to 15 mm.

### Abnormal results

- Up to 15% of the patients tested have false-positive or false-negative results. Because the test is rapid and simple, it may be repeated and findings compared.
- Additional testing, such as a slit-lamp examination with fluorescein or rose Bengal stain, is necessary to corroborate results.
- A positive result confirmed by additional testing indicates a definite tearing deficiency, which may result from aging or, more seriously, from Sjögren's syndrome, a systemic disease of unknown

## Proper filter placement in Schirmer's test

This illustration shows the proper placement of the filter paper for Schirmer's test. The filter paper should be inserted into the inferior conjunctival sac of each eye.

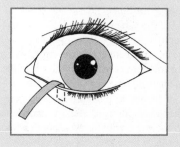

origin most common among postmenopausal women.
- A tearing deficiency may also arise secondarily to systemic diseases, such as lymphoma, leukemia, and rheumatoid arthritis.
- Regardless of the cause, a tearing deficiency is a matter of clinical concern because it can lead to corneal erosions, scarring, and secondary infection.

### Purpose

- To measure tear secretion in the patient with a suspected tearing deficiency

### Patient preparation

- Explain that this test measures tear secretion.
- Tell the patient that the test requires that a strip of filter paper be placed in the lower part of each eye for 5 minutes.
- Reassure the patient that the procedure is painless.
- If the patient wears contact lenses, ask him to remove them before the test. If an anesthetic is instilled, he won't be able to reinsert the lenses for 2 hours after the test.

## Procedure and posttest care

- Confirm the patient's identity using two patient identifiers according to facility policy.
- Seat the patient in the examining chair with his head against the headrest.
- To remove the test strip from the wrapper, bend the rounded wick end at the indentation, and cut open the envelope at the other end.
- Tell the patient to look up, and then gently lower the inferior eyelid.
- Hook the bent end of the strip over the inferior eyelid at the junction of the medial and nasal segments.
- Insert one strip in each eye, and note the time of insertion. Tell the patient not to squeeze or rub his eyes, but to blink normally or to keep his eyes closed lightly.
- After 5 minutes, remove the strips from the patient's eyes, and measure the length of the moistened area from the indentation, using the millimeter scale on the envelope.
- Report the results as a fraction: The numerator is the length of the moistened area, and the denominator is the time the strips were left in place. Also note which eye was tested. Thus, if a strip inserted in the right conjunctival sac for 5 minutes shows 8 mm of moisture, the correct notation is OD (oculus dexter, or right eye), 8 mm/5 minutes.
- To measure the function of the accessory lacrimal glands of Krause and Wolfring, instill one drop of topical anesthetic into each conjunctival sac before inserting the test strips.
- If a topical anesthetic was instilled, advise the patient not to rub his eyes for at least 30 minutes after instillation because this can cause a corneal abrasion. The patient who wears contact lenses shouldn't reinsert them for at least 2 hours.

## Precautions

- To prevent patient discomfort, be careful not to touch the cornea while inserting the test strip.
- Reflex tearing may be caused by the test strip coming in contact with the cornea; this will alter the test results.

# Slit-lamp examination

The slit lamp is an instrument equipped with a special lighting system and a binocular microscope that allows an ophthalmologist to visualize in detail the anterior segment of the eye, including the eyelids, eyelashes, conjunctiva, sclera, cornea, tear film, anterior chamber, iris, crystalline lens, and vitreous face. (See *Understanding biomicroscopic examination*.) To evaluate normally transparent or near-transparent ocular fluids and tissues, the size, shape, intensity, and depth of the light source as well as the magnification of the microscope may be altered. If abnormalities are noted, special devices are attached to the slit lamp to allow more detailed investigation.

## Normal results

- Anterior segment tissues and structures appear normal.

## Abnormal results

- Conditions, such as corneal abrasions and ulcers, lens opacities, iritis, and conjunctivitis as well as irregularly shaped corneas, are present.
- A parchment-like consistency of the lid skin, with redness, minor swelling, and moderate itching, may indicate a hypersensitivity reaction.
- If a corneal abrasion or ulcer is detected, a fluorescein stain may be applied to allow better viewing of the area.

## Purpose

- To detect and evaluate abnormalities of anterior segment tissues and structures

# Understanding biomicroscopic examination

The patient shown at right is undergoing a slit-lamp biomicroscopic examination. The slit lamp directs an intense, narrow beam of light on optic tissue, allowing the ophthalmologist to see the patient's cornea and lens as layers of different optical densities, not transparent structures. This method permits accurate detection of pathologic conditions in the eye's anterior segment.

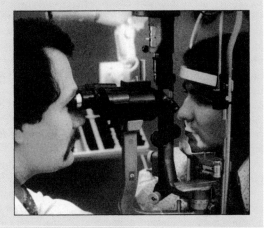

## Patient preparation

- Tell the patient that the slit-lamp examination evaluates the front portion of the eyes and that it requires that he remain still. Reassure him that the examination is painless.
- If the patient wears contact lenses, tell him to remove them for the test, unless the test is being performed to evaluate the fit of the lens.
- If the test calls for dilating eyedrops, check the patient's history for adverse reactions to mydriatics or for the presence of narrow-angle glaucoma before giving the drops. Dilating eyedrops aren't used in routine eye examinations; however, some diseases require pupillary dilation before slit-lamp examination.

## Procedure and posttest care

- Confirm the patient's identity using two patient identifiers according to facility policy.
- Seat the patient in the examining chair. Have him place his feet on the floor, and position his chin on the rest and his forehead against the bar. Dim the lights in the room.
- The ophthalmologist examines the patient's eyes starting with the lids and lashes and progressing to the vitreous face, altering light and magnification as necessary. In some cases, a special camera can be attached to the slit lamp to photograph portions of the eye.
- If dilating drops were instilled, tell the patient that his near vision will be blurred for up to 2 hours.

## Precautions

- Don't give dilating eyedrops to a patient who has angle-closure glaucoma or a history of hypersensitivity reactions to these drops.

## Complications

- When mydriatic drops are used in patients with angle-closure glaucoma, increased intraocular pressure
- Rarely, hypersensitivity to eyedrops

# Tonometry

Tonometry allows indirect measurement of intraocular pressure (IOP) and serves as an effective screen for early detection of glaucoma, which occurs in 2% of people over age 40 and is a common cause of blindness. Indentation tonometry measures this resistance by observing how deeply a known weight depresses the cornea; applanation tonometry provides the same information by measuring the amount of force required to flatten a known area of the cornea. Both procedures necessitate corneal anesthetization and careful examination technique. Patients with IOP problems can now monitor their pressure at home with a portable tonometer. If the IOP is elevated, other tests, such as applanation tonometry, visual field testing, and ophthalmoscopy, must confirm the diagnosis.

## Normal results

- An IOP of 12 to 20 mm Hg, with diurnal variations is normal. The highest point is reached at the time of waking; the lowest point, in the evening.

## Abnormal results

- Elevated IOP requires further testing for glaucoma.
- Because IOP varies diurnally, findings must be supplemented with serial measurements obtained at different times on different days.

## Purpose

- To measure IOP
- To aid in the diagnosis and follow-up evaluation of glaucoma

## Patient preparation

- Explain that this test measures the pressure in the patient's eyes.
- Tell the patient that the test takes only a few minutes and requires that his eyes

be anesthetized, but reassure him that the procedure is painless.
- If he wears contact lenses, instruct him to remove them before the test or until the anesthetic wears off completely.
- Ask the patient to assume a supine position. Make sure he's relaxed, and have him loosen restrictive clothing around his neck. Instruct him not to cough or squeeze his eyelids together.

## Procedure and posttest care

- Confirm the patient's identity using two patient identifiers according to facility policy.
- Ask the patient to look down. Raise his superior eyelid with your thumb, place one drop of the topical anesthetic at the top of the sclera, and have the patient blink.
- Check the tonometer for a zero reading on the steel test block that comes with the instrument. Make sure the plunger moves freely. The first measurement on each eye is obtained with the 5.5-g weight.
- Have the patient look up and stare at a spot on the ceiling. Then ask him to open his mouth, take a deep breath, and exhale slowly for distraction.
- With the thumb and forefinger of one hand, hold the lids of his right eye open against the orbital rim.
- Hold the tonometer vertically with the thumb and forefinger of the other hand, and rest the footplate on the apex of the cornea.
- With the footplate in place, check the indicator needle for a rhythmic transmission caused by the ocular pulse, and then record the calibrated scale reading that converts to a measurement of IOP. If the reading doesn't exceed 4, add an additional weight (7.5, 10, or 15 g) to obtain a reliable result.
- Repeat the procedure on the left eye, and record the time the test is performed.

- Tell the patient not to rub his eyes for at least 20 minutes after the test to prevent corneal abrasion.
- If the patient wears contact lenses, tell him not to reinsert them for at least 2 hours.
- If the tonometer moved across the cornea during the test, tell the patient he may feel a slight scratching sensation in the eye when the anesthetic wears off. This sensation should disappear within 24 hours because most abrasions resulting from tonometry affect only the epithelium, which regenerates in 24 hours.

### Precautions

ALERT

Tonometry should never be performed on a patient with a corneal ulcer or infection, except by a skilled practitioner and only in an emergency such as suspected acute angle-closure glaucoma.

- Avoid resting your fingers on the cornea or pressing on the cornea because this increases IOP.
- Don't touch the patient's lashes; this could trigger a blink response or Bell's phenomenon (upward movement of the eyes with forced closure of the lids), which can cause the footplate to move and scratch the cornea.

# Special procedures

## ▌Ocular ultrasonography

Ocular ultrasonography involves the transmission of high-frequency sound waves through the eye and the measurement of their reflection from ocular structures. An A-scan converts the resulting echoes into waveforms whose crests represent the positions of different structures, providing a linear dimensional picture. The B-scan converts the echoes into patterns of dots that form a two-dimensional, cross-sectional image of the ocular structure.

Because the B-scan is easier to interpret than the A-scan, it's used more commonly to evaluate the structures of the eye and to diagnose abnormalities. However, the A-scan is more valuable in measuring the eye's axial length and characterizing the tissue texture of abnormal lesions. Thus, a combination of A- and B-scans produces the most useful test results.

Illustrating the eyes' structures through ultrasound is especially helpful in evaluating a fundus clouded by an opaque medium such as a cataract. In such a patient, this test can identify pathologies that are normally undetectable through ophthalmoscopy.

Ophthalmologists may also perform this test before surgery—for example, cataract removal—to ensure the integrity of the retina. If an intraocular lens is to be implanted, ultrasound may be used preoperatively to measure the length of the eye and the curvature of the cornea as a guide for the surgeon.

In addition to its diagnostic capabilities, ocular ultrasonography can identify intraocular foreign bodies and determine their position in relation to ocular structures as well as assess the severity of resulting ocular damage.

### Normal results

- The optic nerve and the posterior lens capsule produce echoes that take on characteristic forms on A- and B-scan images.
- The posterior wall of the eye appears as a smooth, concave curve; retrobulbar fat can also be identified.
- The lens and vitreous humor, which don't produce echoes, can also be identified.

- Normal orbital echo patterns depend on the position of the transducer and the position of the patient's gaze during the procedure.

## Abnormal results

- In eyes clouded by a vitreous hemorrhage, the organization of the hemorrhage can be identified by the degree of density that appears on the image. In some instances, the cause of the hemorrhage, the prognosis, and associated abnormalities can also be determined.
- Massive vitreous organization and vitreous bands may also be detected by ultrasonography.
- Retinal detachment, commonly found in a patient with an opaque medium, characteristically produces a dense, sheetlike echo on a B-scan. The extent of retinal or choroidal detachment can be defined by transmitting ultrasound waves through the quadrants of the patient's eye.
- Ocular ultrasonography can be used to diagnose and differentiate intraocular tumors according to size, shape, location, and texture.
- Hemangiomas and cystic lesions produce characteristic ultrasound patterns.
- Other orbital lesions detectable by ultrasound include meningiomas, neurofibromas, gliomas, neurilemomas, and the inflammatory changes associated with Graves' disease.

## Purpose

- To help evaluate the fundus in an eye with an opaque medium such as a cataract
- To help diagnose vitreous disorders and retinal detachment
- To diagnose and differentiate between intraocular and orbital lesions and to follow their progression through serial examinations
- To locate intraocular foreign bodies

## Patient preparation

- Describe the procedure to the patient, and explain that ocular ultrasonography evaluates the eye's structures.
- Tell the patient that he doesn't need to restrict food and fluids.
- Tell the patient who will be performing the test and where it will be done.
- Reassure him that it's safe and painless and takes about 5 to 10 minutes to perform.
- Tell the patient that a small transducer will be placed on his closed eyelid and that the transducer transmits high-frequency sound waves that are reflected by the structures in the eye.
- Explain that he may be asked to move his eyes or change his gaze during the procedure and that his cooperation is required for accurate test results.

## Procedure and posttest care

- Confirm the patient's identity using two patient identifiers according to facility policy.
- The patient is placed in the supine position on an X-ray table.
- For the B-scan, the patient is asked to close his eyes, and a water-soluble gel (such as Goniosol) is applied to his eyelid. The transducer is then placed on the eyelid.
- For the A-scan, the patient's eye is numbed with anesthetizing drops, and a clear plastic eye cup is placed directly on the eyeball. A water-soluble gel is then applied to the eye cup, and the transducer is positioned on the medium.
- The transducer transmits high-frequency sound waves into the patient's eye, and the resulting echoes are transformed into images or waveforms on the oscilloscope screen.
- After the test, the water-soluble gel is removed from the patient's eyelid.

# Orbital computed tomography
## [orbital CT]

Orbital computed tomography (CT) allows visualization of abnormalities not readily seen on standard radiographs, delineating their size, position, and relationship to adjoining structures. A series of tomograms reconstructed by a computer and displayed as anatomic slices on a monitor, the orbital CT scan identifies space-occupying lesions earlier and more accurately than other radiographic techniques and provides three-dimensional images of orbital structures, especially the ocular muscles and the optic nerve.

### Normal results

- Dense orbital bone provides a marked contrast to less-dense periocular fat.
- The optic nerve and the medial and lateral rectus muscles are clearly defined.
- The rectus muscles appear as thin dense bands on each side, behind the eye.
- The optic canals should be equal in size.

### Abnormal results

- Intraorbital and extraorbital space-occupying lesions are present that obscure the normal structures or cause orbital enlargement, indentation of the orbital walls, or bone destruction.
- Infiltrative lesions, such as lymphomas and metastatic carcinomas, appear as irregular areas of density.
- Encapsulated tumors, such as benign hemangiomas and meningiomas, appear as clearly defined masses of consistent density.
- CT scans can also visualize intracranial tumors that invade the orbit, thickening of the optic nerve that may occur with gliomas, meningiomas, and secondary tumors that may cause enlargement of the optic canal.
- CT scans can show early erosion or expansion of the medial orbital wall that may arise from lesions in the ethmoidal cells.
- CT scans can also detect space-occupying lesions in the orbit or paranasal sinuses that cause exophthalmos.
- Thickening of the medial and lateral rectus muscles in proptosis results from Graves' disease.
- Enhancement with a contrast medium may provide information about the circulation through abnormal ocular tissues.

### Purpose

- To evaluate pathologies of the orbit and eye—especially expanding lesions and bone destruction
- To evaluate fractures of the orbit and adjoining structures
- To determine the cause of unilateral exophthalmos

### Patient preparation

- Describe the procedure to the patient, and explain that the orbital CT scan visualizes the anatomy of the eye and its surrounding structures.
- If contrast enhancement isn't scheduled, tell the patient that he doesn't need to restrict food and fluids. If contrast enhancement is scheduled, withhold food and fluids from the patient for 4 hours before the test.
- Tell the patient that a series of X-rays will be taken of his eye, and explain who will perform the test and where it will take place.
- Reassure the patient that the test will cause him no discomfort.
- Tell the patient that he'll be positioned on an X-ray table and that the head of the table will be moved into the scanner,

which will rotate around his head and make loud clacking sounds.

■ If a contrast medium will be used for the procedure, tell the patient that he may feel flushed and warm and may experience a transient headache, a salty or metallic taste, and nausea or vomiting after the contrast medium is injected. Reassure him that these reactions are normal.

■ Make sure that the patient or a responsible family member has signed an informed consent form, if required.

■ Check the patient's history for hypersensitivity reactions to iodine, shellfish, or contrast media, and notify the practitioner of the sensitivities.

■ Instruct the patient to remove jewelry, hairpins, or other metal objects in the X-ray field to allow for precise imaging of the orbital structures.

### Procedure and posttest care

■ Confirm the patient's identity using two patient identifiers according to facility policy.

■ The patient is placed in a supine position on the X-ray table with his head immobilized by straps, if required. Ask him to lie still.

■ The head of the table is moved into the scanner, which rotates around the patient's head, taking radiographs.

■ Information obtained is stored on magnetic tapes, and the images are displayed on a monitor. Photographs may be made if a permanent record is desired.

■ When this series of radiographs has been taken, contrast enhancement is performed. The contrast medium is injected intravenously, and a second series of scans is recorded.

■ If a contrast medium was used, watch for its residual adverse effects, including headache, nausea, or vomiting. After the procedure, advise the patient that he may resume his usual diet.

### Precautions

**ALERT**

Use of contrast enhancement is contraindicated in the patient with hypersensitivity reactions to iodine, shellfish, or contrast media used in other tests.

### Complications

■ Rarely, adverse reaction to the contrast medium

# ▌Orbital radiography
[orbital X-ray]

Orbital radiography evaluates the orbit, the bony cavity that houses the eye and the lacrimal glands, as well as blood vessels, nerves, muscles, and fat. Because portions of the orbit are composed of thin bone that fractures easily, X-rays are commonly taken following facial trauma. They're also useful in diagnosing ocular and orbital pathologies. Special radiographic techniques can reveal foreign bodies in the orbit or eye that are invisible to an ophthalmoscope. In some cases, radiography is used in conjunction with computed tomography scans and ultrasonography to better define an abnormality.

### Normal results

■ Each orbit is composed of a roof, a floor, and medial and lateral walls.

■ The bones of the roof and floor are very thin (the floor can be less than 1 mm thick).

■ The medial walls, which parallel each other, are slightly thicker, except for the portion formed by the ethmoid bone.

■ The lateral walls are the thickest part of the orbit and are strongest at the orbital rim.

■ The superior orbital fissure, at the back of the orbit between the lateral wall and the roof, is actually a gap between the greater and lesser wings of the sphenoid bone.

▪ The optic canal, which carries the optic nerve and ophthalmic artery, is an opening in the lesser wing of the sphenoid bone located at the apex of the orbit.

## Abnormal results

▪ Orbit enlargement indicates the presence of a lesion that has caused proptosis due to increased intraorbital pressure.

▪ Superior orbital fissure enlargement can result from orbital meningioma, from intracranial conditions such as pituitary tumors or, more characteristically, from vascular anomalies.

▪ Optic canal enlargement may result from extraocular extension of a retinoblastoma or, in children, from an optic nerve glioma.

▪ In adults, only prolonged pathology can increase orbital size; but in children, even a rapidly growing lesion can cause orbital enlargement because orbital bones aren't fully developed.

▪ A decrease in the size of the orbit may follow childhood enucleation of the eye or conditions such as congenital microphthalmia.

▪ Destruction of the orbital walls may indicate a malignant neoplasm or an infection.

▪ A benign tumor or cyst produces a clear-cut local indentation of the orbital wall.

▪ Lesions of adjacent structures may also produce radiographic changes due to enlargement and erosion of the orbit.

▪ Increased bone density may be seen in such conditions as osteoblastic metastasis, sphenoid ridge meningioma, or Paget's disease.

▪ To confirm orbital disease, radiographic findings must be supplemented with results from other appropriate tests and procedures.

## Purpose

▪ To help diagnose orbital fractures and diseases

▪ To help locate intraorbital or intraocular foreign bodies

## Patient preparation

▪ Explain that orbital radiography involves taking several X-rays to assess the condition of the bones around the eye.

▪ Describe the test, including who will perform it and where it will take place.

▪ Reassure the patient that the procedure is usually painless unless he has suffered facial trauma, in which case positioning may cause some discomfort. Explain that he'll be asked to turn his head from side to side and to flex or extend his neck.

▪ Instruct the patient to remove all jewelry and other metallic objects from the X-ray field.

## Procedure and posttest care

▪ Confirm the patient's identity using two identifiers per facility policy.

▪ Have the patient recline on the X-ray table or sit in a chair.

▪ Instruct the patient to remain still while the X-rays are taken.

▪ Remember that usually a series of orbital X-rays includes a lateral view, posteroanterior view, submentovertical (base) view, stereo Waters' views (views from both sides), Towne's (half-axial) projection, and optic canal projections. If enlargement of the superior orbital fissure is suspected, apical views are obtained.

▪ The films are first developed and inspected by the radiography department before the patient is released.

# 22
# Ear

## Audiologic tests

### Acoustic immittance

Acoustic immittance tests evaluate middle ear function by measuring the flow of sound energy into the ear (admittance). Not all sound energy that impinges on the tympanic membrane reaches the inner ear; some reflects into the external ear canal. The relationship between incident and reflected sound energy determines the admittance, which depends on the resistance, stiffness, and mass of the auditory system. Normally, stiffness is the predominant factor in the middle ear.

Admittance is commonly measured by two tests: tympanometry and acoustic reflex testing. Each of these tests uses an electronic tone generator, an air pressure manometer, and a tone probe that delivers sound and air pressure stimuli to the ear canal and tympanic membrane through an airtight seal. Tympanometry measures middle ear admittance in response to changes in air pressure in the ear canal; the acoustic reflex test measures the change in admittance produced by contraction of the stapedius muscle in response to an intense sound. Stapedial contraction stiffens the tympanic membrane and ossicular chain, causing a measurable reduction in middle ear admittance. Reflex decay, part of the acoustic reflex test, is a function of the eighth cranial nerve adaptation or fatigue in response to a sustained reflex-eliciting stimulus.

Tympanometry helps diagnose middle ear disease and assesses eustachian tube function. Acoustic reflex testing assesses the seventh (facial) and eighth cranial nerve function and helps establish the site of the lesion. Because admittance tests require little patient cooperation, they are reliable in testing young children and individuals with physical or mental challenges.

#### Normal results
##### Tympanometry
- Four measurements are important on the tympanogram: the ear canal volume, the peak compliance reading, the peak pressure reading, and the slope gradient. These measures are interpreted along with the shape or "type" of the tympanogram and together determine the implication of the tympanometric results.
- A type A tympanogram is a normal finding.

##### Acoustic reflex testing
- Acoustic reflexes present at an intensity of 65 to 100 dB hearing level.
- The sensation level of the reflex is computed by subtracting the hearing threshold for the ear by the frequency

receiving the tone. The sensation level of the reflex should be 65 to 100 dB.

## Abnormal results
### *Tympanometry*
- Any evidence that doesn't reflect a type A tympanogram is considered abnormal.

### *Acoustic reflex testing*
- If the conductive loss is unilateral, presentation of the reflex tone to the involved ear, with measurement contralaterally, may reveal a reflex at an elevated hearing level. The calculated sensation level would be normal in this case. The finding of a reflex when the probe is in an affected ear is negative for conductive involvement.
- If the cochlea is the site of the lesion, reflexes may be present at normal hearing levels, elevated, or absent.
- The more severe the loss, the more likely the finding of an absent reflex.
- Most mild to moderately severe hearing losses have present acoustic reflexes. When the audiologist computes the sensation level of the reflex, it's noted as being reduced if there's significant loss at that frequency.
- Absent acoustic reflexes raise the possibility of a retrocochlear lesion if conductive involvement or severe cochlear loss isn't present.
- Acoustic reflex decay (failure to have a sustained reflex for 5 or more seconds) is also an indicator of possible retrocochlear involvement.
- The patient with nonorganic loss (or pseudohypoacusis, a feigned hearing loss or exaggeration of hearing thresholds) may be discovered during immittance testing. Reflexes present below the admitted threshold are an indicator of a nonorganic problem.

## Purpose
### *Tympanometry*
- To assess the continuity and admittance of the middle ear
- To evaluate the status of the tympanic membrane

### *Acoustic reflex testing*
- To distinguish between cochlear and retrocochlear lesions
- To differentiate eighth nerve or peripheral brain stem lesions from intra-axial brain stem lesions
- To locate seventh nerve lesions relative to stapedius muscle innervation
- To confirm conductive hearing loss
- To help confirm nonorganic loss (feigning or exaggerating hearing loss, also called pseudohypoacusis)

## Patient preparation
- Describe the procedure to the patient, and explain that acoustic immittance tests evaluate the condition of the middle ear.
- Make sure that the patient's ear is free from significant cerumen accumulation.
- Tell the patient that he will feel pressure in the ear, but that the test isn't painful.
- Ask the patient not to move during the test, which takes just a few seconds.

## Procedure and posttest care
**DO'S & DON'TS**

 Check equipment carefully. If the probe tip is clogged with cerumen or debris, the measured admittance won't change, even when the probe isn't coupled to the ear. To clean the probe, carefully insert a wire through each bore, wipe the wire, and then withdraw it.

### For tympanometry

- Otoscopic examination is performed to verify that no impacted cerumen or other obstruction is present in the ear canal.
- The size and shape of the canal are checked to select the appropriate-size probe tip, which is then attached to the probe.
- The probe tip is inserted into the ear canal while pulling upward and backward on the auricle; a proper seal can maintain a negative pressure of +200 daPa. Once a hermetic seal is obtained, the pressure in the ear canal will automatically vary from +200 to –400 daPa.
- A graphic display of the tympanogram is obtained. If the tympanogram has a clear peak, the pressure of the peak is noted and usually printed with the test results. This indicates the pressure within the middle ear cavity. The sound admittance through the middle ear system is noted by the height of the tympanogram, its peak compliance. This value is also typically printed.
- If a flat tympanogram is obtained (no change in admittance), the possibility that the probe tip may have rested against the canal wall or that it was clogged with cerumen must be ruled out with ear canal volume measurements and repeated testing. Measurement error is more likely to be the cause of the flat tympanogram if the ear canal volume is low (0.3 ml or less). The probe tip is removed, cleaned, and reinserted, and the test is repeated.

### For acoustic reflex testing

- The audiologist positions the immittance probe in the patient's ear the same as for tympanometry but uses a device to fix the probe to the patient's head to reduce artifacts that can invalidate test results.
- For threshold testing, stimuli of progressively louder levels are presented until a reflex, if present, is noted.

- Acoustic reflex decay testing involves presentation of a tone, 10 dB above the reflex threshold, at one or more frequencies of 1,000 Hz and below, for a 10-second period. The time that the auditory system sustains the contraction at least half strength is measured. The patient must remain still and quiet during reflex testing.
- Reflexes and reflex decay may be measured ipsilaterally (the loud tone is in the same ear as the probe that measures the contraction) or contralaterally (the loud tone is in the opposite ear from the probe). Ipsilateral reflexes are also called uncrossed reflexes; contralateral reflexes may be called crossed reflexes.

## Precautions

- Obtain medical clearance before performing admittance tests in the patient with head trauma or a possible labyrinthine fistula and on one who has recently had middle ear surgery.
- If you can't obtain a seal even though the probe seems well seated, look for leakage elsewhere in the air system. Check the system by putting the probe in the supplied coupler. If it can't seal, then the tubing has a leak or the equipment is malfunctioning.
- While some screening systems permit acoustic reflex measurements, the results aren't reliable if the probe is hand-held in the ear. Refer to an audiologist as required.

# ▌Auditory brain stem evoked response
### [ABR, brain stem auditory evoked response]

Auditory brain stem evoked response testing is the most common form of auditory evoked potentials testing.

# Auditory brain stem evoked response

These graphs are an example of an auditory brain stem evoked response elicited by 100 ms click stimuli. The patient's auditory neural activity is recorded using surface electrodes. The peaks on the graphs represent activity from cranial nerve VIII and brain stem structures. Traces are repeated for accuracy at each intensity. The morphology and time between labeled peaks is evaluated when assessing the patient's neural integrity. Additionally, the symmetry of left and right ear responses is evaluated (not illustrated). When used to estimate the hearing threshold, the stimuli's intensity is decreased. A prolonged wave V occurs. The lowest intensity eliciting an evoked potential is assumed to be slightly supra-threshold.

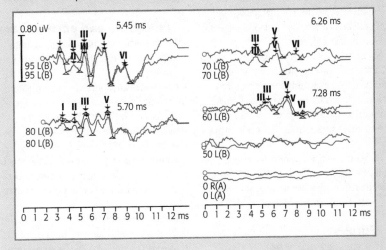

Various forms of auditory evoked responses can be used to evaluate the function of the auditory pathways in a child or adult suspected of having auditory processing deficits.

Electrocochleography (ECoG or ECochG) can be used in the differential diagnosis of Ménière's disease (endolymphatic hydrops), although its diagnostic sensitivity and specificity is considered by some to be lacking, particularly in the early stages of the disease.

## Normal results

■ ABR wave latencies (time of the waveform occurrence after stimulus presentation) occur at predictable times for the patient with normal hearing or with cochlear loss who's hearing signals that are sufficiently above hearing threshold. The latency between wave I and V is about 4.0 ms (no longer than about 4.4 ms). The interaural latency difference of wave V and the I-V interaural latency differences are small, generally less than 0.3 or 0.4 ms. (See *Auditory brain stem evoked response*.)

■ The threshold of the ABR is typically about 10 to 20 dB nHL for click or high-frequency stimuli, and 20 or 30 dB nHL for lower-frequency stimuli.

■ ECoG reveals an amplitude ratio of the summating potential and action potential that's within normal limits for the type of electrode used.

## Abnormal results

- Cochlear loss increases the threshold of the ABR response but doesn't typically alter the wave V latency for stimuli that are well above the threshold.
- The time between waves I and V is unaffected or shortens with cochlear loss; however, establishing wave I may be more difficult.
- Prolongation of the I-V interpeak latency is an indicator of cranial nerve (CN) VIII or lower brain stem disease.
- Asymmetry of the I-V interpeak interval between ears is also a strong sign of a retrocochlear disorder.
- Asymmetry of absolute latency of wave V, abnormal prolongation of V with an increase in the stimulus repetition rate, poor replicability or morphology, and atypical amplitude ratios of waves I to V fail to rule out a retrocochlear abnormality.
- ECoG that shows abnormally large summating potential amplitude, compared with action potential amplitude, is a positive indicator of Ménière's disease.

## Purpose

- To screen neonatal hearing
- To estimate or confirm the extent of hearing loss in infants and toddlers
- To estimate threshold in other difficult-to-test patients, such as those with developmental disabilities and those suspected of nonorganic hearing loss
- To evaluate CN VIII and lower brain stem auditory synchronization, which is abnormal with lesions of this area and with auditory dyssynchronization (auditory neuropathy)

## Patient preparation

- Cerumen removal is required before this test, which is conducted by an audiologist and sometimes at a neurology facility.
- Depending on the age of the child, sedation may be required. Sedated ABR

testing can only be conducted at health care facilities. In other facilities, sleep deprivation of the child may be required to make sure that the patient sleeps during testing.
- The patient should be advised to dress comfortably and be aware that although the test is painless, electrodes will be applied to the skin and will require 1 to 1½ hours to complete. Patients should avoid the use of makeup on the day of the test.

## Procedure and posttest care

- Confirm the patient's identity using two patient identifiers according to facility policy.
- Electrodes are connected to a physiologic amplifier that allows the minute voltages coming from the auditory system to be amplified enough to allow them to be read by the signal-averaging computer. The waveforms are displayed as the amplitude of the response across the time after the presentation of the signals.
- Threshold estimation is typically conducted by an audiologist. In this testing, he varies the intensity of the signal until the threshold of the response is obtained. The response threshold is typically slightly supra-threshold, but threshold estimation is possible if the patient has normal neural synchrony.
- In neurodiagnostic testing for CN VIII and auditory brain stem response, click signals are presented at intensities that are clearly audible and should elicit good synchronization of CN VIII. Typically, the click signals are presented at different rates. More rapid presentations may reveal auditory disease more readily. A click stimulus is presented at a supra-threshold level. The time when wave V occurs in each ear, the time difference between the evoked waves I and V in each ear, and the time difference between these two measures indicate the

probability of retrocochlear disease. Assessment of central auditory processing ability typically involves assessing brain stem potentials and one or more of the potentials generated by the neural structures superior to the brain stem.

- ECoG also involves the presentation of relatively intense signals. The recording electrodes are placed in the ear canal of the patient or on the tympanic membrane. Rarely, a practitioner places the electrode through the tympanic membrane and rests it on the promontory of the middle ear. The cochlear potentials and CN VIII response are recorded.
- If the patient required sedation, he'll need supervision until he completely recovers.

### Precautions

- ECoG using tympanic membrane electrodes requires skill on the part of the audiologist to place the electrode in contact with the tympanic membrane without creating patient discomfort.
- Hearing loss developed in the infant after birth, such as from maternal cytomegalovirus infection, some types of genetic hearing loss, or progressive hearing loss, may interfere with the results.
- Asymptomatic Ménière's disease may lead to high false-negative results via ECoG.

### Complications

- Skin abrasion from electrode placement, irritation, and minor allergic reactions

# ▌Otoscopy

Otoscopy is the direct visualization of the external auditory canal and the tympanic membrane through an otoscope. It's a basic part of physical examination of the ear and should be performed before other auditory or vestibular tests. Otoscopy indirectly provides information about the eustachian tube and the middle ear cavity.

### Normal results

- The tympanic membrane is thin, translucent, shiny, and slightly concave. It appears as a pearl gray or pale pink disk that reflects light in its inferior portion.
- The short process, manubrium mallei, and umbo should be visible but not prominent.
- Light reflex extends inferiorly and anteriorly from the umbo.

### Abnormal results

- Scarring, discoloration, or retraction or bulging of the tympanic membrane indicates a pathologic condition. (See *Common abnormalities of the tympanic membrane,* page 368.)
- Movement of the tympanic membrane in tandem with respiration suggests abnormal patency of the eustachian tube.
- An altered or absent light reflex isn't a reliable indicator of disease because there can be many normal variations of the tympanic membrane and posterior bony ear canal.

### Purpose

- To visualize inner ear structures
- To detect foreign bodies, cerumen, or stenosis in the external canal
- To detect external or middle ear disease, such as an infection or a tympanic membrane perforation

### Patient preparation

- Describe the procedure to the patient, and explain that this test permits visualization of the ear canal and eardrum.
- Reassure the patient that the examination is usually painless.
- Tell the patient that his ear will be pulled upward and backward to straighten the canal to ease insertion of the otoscope.

# Common abnormalities of the tympanic membrane

Visual examination of the tympanic membrane may reveal abnormal findings. This chart lists some of the more common findings as well as their typical causes.

| Abnormal findings | Usual cause |
|---|---|
| Bright red color | Inflammation (otitis media) |
| Yellowish color | Pus or serum behind the tympanic membrane (acute or chronic otitis media) |
| Bubble behind the tympanic membrane | Serous fluid in the middle ear (serous otitis media) |
| Absent light reflection | Bulging tympanic membrane (acute otitis media) |
| Absent or diminishing landmarks | Thickened tympanic membrane (chronic otitis media, otitis externa, or tympanosclerosis) |
| Oval dark areas | Perforated or scarred tympanic membrane (otitis media or trauma) |
| Prominent malleus | Retracted tympanic membrane (nonfunctional eustachian tube) |
| Reduced mobility | Stiffened middle ear system (serous otitis media or, less commonly, middle ear adhesions) |

■ If the patient will undergo pneumatic otoscopy, tell him that he may experience dizziness with nystagmus, a positive fistula sign.

## Procedure and posttest care

■ Confirm the patient's identity using two patient identifiers according to facility policy.
■ When assembling the otoscope, test the lamp, and make sure you attach the largest speculum that fits comfortably into the patient's ear.
■ With the patient seated, tilt his head slightly away from you so that the ear to be examined is pointed upward.
■ Pull the auricle up and back. Insert the otoscope gently into the ear canal with a downward and forward motion. If inser-

tion is difficult, replace the speculum with a smaller one.

**ALERT**

 If the patient is younger than age 3, pull the auricle downward to insert the otoscope.

■ If you still feel resistance, withdraw the otoscope and tell the practitioner.
■ Look through the lens, and gently advance the speculum about 1 to 1.5 cm until you see the tympanic membrane. Obtain as full a view as possible, and note redness, swelling, lesions, discharge, foreign bodies, and scaling in the canal. Check the tympanic membrane for color, scarring, contours, perforation, and a cone of light that appears

at the 5 o'clock position in the right ear and at the 7 o'clock position in the left; this is a reflection of the otoscope lamp.
- Locate the malleus, partially visible through the translucent tympanic membrane. Examine the membrane itself and the surrounding fibrous rim (annulus).

### Precautions
- The otoscope should be advanced slowly and gently through the medial portion of the ear canal to avoid irritation of the canal lining, especially if an infection is suspected.
- Continuing to insert an otoscope against resistance may cause the tympanic membrane to perforate.

### Complications
- Perforation of the tympanic membrane

# Pure tone audiometry and pure tone screening

Pure tone audiometry, performed with an audiometer, provides a record of the thresholds (the lowest intensity levels) at which a patient can hear a set of test tones introduced through earphones or a bone conduction (sound) vibrator. The energy of these pure tones is concentrated at discrete frequencies. The octave frequencies between 125 and 8,000 Hz are used to obtain air conduction thresholds; frequencies between 250 and 4,000 Hz are used to obtain bone conduction thresholds.

Comparison of air and bone conduction thresholds can suggest a conductive, sensorineural, or mixed hearing loss but doesn't indicate the cause of the loss; further audiologic and vestibular tests and X-rays may be needed. Pure tone audiometry results may also suggest a need to consult an audiologist to evaluate communication difficulties.

### Normal results
- Normal levels for adults are 0 to 25 dB.
- Normal levels for children are 0 to 15 dB.

### Abnormal results
- In sensorineural hearing loss, both thresholds are depressed.
- In conductive hearing loss, air thresholds are depressed, but bone thresholds are unchanged.
- In mixed hearing loss, both thresholds are abnormal, with air conduction more depressed than bone conduction.

### Purpose
- To determine the presence, type, and degree of hearing loss
- To assess communication abilities and rehabilitation needs
- To accurately determine pure tone and speech reception threshold

### Patient preparation
- Describe the procedure to the patient, and explain that this test determines the presence and degree of hearing loss. Explain who will perform the test and where it will take place.
- Tell the patient that each ear will be tested, beginning with the ear with the better hearing acuity. Explain that he'll hear tones at various intensities and that he should signal (or press the response button) each time he hears the tone. Emphasize that he should respond even if the tone is faint.
- Just before the test, ask the patient to remove jewelry or apparel that obstructs proper earphone placement.
- Postpone the test if the patient has been exposed to loud noises (loud enough to cause tinnitus or to make face-to-face communication difficult) within the past 16 hours.

### Procedure and posttest care

- Confirm the patient's identity using two patient identifiers according to facility policy.
- Check the patient's ear canal for impacted cerumen using the otoscope.
- Press a finger on the auricle and then the tragus to rule out possible closure of the ear canal under pressure from the earphones. If the canal tends to close, a stiff-walled plastic tube is carefully inserted into the canal. This modification is recorded on the audiogram.
- Position the earphones properly and tighten the headband.
- Present a test tone to the ear with the better hearing acuity.

#### Air conduction testing

- Present a 1,000-Hz tone to the ear with the better hearing acuity. The intensity of the tone is decreased in 10-dB steps until the patient fails to respond. Then intensity is increased in 5-dB steps until he hears the tone again. Sequences of 10-dB decrements and 5-dB increments are repeated until the patient responds to at least two of three presentations at a single level. The threshold level is the lowest decibel level at which the response rate is at least 50%.
- Using this procedure, present tones to the better ear in this order: 1,000 Hz, 2,000 Hz, 4,000 Hz, 8,000 Hz, 1,000 Hz, 500 Hz, and 250 Hz.
- After the better ear has been tested, test the other ear. In each ear, test or retest differences may be +5 dB or –5 dB. If the difference between the first and second threshold at 1,000 Hz is greater than 10 dB, test results are unreliable; equipment should be checked for malfunction, and the patient should be reinstructed and retested.
- Many audiologists sample hearing only at octave points. Others may prefer the detail resulting from testing the mid-octave frequencies. The American Speech-Language-Hearing Association recommends testing the better ear first and that mid-octave points be tested when a difference of 20 dB or greater is seen in the thresholds at adjacent octaves.

#### Bone conduction testing

- The earphones are removed, and the vibrator is placed on the mastoid process of the ear with the better hearing acuity (the auricle shouldn't touch the vibrator).
- Ascending and descending tones are presented, as in air conduction testing, using 250, 500, 1,000, 2,000, and 4,000 Hz.

#### Both tests

- Refer the patient to an audiologist if test results are inconsistent or are confounded by possible crossover.

### Precautions

- Any modifications of standard testing procedure—such as inserting a plastic tube to prevent ear canal collapse—must be recorded on the audiogram.
- Be on the alert for false responses; they can be misleading and influence interpretation of test results. False responses include failure to indicate when a tone has been heard or responding when no tone has been heard.

## ▌Tuning fork

The Weber, Rinne, and Schwabach tuning fork tests are quick, valuable screening tools for detecting hearing loss and obtaining preliminary information as to its type. The Weber test determines whether a patient lateralizes the tone of the tuning fork to one ear. The Rinne test compares air and bone conduction in both ears. The Schwabach test compares the patient's bone conduction response with that of the examiner, who's assumed to have normal hearing.

Test results are most reliable when a low-frequency tuning fork is used; results aren't definitive because they depend on subjective factors, such as the examiner's ability to strike the fork with equal force each time and the patient's ability to report audible tones correctly.

Results of the Weber test may be misleading, and the Rinne test commonly doesn't detect a mild conductive hearing loss (10 to 35 dB). Thus, abnormal test results require confirmation by pure tone audiometry.

## Normal results
- In the Weber test, hearing the same tone equally loudly in both ears (Weber midline result) is normal.
- In the Rinne test, hearing the air-conducted tone louder or longer than the bone-conducted tone (Rinne-positive result) is normal.
- In the Schwabach test, hearing the tone for the same duration as the examiner is normal.

## Abnormal results
### Weber test
- Lateralization of the tone to one ear suggests a conductive loss on that side or a sensorineural loss on the other side.
- Lateralization results if the tone is louder in one ear (Stenger effect) or reaches one ear sooner (phase effect).
- If one ear has a sensorineural loss, the Stenger effect causes lateralization to the unaffected ear; if one ear has a conductive loss, either the Stenger or the phase effect produces lateralization to that ear.
- If a patient's hearing loss is unilateral, the Weber test may suggest the type of loss.

### Rinne test
- Hearing the bone-conducted tone louder or longer than the air-conducted tone indicates a conductive loss.

- In unilateral hearing loss, the tone may be heard louder when conducted by bone, but in the opposite ear; this is a false-negative Rinne test result.
- A sensorineural loss is indicated when the sound is heard louder by air conduction.

### Schwabach test
- Hearing the tone longer than the examiner hears it suggests a conductive loss; conversely, a shorter duration indicates a sensorineural loss.
- A conductive loss attenuates (decreases the energy of) air-conducted sound in a room with ambient noise, enabling the patient with this type of loss to hear bone-conducted sound longer than the examiner can hear it.

## Purpose
- To screen for or confirm hearing loss
- To help distinguish conductive from sensorineural hearing loss

## Patient preparation
- Describe the procedure to the patient, and explain that the tuning fork tests help detect and assess hearing loss. Tell him who will conduct the tests, and reassure him that they're painless.
- Explain to the patient that concentration and prompt responses are essential for accurate testing. Have him use hand signals to indicate whether a tone is louder in his right ear or left ear and when he stops hearing the tone.
- Inform the patient that tuning fork tests aren't definitive and that further testing may be necessary to confirm abnormal results.

## Procedure and posttest care
- Confirm the patient's identity using two patient identifiers according to facility policy.
- Using a low-frequency tuning fork (256 or 512 Hz), practice achieving a

consistent tone by gently striking a prong against your elbow or the heel of your hand, by stroking the prongs upward, or by pinching them together.

- When performing each test, be careful to strike the tuning fork with equal force. Hold the fork at its base to allow the prongs to vibrate freely. Record the name of the test, the result, and the vibrating frequency of the tuning fork.

### Weber test

- Vibrate the fork, and place its base on the midline of the patient's skull at the forehead.
- Ask the patient whether the tone is louder in his left ear or his right ear or is equally loud in both. Describe the results as Weber left, Weber right, or Weber midline, according to his response.

### Rinne test

- Test bone conduction by holding the tuning fork between your thumb and index finger and placing the base of the vibrating fork against the patient's mastoid process.
- Test air conduction by moving the vibrating prongs next to (but not touching) the external ear. Ask the patient which location has the louder or longer sound. Repeat the procedure for the other ear.
- Record results as Rinne-positive if the air-conducted sound is heard louder or longer, or Rinne-negative if the bone-conducted sound is heard louder or longer.

### Schwabach test

- Holding the tuning fork between your thumb and index finger, place the base of the vibrating tuning fork against the patient's left mastoid process, and ask whether he hears the tone. If he does, immediately place the tuning fork on your left mastoid process, and listen for the tone.

- Alternate the tuning fork between the patient's left mastoid process and your own until one of you stops hearing the sound. Record the length of time the patient continues to hear it.
- Repeat the procedure on the right mastoid process.

### All tests

- Refer the patient for further audiologic testing if the tuning fork tests suggest a hearing loss.

## Precautions

- Undetected hearing loss in the examiner may alter the test results.

# Scanning

## Computed tomography of the ear
### [CT of the ear]

Computed tomography (CT) scanning combines the use of a computer and X-rays passed through the body at different angles to produce clear cross-sectional images of body tissues. The test uses high-resolution computed tomography (HRCT) to evaluate patients for cochlear implants, differentiate osseous changes involving the external auditory canal and middle ear, differentiate the osseous structures of the temporal bone and petrous bone, and provide differential diagnoses for middle ear and inner ear problems.

### Normal results

- Normal anatomic structures should be readily identified.

### Abnormal results

- Tympanosclerosis and the osseous changes of the external auditory canal and middle and inner ear structures are abnormal.

## Purpose

- To investigate the cause of bilateral hearing loss
- To confirm cochlear abnormalities
- To differentiate chronic inflammation from cholesteatoma
- To evaluate ossification of the cochlea coils before cochlear implantation
- To depict osseous changes involving the temporal and petrous bone contained in the inner ear
- To accurately define appropriate surgical and therapeutic approaches for patients with middle ear and inner ear disorders
- To assess postsurgical management for patients with middle ear and inner ear disorders

## Patient preparation

- Describe the procedure to the patient. Tell him to remove any metal objects, such as jewelry, before the procedure.
- Check the patient for allergies to iodine products if a contrast medium is to be used. (Contrast medium isn't required for evaluating ossification of the cochlea coils or studying the petrous portion of the temporal bone.) Tell him that a contrast medium will be given intravenously.
- Explain to the patient that he will be secured to the scanner table to eliminate movement.
- Inform him that his body and head will be moved into the scanner, which is an air-conditioned chamber that resembles a giant doughnut. The technician will be able to stay with and communicate with the patient throughout the test, which averages between 15 to 20 minutes.
- Warn the patient that he will hear a humming sound while the machine records the appropriate images.

## Procedure and posttest care

- Confirm the patient's identity using two patient identifiers according to facility policy.
- The protocol for each HRCT depends on the purpose of the test, with most HRCT studies done in the axial and coronal planes.
- The patient is taken to the radiology department and placed on the scanner table with his head toward the machine. The mobile scanner table allows for easy transfer and accurate positioning in the machine.
- A trained technician conducts the study under the supervision of a radiologist.
- The technician explains the details of the procedure to the patient to reassure him and gain his cooperation.
- Numerous low-dosage X-ray beams pass through the patient's body at different angles for a fraction of a second as the scanner rotates around him.
- Detectors in the scanner record the number of X-rays absorbed by different tissues, and a computer transforms these data into an image, which is interpreted by the radiologist.
- The temporal bones are imaged separately in the axial and coronal planes. Because contrast already exists between bone, air, and soft tissue, the use of a contrast medium isn't necessary in most cases.

## Precautions

- If a contrast medium will be used, ask the patient if he has a history of iodine sensitivity.

**Do's & don'ts**

Ask the patient about feelings of claustrophobia. He may require preprocedure medication to alleviate his fears and allow for an accurate study. The ordering practitioner determines this.

---

# Magnetic resonance imaging of the ear

Magnetic resonance imaging (MRI) provides high-quality, cross-sectional images of the body. MRI is used to assess soft tissues, the cranial nerves, and bone.

The use of fast-spin echo (FSE) MRIs and diffusion weighted images for otologic and neurologic assessment, especially when a retrocochlear lesion or other neurologic condition is suspected, is under investigation.

### Normal results
- Anatomic structures should be appear as normal.

### Abnormal results
- Viral labyrinthitis, increased intracranial pressure, paragangliomas, acoustic neuromas, vestibular schwannomas, and other disorders may be found.

### Purpose
- To assess the cause of sudden unilateral sensorineural hearing loss
- To show early nonossified soft-tissue scarring in the membranous labyrinth
- To investigate lesions of the petrous apex
- To diagnose vestibular schwannomas as small as 2 mm
- To visualize cranial nerves VII and VIII, especially when anticipating excision of an auditory neuroma

### Patient preparation
- Explain that MRI is valuable in studying the internal structures of the ear.
- Tell the patient that the MRI machine itself emits a loud, banging noise when it's operating.

- Advise the patient that the test may require the use of an I.V. contrast medium, which seldom causes adverse reactions.
- Tell him that the procedure takes about 15 minutes when contrast medium isn't used. (FSE MRI takes even less time.)
- Have the patient remove all jewelry (including watches and rings) and metal objects, such as hairpins and barrettes.
- Tell him to inform the practitioner if he has a pacemaker, hearing aid, or other electrical device because these items can interfere with the scanner.

### Procedure and posttest care
- The protocol for each MRI depends on the purpose of the test.
- After the patient is prepared and placed on the MRI table, the technician, under the direction of the radiologist, sets the parameter that will provide optimum spatial resolution in a reasonable scan time.
- The patient's head is moved into a large, hollow, cylindrical magnet. The machine surrounds the patient with short bursts of powerful magnetic fields and radio waves.
- These bursts stimulate hydrogen atoms in the patient's system to emit signals, which are detected and analyzed by the computer to create images that resemble "slices" of the patient's body.

### Precautions
- If a contrast medium will be used, ask the patient if he has a history of iodine sensitivity.

#### Do's & don'ts

Ask the patient about feelings of claustrophobia. He may require preprocedure medication to alleviate his fears and allow for an accurate study. The ordering practitioner determines this.

# Vestibular tests

## ▌Electronystagmography and videonystagmography

In electronystagmography (ENG) testing and videonystagmography (VNG) testing, eye movements in response to specific stimuli are recorded and used to evaluate the interactions of the vestibular system and the muscles controlling eye movement in what is known as the vestibulo-ocular reflex. Nystagmus, the involuntary back-and-forth eye movements caused by this reflex, results from the vestibular system's attempts to maintain visual function during head movement.

Nystagmography is a technique for monitoring nystagmus and other eye movements. The eye movements can be monitored using electrodes placed near the eyes. Traditional ENG records the corneoretinal potential—the difference of 1 mV between the positive charge of the cornea and the negative charge of the retina—to record nystagmus through electrodes placed near the eyes. In VNG, goggles are placed over the patient's eyes, and eye movements are recorded with an infrared camera.

The tests seek to determine whether the disorder is peripheral (inner ear or related to cranial nerve VIII involvement) or central (originating from problems of the central nervous system, brain stem, cerebellum, or cerebrum).

### Normal results

For an overview of normal findings, see *Results of electronystagmography,* pages 376 to 379.

### Abnormal results
- Nystagmus after a head turn is prolonged, or nystagmus occurs when the patient isn't turning his head.
- A peripheral lesion may involve the end organ or the vestibular branch of the eighth cranial nerve and may result from conditions such as Ménière's disease, multiple sclerosis, ischemic damage to the cochlea, autoimmune disease, and vestibular ototoxicity and eighth nerve tumors.
- A central lesion may involve the brain stem, cerebellum, cerebrum, or any of the connecting structures and may result from demyelinating diseases, tumors, or circulatory disorders.

### Purpose
- To help identify the cause of dizziness and vertigo
- To confirm the presence and location (central or oculomotor, peripheral, or both) of a lesion
- To assess neurologic disorders

### Patient preparation
- Make sure that the patient's ear canals are free of cerumen before referring him for ENG testing. The caloric testing portion of the ENG can't be conducted safely or accurately if he has cerumen accumulation or a tympanic membrane perforation.
- Inform the patient that tympanometry will be conducted before caloric testing to ensure tympanic membrane integrity.
- Tell the patient that his dizziness problems will be assessed by recording eye movements.
- Inform the patient that the procedure will require about 1½ hours to complete.
- Reassure the patient that the test isn't painful and someone will be present to make sure that he doesn't fall, but explain that some portions may make him briefly dizzy or nauseated. Because of

# Results of electronystagmography

| Test and normal findings | Abnormal findings |
| --- | --- |
| **Saccadic pursuit testing**<br>Square-wave patterns of differing amplitudes mimicking the target, minimal latency, and good accuracy of eye movements | *Ocular dysmetria:* significant undershoots, overshoots, glissades, or pulsion; reduced eye velocity, accuracy, prolonged latency |
| **Gaze testing**<br>No nystagmus with eyes open, weak or no nystagmus with eyes closed | *Spontaneous nystagmus:* significant amount noted when eyes are closed or when tested in complete darkness under goggles while gazing forward |
| | *Gaze nystagmus:* presence of nystagmus only when the eyes are deviated from midline |
| | *Up-beating nystagmus:* upward deviation of eye movement |
| | *Down-beating nystagmus:* downward deviation of eye movement |
| | *Rotary nystagmus:* non-classic benign paroxysmal positional vertigo (BPPV) |
| **Positional testing (head in position)**<br>Eyes open, no nystagmus; eyes closed or wearing light-excluding goggles, no more than weak nystagmus in one or more positions | *Nystagmus:* either changes direction across positions or positioning or remains in the same direction, but isn't spontaneous nystagmus |
| **Positional testing (head in movement toward the position)**<br>Eyes open, no nystagmus; eyes closed or wearing light-excluding goggles, no more than weak nystagmus in one or more positions | *Transient, fatigable torsional eye movement:* during Dix-Hallpike procedure, occurring with subjective dizziness |

## Usual underlying conditions

Central nervous system (CNS) pathology: possible brain stem, cerebellum, or cortex involvement
Nonlocalizing, possibly caused by spontaneous or gaze nystagmus

Nonlocalizing abnormality of the vestibular system: occurs in acute peripheral disorders, is horizontal and initially beats away from the affected ear; possible CNS involvement if present with eyes open, or when viewing a target, or if nystagmus changes direction

CNS involvement (peripheral lesions): spontaneous nystagmus, stronger when patient looks in the direction of the nystagmus fast phase

Cerebellar or brain stem involvement

Cerebellar or cervicomedullary junction involvement

Brain stem or vestibular nuclei

Nonlocalizing: suppression with visual fixation suggestive of peripheral involvement; enhancement of nystagmus or failure to suppress with visual fixation suggestive of central etiology

BPPV: responds well to repositioning maneuvers

*(continued)*

this, advise him not to eat or drink for 3 to 4 hours before the test.

- Suggest that someone accompany the patient to the evaluation, as occasionally the patient doesn't feel well enough to drive after the appointment. Avoid overemphasizing the risk of discomfort because patient anxiety increases the risk of nausea and vomiting during the procedure.
- Encourage the patient to wear comfortable clothing. A woman should wear pants.
- If testing involves traditional ENG with attachment of recording electrodes, inform the patient that his skin will need to be cleaned, so ideally make-up or facial creams shouldn't be used on the day of the test. VNG testing is compromised by mascara, so a woman should refrain from wearing make-up on the day of the test.
- Instruct the patient not to smoke or drink caffeinated beverages the day of the test. He should refrain from taking nonessential medication for 48 hours before the test.
- Ask the patient to bring a list of his medications to the evaluation. He must not use alcoholic beverages, tranquilizers, sleeping pills, antihistamines, antivertigo agents, or opioids for 48 hours before the test because they prevent accurate collection and interpretation of the results. Other medications can create dizziness, which include salicylates, antidepressants, diuretics, stimulants, and certain aminoglycoside antibiotics.
- If the patient wears glasses, tell him to bring them to the test. The patient who wears contact lenses should bring eyeglasses to the examination, if possible.
- Tell the patient that the audiologist will ask for a description of the dizziness and to describe when it began. It's helpful if the patient thinks about what situations create or make the dizziness worse. Also, find out about the progres-

## Results of electronystagmography (continued)

| Test and normal findings | Abnormal findings |
|---|---|
| **Smooth pursuit tracking**<br>Volitional smooth tracking of the target, accuracy within age norms | *Sinusoidal tracking:* with superimposed nystagmus<br><br>*Break-up in tracings or saccades:* jerking, rather than smooth movements; reduced velocity, accuracy, prolonged latency that isn't accounted for by advanced age or poor cooperation |
| **Optokinetic testing**<br>Eye movement follows stimulus at speeds to 30 degrees per second; clear triangular wave pattern; similar pattern for stimuli traveling in both directions | *Significant asymmetry:* not explained by spontaneous or gaze nystagmus<br><br>*Reduced eye velocity:* when compared with age-appropriate norms |
| **Caloric testing**<br>Eyes closed, nystagmus occurring in all conditions; suppressed by visual fixation with cold stimuli, nystagmus beats to opposite ear; with warm stimuli, it beats to same ear (To help recall this phenomenon, use the acronym COWS—cold, opposite, warm, same.) | *Unilateral weakness:* over 20% to 30% difference in maximum slow-phase velocities (averaged across temperatures) between ears<br><br>*Bilateral weakness:* slow-phase velocity of the sum of the four caloric irrigations reduced, typically below 20 degrees (average of each irrigation $\leq$ 5 degrees/second)<br><br>*Directional preponderance:* more than 30% difference in maximum slow-phase velocities for right- versus left-beating nystagmus<br>*Failure to suppress fixation:* visual fixation that fails to reduce nystagmus by at least 40% |

sion of the patient's symptoms by asking him to think about words that might describe the dizziness other than the word "dizzy," such as "spinning," "wobbly," or "unsteady."

### Procedure and posttest care

■ Confirm the patient's identity using two patient identifiers according to facility policy.

■ After the device is set up, light bars are connected to the equipment.
■ The patient is positioned a calibrated distance from the light source and asked to follow the movement of the lights using eye movement only. The eye movements are recorded and graphed.
■ After testing is complete, the patient may resume his usual diet.

## Usual underlying conditions

Nonlocalizing, possibly caused by spontaneous or gaze nystagmus

CNS involvement if peripheral visual problems ruled out

CNS involvement

CNS involvement if peripheral visual problems ruled out

Peripheral lesion of weaker side

Bilateral peripheral or CNS involvement

Nonlocalizing, usually due to underlying spontaneous nystagmus
CNS involvement

### *Oculomotor testing*
#### Saccade testing
■ The patient is asked to watch the movement of a dot on the light bar. The dot position will move varying amounts, which correspond to eye deviations in degrees. The accuracy and velocity of the eye tracking of the rapidly moving light is measured. The traces are analyzed to determine if there's symmetrical

(right versus left and up versus down) eye movement or dysmetria such as excessive overshoot or undershoot. Glissades, a slowing of the eye movement as it approaches a target, is also ruled out.

#### Gaze nystagmus testing
■ The patient is asked to look at the light on the light bar and hold the gaze steady. Gaze is directed left, right, up, and down.
■ The patient is also asked to close his eyes and retain the gaze direction in traditional ENG testing. When VNG recordings are made, the goggles exclude light and the recordings are made with the eyes open. Nystagmus shouldn't occur with the patient's eyes open while he fixates on the target and should be minimal with his eyes closed or when goggles exclude light.

#### Smooth pursuit (sinusoidal) tracking testing
■ The patient watches a moving target as it moves back and forth at varying rates.
■ The eye movement is observed to determine if the patient can track the target accurately.
■ Tracings are analyzed for left-right symmetry and "smoothness" of the eye's tracking (pursuit) of the target.

### *Optokinetics testing*
■ The patient is instructed to look at the light bar as a series of dots moves across the screen, first in one direction (for example, right to left), and then in the other direction.
■ The patient's eyes rapidly move back to center and track another dot. This creates a tracing that looks like nystagmus: the patient follows a dot for a brief period; the eyes rapidly move back to center and track another moving dot. This test assesses the CNS's ability to control rapid eye movement and will be affected by an existing nystagmus.

### Positional and positioning testing

- The patient's eye movements are recorded as he's moved into various body positions and as he remains in these body positions. Recordings note whether nystagmus is present, and if so, the positions that elicit the nystagmus are noted and have diagnostic significance.
- In the Dix-Hallpike test, a diagnostic for benign paroxysmal positional vertigo (BPPV), the patient is seated initially. He's then rapidly moved into a supine, head hanging position, with the head deviated to the side, and then returned to a sitting position.
- If torsional eye movements are observed, time-locked to the subjective report of dizziness, the findings are positive for BPPV. The test is repeated to establish fatigability, also classic in BPPV. The direction of the rotational eye movement assists in diagnosing which semicircular canal is involved and helps to establish the appropriate BPPV repositioning treatment.

### Caloric testing

- The patient lies supine with his head elevated 30 degrees so that the horizontal semicircular canals are perpendicular to the floor.
- The patient's ear is irrigated with water or air (depending upon the system used) for about 60 seconds per irrigation. Four irrigations are completed (both temperatures for each ear).
- Heating and cooling the outer ear causes a change in temperature of the middle ear. The horizontal semicircular canal is located behind the medial wall of the middle ear. The fluid in the semicircular canal moves when the temperature of the fluid is changed, eliciting nystagmus. Thus, for caloric testing, nystagmus is normal.

- The patient is instructed to open his eyes during one portion of each recording. Visual fixation reduces nystagmus if the CNS is normal.
- The symmetry of the nystagmus elicited by irrigation of each ear is assessed. The different temperatures produce different directions of nystagmus. The symmetry of the left beating nystagmus and the right beating nystagmus is analyzed.
- If the patient fails to respond to standard caloric stimulation, ice calorics may be used. A small quantity of ice water or very cold air is introduced into the ear canal to determine if there's residual functioning of that ear's vestibular system.

### Precautions

- If the patient has a back or neck condition that could be aggravated by rapid changes in position, check with the practitioner to determine if any of the positional tests should be omitted.
- Water caloric testing can't be safely used if the patient has a perforated tympanic membrane. Air caloric test results won't be accurate.

### Complications

- Dizziness

# Posturography

Balance involves the coordination of input from the vestibular system, from vision, and from proprioception. Posturography assesses the patient's ability to retain equilibrium when vision and proprioceptive input is removed.

### Normal results

- Dynamic platform posturography sensory organization test results indicate whether the patient has a preference for visual, proprioceptive, or vestibular inputs. The analysis determines whether the patient is using ankle or hip strategies to compensate for platform or visual surround motion. This information can be used by the physical therapist in planning and monitoring treatment and can be used as a prognostic indicator.

■ Dynamic posturography provides age-norm scores to determine a patient's stability. A score of 100% indicates good stability; 0% indicates that the patient would have fallen had the patient not have been in the harness.

■ Scores for the somatosensory, visual, and vestibular contributions to balance are also given.

■ All tests are interpreted in light of age-appropriate norms.

### Abnormal results

■ Scores that don't meet age-appropriate norms are considered abnormal.

■ The results of the limit of stability test have implications for analyzing the risk of a fall.

**DRUG CHALLENGE**

Medications, such as vestibular suppressants or centrally acting medicines (may affect balance)

### Purpose

■ To objectively determine the functional impairment associated with dizziness

■ To determine the relative strengths and weaknesses of the vestibular system for establishing and monitoring the progress of a rehabilitation plan

### Patient preparation

■ Advise the patient not to smoke or drink caffeinated beverages the day of the test.

■ Ask the patient to bring a list of his medications to the evaluation. He must not take alcoholic beverages; tranquilizers; sleeping pills; antihistamines; antivertigo agents; opioids; and other medications that can create dizziness, including salicylates, antidepressants, diuretics, stimulants, and certain aminoglycoside antibiotics for 48 hours before the test because they prevent accurate interpretation of the results.

■ Inform the patient that during the test he will stand on a platform. The platform can move, and the visual field in front will move.

■ Tell the patient that the test assesses how vision and motion affect his sense of balance. Assure him that he won't fall during the test.

■ Suggest that the patient wear comfortable, loose-fitting clothing; advise a woman to wear pants.

### Procedure and posttest care

■ Confirm the patient's identity using two patient identifiers according to facility policy.

■ Procedures are somewhat specific to the equipment manufacturer. A battery of tests is typically administered.

■ After testing is complete, the patient may resume his usual diet and medications.

### *Sensory organization test*

■ The patient is placed in a harness, standing on a platform, while looking forward toward a screen that encompasses the entire visual field.

■ The sensor on the platform measures the patient's sway and the strength and latency of leg movements that occur when the platform or visual field moves. Six test conditions include:

– The patient sees the screen in front, and the platform is fixed. (Eyes open Rhomberg test)

– The patient closes his eyes. The platform remains fixed. (Eyes closed Rhomberg test)

– The visual field around the patient moves. The platform remains fixed. The patient receives proprioceptive

and vestibular input that differs from
that of the visual system. The patient
with deficits in these areas experiences
greater imbalance.
– The platform moves. The visual field
remains fixed. The patient receives
proprioceptive and vestibular input
that differs from that of the visual system.
– The patient's eyes are closed. The
platform moves. Proprioception and
vestibular input are assessed.
– The platform and screen in front
move in concert. The three sensory
systems work together to maintain balance.
▪ The test evaluates the person's ability
to integrate information across the sens-
es and to suppress information that results in sensory conflicts.

### Motor control test
▪ The platform makes a series of jerky
motions, and the patient's responses are
measured.

### Adaptation test
▪ The platform is tilted up or down, and
the patient's ability to compensate for
this movement during repetition of the
platform tilt is analyzed.

### Limit of stability test
▪ The patient leans as far as possible in
different directions, and his responses
are measured.

## Precautions
▪ The person conducting the posturography places the patient in a body harness to prevent falls.

# V

# Body system tests

# Respiratory system

## Endoscopy

### Bronchoscopy

Bronchoscopy allows direct visualization of the larynx, trachea, and bronchi through a flexible fiber-optic bronchoscope or a rigid metal bronchoscope. A more recent approach is the use of virtual bronchoscopy. (See *Virtual bronchoscopy*.) Although a flexible fiber-optic bronchoscope allows a wider view and is used more commonly, the rigid metal bronchoscope is required to remove foreign objects, excise endobronchial lesions, and control massive hemoptysis. A brush, biopsy forceps, or catheter may be passed through the bronchoscope to obtain specimens for cytologic examination.

#### Normal results
- The bronchi appear structurally similar to the trachea.
- The right bronchus is slightly larger and more vertical than the left.
- Smaller segmental bronchi branch off the main bronchi.

#### Abnormal results
- Bronchial wall abnormalities include inflammation, swelling, protruding cartilage, ulceration, enlargement of the mucous gland orifices or submucosal lymph nodes, and tumors.
- Endotracheal abnormalities include stenosis, compression, ectasia (dilation of tubular vessel), irregular bronchial branching, and abnormal bifurcation due to diverticulum.
- Abnormal substances in the trachea or bronchi include blood, secretions, calculi, and foreign bodies.
- Results of tissue and cell studies may indicate interstitial pulmonary disease, bronchogenic carcinoma, tuberculosis, or other pulmonary infections.

#### Purpose
- To visually examine a tumor, an obstruction, secretions, bleeding, or a foreign body in the tracheobronchial tree
- To help diagnose bronchogenic carcinoma, tuberculosis, interstitial pulmonary disease, and fungal or parasitic pulmonary infection by obtaining a specimen for bacteriologic and cytologic examination
- To remove foreign bodies, malignant or benign tumors, mucus plugs, and excessive secretions from the tracheobronchial tree

# Virtual bronchoscopy

Using a computer and data from a spiral computed tomography (CT) scan, physicians can now examine the respiratory tract noninvasively with virtual bronchoscopy. Although still in its early stages, researchers believe that this test can enhance screening, diagnosis, preoperative planning, surgical technique, and postoperative follow-up.

Unlike its counterpart—conventional bronchoscopy—virtual bronchoscopy is noninvasive, doesn't require sedation, and provides images for examination beyond the segmental bronchi, thus allowing for possible diagnosis of areas that may be stenosed, obstructed, or compressed from an external source. The images obtained from the CT scan include views of the airways and lung parenchyma. Anatomic structures and abnormalities can be precisely identified and therefore can be helpful in locating potential biopsy sites to be obtained with conventional bronchoscopy and provide simulation for planning the optimal surgical approach.

Virtual bronchoscopy does have disadvantages. This technique doesn't allow for actual biopsies to be obtained from tissue sources. It also can't demonstrate details of the mucosal surface, such as color or texture. Moreover, if an area contains viscous secretions, such as mucus or blood, visualization becomes difficult.

More research on this technique is needed. However, researchers believe that virtual bronchoscopy may play a major role in the screening and early detection of certain cancers, thus allowing for treatment at an earlier, possibly curable stage.

## Patient preparation

- Explain that bronchoscopy is used to examine the lower airways.
- Describe the procedure, and instruct the patient to fast for 6 to 12 hours before the test.
- Tell the patient who will perform the test, where it will be done, and that the room will be darkened.
- Tell the patient that a chest X-ray and blood studies will be performed before the bronchoscopy and afterward, if appropriate.
- Advise the patient that he may receive an I.V. sedative to help him relax.
- If the procedure isn't being performed under general anesthesia, inform the patient that a local anesthetic will be sprayed into his nose and mouth to suppress the gag reflex. Warn him that the spray has an unpleasant taste and that he may experience discomfort during the procedure.

- Reassure the patient that his airway won't be blocked during the procedure and that oxygen will be given through the bronchoscope.
- Make sure that the patient or a responsible family member has signed an informed consent form.
- Check the patient's history for hypersensitivity to the anesthetic.
- Obtain the patient's baseline vital signs.
- Give the preoperative sedative as ordered.
- Have the patient remove his dentures, if appropriate, before he receives a sedative.

## Procedure and posttest care

- Confirm the patient's identity using two patient identifiers according to facility policy.
- Place the patient in the supine position or have him sit upright in a chair.

- Tell the patient to remain relaxed with his arms at his sides and to breathe through his nose.
- Provide supplemental oxygen by nasal cannula, if necessary.
- After the local anesthetic is sprayed into the patient's throat and it takes effect, assist as appropriate as a bronchoscope is introduced through the patient's mouth or nose. When the scope is just above the vocal cords, about 3 to 4 ml of 2% to 4% lidocaine is flushed through the inner channel of the scope to the vocal cords to anesthetize deeper areas. The practitioner inspects the anatomic structure of the trachea and bronchi, observes the color of the mucosal lining, and notes masses or inflamed areas.
- As indicated, provide biopsy forceps that may be used to remove a tissue specimen from a suspect area, a bronchial brush to obtain cells from the surface of a lesion, and a suction apparatus to remove foreign bodies or mucus plugs. Bronchoalveolar lavage may be performed to diagnose the infectious causes of infiltrates in an immunocompromised patient or to remove thickened secretions.
- After collection, place the specimens in their respective, properly labeled containers in accordance with laboratory and pathology guidelines, and send them to the laboratory at once.
- Be aware that bronchoscopy may require fluoroscopic guidance for distal evaluation of lesions for a transbronchial biopsy in alveolar areas.
- Check the patient's vital signs according to facility policy, or at least every 15 minutes until the patient is stable and then every 30 minutes for 4 hours, every hour for the next 4 hours, and then every 4 hours for 24 hours. Immediately notify the practitioner of adverse reactions to the anesthetic or sedative.

- Place the conscious patient in semi-Fowler's position; place the unconscious patient on his side with his head slightly elevated to prevent aspiration.
- Provide an emesis basin and instruct the patient to spit out saliva rather than swallow it. Observe sputum for blood and report excessive bleeding immediately.
- Tell the patient who has had a biopsy to refrain from clearing his throat and coughing, which may dislodge the clot at the biopsy site and cause hemorrhaging.
- Immediately report subcutaneous crepitus around the patient's face and neck because this may indicate tracheal or bronchial perforation.

### ALERT

 Watch for, listen for, and immediately report symptoms of respiratory difficulty resulting from laryngeal edema or laryngospasm, such as laryngeal stridor and dyspnea. Observe for signs of hypoxemia, pneumothorax, bronchospasm, and bleeding.

- Restrict food and fluids to avoid aspiration until the gag reflex returns (usually in 1 to 2 hours). Then the patient may resume his usual diet, beginning with sips of clear liquid or ice chips.
- Reassure the patient that hoarseness, loss of voice, and sore throat are temporary. Provide lozenges or a soothing liquid gargle to ease discomfort when his gag reflex returns.

### Precautions
- A patient with respiratory failure who can't breathe adequately by himself should be placed on a ventilator before bronchoscopy.

### Complications
- Tracheal or bronchial perforation
- Pneumothorax

- Laryngeal edema
- Hypoxemia
- Cardiac arrhythmias
- Bleeding
- Laryngospasm

# Direct laryngoscopy

Direct laryngoscopy allows visualization of the larynx by the use of a fiber-optic endoscope or laryngoscope passed through the mouth and pharynx to the larynx. It's indicated for children, patients with strong gag reflexes due to anatomic abnormalities, and those who have had no response to short-term therapy for symptoms of pharyngeal or laryngeal disease, such as stridor and hemoptysis. Secretions or tissue may be removed during this procedure for further study. The test is usually contraindicated in patients with epiglottiditis, but may be performed on them in an operating room with resuscitative equipment available.

## Normal results
- No evidence of inflammation, lesions, strictures, or foreign bodies is present.

## Abnormal results
- The combined results of direct laryngoscopy, biopsy, and radiography may indicate laryngeal carcinoma.
- Results of direct laryngoscopy may show benign lesions, strictures, or foreign bodies and, with a biopsy, may distinguish laryngeal edema from a radiation reaction or tumor.
- Vocal cord dysfunction may be detected.

## Purpose
- To detect lesions, strictures, or foreign bodies
- To remove benign lesions or foreign bodies from the larynx
- To help diagnose laryngeal cancer

- To examine the larynx when indirect laryngoscopy is inadequate

## Patient preparation
- Explain that direct laryngoscopy is used to detect laryngeal abnormalities.
- Instruct the patient to fast for 6 to 8 hours before the test.
- Tell the patient who will perform the procedure and where it will be done.
- Inform the patient that he'll receive a sedative to help him relax, medication to reduce secretions and, during the procedure, a general or local anesthetic. Reassure him that this procedure won't obstruct his airway.
- Make sure that the patient or a responsible family member has signed an informed consent form.
- Check the patient's history for hypersensitivity to the anesthetic.
- Obtain the patient's baseline vital signs.
- Instruct the patient to remove dentures, contact lenses, and jewelry and to void before giving him a sedative.
- Give the sedative and other medication (usually 30 minutes to 1 hour before the test) as ordered.

## Procedure and posttest care
- Confirm the patient's identity using two patient identifiers according to facility policy.
- Place the patient in the supine position.
- Encourage the patient to breathe through his nose and to relax with his arms at his sides.
- Assist as appropriate when a general anesthetic is given or when the patient's mouth and throat are sprayed with a local anesthetic.
- A laryngoscope is introduced through the patient's mouth, the larynx is examined for abnormalities, and a specimen or secretions may be removed for further study; minor surgery, such as re-

moval of polyps or nodules, may be performed at this time.

- Place the specimens in their respective containers. Specimen collection should be done in accordance with laboratory and pathology guidelines.
- Place the conscious patient in semi-Fowler's position; place the unconscious patient on his side with his head slightly elevated to prevent aspiration.
- Check the patient's vital signs according to facility protocol, or every 15 minutes until the patient is stable and then every 30 minutes for 2 hours, every hour for the next 4 hours, and then every 4 hours for 24 hours. Immediately report to the practitioner any adverse reaction to the anesthetic or sedative (tachycardia, palpitations, hypertension, euphoria, excitation, and rapid, deep respirations).
- Apply an ice collar to minimize laryngeal edema.
- Provide an emesis basin, and instruct the patient to spit out saliva rather than swallow it. Observe sputum for blood and report excessive bleeding immediately.
- Instruct the patient to refrain from clearing his throat and coughing to prevent hemorrhaging at the biopsy site.
- Advise the patient to avoid smoking until his vital signs are stable and there's no evidence of complications.
- Immediately report subcutaneous crepitus around the patient's face and neck, which may indicate tracheal perforation.
- Listen to the patient's neck with a stethoscope for signs of stridor and airway obstruction.

### ACTION STAT!

 Observe the patient with epiglottiditis for signs of airway obstruction, and immediately report signs of respiratory difficulty. Keep emergency resuscitation equipment

available; keep a tracheotomy tray nearby for 24 hours.

- Restrict food and fluids to avoid aspiration until the gag reflex returns (usually within 2 hours). Then the patient may resume his usual diet, beginning with sips of water.
- Reassure the patient that voice loss, hoarseness, and sore throat are temporary. Provide throat lozenges or a soothing liquid gargle when his gag reflex returns.

### Complications

- Tracheal perforation or airway obstruction
- Adverse reactions to the anesthetic
- Bleeding

## Mediastinoscopy

Using an exploring speculum with built-in fiber light and side slit, mediastinoscopy allows direct viewing of mediastinal structures. It also permits palpation and biopsy of paratracheal and carinal lymph nodes. This surgical procedure is indicated when other tests, such as sputum cytology, lung scans, radiography, and bronchoscopic biopsy, fail to confirm the diagnosis.

Scarring of the area from previous mediastinoscopy contraindicates this procedure.

### Normal results

- Lymph nodes appear as small, smooth, flat oval bodies of lymphoid tissue.

### Abnormal results

- Malignant lymph nodes usually indicate inoperable, but not always untreatable, lung or esophageal cancer or lymphomas (such as Hodgkin's disease).

## Purpose

- To detect bronchogenic carcinoma, lymphoma (including Hodgkin's disease), and sarcoidosis
- To determine stages of lung cancer

## Patient preparation

- Explain that mediastinoscopy is used to evaluate the lymph nodes and other structures in the chest. Review his history for previous mediastinoscopy because scarring from a previous mediastinoscopy contraindicates the test.
- Describe the procedure to the patient, and answer his questions.
- Instruct the patient to fast after midnight before the test.
- Tell the patient who will perform the procedure, where it will be done, that he'll be given general anesthesia, and that the procedure takes about 1 hour.
- Tell the patient that he may have temporary chest pain, tenderness at the incision site, or a sore throat (from intubation).
- Reassure the patient that complications are rare.
- Make sure that the patient or a responsible family member has signed an informed consent form.
- Check the patient's history for hypersensitivity to the anesthetic.
- Give a sedative the night before the test and again before the procedure as ordered.

## Procedure and posttest care

- Confirm the patient's identity using two patient identifiers according to facility policy.
- After the endotracheal tube is in place, a small transverse suprasternal incision is made.
- Using finger dissection, the surgeon forms a channel and palpates the lymph nodes.
- The mediastinoscope is inserted, and tissue specimens are collected and sent to the laboratory for frozen section examination.
- If analysis confirms malignancy of a resectable tumor, thoracotomy and pneumonectomy may follow immediately.
- Monitor the patient's postoperative vital signs, and check his dressings for bleeding and fluid drainage.
- Observe the patient for complications.
- Give the prescribed analgesic as needed.

## Complications

- Pneumothorax
- Perforated esophagus
- Mediastinitis
- Infection
- Hemorrhage
- Left recurrent laryngeal nerve damage
- Cardiac tamponade

# Thoracoscopy

In thoracoscopy, an endoscope is inserted directly into the chest wall to view the pleural space, thoracic walls, mediastinum, and pericardium. It's used for diagnostic and therapeutic purposes and can sometimes replace traditional thoracotomy. Thoracoscopy reduces morbidity (by reducing the use of open chest surgery) and postoperative pain, decreases surgical and anesthesia time, and allows faster recovery.

## Normal results

- Pleural cavity contains a small amount of lubricating fluid that facilitates movement of the lung and chest wall.
- The parietal and visceral layers are lesion-free and can separate from each other.

## Abnormal results

- Lesions adjacent to or involving the pleura or mediastinum suggest possible malignancy, and biopsies can be taken.

- Blebs can be removed by wedge resection to reduce the risk of repeat episodes of spontaneous pneumothorax.
- The presence of increased pleural fluid indicates pleural effusion; specimens can be obtained for analysis and diagnosis of the cause.

### Purpose

- To diagnose pleural disease
- To obtain biopsy specimens
- To treat pleural conditions, such as cysts, blebs, and effusions
- To perform wedge resections

### Patient preparation

- Explain that thoracoscopy permits visual examination of the chest wall to view the pleural space, thoracic wall, mediastinum, and pericardium.
- Describe the procedure. Caution the patient that an open thoracotomy may still be needed for diagnosis or treatment and that general anesthesia may be required.
- Instruct the patient not to eat or drink for 10 to 12 hours before the procedure.
- Make sure that the appropriate preoperative tests (such as pulmonary function and coagulation tests, electrocardiography, and chest X-ray) have been performed and that an informed consent form has been signed.
- Tell the patient that he'll have a chest tube and drainage system in place after surgery. Reassure him that analgesics will be available and that complications are rare.

### Procedure and posttest care

- Confirm the patient's identity using two patient identifiers according to facility policy.
- The patient is anesthetized, and a double-lumen endobronchial tube is inserted.

- The lung on the operative side is collapsed, and a small intercostal incision is made through which a trocar is inserted.
- A lens is then inserted to view the area and assess thoracoscopy access.
- Two or three more small incisions are made, and trocars are placed to insert suction and dissection instruments.
- The camera lens and instruments are moved from site to site as needed.
- After thoracoscopy, the lung is reexpanded, a chest tube is placed through one incision site, and a water-sealed drainage system is attached. The other incisions are closed with adhesive strips and dressed.
- Monitor the patient's postoperative vital signs as per facility policy or every 15 minutes for 1 hour, every 30 minutes for 2 hours, every hour for 2 hours, and then every 4 hours.
- Assess the patient's respiratory status and the patency of the chest drainage system.
- Give analgesics as needed for pain, and monitor the patient for adverse effects.

### Precautions

- Thoracoscopy is contraindicated in the patient who has coagulopathies or lesions near major blood vessels, who has had previous thoracic surgery, or who can't be adequately oxygenated with one lung.

### Complications

- Hemorrhage
- Nerve injury
- Perforation of the diaphragm
- Air emboli
- Tension pneumothorax

# *Fluid analysis*

## ▌ **Pleural fluid analysis**

The pleura, a two-layer membrane that covers the lungs and lines the thoracic cavity, maintains a small amount of lubricating fluid between its layers to minimize friction during respiration. Increased fluid in this space may result from such diseases as cancer or tuberculosis or from blood or lymphatic disorders and can cause respiratory difficulty.

In pleural fluid aspiration (thoracentesis), the thoracic wall is punctured to obtain a specimen of pleural fluid for analysis or to relieve pulmonary (and possibly cardiac) compression and resultant respiratory distress.

### **Normal results**

▪ Pressure is negative, and there is less than 20 ml of serous fluid.

### **Abnormal results**

▪ Pleural effusion results from the abnormal formation or reabsorption of pleural fluid.
▪ Pleural fluid is either a transudate (a low-protein fluid leaked from normal blood vessels) or an exudate (a protein-rich fluid leaked from blood vessels with increased permeability); either may contain blood (hemothorax), chyle (chylothorax), or pus (empyema) and necrotic tissue. Blood-tinged fluid may indicate a traumatic tap; if so, the fluid should clear as aspiration progresses.
▪ Transudative effusion generally results from diminished colloidal pressure, increased negative pressure within the pleural cavity, ascites, systemic and pulmonary venous hypertension, heart failure, hepatic cirrhosis, and nephritis.
▪ Exudative effusion results from disorders that increase pleural capillary permeability (possibly with changes in hydrostatic or colloid osmotic pressures), lymphatic drainage interference, infections, pulmonary infarctions, and neoplasms. It is associated with depressed glucose levels, elevated lactate dehydrogenase (LD) isoenzymes, and rheumatoid arthritis cells; negative smears, cultures, and cytologic examination may indicate pleurisy associated with rheumatoid arthritis.
▪ The most common pathogens that appear in pleural fluid culture studies are *Mycobacterium tuberculosis, Staphylococcus aureus, Streptococcus pneumoniae* and other streptococci, *Haemophilus influenzae* and, in the case of a ruptured pulmonary abscess, anaerobes such as Bacteroides.
▪ A high percentage of neutrophils suggests septic inflammation; predominating lymphocytes suggest tuberculosis or fungal or viral effusions.
▪ Serosanguineous fluid may indicate pleural extension of a malignant tumor.
▪ Elevated LD in a nonpurulent, nonhemolyzed, nonbloody effusion may also suggest malignancy.
▪ Pleural fluid glucose levels 30 to 40 mg/dl lower than blood glucose levels may indicate a malignant tumor, a bacterial infection, nonseptic inflammation, or metastasis.
▪ Increased amylase levels occur in pleural effusions associated with pancreatitis.

**DRUG CHALLENGE**

 Antimicrobial therapy before fluid aspiration for culture (possible decrease in numbers of bacteria, making it difficult to isolate the infecting organism)

### **Purpose**

▪ To determine the cause and nature of pleural effusion
▪ To permit better radiographic visualization of a lung with large effusions

## Patient preparation

- Explain that pleural fluid analysis assesses the space around the lungs for fluid.
- Inform the patient that he doesn't need to restrict food and fluids.
- Make sure that the patient or a responsible family member has signed an informed consent form.
- Tell the patient who will perform the test and where it will be done.
- Explain that chest X-rays or an ultrasound study may precede the test to help locate the fluid.
- Check the patient's history for hypersensitivity to local anesthetics.
- Warn the patient that he may feel a stinging sensation on injection of the anesthetic and some pressure during withdrawal of the fluid.
- Advise the patient not to cough, breathe deeply, or move during the test to minimize the risk of injury to the lung.

## Procedure and posttest care

- Confirm the patient's identity using two patient identifiers according to facility policy.
- Record the patient's baseline vital signs.
- If necessary, clip the hair around the needle insertion site.
- Position the patient to widen intercostal spaces and to allow easier access to the pleural cavity. He must be well-supported and comfortable, preferably seated at the edge of the bed with a chair or stool supporting his feet and his head and arms resting on a padded overbed table. If the patient can't sit up, he may be positioned on his unaffected side, with the arm on the affected side elevated above his head.
- Remind the patient not to cough, breathe deeply, or move suddenly during the procedure.

- After positioning, the practitioner disinfects the skin, drapes the area, injects a local anesthetic into the subcutaneous tissue, and inserts the thoracentesis needle above the rib to avoid lacerating intercostal vessels. When the needle reaches the pocket of fluid, the 50-ml syringe is attached, and the stopcock and clamps are opened on the tubing to aspirate the fluid into the container.
- During aspiration, observe the patient for signs of respiratory distress, such as weakness, dyspnea, pallor, cyanosis, changes in heart rate, tachypnea, diaphoresis, blood-tinged frothy mucus, and hypotension.
- After the needle is withdrawn, apply slight pressure and a small adhesive bandage to the puncture site.
- Label the specimen container, and record the date and time of the test and the amount, color, and character of the fluid (clear, frothy, purulent, bloody) on the laboratory request.
- Note any signs of distress exhibited during the procedure.
- Record the exact location from which the fluid was removed to aid diagnosis.
- Reposition the patient comfortably on the affected side. Tell him to remain on this side for at least 1 hour to seal the puncture site. Elevate the head of the bed to facilitate breathing.
- Monitor the patient's vital signs every 30 minutes for 2 hours and then every 4 hours until they're stable.
- Tell the patient to call a nurse immediately if he experiences difficulty breathing.

ALERT

Watch for signs of pneumothorax, tension pneumothorax, fluid reaccumulation and, if a large amount of fluid was withdrawn, pulmonary edema or cardiac distress due to mediastinal shift. Usually, a posttest X-ray is ordered to detect these complications before clinical symptoms appear.

---

■ Check the puncture site for fluid leakage. A large amount of leakage is abnormal. Also check the site and surrounding area for subcutaneous emphysema.

### Precautions
■ Keep in mind that thoracentesis is contraindicated in the patient who has a history of bleeding disorders or anticoagulant therapy.
■ Use strict sterile technique.

### Complications
■ Pneumothorax or tension pneumothorax.

# Sweat test
## [iontophoretic sweat test]

The sweat test is a quantitative measurement of electrolyte concentrations (primarily sodium and chloride) in sweat, usually performed using pilocarpine iontophoresis (pilocarpine is a sweat inducer). Although this test is primarily used to confirm cystic fibrosis (CF) in children, it's also performed in adults to determine if they're homozygous or heterozygous for CF.

### Reference values
■ Sodium levels range from 10 to 30 mEq/L (SI, 10 to 30 mmol/L).
■ Chloride levels range from 10 to 35 mEq/L (SI, 10 to 35 mmol/L).
■ In women, sweat electrolyte levels fluctuate cyclically; chloride levels usually peak 5 to 10 days before onset of menses, and most women retain fluid before menses.
■ Men also show fluctuations up to 70 mEq/L (SI, 70 mmol/L).

### Abnormal results
■ Sodium levels of 50 to 60 mEq/L (SI, 50 to 60 mmol/L) strongly suggests CF. Levels above 60 mEq/L (SI, > 60 mmol/L) with typical clinical features confirm the diagnosis.
■ A few conditions other than CF result in elevated sweat electrolyte levels—most notably, untreated adrenal insufficiency as well as type I glycogen storage disease, vasopressin-resistant diabetes insipidus, meconium ileus, and renal failure.
■ CF is the only condition that raises sweat electrolyte levels above 80 mEq/L (SI, 80 mmol/L).

### Purpose
■ To confirm CF
■ To exclude the diagnosis in siblings of the patient with CF

### Patient preparation
■ Explain the sweat test to the child (if he's old enough to understand), using clear, simple terms.
■ Inform the child and his parents that there are no restrictions on diet, medication, or activity before the test.
■ Tell the child who will perform the test and where.
■ Tell the child that he may feel a slight tickling sensation during the procedure, but won't feel any pain.
■ Encourage the parents to assist with preparations and to stay with their child during the test. Their presence will minimize the child's anxiety.

### Procedure and posttest care
■ Confirm the patient's identity using two patient identifiers according to facility policy.
■ Wash the area that will undergo iontophoresis with distilled water, and dry it. (The flexor surface of the right forearm is commonly used or, when the patient's arm is too small to secure elec-

trodes [as with an infant], the right thigh.)

■ Place a gauze pad saturated with premeasured pilocarpine solution on the positive electrode; place the pad saturated with normal saline solution on the negative electrode.

■ Apply both electrodes to the area to undergo iontophoresis, and secure them with straps. Lead wires to the analyzer are given a current of 4 mA in 15 to 20 seconds. Iontophoresis will continue at 15- to 20-second intervals for 5 minutes.

■ Try to distract the child with a book, television, toy, or another diversion if he becomes nervous or frightened during the test.

■ Remove both electrodes after iontophoresis.

■ Discard the pads, clean the skin with distilled water, and then dry it.

■ Using forceps, place a dry gauze pad or filter paper (previously weighed on a gram scale) on the area that underwent iontophoresis.

■ Cover the pad or filter paper with a slightly larger piece of plastic, and seal the edges of the plastic with waterproof adhesive tape.

■ Leave the gauze pad or filter paper in place for about 30 to 40 minutes. (The appearance of droplets on the plastic usually indicates induction of an adequate amount of sweat.)

■ Remove the pad or filter paper with the forceps, place it immediately in the weighing bottle, and insert the stopper in the bottle. (The difference between the first and second weights indicates the weight of the sweat specimen collected.)

■ Wash the area that underwent iontophoresis with soap and water, and dry it thoroughly. If the area looks red, reassure the patient that this is normal and will disappear within a few hours.

■ Tell the patient or his parents that he may resume his usual activities.

### Precautions

■ Never perform iontophoresis on the chest, especially in a child, because the current can induce cardiac arrest.

■ Use battery-powered equipment to prevent electric shock, if possible.

■ Stop the test immediately if the patient complains of a burning sensation, which usually indicates that the positive electrode is exposed or positioned improperly. Adjust the electrode and continue the test.

■ Make sure at least 100 mg of sweat is collected for analysis.

■ Dehydration or edema in the patient may alter the test results.

### Complications

■ Electric shock

# Function tests

## Pulmonary function tests
### [PFTs]

Pulmonary function tests (volume, capacity, and flow rate tests) are a series of measurements that evaluate ventilatory function through spirometric measurements; they're performed on patients with suspected pulmonary dysfunction.

Of the seven tests used to determine volume, tidal volume ($V_T$) and expiratory reserve volume (ERV) are direct spirographic measurements; minute volume, carbon dioxide response, inspiratory reserve volume, and residual volume are calculated from the results of other pulmonary function tests; and thoracic gas volume (TGV) is calculated from body plethysmography.

Of the pulmonary capacity tests, vital capacity (VC), inspiratory capacity (IC), functional residual capacity (FRC), total lung capacity, and forced expiratory flow may be measured directly or calculated from the results of other tests. Forced vital capacity (FVC), flow-volume curve, forced expiratory volume (FEV), peak expiratory flow rate, and maximal voluntary ventilation (MVV) are direct spirographic measurements. Diffusing capacity for carbon monoxide ($DL_{CO}$) is calculated from the amount of carbon monoxide exhaled.

## Reference values

■ The following values are predicted for each patient based on age, height, weight, and sex and are expressed as a percentage; results are considered abnormal if they're less than 80% of these values:

– $V_T$, 5 to 7 ml/kg of body weight
– ERV, 25% of VC
– IC, 75% of VC
– $FEV_1$, 83% of VC (after 1 second)
– $FEV_2$, 94% of VC (after 2 seconds)
– $FEV_3$, 97% of VC (after 3 seconds).

## Abnormal results

■ See *Interpreting pulmonary function test results*, pages 396 to 399.

**DRUG CHALLENGE**

Opioid analgesics or sedatives (possible decrease in inspiratory and expiratory forces); bronchodilators (possible temporary improvement in pulmonary function)

## Purpose

■ To determine the cause of dyspnea
■ To assess the effectiveness of specific therapeutic regimens
■ To determine whether a functional abnormality is obstructive or restrictive
■ To measure pulmonary dysfunction

■ To evaluate a patient before surgery
■ To evaluate a person as part of a job screening (firefighting, for example)

## Patient preparation

■ Explain that pulmonary function tests evaluate pulmonary function. Instruct the patient to eat only a light meal and not to smoke for 12 hours before the tests.
■ Describe the tests and equipment. Explain who will perform the tests, where they will take place, and how long they will last.
■ Describe the operation of a spirometer.
■ Advise the patient that the accuracy of the tests depends on his cooperation.
■ Assure the patient that the procedures are painless and that he'll be able to rest between tests.
■ Inform the laboratory if the patient is taking an analgesic that depresses respiration.
■ As ordered, withhold bronchodilators for 8 hours.
■ Just before the test, tell the patient to void and to loosen tight clothing. If he wears dentures, tell him to wear them during the test to help form a seal around the mouthpiece. Advise him to put on the noseclip so that he can adjust to it before the test.

## Procedure and posttest care

■ Confirm the patient's identity using two patient identifiers according to facility policy.
■ When measuring $V_T$, tell the patient to breathe normally into the mouthpiece 10 times.
■ When measuring ERV, tell the patient to breathe normally for several breaths and then to exhale as completely as possible.
■ When measuring VC, tell the patient to inhale as deeply as possible and to exhale into the mouthpiece as completely

*(Text continues on page 400.)*

# Interpreting pulmonary function test results

Pulmonary function test results are interpreted after data are collected and calculated. The implications are reviewed in the chart below.

| Pulmonary function test | Method of calculation | Implications |
|---|---|---|
| **Tidal volume ($V_T$):** Amount of air inhaled or exhaled during normal breathing | Determining the spirographic measurement for 10 breaths and then dividing by 10 | Decreased $V_T$ may indicate restrictive disease and requires further testing, such as full pulmonary function studies or chest X-rays. |
| **Minute volume (MV):** Total amount of air expired per minute | Multiplying $V_T$ by the respiratory rate | Normal MV can occur in emphysema; decreased MV may indicate other diseases such as pulmonary edema. Increased MV can occur with acidosis, increased carbon dioxide ($CO_2$), decreased partial pressure of arterial oxygen, exercise, and low compliance states. |
| **Carbon dioxide ($CO_2$) response:** Increase or decrease in MV after breathing various $CO_2$ concentrations | Plotting changes in MV against increasing inspired $CO_2$ concentrations | Reduced $CO_2$ response may occur in emphysema, myxedema, obesity, hypoventilation syndrome, and sleep apnea. |
| **Inspiratory reserve volume (IRV):** Amount of air inspired over above-normal inspiration | Subtracting $V_T$ from inspiratory capacity (IC) | Abnormal IRV alone doesn't indicate respiratory dysfunction; IRV decreases during normal exercise. |
| **Expiratory reserve volume (ERV):** Amount of air exhaled after normal expiration | Direct spirographic measurement | ERV varies, even in healthy people, but usually decreases in obese people. |

## Interpreting pulmonary function test results *(continued)*

| Pulmonary function test | Method of calculation | Implications |
|---|---|---|
| **Residual volume (RV):** Amount of air remaining in the lungs after forced expiration | Subtracting ERV from functional residual capacity (FRC) | RV > 35% of total lung capacity (TLC) after maximal expiratory effort may indicate obstructive disease. |
| **Vital capacity (VC):** Total volume of air that can be exhaled after maximum inspiration | Direct spirographic measurement or adding $V_T$, IRV, and ERV | Normal or increased VC with decreased flow rates may indicate any condition that causes a reduction in functional pulmonary tissue such as pulmonary edema. Decreased VC with normal or increased flow rates may indicate decreased respiratory effort resulting from neuromuscular disease, drug overdose, or head injury; decreased thoracic expansion; or limited diaphragm movement. |
| **Inspiratory capacity (IC):** Amount of air that can be inhaled after normal expiration | Direct spirographic measurement or adding IRV and $V_T$ | Decreased IC indicates restrictive disease. |
| **Thoracic gas volume (TGV):** Total volume of gas in the lungs from ventilated and nonventilated airways | Body plethysmography | Increased TGV indicates air trapping, which may result from obstructive disease. |
| **Functional residual capacity (FRC):** Amount of air remaining in the lungs after normal expiration | Nitrogen washout, helium dilution technique, or adding ERV and RV | Increased FRC indicates overdistention of the lungs, which may result from obstructive pulmonary disease. |

*(continued)*

## Interpreting pulmonary function test results *(continued)*

| Pulmonary function test | Method of calculation | Implications |
|---|---|---|
| **Total lung capacity (TLC):** Total volume of the lungs when maximally inflated | Adding $V_T$, IRV, ERV, and RV; FRC and IC; or VC and RV | Low TLC indicates restrictive disease; high TLC indicates overdistended lungs caused by obstructive disease. |
| **Forced vital capacity (FVC):** Amount of air exhaled forcefully and quickly after maximum inspiration | Direct spirographic measurement; expressed as a percentage of the total volume of gas exhaled | Decreased FVC indicates flow resistance in the respiratory system from obstructive disease such as chronic bronchitis, or from restrictive disease such as pulmonary fibrosis. |
| **Flow-volume curve (also called flow-volume loop):** Greatest rate of flow ($V_{max}$) during FVC maneuvers versus lung volume change | Direct spirographic measurement at 1-second intervals; calculated from flow rates (expressed in liters per second) and lung volume changes (expressed in liters) during maximal inspiratory and expiratory maneuvers | Decreased flow rates at all volumes during expiration indicate obstructive disease of the small airways such as emphysema. A plateau of expiratory flow near TLC, a plateau of inspiratory flow at mid-VC, and a square wave pattern through most of VC indicate obstructive disease of large airways. Normal or increased PEFR, decreased flow with decreasing lung volumes, and markedly decreased VC indicate restrictive disease. |
| **Forced expiratory volume (FEV):** Volume of air expired in the 1st, 2nd, or 3rd second of an FVC maneuver | Direct spirographic measurement; expressed as a percentage of FVC | Decreased $FEV_1$ and increased $FEV_2$ and $FEV_3$ may indicate obstructive disease; decreased or normal $FEV_1$ may indicate restrictive disease. |

# Interpreting pulmonary function test results *(continued)*

| Pulmonary function test | Method of calculation | Implications |
|---|---|---|
| **Forced expiratory flow (FEF):** Average rate of flow during the middle half of FVC | Calculated from the flow rate and the time needed for expiration of the middle 50% of FVC | Low FEF (25% to 75%) indicates obstructive disease of the small and medium-size airways. |
| **Peak expiratory flow rate (PEFR):** $V_{max}$ during forced expiration | Calculated from the flow-volume curve or by direct spirographic measurement using a pneumotachometer or electronic tachometer with a transducer to convert flow to electrical output display | Decreased PEFR may indicate a mechanical problem, such as upper airway obstruction, or obstructive disease. PEFR is usually normal in restrictive disease but decreases in severe cases. Because PEFR is effort dependent, it's also low in a person who has poor expiratory effort or doesn't understand the procedure. |
| **Maximal voluntary ventilation (MVV) (also called maximum breathing capacity):** The greatest volume of air breathed per unit of time | Direct spirographic measurement | Decreased MVV may indicate obstructive disease; normal or decreased MVV may indicate restrictive disease such as myasthenia gravis. |
| **Diffusing capacity for carbon monoxide ($DL_{CO}$):** Milliliters of carbon monoxide diffused per minute across the alveolocapillary membrane | Calculated from analysis of the amount of carbon monoxide exhaled compared with the amount inhaled | Decreased $DL_{CO}$ due to a thickened alveolocapillary membrane occurs in interstitial pulmonary diseases, such as pulmonary fibrosis, asbestosis, and sarcoidosis; $DL_{CO}$ is reduced in emphysema because of alveolocapillary membrane loss. |

as possible. This procedure is repeated three times, and the test result showing the largest volume is used.

■ When measuring IC, tell the patient to breathe normally for several breaths and then to inhale as deeply as possible.

■ When measuring FRC, tell the patient to breathe normally into a spirometer that contains a known concentration of an insoluble gas (usually helium or nitrogen) in a known volume of air. After a few breaths, the concentrations of gas in the spirometer and in the lungs reach equilibrium. Then the point of equilibrium and the concentration of gas in the spirometer are recorded.

■ When measuring TGV, be aware that the patient is put in an airtight box (or body plethysmograph) and told to breathe through a tube connected to a transducer. At end-expiration, the tube is occluded, the patient is told to pant, and changes in intrathoracic and plethysmographic pressures are measured. The results are used to calculate total TGV and FRC.

■ When measuring FVC and FEV, tell the patient to inhale as slowly and deeply as possible and then exhale into the mouthpiece as quickly and completely as possible. This procedure is repeated three times, and the largest volume is recorded. The volume of air expired at 1 second ($FEV_1$), at 2 seconds ($FEV_2$), and at 3 seconds ($FEV_3$) during all three repetitions is also recorded.

■ When measuring MVV, tell the patient to breathe into the mouthpiece as quickly and deeply as possible for 15 seconds.

■ When measuring $DL_{CO}$, the patient inhales a gas mixture with a low concentration of carbon monoxide and then holds his breath for 10 seconds before exhaling.

■ After the tests, instruct the patient to resume his usual activities, diet, and medications as ordered.

### Precautions

■ Pulmonary function tests are contraindicated in the patient with acute coronary insufficiency, angina, or recent myocardial infarction.

### Complications

■ Respiratory distress or bronchospasm

## Radiography

 ## Chest radiography
[chest X-ray, CXR]

In chest radiography, X-rays or electromagnetic waves penetrate the chest and cause an image to form on specially sensitized film. Normal pulmonary tissue is radiolucent, whereas abnormalities—such as infiltrates, foreign bodies, fluids, and tumors—appear as densities on the film. A chest X-ray is most useful when compared with previous films to detect changes.

### Normal and abnormal results

■ For an overview of normal and abnormal chest radiography findings, see *Selected clinical implications of chest X-ray films.*

■ For an accurate diagnosis, radiography findings must be correlated with the results of additional radiologic and pulmonary tests as well as physical assessment findings.

### Purpose

■ To detect pulmonary disorders, such as pneumonia, atelectasis, pneumothorax, pulmonary bullae, pleurisy, and tumors

■ To detect mediastinal abnormalities, such as tumors, and cardiac disease such as heart failure

# Selected clinical implications of chest X-ray films

| Normal anatomic location and appearance | Possible abnormality | Implications |
|---|---|---|
| **Trachea** Visible midline in the anterior mediastinal cavity; translucent tubelike appearance | ▪ Deviation from midline | ▪ Tension pneumothorax, atelectasis, pleural effusion, consolidation, mediastinal nodes or, in children, enlarged thymus |
| | ▪ Narrowing with hourglass appearance and deviation to one side | ▪ Substernal thyroid or stenosis secondary to trauma |
| **Heart** Visible in the anterior left mediastinal cavity; solid appearance due to blood contents; edges may be clear in contrast with surrounding air density of the lung | ▪ Shift ▪ Hypertrophy of right heart ▪ Cardiac borders obscured by stringy densities ("shaggy heart") | ▪ Atelectasis, pneumothorax ▪ Cor pulmonale, heart failure ▪ Cystic fibrosis |
| **Aortic knob** Visible as water density; formed by the arch of the aorta | ▪ Solid densities, possibly indicating calcifications ▪ Tortuous shape | ▪ Atherosclerosis ▪ Atherosclerosis |
| **Mediastinum (mediastinal shadow)** Visible as the space between the lungs; shadowy appearance that widens at the hilum of the lungs | ▪ Deviation to nondiseased side; deviation to diseased side by traction ▪ Gross widening | ▪ Pleural effusion or tumor, fibrosis or collapsed lung ▪ Neoplasms of esophagus, bronchi, lungs, thyroid, thymus, peripheral nerves, lymphoid tissue; aortic aneurysm; mediastinitis; cor pulmonale |
| **Ribs** Visible as thoracic cavity encasement | ▪ Break or misalignment ▪ Widening of intercostal spaces | ▪ Fractured sternum or ribs ▪ Emphysema |
| **Spine** Visible midline in the posterior chest; straight bony structure | ▪ Spinal curvature ▪ Break or misalignment | ▪ Scoliosis, kyphosis ▪ Fractures |

*(continued)*

# Selected clinical implications of chest X-ray films *(continued)*

| Normal anatomic location and appearance | Possible abnormality | Implications |
|---|---|---|
| **Clavicles**<br>Visible in upper thorax; intact and equidistant in properly centered X-ray films | ▪ Break or misalignment | ▪ Fractures |
| **Hila (lung roots)**<br>Visible above the heart, where pulmonary vessels, bronchi, and lymph nodes join the lungs; appear as small, white, bilateral densities | ▪ Shift to one side<br>▪ Accentuated shadows | ▪ Atelectasis<br>▪ Pneumothorax, emphysema, pulmonary abscess, tumor, enlarged lymph nodes |
| **Mainstem bronchus**<br>Visible; part of the hila with translucent tubelike appearance | ▪ Spherical or oval density | ▪ Bronchogenic cyst |
| **Bronchi**<br>Usually not visible | ▪ Visible | ▪ Bronchial pneumonia |
| **Lung fields**<br>Usually not visible throughout, except for the blood vessels | ▪ Visible<br>▪ Irregular | ▪ Atelectasis<br>▪ Resolving pneumonia, infiltrates, silicosis, fibrosis, metastatic neoplasm |
| **Hemidiaphragm**<br>Rounded, visible; right side ⅜″ to ¾″ (1 to 2 cm) | ▪ Elevation of diaphragm (difference in elevation can be measured on inspiration and expiration to detect movement)<br>▪ Flattening of diaphragm<br>▪ Unilateral elevation of either side<br>▪ Unilateral elevation of left side only | ▪ Active tuberculosis, pneumonia, pleurisy, acute bronchitis, active disease of the abdominal viscera, bilateral phrenic nerve involvement, atelectasis<br>▪ Asthma, emphysema<br><br>▪ Possible unilateral phrenic nerve paresis<br>▪ Perforated ulcer (rare), gas distention of stomach or splenic flexure of colon, free air in abdomen |

- To determine the correct placement of pulmonary catheters, endotracheal tubes, and other chest tubes
- To determine the location and size of lesions or foreign bodies (coins, broken central lines) that were swallowed or aspirated
- To help assess pulmonary status
- To evaluate the patient's response to interventions

### Patient preparation

- Explain that chest radiography assesses respiratory status.
- Tell the patient that he doesn't need to restrict food and fluids.
- Describe the test, including who will perform it and when it will take place.
- Provide a gown without snaps, and instruct the patient to remove jewelry and other metallic objects that may be in the X-ray field.
- Explain to the patient that he'll be asked to take a deep breath and to hold it momentarily while the film is being taken to provide a clearer view of pulmonary structures.

### Procedure and posttest care

- Confirm the patient's identity using two patient identifiers according to facility policy.
- If a stationary X-ray machine is used, the patient stands or sits in front of the machine so films can be taken of the posteroanterior and left lateral views.
- If a portable X-ray machine is used at the patient's bedside, the patient is moved to the top of the bed, if his tolerance permits. The head of the bed is elevated for maximum upright positioning.
- Place cardiac monitoring lead wires, I.V. tubing from central lines, pulmonary artery catheter lines, and safety pins as far from the X-ray field as possible.

### Precautions

- Chest radiography is usually contraindicated during the first trimester of pregnancy; however, when radiography is absolutely necessary, a lead apron placed over the patient's abdomen can shield the fetus.
- If the patient is intubated, check that no tubes have been dislodged during positioning.
- To avoid exposure to radiation, leave the room or the immediate area while the films are being taken. If you must stay in the area, wear a lead-lined apron or protective clothing.
- Portable films are usually less reliable than stationary radiographs.

### Complications

- Dislodgement of tubes or wires during positioning

# Chest tomography

Also called laminagraphy, planigraphy, stratigraphy, or body section roentgenography, chest tomography provides clearly focused radiographic images of selected body sections otherwise obscured by shadows of overlying or underlying structures. In this procedure, the X-ray tube and film move around the patient in opposite directions (a motion called the linear tube sweep), producing exposures in which a selected body plane appears sharply defined and the areas above and below it are blurred. Some facilities have spiral computed tomography (CT) available. (See *Spiral CT,* page 404.) It's used to further evaluate chest lesions when other tests are inconclusive.

### Normal results

- Normal results reveal structures equivalent to those seen on a normal chest radiograph film.

# Spiral CT

The spiral (helical) computed tomography (CT) scan is produced while the X-ray tube rotates continuously around the patient, forming a spiral path through the patient. This path represents a contiguous volumetric data set, covering a specific volume of the patient's anatomy with no spatial or temporal gaps. The patient continuously moves through the slip-ring gantry, and no two data points are taken in exactly the same plane.

Benefits include increased speed (spiral CT is typically 8 to 10 times faster than conventional CT), improved image quality and diagnostic accuracy, and reduced radiation exposure. The improved speed—the scan can usually be obtained during a single breath hold—is especially beneficial for elderly, pediatric, and critically ill patients, in whom scanning commonly proves difficult.

There are disadvantages. Spiral CT delivers a limited amount of milliamperes, which can result in a grainier image than conventional CT (more common in larger patients). In addition, artifacts ("pseudothrombi") can be created in the infrahepatic inferior vena cava by the admixture of unopacified blood and contrast medium flowing in from the renal veins. These disadvantages are being resolved with improved equipment and technique.

## Abnormal results

- Central calcification in a nodule suggests a benign lesion; an irregularly bordered tumor suggests malignancy.
- A sharply defined tumor suggests granuloma or nonmalignancy.
- Evaluation of the hilum can help differentiate blood vessels from nodes, detect tumor extension into the hilar lung area, and identify bronchial dilation, stenosis, and endobronchial lesions.

- Extension of a mediastinal lesion to the ribs or spine is abnormal.

### Purpose

- To demonstrate pulmonary densities (for cavitation, calcification, and presence of fat), tumors (especially those obstructing the bronchial lumen), or lesions (especially those located deep within the mediastinum such as at lymph nodes at the hilum)
- To evaluate severity of disease such as emphysema

### Patient preparation

- Explain that chest tomography helps evaluate lesions inside the chest.
- Describe the test, including who will perform it and where it will take place.
- Tell the patient that he doesn't need to restrict food and fluids.
- Warn the patient that the equipment is noisy because of rapidly moving metal-on-metal parts and that the X-ray tube swings overhead.
- Advise the patient to breathe normally during the test, but to remain immobile; tell him that foam wedges will be used to help him maintain a comfortable, motionless position.
- Tell the patient to close his eyes to prevent involuntary movement.
- Instruct the patient to remove all jewelry and metallic objects within the X-ray field.

### Procedure and posttest care

- Confirm the patient's identity using two patient identifiers according to facility policy.
- The patient is placed in a supine position or in different degrees of lateral rotation on the X-ray table. The X-ray tube then swings over the patient, taking numerous films from different angles.
- For lung tomography, the X-ray tube is usually moved in a linear direction, but may be moved in a hypocycloid, circu-

lar, elliptic, trispiral, or figure-eight pattern. Multidirectional films help diagnose mediastinal lesions or tumors.

### Precautions
▪ Tomography is contraindicated during pregnancy.
▪ To avoid exposure to radiation, leave the room or the immediate area during the test; if you must stay in the area, wear a lead-lined apron.

# Paranasal sinus radiography

In paranasal sinus radiography, X-rays or electromagnetic waves penetrate the paranasal sinuses and react on specially sensitized film, forming a film image that differentiates sinus structures.

When surrounding facial structures that are superimposed on the paranasal sinuses interfere with visualization of relevant areas, computed tomography scanning may be performed to provide further information.

### Normal results
▪ Paranasal sinuses are radiolucent and filled with air, which appears black on films.

### Abnormal results
▪ For an overview of abnormal results, see *Abnormal findings in paranasal sinus radiography,* page 406.

### Purpose
▪ To detect unilateral or bilateral abnormalities, possibly indicating trauma or disease
▪ To confirm diagnosis of neoplastic or inflammatory paranasal sinus disease
▪ To determine the location and size of a malignant neoplasm

### Patient preparation
▪ Explain that paranasal sinus radiography helps evaluate abnormalities of the paranasal sinuses.
▪ Describe the test, including who will perform it and where it will take place.
▪ Tell the patient that his head may be immobilized in a foam vise during the test to help him maintain the correct position, but that the vise doesn't hurt.
▪ Explain to the patient that he'll be asked to sit upright and avoid moving while the X-rays are being taken to prevent blurring of the image and to allow visualization of air-fluid levels, if present. Emphasize the importance of his cooperation.
▪ Instruct the patient to remove dentures, all jewelry, and metallic objects in the X-ray field.

### Procedure and posttest care
▪ Confirm the patient's identity using two patient identifiers according to facility policy.
▪ Have the patient sit upright (his head may be placed in a foam vise) between the X-ray tube and a film cassette.
▪ During the test, the X-ray tube is positioned at specific angles and the patient's head is placed in various standard positions while his paranasal sinuses are filmed from different angles. If necessary, assist with positioning the patient.

### Precautions
▪ Paranasal sinus radiography is usually contraindicated during pregnancy; however, when it's absolutely necessary, a lead-lined apron placed over the patient's abdomen can shield the fetus.
▪ To avoid exposure to radiation, leave the room or the immediate area during the test; if you must stay in the area, wear a lead-lined apron.
▪ If the patient is wearing dentures, jewelry, or other metallic objects in the X-ray field, it may cause poor imaging.

# Abnormal findings in paranasal sinus radiography

| Disorder | Abnormal findings |
|---|---|
| Paranasal sinus trauma or fracture | ▪ Edema or hemorrhage in mucous membrane lining or sinus cavity<br>▪ Clouded sinus air cells<br>▪ Air-fluid level<br>▪ Radiolucent, linear bone defects<br>▪ Irregular, overriding bone edges<br>▪ Depression or displacement of bone fragments<br>▪ Foreign bodies |
| Acute sinusitis | ▪ Swollen, inflamed mucous membrane<br>▪ Inflammatory exudate<br>▪ Hazy to opaque sinus air cells<br>▪ Air-fluid level |
| Chronic sinusitis | ▪ Thickening or sclerosis of bony wall of affected sinus |
| Wegener's granulomatosis | ▪ Clouded to opaque sinus air cells<br>▪ Destruction of bony sinus wall |
| Malignant neoplasm | ▪ Rounded or lobulated soft-tissue mass, projecting into sinus<br>▪ Destruction of bony sinus wall |
| Benign bone tumor | ▪ Distortion of bony sinus wall in specific patterns |
| Cyst, polyp, or benign tumor | ▪ Rounded or lobulated soft-tissue mass, projecting into sinus |
| Mucocele | ▪ Clouded sinus air cells<br>▪ Destruction of bony sinus wall resulting in various degrees of radiolucency |

# Pulmonary angiography
[pulmonary arteriography]

Pulmonary angiography is the radiographic examination of the pulmonary circulation following injection of a radiopaque iodine contrast agent into the pulmonary artery or one of its branches.

## Normal results
▪ Contrast agent flows symmetrically and without interruption through the pulmonary circulatory system.

## Abnormal results
▪ Interruption of blood flow may result from emboli and from other types of pulmonary vascular abnormalities or tumors.

## Purpose

- To detect pulmonary embolism in a patient who is equivocal
- To evaluate pulmonary circulation abnormalities
- To evaluate pulmonary circulation preoperatively in the patient with congenital heart disease
- To locate a large embolus before surgical removal

## Patient preparation

- Describe the pulmonary angiography procedure to the patient. Explain that this test permits evaluation of the blood vessels to help identify the cause of his symptoms.
- Instruct the patient to fast for 8 hours before the test or as prescribed. Tell him who will perform the test, where it will take place, and that laboratory work for kidney function and coagulation may precede the test.
- Tell the patient that a small puncture will be made in the blood vessel of his right arm where blood samples are usually drawn, or in the right groin at the femoral vein, and that a local anesthetic will be used to numb the area. Inform him that a small catheter will then be inserted into the blood vessel and passed into the right side of the heart to the pulmonary artery.
- Tell the patient the contrast medium will then be injected into this artery. Warn him that he may feel flushed, experience an urge to cough, or experience a salty taste for about 3 to 5 minutes after the injection.
- Inform the patient that his heart rate will be monitored continuously during the procedure and that he should tell the physician or nurse if he has concerns.
- Make sure that the patient or a responsible family member has signed an informed consent form. Check the patient's history for hypersensitivity to anesthetics, iodine, seafood, or radiographic contrast agents.
- Obtain or check laboratory tests (including prothrombin time, partial thromboplastin time, platelet count, and blood urea nitrogen [BUN] and serum creatinine levels), and notify the radiologist of any abnormal results. I.V. hydration may need to be considered depending on the patient's renal and cardiac status. The radiologist may want to discontinue a heparin drip 3 to 4 hours before the test.

## Procedure and posttest care

- Confirm the patient's identity using two patient identifiers according to facility policy.
- After the patient is placed in a supine position, the local anesthetic is injected, and the cardiac monitor is attached to the patient. Blood pressure and pulse oximeter are monitored as per facility protocol.
- A puncture is made at the procedure site, and a catheter is introduced into the antecubital or femoral vein. As the catheter passes through the right atrium, the right ventricle, and the pulmonary artery, pressures are measured and blood samples are drawn from various regions of the pulmonary circulation.
- The contrast medium is injected and circulates through the pulmonary artery and lung capillaries while X-rays are taken.
- Apply pressure over the catheter insertion site for 15 to 20 minutes or until bleeding stops.
- Maintain bed rest for about 6 hours.
- Observe the site for bleeding and swelling.

### ACTION STAT!

 If the catheter insertion site begins to bleed, maintain pressure at the insertion site for 10 minutes, and notify the practitioner.

- Check the patient's blood pressure and pulse rate and the catheter insertion site (arm or groin) every 15 minutes for 1 hour, every hour for 4 hours, and then every 4 hours for 16 hours.
- Observe the patient for signs of myocardial perforation or rupture by monitoring vital signs.
- Be alert for signs of acute renal failure, such as sudden onset of oliguria, nausea, and vomiting. Check BUN and serum creatinine levels.
- Check the catheter insertion site for inflammation or hematoma formation, and report symptoms of a delayed hypersensitivity response to the contrast agent or to the local anesthetic (dyspnea, itching, tachycardia, palpitations, hypotension or hypertension, excitation, or euphoria).
- Advise the patient about any restriction of activity. Tell him that he may resume his usual diet after the test (encourage him to drink lots of fluids), or give I.V. fluids, as ordered, to flush the contrast agent from his body.

### Precautions

- Pulmonary angiography is contraindicated during pregnancy.
- Monitor the patient for ventricular arrhythmias due to myocardial irritation from passage of the catheter through the heart chambers.
- Observe for signs of hypersensitivity to the contrast agent, such as dyspnea, nausea, vomiting, sweating, increased heart rate, and numbness of extremities.

<small>**Do's & don'ts**</small>

 Keep emergency equipment available in case of a hypersensitivity reaction to the contrast agent.

- Measure pulmonary artery pressures. Right ventricular end-diastolic pressure is usually less than or equal to 20 mm

Hg, and pulmonary artery systolic pressure is usually less than or equal to 70 mm Hg. Pressures greater than this increase the risk of mortality associated with this procedure.

### Complications

- Myocardial perforation or rupture, ventricular arrhythmias and conduction defects, cardiac valve damage, or right-sided heart failure
- Acute renal failure.
- Bleeding, hematoma formation, infection, or an adverse reaction to the contrast medium.

# Scanning

## Lung perfusion scan

A lung perfusion scan produces an image of pulmonary blood flow after I.V. injection of a radiopharmaceutical, either human serum albumin microspheres or macroaggregated albumin bonded to technetium.

### Normal results

- The lung shows a uniform uptake pattern.
- Areas with normal blood perfusion, called *hot spots*, show a high uptake of the radioactive substance.

### Abnormal results

- Areas of low radioactive uptake, called *cold spots*, indicate poor perfusion.
- Decreased regional blood flow that occurs without vessel obstruction may indicate pneumonitis.

### Purpose

- To assess arterial perfusion of the lungs
- To detect pulmonary emboli
- To evaluate pulmonary function before lung resection

## Patient preparation

- Explain that the lung perfusion scan helps evaluate respiratory function.
- Tell the patient that he doesn't need to restrict food and fluids.
- Describe the test to the patient, including who will perform it and where it will take place.
- Tell the patient that a radiopharmaceutical will be injected into a vein in his arm and that he'll then sit in front of a camera or lie under it. Explain that neither the camera nor the uptake probe emits radiation and that the amount of radioactivity in the radiopharmaceutical is minimal.
- Assure the patient that he'll be comfortable during the test and that he doesn't have to remain perfectly still.
- On the test request, note if the patient has conditions, such as chronic obstructive pulmonary disease (COPD), vasculitis, pulmonary edema, tumor, sickle cell disease, or parasitic disease.
- Make sure that the patient or a responsible family member has signed an informed consent form, if required.

## Procedure and posttest care

- Confirm the patient's identity using two patient identifiers according to facility policy.
- With the patient supine and taking moderately deep breaths, the radiopharmaceutical is injected I.V. slowly over 5 to 10 seconds to allow more even distribution of pulmonary blood flow.
- After the injection, the gamma camera takes a series of single stationary images in the anterior, posterior, oblique, and both lateral chest views.
- Images, which are projected on an oscilloscope screen, show the distribution of radioactive particles.
- If a hematoma develops at the injection site, apply warm soaks.

## Precautions

- A lung scan is contraindicated in the patient who's hypersensitive to the radiopharmaceutical.
- Conditions, such as COPD, vasculitis, pulmonary edema, tumor, sickle cell disease, and parasitic disease may cause possible poor imaging.

## Complications

- Hematoma at the injection site
- Sensitivity to the radiopharmaceutical used in the procedure

# Lung ventilation scan

The lung ventilation scan is performed after the patient inhales a mixture of air and radioactive gas that delineates areas of the lung ventilated during respiration. The scan records gas distribution during three phases: the buildup of radioactive gas (wash-in phase), the time after rebreathing when radioactivity reaches a steady level (equilibrium phase), and after removal of the radioactive gas from the lungs (wash-out phase).

## Normal results

- The test should indicate an equal distribution of gas in both lungs and normal wash-in and wash-out phases.

## Abnormal results

- Unequal gas distribution in both lungs indicates poor ventilation or airway obstruction in areas with low radioactivity.
- When compared with a lung scan (perfusion scan), in vascular obstructions—such as pulmonary embolism—the perfusion to the embolized area is decreased, but the ventilation to this area is maintained.
- In parenchymal disease, such as pneumonia, ventilation is abnormal within the areas of consolidation.

## Purpose
- To help diagnose pulmonary emboli
- To identify areas of the lung capable of ventilation
- To help evaluate regional respiratory function
- To locate regional hypoventilation, which may indicate atelectasis, obstructing tumors, or chronic obstructive pulmonary disease

## Patient preparation
- Describe the lung ventilation scan to the patient, and explain that this test helps evaluate respiratory function.
- Tell the patient that he doesn't need to restrict food and fluids.
- Tell the patient who will perform the test and where it will take place.
- Ask the patient to remove all jewelry and metal objects from the scanning field.
- Explain to the patient that he'll be asked to hold his breath for a short time after inhaling a gas and to remain still while a machine scans his chest.
- Reassure the patient that a minimal amount of radioactive gas is used.
- Make sure that the patient or a responsible family member has signed an informed consent form, if required.

## Procedure and posttest care
- Confirm the patient's identity using two patient identifiers according to facility policy.
- After the patient inhales air mixed with a small amount of radioactive gas through a mask, its distribution in the lungs is monitored on a nuclear scanner.
- The patient's chest is scanned as he exhales.

## Precautions
- Watch for leaks in the closed system of radioactive gas, such as through the mask, which can contaminate the surrounding atmosphere.

## Complications
- Panic attacks from wearing the tight-fitting mask in this procedure

# Thoracic computed tomography

Thoracic computed tomography (CT) provides cross-sectional views of the chest by passing an X-ray beam from a computerized scanner through the body at different angles. CT scanning may be done with or without an injected contrast medium, which is primarily used to highlight blood vessels and to allow greater visual discrimination.

This test provides a three-dimensional image and is especially useful in detecting small differences in tissue density. The thoracic CT scan may replace mediastinoscopy in the diagnosis of mediastinal masses and Hodgkin's disease; its value in the evaluation of pulmonary pathology is proven.

## Normal results
- Black and white areas on a thoracic CT scan refer, respectively, to air and bone densities.
- Shades of gray correspond to water, fat, and soft-tissue densities.

## Abnormal results
- Abnormal thoracic CT scan results include tumors, nodules, cysts, aortic aneurysms, enlarged lymph nodes, pleural effusion, and accumulations of blood, fluid, or fat.

## Purpose
- To locate suspected neoplasms (such as in Hodgkin's disease), especially with mediastinal involvement
- To differentiate coin-size calcified lesions (indicating tuberculosis) from tumors
- To differentiate emphysema or bronchopleural fistula from lung abscess

- To distinguish tumors adjacent to the aorta from aortic aneurysms
- To detect the invasion of a neck mass in the thorax
- To evaluate primary malignancy that may metastasize to the lungs, especially in the patient with a primary bone tumor, soft-tissue sarcoma, or melanoma
- To evaluate the mediastinal lymph nodes
- To evaluate the severity of lung disease such as emphysema
- To detect a dissection or leak of an aortic aneurysm or aortic arch aneurysm
- To plan radiation treatment

### Patient preparation

- Explain that the thoracic CT provides cross-sectional views of the chest and distinguishes small differences in tissue density.
- If a contrast medium won't be used, inform the patient that he doesn't need to restrict food and fluids. If the test is to be performed with contrast enhancement, instruct him to fast for 4 hours before the test.
- Tell the patient who will perform the test and where it will take place.
- Inform the patient that he'll be positioned on an X-ray table that moves into the center of a large ring-shaped piece of X-ray equipment and that the equipment may be noisy.
- Inform the patient that a contrast medium may be injected into a vein in his arm. If so, he may experience nausea, warmth, flushing of the face, and a salty or metallic taste. Reassure him that these symptoms are normal and that radiation exposure is minimal.
- Tell the patient not to move during the test, but to breathe normally until told to follow specific breathing instructions. Instruct him to remove all jewelry and metallic objects in the X-ray field.

- Check the patient's history for hypersensitivity to iodine, shellfish, or contrast media.
- Make sure that the patient or a responsible family member has signed an informed consent form, if required.

### Procedure and posttest care

- Confirm the patient's identity using two patient identifiers according to facility policy.
- After the patient is placed in a supine position on the X-ray table and the contrast medium has been injected, the machine scans the patient at different angles while the computer calculates small differences in the densities of various tissues, water, fat, bone, and air.
- This information is displayed as a printout of numerical values and as a projection on a monitor. Images may be recorded for further study.

**ALERT**

Watch the patient for signs of delayed hypersensitivity to the contrast medium (itching, hypotension or hypertension, or respiratory distress).

- After the test, encourage the patient to drink lots of fluids.

### Precautions

- Thoracic CT scanning is contraindicated during pregnancy.
- The test is also contraindicated—if a contrast medium is used—in a person who has a history of hypersensitivity reactions to iodine, shellfish, or contrast media.

### Complications

- Adverse effects from contrast medium

# Skeletal system

## 24

24

## Radiography and nuclear medicine

### ▌Arthrography

Arthrography allows radiographic examination of a joint after injection of a radiopaque dye, air, or both (double-contrast arthrogram) to outline soft-tissue structures and the contour of the joint. The joint is put through its range of motion while a series of radiographs are taken.

#### Normal results
■ A knee arthrogram shows characteristic wedge-shaped shadow, pointed toward the interior of the joint, which indicates a normal medial meniscus.
■ A shoulder arthrogram shows the bicipital tendon sheath, redundant inferior joint capsule, and subscapular bursa intact.

#### Abnormal results
■ Medial meniscal tears and lacerations are detected.
■ Extrameniscal lesions, such as osteochondritis dissecans, chondromalacia patellae, osteochondral fractures, cartilaginous abnormalities, synovial abnormalities, tears of the cruciate ligaments, and disruption of the joint capsule and collateral ligaments are observed.

■ Shoulder abnormalities, such as adhesive capsulitis, bicipital tenosynovitis or rupture, and rotator cuff tears are present.
■ Damage from recurrent dislocations is observed.

#### Purpose
■ To identify acute or chronic tears or other abnormalities of the joint capsule or supporting ligaments of the knee, shoulder, ankle, hips, or wrist
■ To detect internal joint derangements
■ To locate synovial cysts

#### Patient preparation
■ Describe arthrography to the patient, and answer any questions he may have. Explain that this test permits examination of a joint.
■ Inform the patient that he need not restrict food and fluids.
■ Tell the patient who will perform the procedure and where it will take place.
■ Explain that the fluoroscope allows the physician to track the contrast medium as it fills the joint space.
■ Inform the patient that standard X-ray films will also be taken after diffusion of the contrast medium.
■ Tell the patient that although the joint area will be anesthetized, he may experience a tingling sensation or pressure in the joint when the contrast medium is injected.

- Instruct the patient to remain as still as possible during the procedure, except when following instructions to change position.
- Stress to the patient the importance of his cooperation in assuming various positions because films must be taken as quickly as possible to ensure optimum quality.
- Check the patient's history to determine if he's hypersensitive to local anesthetics, iodine, seafood, or dyes used for other diagnostic tests.

### Procedure and posttest care

- Confirm the patient's identity using two patient identifiers according to facility policy.

#### Knee arthrography

- The knee is cleaned with an antiseptic solution, and the area around the puncture site is anesthetized. (It isn't usually necessary to anesthetize the joint space itself.)
- A 2″ needle is then inserted into the joint space between the patella and femoral condyle, and fluid is aspirated. The aspirated fluid is usually sent to the laboratory for analysis.
- While the needle is still in place, the aspirating syringe is removed and replaced with a syringe containing dye.
- If fluoroscopic examination demonstrates correct placement of the needle, the dye is injected into the joint space.
- After the needle is removed, the site is rubbed with a sterile sponge, and the wound may be sealed with collodion.
- The patient is asked to walk a few steps or to move his knee through a range of motion to distribute the dye in the joint space. A film series is taken quickly with the knee held in various positions.
- If the films are clean and demonstrate proper dye placement, the knee is bandaged, possibly with an elastic bandage.

- Tell the patient to keep the bandage in place for several days, and teach him how to rewrap it.

#### Shoulder arthrography

- The skin is prepared, and a local anesthetic is injected subcutaneously just in front of the acromioclavicular joint.
- Additional anesthetic is injected directly onto the head of the humerus.
- The short lumbar puncture needle is inserted until the point is embedded in the joint cartilage.
- The stylet is removed, a syringe of contrast medium is attached and, using fluoroscopic guidance, about 1 ml of dye is injected into the joint space, as the needle is withdrawn slightly.
- If fluoroscopic examination demonstrates correct needle placement, the rest of the dye is injected while the needle is slowly withdrawn, and the site is wiped with a sterile sponge.
- A film series is taken quickly to achieve maximum contrast.

#### Both types

- Tell the patient to rest the joint for at least 12 hours.
- Inform the patient that he may experience some swelling or discomfort or may hear crepitant noises in the joint after the test, but that these symptoms usually disappear after 1 or 2 days; tell him to report persistent symptoms.
- Advise the patient to apply ice to the joint if swelling occurs and to take a mild analgesic for pain.
- Instruct the patient to report any signs of infection at the needle insertion site, such as warmth, redness, swelling, or foul-smelling drainage.

### Precautions

- Arthrography is contraindicated during pregnancy and in the patient with active arthritis, joint infection, or previous sensitivity to radiopaque media.

## Complications

- Hypersensitivity reactions to contrast medium
- Infection
- Persistent joint swelling or crepitus

# Bone densitometry
[DEXA scan]

Bone densitometry assesses bone mass quantitatively. This noninvasive technique, also known as dual energy X-ray absorptiometry, uses an X-ray tube to measure bone mineral density, but exposes the patient to only minimal radiation. The images detected are computer-analyzed to determine bone mineral status. The computer calculates the size and thickness of the bone as well as its volumetric density to determine its potential resistance to mechanical stress. It may be performed in the radiology department of a hospital, a physician's office, or a clinic.

The value and reliability of bone densitometry as a predictor of fractures are under investigation. Also, large-scale studies are being conducted to establish an "at-risk" level of bone density to help predict fractures.

### Normal results

- Computer-analyzed results of the bone densitometry scan are within normal limits for the patient's age, sex, and height. (See *Bone densitometry*.)
- The patient's rate of bone loss can be trended over time.
- T-score above −1 is normal.

### Abnormal results

- T-score between −1 and −2.5 may suggest osteopenia.
- T-score at or below −2.5 may suggest osteoporosis.

### Purpose

- To determine bone mineral density
- To identify the risk of osteoporosis
- To evaluate clinical response to therapy for reducing the rate of bone loss

### Patient preparation

- Reassure the patient that the bone densitometry test is painless and that the exposure to radiation is minimal.
- Tell the patient that the test will take from 10 minutes to 1 hour, depending on the areas to be scanned.
- Tell the patient who will perform the test and where it will take place.

### Procedure and posttest care

- Instruct the patient to remove all metallic objects from the area to be scanned.
- The patient is positioned on a table under the scanning device, with the radiation source below and the detector above. The detector measures the bone's

## Bone densitometry

These illustrations show the difference between normal bone and a bone with osteoporosis. The osteoporotic bone has much less density, making it less resistant to trauma.

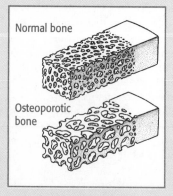

Normal bone

Osteoporotic bone

© 2007 Lippincott Williams & Wilkins. Courtesy of Neil O. Hardy, Westpoint, Connecticut.

radiation absorption and produces a digital readout.

## Precautions

- Bone densitometry is contraindicated during pregnancy.
- Osteoarthritis, fractures, the size of the region being scanned, and the fat tissue distribution all influence the accuracy of the test results.

 # Bone scan

A bone scan involves imaging the skeleton by a scanning camera after I.V. injection of a radioactive tracer compound. The tracer of choice, radioactive technetium diphosphonate, collects in bone tissue in increased concentrations at sites of abnormal metabolism. When scanned, these sites appear as hot spots that are typically detectable months before an X-ray can reveal a lesion. To promote early detection of lesions, this test may be performed with a gallium scan.

### Normal results

- The tracer concentrates in bone tissue at sites of new bone formation or increased metabolism.
- The epiphyses of growing bone are normal sites of high concentration.

### Abnormal results

- Increased uptake of the tracer where bone formation is occurring faster than in surrounding bone may suggest bone cancer, infection, fracture, or other disorders, when considered in light of the patient's medical and surgical history, X-rays, and other laboratory tests.

**DRUG CHALLENGE**

 Antihypertensives (invalidate test results)

## Purpose

- To detect or to rule out malignant bone lesions when radiographic findings are normal but cancer is confirmed or suspected
- To detect occult bone trauma due to pathologic fractures
- To monitor degenerative bone disorders
- To detect infection
- To evaluate unexplained bone pain
- To stage cancer

### Patient preparation

- Describe the bone scan procedure to the patient. Explain that this test may detect skeletal abnormalities sooner than is possible with ordinary X-rays.
- Tell the patient who will perform the test, where it will take place, and that he may have to assume various positions on a scanner table. Emphasize that he must keep still for the scan.
- Assure the patient that the scan itself is painless and that the isotope, although radioactive, emits less radiation than a standard X-ray machine.
- Make sure that the patient or a responsible family member has signed an informed consent form, if required.
- If a bone scan is ordered to diagnose cancer, evaluate the patient's emotional state and offer support.
- Give prescribed analgesics.
- After the patient receives an I.V. injection of the tracer and imaging agent, encourage him to increase his intake of fluids for the next 1 to 3 hours to facilitate renal clearance of the circulating free tracer.

### Procedure and posttest care

- Confirm the patient's identity using two patient identifiers according to facility policy.
- The patient receives an I.V. injection of tracer and imaging agent. Encourage in-

creased fluids for the next 1 to 3 hours to facilitate renal clearance.

■ Instruct the patient to void immediately before the procedure (otherwise, a urinary catheter may be inserted to empty the bladder), and then position him on the scanner table.

■ As the scanner head moves back and forth over the patient's body, it detects low-level radiation emitted by the skeleton and translates this into a film, paper chart, or both to produce two-dimensional pictures of the area scanned.

■ If appropriate, assist with repositioning the patient several times during the test to obtain adequate views. (The scanner takes as many views as needed to cover the specified area.)

■ Anticipate the need to sedate children who can't hold still for the scan.

■ Check the injection site for redness or swelling. If a hematoma develops, apply warm soaks.

■ Don't schedule other radionuclide tests for 24 to 48 hours.

■ Instruct the patient to drink lots of fluids and to empty his bladder frequently for the next 24 to 48 hours.

■ Provide analgesics for pain resulting from positioning on the scanning table as needed.

### Precautions

■ To avoid exposing the fetus or infant to radiation, a bone scan is contraindicated during pregnancy or lactation.

### Complications

■ Allergic reaction to the radionuclide used in the test
■ Infection at the injection site

# Scanning

## Skeletal computed tomography

Skeletal computed tomography (CT) provides a series of tomograms, translated by a computer and displayed on a monitor, representing cross-sectional images of various layers (or slices) of bone. This technique can reconstruct cross-sectional, horizontal, sagittal, and coronal plane images.

Taking collimated (parallel) radiographs increases the number of radiation density calculations the computer makes, thereby improving the degree of resolution and thus specificity and accuracy. Hundreds of thousands of readings of radiation levels absorbed by tissues may be combined to depict anatomic slices of varying thickness.

### Normal results

■ No pathology is found in the bones or joints.
■ Crisp images of the structure are obtained while blurring or eliminating details of surrounding structures.

### Abnormal results

■ Primary bone tumors and soft-tissue tumors as well as skeletal metastasis are present.
■ Joint abnormalities that are difficult to detect by other methods are detected.

### Purpose

■ To determine the existence and extent of primary bone tumors, skeletal metastases, soft-tissue tumors, injuries to ligaments or tendons, and fractures
■ To diagnose joint abnormalities difficult to detect by other methods

## Patient preparation

- Explain that skeletal CT allows visualization of bones and joints. If a contrast medium isn't ordered, tell the patient that he doesn't need to restrict food and fluids. If a contrast medium is ordered, instruct him to fast for 4 hours before the test.
- Explain to the patient who will perform the procedure and where it will take place. Reassure him that the procedure is painless.
- Explain to the patient that he'll be positioned on an X-ray table inside a CT scanner and asked to lie still; the computer-controlled scanner will revolve around him taking multiple scans. Stress that he should lie as still as possible because movement may cause distorted images.
- If a contrast medium is used, tell the patient that he may feel flushed and warm and may experience a transient headache, a salty or metallic taste, and nausea or vomiting after its injection. Reassure him that these reactions are normal.
- Instruct the patient to wear a radiologic examining gown and remove all metal objects and jewelry in the X-ray field.

**A**LERT

Check the patient's history for hypersensitivity reactions to iodine, shellfish, or contrast media. Mark such reactions in the chart, and notify the practitioner, who may order prophylactic medications or choose not to use a contrast medium.

- If the patient appears restless or apprehensive about the procedure, a mild sedative may be prescribed.
- Make sure that the patient or a responsible family member has signed an informed consent form, if required.

## Procedure and posttest care

- Confirm the patient's identity using two patient identifiers according to facility policy.
- Place the patient in a supine position on an X-ray table, and tell him to lie as still as possible.
- The table is slid into the circular opening of the CT scanner. The scanner revolves around the patient, taking radiographs at preselected intervals.
- After the first set of scans is taken, the patient is removed from the scanner, and a contrast medium is given if necessary.
- Observe the patient for signs and symptoms of a hypersensitivity reaction, including pruritus, rash, and respiratory difficulty, for 30 minutes after the contrast medium has been injected.
- After contrast medium I.V. injection, the patient is moved back into the scanner and another series of scans is taken. The images obtained from the scan are displayed on a monitor during the procedure and stored on magnetic tape to create a permanent record for subsequent study.
- If contrast media is used, observe for a delayed allergic reaction, and treat as necessary. (Diphenhydramine [Benadryl] is the drug of choice.)
- Encourage fluids to assist in eliminating the contrast medium.
- Tell the patient that he may resume his usual diet and activities, if appropriate.
- Provide comfort measures and pain medication as ordered because of prolonged positioning on the table.

## Precautions

- This procedure is contraindicated during pregnancy.
- This test is contraindicated in a patient who's hypersensitive to iodine, shellfish, or contrast media, or in a patient with renal insufficiency (if he isn't on dialysis).

- The patient may experience strong feelings of claustrophobia or anxiety when inside the CT body scanner. In this case, a mild sedative may be ordered to help reduce anxiety.

### Complications
- Hypersensitivity reaction to the contrast medium

# Skeletal magnetic resonance imaging

A noninvasive technique, skeletal magnetic resonance imaging (MRI) produces clear and sensitive images of bone and soft tissue. The scan provides superior contrast of body tissues and allows imaging of multiple planes, including direct sagittal and coronal views in regions that can't be easily visualized with X-rays or computed tomography scans. MRI eliminates any risks associated with exposure to X-ray beams and causes no known harm to cells.

### Normal results
- No pathology is observed in bone, muscles, and joints.

### Abnormal results
- Structural abnormalities suggest possible primary and metastatic tumors and various disorders.

### Purpose
- To evaluate bony and soft-tissue tumors
- To identify changes in bone marrow composition
- To identify spinal disorders

### Patient preparation
- Make sure the scanner can accommodate the patient's weight and abdominal girth.
- Explain to the patient that skeletal MRI assesses bone and soft tissue. Tell

him who will perform the test and where it will take place.
- Explain that although MRI is painless and involves no exposure to radiation from the scanner, a contrast medium may be used, depending on the type of tissue being studied.
- If the patient is claustrophobic or if extensive time is required for scanning, explain to him that a mild sedative may be given to reduce anxiety. Open scanners have been developed for use on the patient with extreme claustrophobia or morbid obesity, but tests using such machines take longer.
- Tell the patient that he must lie flat, and describe the test procedure.
- Explain to the patient that he'll hear the scanner clicking, whirring, and thumping as it moves inside its housing.
- Reassure the patient that he'll be able to communicate with the technician at all times.
- Instruct the patient to remove all metallic objects, including jewelry, hairpins, or watches.
- Ask whether the patient has any surgically implanted joints, pins, clips, valves, pumps, or pacemakers containing metal that could be attracted to the strong MRI magnet. If he does, he won't be able to have the test.
- Make sure that the patient or a responsible family member has signed an informed consent form, if required.

### Procedure and posttest care
- Confirm the patient's identity using two patient identifiers according to facility policy.
- At the scanner room door, check the patient one last time for metal objects.
- The patient is placed on a narrow, padded, nonmetallic table that moves into the scanner tunnel. Fans continuously circulate air in the tunnel, and a call bell or intercom is used to maintain verbal contact.

- Remind the patient to remain still throughout the procedure.
- While the patient lies within the strong magnetic field, the area to be studied is stimulated with radiofrequency waves.
- If the test is prolonged with the patient lying flat, monitor him for orthostatic hypotension.
- Provide comfort measures and pain medication as needed and ordered because of prolonged positioning in the scanner.
- After the test, tell the patient that he may resume his usual activity.
- Provide emotional support to the patient with claustrophobia or anxiety over his diagnosis.

### Precautions

- MRI can't be performed on a patient with a pacemaker, intracranial aneurysm clip, or other ferrous metal implants. Ventilators, I.V. infusion pumps, oxygen tanks, and other metallic or computer-based equipment must be kept out of the MRI area.
- If the patient is unstable, make sure an I.V. line without metal components is in place and that all equipment is compatible with MRI imaging. If necessary, monitor the patient's oxygen saturation, cardiac rhythm, and respiratory status during the test. An anesthesiologist may be needed to monitor a heavily sedated patient.
- Make sure that the technician maintains verbal contact with the conscious patient.

### Complications

- Anxiety and claustrophobia
- Orthostatic hypertension after the test

# Endoscopy and joint aspiration

## ▌Arthroscopy

Arthroscopy is the visual examination of the interior of a joint (most commonly a major joint, such as a shoulder, hip, or knee) with a specially designed fiber-optic endoscope that's inserted through a cannula in the joint cavity. It usually follows and confirms a diagnosis made through physical examination, radiography, and arthrography.

Arthroscopy may be performed under local anesthesia, but it's usually performed under a spinal or general anesthesia, particularly when surgery is anticipated. A camera may be attached to the arthroscope to photograph areas for later study. (See *Arthroscopy of the knee,* page 420.)

### Normal results

- The diarthrodial joint is surrounded by muscles, ligaments, cartilage, and tendons and lined with a synovial membrane.
- In children, the menisci are smooth and opaque, with their thick outer edges attached to the joint capsule and their inner edges lying snugly against the condylar surfaces, unattached.
- Articular cartilage appears smooth and white; ligaments and tendons appear cablelike and silvery.
- The synovium is smooth and marked by a fine vascular network.
- Degenerative changes begin during adolescence.

### Abnormal results

- Meniscal disease, such as a torn medial or lateral meniscus or other meniscal injuries; patellar disease, such as chondromalacia, dislocation, subluxation, parapatellar synovitis or fracture; condylar

# Arthroscopy of the knee

With the patient's knee flexed about 40 degrees, the arthroscope is introduced into the joint. The physician flexes, extends, and rotates the knee to view the joint space. Counterclockwise from the top right, these illustrations show a normal patellofemoral joint with smooth joint surfaces; the articular surface of the patella, showing chondromalacia; and a tear in the anterior cruciate ligament.

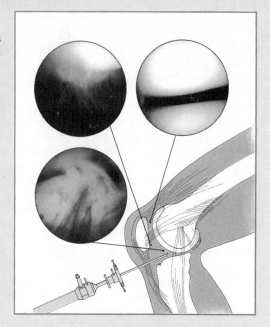

disease, such as degenerative articular cartilage, osteochondritis dissecans, and loose bodies may be detected.
- Extrasynovial disease, such as torn anterior cruciate or tibial collateral ligaments, Baker's cyst, and ganglionic cyst may also be revealed.
- Synovial disease, such as synovitis, rheumatoid and degenerative arthritis, and foreign bodies associated with gout, pseudogout, and osteochondromatosis may be detected.

## Purpose
- To detect and diagnose meniscal, patellar, condylar, extrasynovial, and synovial diseases
- To monitor disease progression
- To perform joint surgery
- To monitor the effectiveness of therapy

## Patient preparation
- Explain to the patient that arthroscopy is used to examine the interior of the joint, to evaluate joint disease, or to monitor his response to therapy as appropriate.
- Describe the procedure to the patient, and answer his questions.
- If surgery or another treatment is anticipated, explain that this may be accomplished during arthroscopy.
- Instruct the patient to fast after midnight before the procedure.
- Tell him who will perform the procedure and where it will be done.
- If local anesthesia will be used, tell the patient that he may experience slight discomfort from the injection of the local anesthetic and the pressure of the tourniquet on his leg. The patient will also feel a thumping sensation as the cannula is inserted in the joint capsule.

- Make sure that the patient or a responsible family member has signed an informed consent form.
- Check the patient's history for hypersensitivity to the anesthetic.
- Be aware that the surgical site is prepared by shaving the area 5″ (12.7 cm) above and below the joint and a sedative is given, as ordered. The patient is positioned and draped according to facility policy.

### Procedure and posttest care

- Confirm the patient's identity using two patient identifiers according to facility policy.
- Arthroscopic techniques vary depending on the surgeon and the type of arthroscope used.
- The patient's leg is elevated and wrapped with an elastic bandage to drain as much blood from the leg as possible, or a mixture of lidocaine with epinephrine and normal saline is instilled into the patient's knee to distend the knee and help reduce bleeding.
- The local anesthetic is given, a small incision is made, and a cannula is passed through the incision and positioned in the joint cavity.
- The arthroscope is then inserted, and the knee structures are visually examined and photographed for further study.
- After visual examination, a synovial biopsy or appropriate surgery is performed as indicated.
- When the examination is completed, the arthroscope is removed, the joint is irrigated, the cannula is removed, and an adhesive strip and compression dressing are applied over the incision site.
- Watch the patient for fever, swelling, increased pain, and localized inflammation at the incision site. If the patient reports discomfort, provide an analgesic as ordered.

- Monitor the patient's circulation and sensation in his leg.
- Advise the patient to elevate the leg and apply ice for the first 24 hours.
- Instruct the patient to report fever, bleeding, drainage, or increased swelling or pain in the joint.
- Advise the patient to bear only partial weight, using crutches, a walker, or a cane for 48 hours.
- If an immobilizer is ordered, teach the patient how to apply it.
- Tell the patient that showering is permitted after 48 hours, but a tub bath should be avoided until after the postoperative visit.
- Tell the patient that he may resume his usual diet as ordered.

### Precautions

- Arthroscopy is contraindicated in a patient with fibrous ankylosis with flexion of less than 50 degrees.
- The procedure is contraindicated when a patient with local skin or wound infections has a risk of subsequent joint involvement.

### Complications

- Hematoma, infection, joint injury, and thrombophlebitis

# ■ Synovial fluid analysis

In synovial fluid aspiration, or arthrocentesis, a sterile needle is inserted into a joint space—most commonly the knee—to obtain a fluid specimen for analysis. This procedure is indicated for the patient with undiagnosed articular disease and symptomatic joint effusion, a condition marked by the excessive accumulation of synovial fluid. Although rare, complications associated with synovial fluid aspiration include joint infection and hemorrhage leading to hemarthrosis (accumulation of blood within the joint).

## Normal results

▪ Routine examination includes gross analysis for color, clarity, quantity, viscosity, pH, and the presence of a mucin clot as well as microscopic analysis for WBC count and differential.

▪ Special examination includes microbiological analysis for formed elements (including crystals) and bacteria, serologic analysis, and chemical analysis for such components as glucose, protein, and enzymes.

## Abnormal results

▪ Various joint diseases, including noninflammatory disease (traumatic arthritis and osteoarthritis), inflammatory disease (systemic lupus erythematosus, rheumatic fever, pseudogout, gout, and rheumatoid arthritis), and septic disease (tuberculous and septic arthritis) may be detected.

## Purpose

▪ To aid differential diagnosis of arthritis, particularly septic or crystal-induced arthritis
▪ To identify the cause and nature of joint effusion
▪ To relieve the pain and distention resulting from the accumulation of fluid within the joint
▪ To give a drug locally (usually corticosteroids)

## Patient preparation

▪ Describe synovial fluid analysis to the patient, and answer his questions.
▪ Explain that this test helps determine the cause of joint inflammation and swelling and also helps relieve the associated pain.
▪ Instruct the patient to fast for 6 to 12 hours before the test if glucose testing of synovial fluid is ordered; otherwise, in-

form him that he need not restrict food and fluids.
▪ Tell the patient who will perform the test and where it will be done.
▪ Warn the patient that although he'll receive a local anesthetic, he may still feel slight pain when the needle penetrates the joint capsule.
▪ Make sure that the patient or a responsible family member has signed an informed consent form.
▪ Check the patient's history for hypersensitivity to iodine compounds (such as povidone-iodine), procaine, lidocaine, or other local anesthetics.
▪ Give a sedative as ordered.

## Procedure and posttest care

▪ Confirm the patient's identity using two patient identifiers according to facility policy.
▪ Position the patient, and explain that he'll need to maintain this position throughout the procedure.
▪ Clean the skin over the puncture site with surgical detergent and alcohol.
▪ Paint the site with tincture of povidone-iodine and allow it to air-dry for 2 minutes.
▪ After the local anesthetic is given, the aspirating needle is quickly inserted through the skin, subcutaneous tissue, and synovial membrane into the joint space.
▪ As much fluid as possible is aspirated into the syringe; at least 15 ml should be obtained, although a smaller amount is usually adequate for analysis.
▪ Assist as appropriate to maintain the joint (except for the area around the puncture site) wrapped with an elastic bandage to compress the free fluid into this portion of the sac, ensuring maximal fluid collection.
▪ If a corticosteroid is being injected, prepare the dose as necessary. For instillation, the syringe is detached, leaving the needle in the joint, and the syringe

containing the steroid is attached to the needle instead.

■ After the steroid is injected and the needle withdrawn, wipe the puncture site with an alcohol pad.

■ Apply pressure to the puncture site for about 2 minutes to prevent bleeding, and then apply a sterile dressing.

■ If synovial fluid glucose levels are being measured, perform a venipuncture to obtain a specimen for blood glucose analysis.

■ Apply ice or cold packs to the affected joint for 24 to 36 hours after aspiration to decrease pain and swelling. Use pillows for support. If a large quantity of fluid was aspirated, apply an elastic bandage to stabilize the joint.

■ If the patient's condition permits, tell him that he may resume his usual activity immediately after the procedure. However, warn him to avoid excessive use of the affected joint for a few days even if pain and swelling subside.

■ Watch for increased pain or fever; these symptoms may indicate joint infection.

■ Be careful when handling the dressings and linens of the patient with drainage from the joint space, especially if septic arthritis is confirmed or suspected.

■ Tell the patient that he may resume his usual diet as ordered.

### For cultures
■ Obtain 2 to 5 ml of synovial fluid and, if possible, inoculate the medium immediately. Otherwise, add one or two drops of heparin to the specimen.

### For cytologic analysis
■ Add 5 mg of EDTA or one or two drops of heparin to 2 to 5 ml of synovial fluid.

### For glucose analysis
■ Add potassium oxalate, as specified by the laboratory, to 3 to 5 ml of fluid.

### For crystal examination
■ Add heparin if specified by the laboratory.

### For other studies
■ For general appearance and clot evaluation, obtain 2 to 5 ml of synovial fluid, but don't add an anticoagulant.

■ Send the properly labeled specimens to the laboratory immediately after collection—gonococci are particularly labile. If a white blood cell count is being obtained as well, clearly label the specimen "Synovial Fluid" and "Caution: Don't Use Acid Diluents."

## Precautions
■ Wear gloves when handling all specimens.

■ Don't perform the test in areas of skin or wound infections.

■ Use strict sterile technique throughout aspiration to prevent contamination of the joint space or the synovial fluid specimen.

■ Add an anticoagulant to the specimen, according to the laboratory tests requested. Gently invert the tube several times to mix the specimen and anticoagulant adequately.

## Complications
■ Bleeding, hematoma, or infection

# Reproductive system

## Tissue analysis

### Amniotic fluid analysis

Amniocentesis is the percutaneous transabdominal puncture of the uterus to obtain a 10- to 20-ml sample of amniotic fluid for laboratory analysis. It may be used to detect certain birth defects, such as Down syndrome or spina bifida; to determine fetal maturity; to detect hemolytic disease of the newborn; or, through karyotyping, to detect gender and chromosomal abnormalities. This test can be performed only when the amniotic fluid level reaches 150 ml, usually after 16 weeks' gestation.

Amniocentesis is indicated if the patient is older than age 35; has a family history of genetic, chromosomal, or neural tube defects; or has had a miscarriage. Although adverse effects are rare, potential complications include spontaneous abortion, trauma to the fetus or placenta, bleeding, premature labor, infection, and Rh sensitization from fetal bleeding into the maternal circulation. Because of the severity of possible complications, amniocentesis is contraindicated as a general screening test. Abnormal test results or failure of the tissue cultures to grow may necessitate test repetition.

Another method of detecting fetal chromosomal and biochemical disorders in early pregnancy is chorionic villi sampling. (See *Chorionic villi sampling,* pages 426 and 427.)

#### Normal results

- Normal amniotic fluid is clear, but may contain white flecks of vernix caseosa when the fetus is near term.
- The type II cells lining the fetal lung alveoli produce lecithin slowly in early pregnancy and then markedly increase production around the 35th week.
- For an analysis of the appearance and components of amniotic fluid, see *Findings in amniotic fluid analysis,* page 428.

#### Abnormal results

- Blood, which is found in about 10% of amniocenteses, results from a faulty tap and doesn't indicate an abnormality.
- "Port wine" fluid, on the other hand, may be a sign of abruptio placentae, and blood of fetal origin may indicate damage to the fetal, placental, or umbilical cord vessels by the amniocentesis needle.
- Large amounts of bilirubin, a breakdown product of red blood cells, may indicate hemolytic disease of the new-

born. Normally, the bilirubin level increases from 14 to 24 weeks' gestation, then declines as the fetus matures, essentially reaching zero at term.

■ Meconium in the amniotic fluid produces a peak of 410 mμ on the spectrophotometric analysis. If meconium is present during labor, the neonate's nose and throat require thorough cleaning to prevent meconium aspiration.

■ Creatinine, a product of fetal urine, increases in the amniotic fluid as the fetal kidneys mature. Generally, the creatinine value exceeds 2 mg/dl in a mature fetus.

■ Alpha-fetoprotein (AFP) is a fetal alpha globulin produced first in the yolk sac and later in the parenchymal cells of the liver and GI tract. Fetal serum AFP levels are about 150 times higher than amniotic fluid levels; maternal serum AFP levels are far lower than amniotic fluid levels. High amniotic fluid levels indicate neural tube defects, but the AFP level may remain normal if the defect is small and closed. Elevated AFP levels may also occur in multiple pregnancy; in disorders such as omphalocele, congenital nephrosis, esophageal or duodenal atresia, cystic fibrosis, exomphalos, Turner's syndrome, and fetal bladder neck obstruction with hydronephrosis; and in impending fetal death.

■ The amount of uric acid in the amniotic fluid increases as the fetus matures, but these levels fluctuate widely and can't accurately predict maturity. Laboratory studies indicate that severe erythroblastosis fetalis, familial hyperuricemia, and Lesch-Nyhan syndrome tend to increase the uric acid level.

■ Estrone, estradiol, estriol, and estriol conjugates appear in amniotic fluid in varying amounts. Levels of estriol, the most prevalent estrogen, increase substantially at term. Severe erythroblastosis fetalis decreases the estriol level.

■ The sphingomyelin level parallels that of lecithin until the 35th week, when it gradually decreases. Measuring the ratio of lecithin to sphingomyelin (L/S) confirms fetal pulmonary maturity (L/S ratio > 2) or suggests a risk of respiratory distress (L/S ratio < 2).

■ Phosphatidylglycerol levels are present with pulmonary maturity; an absence of phosphatidylinositol indicates pulmonary immaturity.

■ A glucose level greater than 45 mg/dl (SI, > 2.6 mmol/L) indicates poor maternal and fetal control.

■ Laboratory analysis can identify at least 25 different enzymes (usually in low concentrations) in amniotic fluid. The enzymes have few known clinical implications, although elevated acetylcholinesterase levels may occur with neural tube defects, exomphalos, and other serious malformations.

### Purpose

■ To detect fetal abnormalities, particularly chromosomal and neural tube defects

■ To detect hemolytic disease of the newborn

■ To diagnose metabolic disorders, amino acid disorders, and mucopolysaccharidosis

■ To determine fetal age and maturity, especially pulmonary maturity

■ To assess fetal health by detecting the presence of meconium or blood or measuring amniotic levels of estriol and fetal thyroid hormone

■ To identify fetal gender when one or both parents are carriers of a sex-linked disorder

### Patient preparation

■ Describe the procedure to the patient and explain that amniocentesis detects fetal abnormalities.

■ Assess her understanding of the test and answer her questions.

# Chorionic villi sampling

Chorionic villi sampling (CVS) is a prenatal test for quick detection of fetal chromosomal and biochemical disorders that's performed during the first trimester of pregnancy. Preliminary results may be available within hours; complete results, within a few days. In contrast, amniocentesis can't be performed before 16 weeks' gestation, and the results aren't available for at least 2 weeks. CVS can detect fetal abnormalities as much as 10 weeks sooner than amniocentesis.

Chorionic villi are fingerlike projections that surround the embryonic membrane and eventually give rise to the placenta. Cells obtained from an appropriate sample are of fetal, rather than maternal, origin and thus can be analyzed for fetal abnormalities.

## Collection time

Samples are best obtained between the 8th and 10th weeks of pregnancy. Before 7 weeks, the villi cover the embryo and make selective sampling difficult. After 10 weeks, maternal cells begin to grow over the villi, and the amniotic sac begins to fill the uterine cavity, making the procedure difficult and potentially dangerous.

## Collection method

To collect a sample, the patient is placed in the lithotomy position. The physician checks the placement of the patient's uterus bimanually and then inserts a Graves speculum and swabs the cervix with an antiseptic solution. If necessary, he may use a tenaculum to straighten an acutely flexed uterus, permitting cannula insertion. Guided by ultrasound and

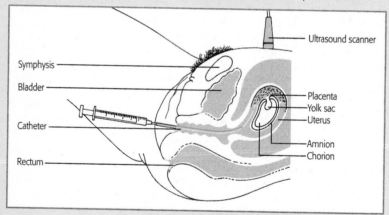

Symphysis

Bladder

Catheter

Rectum

Ultrasound scanner

Placenta
Yolk sac
Uterus

Amnion
Chorion

- Inform her that she doesn't need to restrict food and fluids.
- Tell her that the test requires a specimen of amniotic fluid, who will perform the test, and when it will take place.
- Advise her that normal test results can't guarantee a normal fetus because some fetal disorders are undetectable.

- Make sure that the patient has signed an informed consent form.
- Explain to the patient that she'll feel a stinging sensation when the local anesthetic is injected.
- Provide emotional support before and during the test.

possibly endoscopy, he directs the catheter through the cannula to the villi. Suction is applied to the catheter to remove about 30 mg of tissue from the villi. The sample is withdrawn, placed in a Petri dish, and examined with a dissecting microscope. Part of the specimen is then cultured for further testing.

### Interpretation

CVS can be used to detect about 200 diseases prenatally. For example, direct analysis of rapidly dividing fetal cells can detect chromosome disorders, deoxyribonucleic acid analysis can detect hemoglobinopathies, and lysosomal enzyme assays can screen for lysosomal storage disorders such as Tay-Sachs disease.

The test appears to provide reliable results, except when the sample contains too few cells or the cells fail to grow in culture. Patient risks for this procedure appear to be similar to those for amniocentesis: a small chance of spontaneous abortion, cramps, infection, and bleeding. However, recent research reports an incidence of limb malformations in neonates when CVS has been performed.

Unlike amniocentesis, CVS can't detect complications in cases of Rh sensitization, uncover neural tube defects, or determine pulmonary maturity. However, it may prove to be the best way to detect other serious fetal abnormalities early in pregnancy.

■ Ask the patient to void just before the test to minimize the risk of puncturing the bladder and aspirating urine instead of amniotic fluid.

### Procedure and posttest care

■ Confirm the patient's identity using two patient identifiers according to facility policy.

■ A pool of amniotic fluid is located after determining fetal and placental position, usually through palpation and ultrasonic visualization.

■ The skin is prepared with antiseptic and alcohol, and then 1 ml of 1% lidocaine is injected with a 25G needle, first intradermally and then subcutaneously.

■ Next, a 20G spinal needle with a stylet is inserted into the amniotic cavity, and the stylet is withdrawn.

■ A 10-ml syringe is attached to the needle, and then the fluid is aspirated and placed in an amber or foil-covered test tube.

■ The needle is withdrawn and an adhesive bandage is placed over the needle insertion site.

■ Monitor fetal heart rate and maternal vital signs every 15 minutes for at least 30 minutes.

■ Position the patient on her left side if she sweats profusely or feels faint or nauseated to counteract uterine pressure on the vena cava.

#### DO'S & DON'TS

Instruct the patient before she's discharged to immediately report abdominal pain or cramping, chills, fever, vaginal bleeding or leakage of serous vaginal fluid, or fetal hyperactivity or unusual fetal lethargy.

### Precautions

■ Instruct the patient to fold her hands behind her head to prevent her from accidentally touching the sterile field and causing contamination.

■ Infectious mononucleosis, cirrhosis, hepatic cancer, teratoma, endodermal sinus tumor, gastric carcinoma, pancreatic carcinoma, and subacute hereditary tyrosinemia may cause a possible increase in AFP levels.

# Findings in amniotic fluid analysis

| Test | Normal findings | Fetal implications of abnormal findings |
|---|---|---|
| Color | Clear, with white flecks of vernix caseosa in a mature fetus | Blood of maternal origin (usually harmless); "port wine" fluid indicating abruptio placentae; fetal blood indicating damage to the fetal, placental, or umbilical cord vessels |
| Bilirubin | Early: < 0.075 mg/dl (SI, < 1.3 µmol/L) Term: < 0.025 mg/dl (SI, < 0.41 µmol/L) | High levels indicating hemolytic disease of the neonate in isoimmunized pregnancy |
| Meconium | Absent (except in breech presentation) | Presence indicating fetal hypotension or distress |
| Creatinine | > 2 mg/dl (SI, 177 µmol/L) | Decreased levels indicating immature fetus (less than 37 weeks) |
| Lecithin-sphingomyelin ratio | > 2 | < 2 indicating pulmonary immaturity |
| Phosphatidyl-glycerol | Present | Absence indicating pulmonary immaturity |
| Glucose | < 45 mg/dl (SI, 2.3 mmol/L) | Excessive increases at term or near term indicating hypertrophy of fetal pancreas |
| Alpha-fetoprotein | Variable, depending on gestation age and laboratory technique | Inappropriate increases indicating neural tube defects, such as spina bifida or anencephaly, impending fetal death, congenital nephrosis, or contamination by fetal blood |
| Bacteria | Absent | Presence indicating chorioamnionitis |
| Chromosome | Normal karyotype | Abnormal karyotype indicating fetal gender and chromosome disorders |
| Acetyl-cholinesterase | Absent | Presence indicating neural tube defects, exomphalos, or other serious malformations |

## Complications

- Spontaneous abortion, fetal or placental trauma
- Bleeding
- Premature labor
- Infection
- Rh sensitization from fetal bleeding into maternal circulation

# Chromosome analysis
[chromosome karyotype]

Chromosome analysis studies the relationship between the microscopic appearance of chromosomes and an individual's phenotype—the expression of the genes in physical, biochemical, or physiologic traits.

Only rapidly dividing cells, such as bone marrow or neoplastic cells, permit direct, immediate study. In other cells, mitosis is stimulated by the addition of phytohemagglutinin. Indications for the test determine the specimen required (blood, bone marrow, amniotic fluid, skin, or placental tissue) and the specific analytic procedure. Umbilical cord sampling may also be used to perform chromosome analysis. (See *Percutaneous umbilical blood sampling.*)

### Normal results

- 46 chromosomes: 22 pairs of nonsex chromosomes (autosomes) and 1 pair of sex chromosomes (Y for the male-determining chromosome, X for the female-determining chromosome). On a karyotype, chromosomes are arranged according to size and the location of their primary constrictions, or centromeres.
- The centromere may be medial (metacentric), slightly to one end of the chromosome (submetacentric), or entirely to one end (acrocentric).
- The largest chromosomes are displayed first; the others are arranged in order of decreasing size, with the two sex chromosomes traditionally placed last. By convention, the centromere is always placed at the top in a karyotype. Thus, if the two pairs of chromosomal arms are of unequal length, the arm above the centromere will be shorter. The letter "p" designates the short arm; the letter "q," the long arm.
- Special stains identify individual chromosomes and locate and enumerate particular portions of chromosomes.

### Abnormal results

- Chromosomal abnormalities may be numerical or structural.
- Any numerical deviation from the norm of 46 chromosomes is called *aneuploidy.*

## Percutaneous umbilical blood sampling

Useful in chromosome analysis, percutaneous umbilical blood sampling (PUBS) provides a fetal blood sample for karyotype, direct Coombs' test, or complete blood count. PUBS, sometimes called cordocentesis, can also be used to determine fetal blood type, check blood gas levels and acid-base status, and identify and treat isoimmunization.

To obtain a percutaneous umbilical blood sample, a needle is inserted transabdominally (using ultrasound guidance) into a fetal umbilical vessel. A blood sample is then tested to make sure that fetal and not maternal blood has been drawn. Possible complications include blood leakage at the puncture site, fetal bradycardia, and infection.

- Fewer than 46 chromosomes is called *hypoploidy;* more than 46, *hyperploidy.*
- Special designations exist for whole multiples of the haploid number 23: diploidy for the normal somatic number of 46, triploidy for 69, tetraploidy for 92, and so forth. Fetuses with this condition are usually spontaneously aborted or, if they live, have severe mental retardation and various other health problems.
- When the deviation occurs within a single pair of chromosomes, the suffix "–somy" is used, as in trisomy for the presence of three chromosomes instead of the usual pair or monosomy for the presence of only one chromosome.
- Aneuploidy most commonly follows failure of the chromosomal pair to separate (nondisjunction) during anaphase, the mitotic stage that follows metaphase. It may also result from anaphase lag, in which one of the normally separated

# Chromosome analysis findings

| Specimen and indication | Result |
|---|---|
| **Blood** | |
| • To evaluate abnormal appearance or development, suggesting chromosomal irregularity | • Abnormal chromosome number (aneuploidy) or arrangement |
| • To evaluate couples with a history of miscarriages or to identify balanced translocation carriers having unbalanced offspring | • Normal chromosomes<br>• Parental balanced translocation carrier |
| • To detect chromosomal rearrangements in rare genetic diseases predisposing the patient to malignant neoplasms | • Chromosomal rearrangements, gaps, and breaks |
| **Blood or bone marrow** | |
| • To identify Philadelphia chromosome and confirm chronic myelogenous leukemia | • Translocation of chromosome 22q (long arm) to another chromosome (often chromosome 9)<br>• Aneuploidy (usually due to abnormalities in chromosomes 8 and 12)<br>• Trisomy 21 |
| **Skin** | |
| • To evaluate abnormal appearance or development, suggesting chromosomal irregularity | • All chromosomal abnormalities possible |
| **Amniotic fluid** | |
| • To evaluate the developing fetus with possible chromosomal abnormality | • All chromosomal abnormalities possible |
| **Placental tissue** | |
| • To evaluate products of conception after a miscarriage to determine if the abnormality is fetal or placental in origin | • All chromosomal abnormalities possible |
| **Tumor tissue** | |
| • For research purposes only | • Many chromosomal abnormalities possible |

## Implication

■ Identifies specific chromosomal abnormality

■ Miscarriage unrelated to parental chromosomal abnormality
■ Increased risk of repeated abortion or unbalanced offspring indicates need for amniocentesis in future pregnancies

■ Occurs in Bloom's syndrome, Fanconi's syndrome, telangiectasia; patient predisposed to malignant neoplasms

■ Aids in the diagnosis of chronic myelogenous leukemia

■ Occurs in acute myelogenous leukemia

■ Occasionally occurs in chronic lymphocytic leukemia cells

■ Same as chromosomal abnormality in blood; rarely, mosaic individual has normal blood but abnormal skin chromosomes

■ Same as chromosomal abnormality in blood or fetus

■ More than 50% of aborted tissue is chromosomally abnormal

■ Although malignant tumors aren't associated with specific chromosomal aberrations, most are aneuploid, usually hyperploid

chromosomes fails to move to a pole and is left out of the daughter cells.
■ If nondisjunction or anaphase lag occurs during meiosis, the cells of the zygote will all be the same. Errors in mitotic division after zygote formation will produce more than one cell line (mosaicism).
■ Structural chromosomal abnormalities result from chromosome breakage.
■ Intrachromosomal rearrangement occurs within a single chromosome in these forms:
  –deletion—loss of an end (terminal) or middle (interstitial) portion of a chromosome
  –inversion—end-to-end reversal of a chromosome segment, which may be pericentric inversion (including the centromere) or paracentric inversion (occurring in only one arm of the chromosome)
  –ring chromosome formation—breakage of both ends of a chromosome and reunion of the ends
  –isochromosome formation—abnormal splitting of the centromere in a transverse rather than a longitudinal plane.
■ Implications of chromosome analysis results depend on the specimen and indications for the test. (See *Chromosome analysis findings.*)

### DRUG CHALLENGE

 Chemotherapy (possible abnormal results due to chromosome breaks)

## Purpose
■ To identify chromosomal abnormalities, such as hypoploidy or hyperploidy, as the underlying cause of malformation, maldevelopment, or disease

## Patient preparation

- Explain to the patient or his parents, if appropriate, the purpose of the chromosome analysis.
- Tell the patient who will perform the test and what kind of specimen will be required.
- Inform the patient when results will be available, according to the specimen required.

## Procedure and posttest care

- Confirm the patient's identity using two patient identifiers according to facility policy.
- Collect a blood sample (in a 5- to 10-ml heparinized tube), or assist with collection of a tissue specimen, 1 ml of bone marrow, or at least 20 ml of amniotic fluid.
- Provide appropriate posttest care, depending on the procedure used to collect the specimen.
- Explain the test results and their implications to the patient or his parents, if he's a child, with a chromosomal abnormality.
- Recommend appropriate genetic or other counseling and follow-up care if necessary, such as an infant stimulation program for a patient with Down syndrome.

## Precautions

- Keep all specimens sterile, especially those requiring a tissue culture.
- To facilitate interpretation of test results, send the specimen to the laboratory immediately after collection, with a brief patient history and the indication for the test.
- Refrigerate the specimen if transport is delayed, but never freeze it.

**ALERT**

Before a skin biopsy, make sure the povidone-iodine solution is thoroughly removed with alco-

hol. This solution could prevent cell growth.

# Colposcopy

In colposcopy, the cervix and vagina are visually examined by an instrument containing a magnifying lens and a light (colposcope). This test is primarily used to evaluate abnormal cytology or grossly suspicious lesions and to examine the cervix and vagina after a positive Papanicolaou (Pap) test result.

During the examination, a biopsy may be performed and photographs taken of suspicious lesions with the colposcope and its attachments.

## Normal results

- Surface contour of the cervical vessels is smooth and pink.
- Columnar epithelium appears grape-like.
- Different tissue types are sharply demarcated.

## Abnormal results

- White epithelium (leukoplakia) or punctate and mosaic patterns may indicate underlying cervical intraepithelial neoplasia.
- Keratinization in the transformation zone may indicate cervical intraepithelial neoplasia or invasive carcinoma.
- Atypical vessels may indicate invasive carcinoma.
- Other abnormalities include inflammatory changes (usually from infection), atrophic changes (usually from aging or, less commonly, the use of hormonal contraceptives), erosion (probably from increased pathogenicity of vaginal flora due to changes in vaginal pH), and papilloma and condyloma (possibly from viruses).

## Purpose

- To help confirm cervical intraepithelial neoplasia or invasive carcinoma after a positive Pap test result
- To evaluate vaginal or cervical lesions
- To monitor conservatively treated cervical intraepithelial neoplasia
- To monitor the patient whose mother received diethylstilbestrol during pregnancy

## Patient preparation

- Explain to the patient that the colposcopy magnifies the image of the vagina and cervix, providing more information than a routine vaginal examination.
- Inform the patient that she doesn't need to restrict food and fluids.
- Tell the patient who will perform the examination, where it will be done, and that it's safe and painless.
- Tell the patient that a biopsy may be performed during colposcopy and that this may cause minimal but easily controlled bleeding and mild cramping.
- Make sure that the patient has signed an informed consent form.

## Procedure and posttest care

- Confirm the patient's identity using two patient identifiers according to facility policy.
- The practitioner puts on gloves. With the patient in the lithotomy position, the practitioner inserts the speculum and, if indicated, performs a Pap test. Help the patient relax during insertion by telling her to breathe through her mouth and concentrate on relaxing her abdominal muscles.
- The cervix is gently swabbed with acetic acid solution to remove mucus.
- After the cervix and vagina are examined, biopsy is performed on areas that appear abnormal.
- Bleeding is stopped by applying pressure, hemostatic solutions, or by cautery.

- After a biopsy, instruct the patient to abstain from intercourse and to avoid inserting anything in her vagina (including a tampon) until healing of the biopsy site is confirmed (in about 10 days).

## Complications

- Bleeding (especially in pregnant patients)
- Infections

# Loop electrosurgical excision procedure
### [LEEP]

Loop electrosurgical excision procedure (LEEP) is a method for obtaining tissue specimens of the cervix for biopsy and removing abnormal tissue from the cervix and high in the endocervical canal. This procedure is usually done after a Papanicolaou (Pap) smear and colposcopy as follow-up to ensure the accuracy of results and for further investigation of abnormal tissue as a means to exclude the diagnosis of invasive cancer and to determine the extent of noninvasive lesions. Complications associated with LEEP include heavy bleeding, severe cramping, infection, and accidental cutting or burning of normal tissue. Cervical stenosis is also a possible risk.

## Normal results

- Normal squamous cells of the cervix that flatten as they grow are present.

## Abnormal results

- Dysplastic cervical cells or more extensive invasion of the cancerous cells are detected deeper in the cervix.

## Purpose

- To confirm results of colposcopy and Pap smear
- To identify lesions as benign or cancerous, invasive or noninvasive

- To remove cervical dysplasia and non-invasive cervical cancers

### Patient preparation

- Describe the procedure to the patient, and explain that it provides a cervical tissue specimen for microscopic study and treats abnormal tissue growth.
- Make sure the patient has signed an informed consent form.
- Help allay the patient's anxiety about a possible diagnosis of cervical cancer.
- Tell the patient who will perform the procedure and where it will be done.
- Tell the patient that she may experience mild discomfort during and after the procedure and that she may have some vaginal bleeding afterward.
- Advise the outpatient to have someone accompany her home after the procedure.

### Procedure and posttest care

- Confirm the patient's identity using two patient identifiers according to facility policy.
- Place the patient in the lithotomy position, and encourage her to relax.
- The physician inserts a vaginal speculum and applies a local anesthetic to the area.
- The cervix is cleaned with a mild vinegar solution (3% acetic acid solution) or iodine to remove any debris or mucus. The solution also aids in identifying normal and abnormal tissues.
- The physician inserts a thin wire loop attached to a high-frequency current, uses the loop to remove the suspected tissue, and sends the tissue to the laboratory.
- The physician applies a cervical paste to the area where tissue was removed to reduce bleeding.
- Inform the patient that she may experience some vaginal bleeding and mild cramping after the procedure; inform her that she may experience brown-black vaginal discharge or a white watery discharge for about 1 week after the procedure, with possible spotting for up to 4 weeks. Encourage her to wear a perineal pad and change it frequently.

 Instruct the patient to notify her practitioner if she experiences fever, bleeding greater than a normal menstrual flow, increasing pelvic pain or severe abdominal pain, or a foul-smelling or malodorous vaginal discharge.

- Advise the patient not to douche, use tampons or bubble baths, or engage in sexual intercourse for about 3 to 4 weeks.
- Urge the patient to return for follow-up with her practitioner as indicated for information about results.

### Precautions

- LEEP is contraindicated in patients with active menstrual bleeding and pregnant patients.

 # Papanicolaou test
### [Pap, Pap smear, ThinPrep Pap test]

The Papanicolaou test is a widely known cytologic test for early detection of cervical cancer. A physician or specially trained nurse scrapes secretions from the patient's cervix and spreads them on a slide, which is sent to the laboratory for cytologic analysis.

Although cervical scrapings are the most common test specimen, the test may involve cytologic evaluation of the vaginal pool, prostatic secretions, urine, gastric secretions, cavity fluids, bronchial aspirations, sputum, or solid tumor cells obtained by fine needle aspiration. The American Cancer Society recommends a Pap test every year for women ages 21 to 30. After age 30, if the patient has had three consecutive negative test results and isn't in a high-risk category, she may undergo screening every 3 years. Women older than age 70 with no abnormal tests in the previous 10-year period and with an intact cervix may stop screening tests. If a Pap test is positive or suggests malignancy, cervical biopsy can confirm the diagnosis.

## Normal results

■ No malignant cells or other abnormalities are present.

## Abnormal results

■ Malignant cells usually have relatively large nuclei and only small amounts of cytoplasm. They show abnormal nuclear chromatin patterns and marked variation in size, shape, and staining properties and may have prominent nucleoli.
■ A Pap smear may be graded in different ways, so check your laboratory's reporting format.
  – In the Bethesda system, the current standardized method, potentially premalignant squamous lesions fall into three categories: atypical squamous cells of undetermined significance, low-grade squamous intraepithelial lesions, and high-grade squamous intraepithelial lesions.
  – The low-grade category includes mild dysplasia and the changes of the human papillomavirus.
  – The high-grade category includes moderate to severe dysplasia and carcinoma in situ.
■ To confirm a suggestive or positive cytology report, the test may be repeated or followed by a biopsy. (See *Testing for cervical cancer,* page 436.)

## Purpose

■ To detect malignant cells
■ To detect inflammatory tissue changes
■ To assess the patient's response to chemotherapy and radiation therapy
■ To detect viral, fungal and, occasionally, parasitic invasion

## Patient preparation

■ Explain that the Pap test allows for the study of cervical cells.
■ Stress its importance as an aid for detection of cancer at a stage when the disease is commonly asymptomatic and still curable.
■ The test shouldn't be scheduled during the menstrual period; the best time is midcycle.
■ Instruct the patient to avoid having intercourse for 24 hours, not to douche for 48 hours, and not to insert vaginal medications for 1 week before the test because doing so can wash away cellular deposits and change the vaginal pH.
■ Tell the patient that the test requires that the cervix be scraped, who will perform the procedure and when, and that she may experience slight discomfort but no pain from the speculum (but may feel some pain when the cervix is scraped).
■ Inform her that the procedure takes 5 to 10 minutes or slightly longer if the vagina, pelvic cavity, and rectum are examined bimanually.
■ Obtain an accurate patient history, and ask these questions: When did you last have a Pap test? Have you ever had an abnormal Pap test? When was your last menstrual period? Are your periods regular? How many days do they last? Is bleeding heavy or light? Have you taken or are you presently taking hormones or oral contraceptives? Do you use an intrauterine device? Do you have any vaginal discharge, pain, or itching? Which, if any, gynecologic disorders have occurred in your family? Have you ever had gynecologic surgery, chemotherapy, or radiation therapy? If so, describe it

# Testing for cervical cancer

To analyze cervical cells, the ThinPrep test may be collected in the same manner as a Papanicolaou (Pap) test using a cytobrush and plastic spatula. The specimens are deposited in a bottle provided with a fixative and sent to the laboratory. A filter is then inserted into the bottle and excess mucus, blood, and inflammatory cells are filtered out by centrifuge. Remaining cells are then placed on a slide in a uniform, thin layer and read as a Pap test. This causes fewer slides to be classified as unreadable, significantly reducing the incidence of false negatives and the need for repeat tests.

When using the ThinPrep test, screening can also be easily done for the human papillomavirus (HPV), of which certain strains have been identified as the primary cause of cervical cancer. The Digene hc2 HPV deoxyribonucleic acid (DNA) test has been approved by the Food and Drug Administration to determine if those identified at high risk for developing cervical cancer have been exposed to HPV. The specimen is collected as a Pap smear but is dispersed with ThinPrep solution. Separate aliquots are used for each test, from brushings of the endocervix. The brush is then inserted into the specialized tube, snapped off at the shaft, and capped securely. The target solution in the tube disrupts the virus and releases target DNA, which combines with specific ribonucleic acid (RNA) probes creating RNA:DNA hybrids. The hybrids are captured, bound, and able to be magnified and measured using a luminometer.

If the patient is found to be positive for HPV, it means she has been infected with the virus. Depending on the type of HPV found through DNA testing, the patient harboring high-risk HPV strains has a higher risk of developing cervical cancer. It's recommended that the patient undergo colposcopy in which the cervix is viewed under microscope and a biopsy is taken from the tissue sample.

fully. Note the pertinent patient history data on the laboratory request.

- Provide emotional support if the patient is anxious; tell her that test results should be available in a few weeks.
- Ask the patient to empty her bladder before the test is performed.

## Procedure and posttest care

- Confirm the patient's identity using two patient identifiers according to facility policy.
- Instruct the patient to disrobe from the waist down and to drape herself.
- Ask the patient to lie on the examining table and to place her heels in the stirrups. (She may be more comfortable if she keeps her shoes or socks on.) Tell her to slide her buttocks to the edge of the table. Adjust the drape to minimize exposure.

- To avoid startling the patient, tell her when the examination will begin.
- The practitioner puts on gloves and inserts an unlubricated speculum into the vagina. To make insertion easier, the speculum may be moistened with saline solution or warm water.
- After the practitioner locates the cervix, he collects secretions from the cervix and material from the endocervical canal. He places the endocervical brush inside the endocervix and rolls it firmly inside the canal. If using a Pap stick (wooden spatula), it's placed against the cervix with the longest protrusion in the cervical canal, and then rotated clockwise 360 degrees firmly against the cervix.
- The practitioner then spreads the specimen on the slide according to laboratory recommendations and immediately

immerses the slide in (or sprays it with) a fixative.

■ Alternatively, posterior vaginal pool secretions and pancervical material may be collected and smeared on a single slide, which must be fixed immediately according to laboratory instructions.

■ Label the specimen appropriately, including the date, the patient's name, age, the date of her last menstrual period, and the collection site and method.

■ A bimanual examination may follow after the removal of the speculum. Help the patient up and ask her to dress when the examination is completed.

■ Supply the patient with a sanitary napkin if cervical bleeding occurs.

■ Tell the patient when to return for her next Pap test.

### Precautions

■ Make sure the cervical specimen is aspirated and scraped from the cervix. A vaginal pool sample isn't recommended for cervical or endometrial cancer screening.

■ The specimen should be thick enough that it isn't transparent.

■ Scrapings taken directly from the lesion are preferred if vaginal or vulval lesions are present.

■ Use a small pipette, if necessary, in a patient whose uterus is involuting or atrophying from age, to aspirate cells from the squamocolumnar junction and the cervical canal.

### Complications

■ Bleeding

# ▌Semen analysis

Semen analysis is a simple, inexpensive, and reasonably definitive test that's used in many applications, including evaluating a man's fertility. Fertility analysis usually includes measuring seminal fluid volume, performing sperm counts, and microscopic examination of spermatozoa. Sperm are counted in much the same way that white blood cells, red blood cells, and platelets are counted in a blood sample. Motility and morphology are studied microscopically after staining a drop of semen.

If analysis detects an abnormality, additional tests (for example, liver, thyroid, pituitary, or adrenal function tests) may be performed to identify the underlying cause and to screen for metabolic abnormalities (such as diabetes mellitus). Significant abnormalities—such as greatly decreased sperm count or motility or a marked increase in morphologically abnormal forms—may require testicular biopsy.

Semen analysis can also be used to detect semen on a rape victim, to identify the blood group of an alleged rapist, or to prove sterility in a paternity suit. (See *Identifying semen for medicolegal purposes,* page 438.)

### Normal results

■ The volume of semen ranges from 0.7 to 6.5 ml.

■ The semen volume of many men in infertile couples is increased.

■ Abstinence for 1 week or more results in progressively increased semen volume. (With abstinence of up to 10 days, sperm counts increase, sperm motility progressively decreases, and sperm morphology stays the same.)

■ Liquefied semen is generally highly viscid, translucent, and gray-white, with a musty or acrid odor. After liquefaction, specimens of normal viscosity can be poured in drops.

■ Semen is slightly alkaline with a pH of 7.3 to 7.9.

■ It coagulates immediately and liquefies within 20 minutes.

■ The normal sperm count is 20 million/ml to 150 million/ml and can be greater.

# Identifying semen for medicolegal purposes

Spermatozoa (or their fragments) persist in the vagina for more than 72 hours after sexual intercourse. This allows detection and positive identification of semen from vaginal aspirates or smears or from stains on clothing, other fabrics, skin, or hair, which is commonly necessary for medicolegal purposes, usually in connection with rape or homicide investigations. Spermatozoa taken from the vagina of an exhumed body that has been properly embalmed and remains reasonably intact can also be identified.

To determine which stains or fluids require further investigation, clothing or other fabrics can be scanned with ultraviolet light to detect the typical greenwhite fluorescence of semen. Soaking appropriate samples of clothing, fabric, or hair in physiologic saline solution elutes the semen and spermatozoa. Deposits of dried semen can be gently sponged from the victim's skin.

The two most common tests to identify semen are the determination of acid phosphatase concentration (the more sensitive test) and microscopic examination for the presence of spermatozoa. Acid phosphatase appears in semen in significantly greater concentrations than in other body fluids. In microscopic examination, spermatozoa or head fragments can be identified on stained smears prepared directly from vaginal scrapings or aspirates or from the concentrated sediment of eluates or lavages.

Like other body fluids, semen contains the soluble A, B, and H blood group substances in about 80% of males who are genetically determined secretors (males who have the dominant secretor gene in a homozygous or heterozygous state). Thus, the male who has group A blood and is a secretor has soluble blood group A substance in his seminal fluid and group A substance on the surface of his red blood cells. This fact can be of considerable medicolegal importance. Semen analysis can demonstrate that the semen of a suspect in a rape or homicide investigation is different from or consistent with semen found in or on the victim's body.

■ Forty percent of spermatozoa have normal morphology, and 20% or more of spermatozoa show progressive motility within 4 hours of collection.
■ The normal postcoital cervical mucus test shows 10 to 20 motile spermatozoa per microscopic high-power field and spinnbarkeit (a measurement of the tenacity of the mucus) of at least 4″ (10 cm). These findings indicate adequate spermatozoa and receptivity of the cervical mucus. Shaking or dead sperm may indicate antisperm antibodies.

## Abnormal results
■ Abnormal semen isn't synonymous with infertility.

■ Only one viable spermatozoon is needed to fertilize an ovum. Although a normal sperm count is 20 million/ml or more, many men with sperm counts below 1 million/ml have fathered normal children. Only men who can't deliver *any* viable spermatozoa in their ejaculate during sexual intercourse are absolutely sterile.
■ Subnormal sperm counts, decreased sperm motility, and abnormal morphology are usually associated with decreased fertility.

## Purpose

- To evaluate male fertility in an infertile couple
- To substantiate the effectiveness of a vasectomy
- To detect semen on the body or clothing of a suspected rape victim or elsewhere at the crime scene
- To identify blood group substances to exonerate or incriminate a criminal suspect
- To rule out paternity on grounds of complete sterility

## Patient preparation
### For fertility evaluation

- Provide written instructions, and inform the patient that the most desirable specimen requires masturbation, ideally in a physician's office or laboratory.
- Tell the patient to follow the instructions given to him regarding the period of sexual continence before the test because this may increase his sperm count. Some physicians specify a fixed number of days, usually between 2 and 5; others advise a period of continence equal to the usual interval between episodes of sexual intercourse.
- If the patient prefers to collect the specimen at home, emphasize the importance of delivering the specimen to the laboratory within 1 hour after collection. Warn him not to expose the specimen to extreme temperatures or to direct sunlight (which can also increase its temperature). Ideally, the specimen should remain at body temperature until liquefaction is complete (about 20 minutes). To deliver a semen specimen during cold weather, suggest that the patient keep the specimen container in a coat pocket on the way to the laboratory to protect the specimen from exposure to cold.
- Alternatives to collection by masturbation include coitus interruptus or the use of a condom. For collection by coitus interruptus, instruct the patient to withdraw immediately before ejaculation and to deposit the ejaculate in a suitable specimen container. For collection by condom, tell the patient to first wash the condom with soap and water, rinse it thoroughly, and allow it to dry completely. (Powders or lubricants applied to the condom may be spermicidal.) Special sheaths that don't contain spermicide are also available for semen collection. After collection, instruct him to tie the condom, place it in a glass jar, and promptly deliver it to the laboratory.
- Fertility may also be determined by collecting semen from the woman after coitus to assess the ability of the spermatozoa to penetrate the cervical mucus and remain active. For the postcoital cervical mucus test, instruct the patient to report for examination 1 to 2 days before ovulation as determined by basal temperature records. A urine luteinizing hormone-releasing hormone test may help predict ovulation in the patient with an irregular cycle. Instruct the couple to abstain from intercourse for 2 days and then to have sexual intercourse 2 to 8 hours before the examination. Remind them to avoid using lubricants. Explain to the patient scheduled for this test that the procedure takes only a few minutes. Tell her that she'll be placed in the lithotomy position and that a speculum will be inserted into the vagina to collect the specimen. She may feel some pressure, but no pain.

### For semen collection from a rape victim

- Explain to the patient that the practitioner will try to obtain a semen specimen from her vagina.
- Prepare the victim for insertion of the speculum as you would the patient scheduled for postcoital examination.

#### DO'S & DON'TS

Handle the victim's clothes as little as possible. If her clothes are moist, put them in a paper bag—not a plastic bag (which causes seminal stains and secretions to mold). Label the bag properly, and send it to the laboratory immediately.

- Provide emotional support by speaking to the patient calmly and reassuringly. Encourage her to express her fears and anxieties. Listen sympathetically.
- If the patient is scheduled for vaginal lavage, tell her to expect a cold sensation when saline solution is instilled to wash out the specimen.
- Help the patient relax by instructing her to breathe deeply and slowly through her mouth.
- Instruct the victim to urinate just before the test, but warn her not to wipe the vulva afterward because this may remove semen.

### Procedure and posttest care

- Confirm the patient's identity using two patient identifiers according to facility policy.
- Obtain a semen specimen for a fertility study by asking the patient to collect semen in a clean plastic specimen container.
- A specimen is obtained from the vagina of a rape victim by direct aspiration, saline lavage, or a direct smear of vaginal contents using a Pap stick or, less desirably, a cotton applicator stick. Dried smears are usually collected from the suspected rape victim's skin by gently washing the skin with a small piece of gauze moistened with physiologic saline solution.

- Prepare direct smears on glass microscopic slides after labeling the frosted end. Immediately place smeared slides in Coplin jars containing 95% ethanol.
- Before postcoital examination, the practitioner wipes excess mucus from the external cervix and collects the specimen by direct aspiration of the cervical canal using a 1-ml tuberculin syringe without a cannula or needle.
- Inform a patient who's undergoing infertility studies that test results should be available in 24 hours.
- Refer the suspected rape victim to an appropriate specialist for counseling—a gynecologist, psychiatrist, clinical psychologist, nursing specialist, member of the clergy, or representative of a community support group such as Women Organized Against Rape.

### Precautions

- If the patient prefers to collect the specimen during coitus interruptus, tell him he must prevent any loss of semen during ejaculation.
- Deliver all specimens, regardless of the source or method of collection, to the laboratory within 1 hour.
- Protect semen specimens for fertility studies from extremes of temperature and direct sunlight during delivery to the laboratory.

#### DO'S & DON'TS

Never lubricate the vaginal speculum. Oil or grease hinders examination of spermatozoa by interfering with smear preparation and staining and by inhibiting sperm motility through toxic ingredients. Instead, moisten the speculum with water or physiologic saline solution.

▪ Use extreme caution in securing, labeling, and delivering all specimens to be used for medicolegal purposes. You may be asked to testify as to when, where, and from whom the specimen was obtained; the specimen's general appearance and identifying features; steps taken to ensure the specimen's integrity; and when, where, and to whom the specimen was delivered for analysis. If your facility or clinic uses routing requests for such specimens, fill them out carefully and place them in the permanent medicolegal file.

# Sexual assault testing

Each facility or agency has a specific protocol for specimen collection in cases involving sexual assault. Specimens can be collected from various sources, including blood, hair, nails, tissues, and body fluids such as urine, semen, saliva, and vaginal secretions. Evidence can be obtained also from the results of diagnostic tests, such as computed tomography and radiography. Regardless of the protocol or specimen source, accurate and precise specimen collection is essential in conjunction with thorough, objective documentation because in many cases, this information will be used as evidence in legal proceedings.

Many institutions have a Sexual Assault Nurse Examiner (SANE) available to care for patients who are victims of sexual assault. SANEs are skilled rape crisis professionals who can evaluate the victim and collect specimens. They may also be called upon at a later date to testify in legal proceedings.

## Normal results
▪ Not applicable

## Abnormal results
▪ Not applicable

## Purpose
▪ To collect specimens for sexual assault testing

## Patient preparation
▪ Assess the patient's ability to undergo the specimen collection procedure.
▪ Explain the procedures that the patient will undergo, what specimens will be collected and from where, and provide emotional support throughout.
▪ Obtain consent from the patient or family for specimens to be obtained.
▪ Ask the patient if she would like someone, such as a family member, friend, or other person to stay with her during the specimen collection.
▪ Ensure patient privacy throughout the collection procedure.

## Procedure and posttest care
### Specimen collection
General guidelines for collecting specimens
If you're responsible for collecting specimens in a sexual assault, follow these important guidelines:
▪ Be knowledgeable about your facility's policy and procedures for specimen collection in sexual assault cases.
▪ When obtaining specimens, be sure to collect them from the victim and, if possible, from the suspect.
▪ Check with local law enforcement agencies about additional specimens that may be needed; for example, trace evidence, such as soot, grass, gravel, glass, or other debris.
▪ Wear gloves and change them frequently; use disposable equipment and instruments if possible.
▪ Avoid coughing, sneezing, or talking over specimens or touching your face, nose, or mouth when collecting specimens.
▪ Include the victim's clothing as part of the collection procedure.

■ Place all items collected in a paper bag.

■ Document each item or specimen collected; have another person witness each collection and document it.
■ Obtain photographs of all injuries for documentation.
■ Include written documentation of the victim's physical and psychological condition on first encounter, throughout specimen collection, and afterward.
■ When possible, obtain a special Sexual Assault Evidence Collection Kit, which contains the necessary items for specimen collection based on the evidence required by the local crime laboratory. In addition, the kit contains a form that's to be completed, signed, and dated by the examiner. When collecting specimens for moist secretions, typically a one-swab technique is used; if secretions are dry, then a two-swab technique is used.
■ Before obtaining any specimens, inspect the genital area using a Wood's lamp. This device uses long-wave ultraviolet light to scan the area for secretions and helps identify areas of trauma.

### Clothing for specimen collection
■ Ask the patient to stand on a clean piece of examination paper if he or she is able to stand; if the patient can't stand, then have the patient remain on the examination table or bed.
■ Have the patient remove each article of clothing, one at a time, and place each article in a separate, clean paper bag.
■ If the clothing is wet, allow it to dry first before placing the item into the paper bag.

■ Fold the examination paper onto itself and place it into a clean paper bag.
■ Fold over, seal, label, and initial each bag.

### Vaginal or cervical secretion collection
■ Swab the vaginal area thoroughly with four swabs; swab the cervical area with two swabs, making sure to keep the vaginal swabs separate from the cervical swabs.
■ Run the vaginal swabs over a slide (supplied in the kit) and allow the slide and swabs to air dry; do the same for the cervical swabs.
■ Place the vaginal swabs in the swab container and close it; place the slide in the cardboard sleeve, close it and tape it shut; repeat this procedure for the cervical swabs.
■ Place the swab container and cardboard sleeve into the envelope, and seal it securely.
■ Complete the information as provided on the front of the envelope; if both vaginal and cervical swabs are obtained, use a separate envelope for each.

### Anal secretion collection
■ Moisten a single swab with sterile water.
■ Insert the swab gently into the patient's rectum about 1¼" (3 cm).
■ Rotate the swab gently and then remove it.
■ Allow the swab to air dry and then place it in an envelope.
■ Seal and label the envelope appropriately.

### Penile secretion collection

- Moisten a single swab with sterile water.
- Swab the entire external surface of the penis.
- Repeat this at least one more time (so that at least two swabs are obtained).
- Allow the swabs to air-dry and then place each in a separate envelope.
- Seal and label the envelopes appropriately.

### Pubic hair collection

- Use the comb provided in the kit and comb through the pubic hair.
- Collect about 20 to 30 pubic hairs and place them in the envelope.
- Alternatively, obtain 20 to 30 plucked hairs from the patient; allow the patient the option of plucking own pubic hair.
- Place the hair in the envelope, seal and label it appropriately.

### Blood samples

- After performing a venipuncture, obtain at least 5 ml of blood in an EDTA tube.
- Write the patient's name and date on the label of the tube.
- Remove the DNA stain card from the kit and label it with the patient's name.
- Using the blood collected in this tube, withdraw 1 ml of blood and apply blood to each of the four circles on the card, completely filling each circle if possible.
- Let the card air dry and then place the card in the envelope.
- Seal and label the envelope appropriately.
- Place the blood tube into the tube holder supplied in the kit and seal the holder with tape supplied in the kit (may be referred to as evidence tape).
- Place the tube and holder in the zippered bag provided.

- Collect additional blood samples to test for pregnancy; sexually transmitted diseases, such as gonorrhea, chlamydia, and syphilis; or toxicology as appropriate and send to the laboratory immediately.

### Urine specimens

- Obtain a random urine specimen from the patient; if necessary, obtain the urine specimen via catheterization.

## *Specimen storage and transport*

- Refrigerate blood samples obtained.
- Place all other specimens in the specimen kit and keep the kit at room temperature.
- Give all the specimens to the police when they arrive.

## *Specimen care after collection*

- Be sure to follow the directions in the kit precisely to ensure that the chain of evidence is followed.
- Document all specimens collected, including type, location, time and patient's name, identification number and any other relevant information. Include photographs as appropriate, making sure to also include relevant information on the photo.
- Provide follow-up counseling and support to the patient.
- If necessary, administer ordered medications, such as tetanus or antibiotics.
- Make sure that the patient has a support person to accompany home.
- Arrange for referral to local support group or follow up with a trained counselor.

# Endoscopy

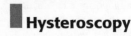

## Hysteroscopy

In hysteroscopy, a small-diameter endoscope is used to visualize the interior of the uterus. Performed in the physician's office or a short procedure unit under local or general anesthesia, this procedure has become widely used to investigate abnormal uterine bleeding. It also aids in the removal of polyps and in the diagnosis and treatment of other uterine abnormalities. Other investigational uses for hysteroscopy are being studied, and it is also approved by the U.S. Food and Drug Administration for total sterilization.

### Normal results
- The interior of the uterus is normal in size and shape and free from adhesions and lesions.

### Abnormal results
- The physician may detect polyps, uterine wall tumors, and other uterine abnormalities.

### Purpose
- To investigate abnormal uterine bleeding
- To remove polyps
- To evaluate an infertile patient
- To remove embedded intrauterine devices
- To aid in the diagnosis and treatment of intrauterine adhesions
- To diagnose uterine fibroids
- To resect fibroids and ablate the endometrium
- To provide total sterilization

### Patient preparation
- Explain that hysteroscopy helps detect abnormalities in the uterus.

- Tell the patient that the physician will perform this procedure in his office, usually using a local anesthetic. (However, if the patient's problems appear extensive, an in-hospital operative hysteroscopy would be indicated.)
- Inform the patient that the test should take place within the first week after the end of her menstrual cycle. Ask her when her last Papanicolaou test was performed, and obtain the results.
- Tell the patient that the physician will perform a complete pelvic examination before the hysteroscopy and that cultures of the vagina and cervix will be taken if necessary.
- Inform the patient that she'll be asked to empty her bladder before the test.
- Tell the patient that she may have some vaginal bleeding and mild abdominal cramping after the test.
- Explain to the patient that the physician may inflate her uterus with carbon dioxide gas so that he can see the interior of the uterus better. This gas will be absorbed and dispersed by her body and may cause upper abdominal or shoulder pain lasting 24 to 36 hours after the test.
- Recommend to the patient that she have a friend or relative drive her home.
- Make sure that the patient or a responsible family member has signed an informed consent form.
- Check the patient's history for hypersensitivity to the anesthetic.
- Make sure laboratory work is completed and results are reported before the test.

### Procedure and posttest care
- Confirm the patient's identity using two patient identifiers according to facility policy.
- Place the patient in a modified dorsal lithotomy position with her legs held in the stirrups.
- The physician will expose the cervix using the smallest speculum possible,

and then will suffuse the cervix with 1% lidocaine. Depending on the purpose of the procedure, a paracervical block, an anxiolytic, or an analgesic may also be used. In some cases, a regional or general anesthetic may be used.

- The physician will gently sound the endocervical canal and uterine cavity and will dilate the canal, as necessary, to insert the hysteroscope. (Modern hysteroscopes are 10″ [25 cm] long.) Visualization of the uterine cavity begins at the level of the internal os.
- The two primary types of hysteroscopy are contact and panoramic. In contact hysteroscopy, the uterus isn't distended and only the area in direct contact with the hysteroscope can be viewed. In panoramic hysteroscopy, the more common type, an external illumination source and media (such as carbon dioxide gas) for distention are needed. This method allows visualization of the tissue from a distance.
- Monitor the patient's vital signs.
- The patient may have slight vaginal bleeding and lower abdominal cramping. Provide a sanitary pad, if needed.
- Severe cramps, dyspnea, and upper abdominal and right shoulder pain can develop if carbon dioxide passes into the peritoneal cavity. Reassure the patient that some abdominal and shoulder pain is normal and should disappear within 24 to 36 hours. Recommend that she have a friend or relative drive her home.
- Provide analgesics, as needed.

### Precautions

- Hysteroscopy requires experience in topographic interpretation of the uterus and skill in manipulating the required instruments.
- During the procedure, monitor the patient's vital signs and discomfort level.

### Complications

- Severe cramps, dyspnea, upper abdominal and right shoulder pain
- Adverse reaction to drugs
- Infection

# Laparoscopy

Laparoscopy permits visualization of the peritoneal cavity by the insertion of a small fiber-optic telescope (laparoscope) through the anterior abdominal wall. This surgical technique may be used diagnostically to detect abnormalities, such as cysts, adhesions, fibroids, and infection. It can also be used therapeutically to perform procedures, such as adhesion lysis; ovarian biopsy; tubal sterilization; removal of ectopic pregnancies, fibroids, hydrosalpinx, and foreign bodies; and fulguration of endometriotic implants.

### Normal results

- The uterus and fallopian tubes are of normal size and shape, free from adhesions, and mobile.
- The ovaries are of normal size and shape.
- Cysts and endometriosis are absent.
- Dye injected through the cervix flows freely from the fimbria.

### Abnormal results

- An ovarian cyst appears as a bubble on the surface of the ovary. The cyst may be clear if filled with follicular fluid or serous or mucous material, or it may be red, blue, or brown if filled with blood.
- Adhesions may appear as thick and fibrous tissue or as almost transparent strands of tissue.
- Endometriosis may resemble small, blue powder burns on the peritoneum or the serosa of any pelvic or abdominal structure; however, clear, red lesions are also possible.

- Fibroids appear as lumps on the uterus, hydrosalpinx as an enlarged fallopian tube.
- Ectopic pregnancy appears as an enlarged or ruptured fallopian tube.
- In pelvic inflammatory disease (PID), infection or abscess is evident.

### Purpose
- To identify the cause of pelvic pain
- To help detect endometriosis, ectopic pregnancy, and PID
- To evaluate pelvic masses or the fallopian tubes of the infertile patient
- To stage carcinoma in selected cases

### Patient preparation
- Explain that laparoscopy is used to detect abnormalities of the uterus, fallopian tubes, and ovaries.
- Instruct the patient to fast for at least 8 hours before surgery.
- Tell the patient who will perform the procedure and where it will take place.
- Tell the patient whether she'll receive a general anesthetic and whether the procedure will require an outpatient visit or overnight hospitalization.
- Warn the patient that she may experience pain at the puncture site and in the shoulder.
- Make sure that the patient or a responsible family member has signed an informed consent form.
- Check the patient's history for hypersensitivity to the anesthetic.
- Make sure laboratory work is completed and results are reported before the test.
- Instruct the patient to empty her bladder just before the test.

### Procedure and posttest care
- Confirm the patient's identity using two patient identifiers according to facility policy.
- The patient is anesthetized and placed in the lithotomy position.

- The physician catheterizes the bladder and then performs a bimanual examination of the pelvic area to detect abnormalities that may contraindicate the test and to ensure that the bladder is empty.
- The tenaculum is placed on the cervix and a uterine manipulator is inserted; an incision is made at the inferior rim of the umbilicus.
- The Veress needle is inserted into the peritoneal cavity, and 2 to 3 L of carbon dioxide or nitrous oxide is insufflated to distend the abdominal wall and provide an organ-free space for trocar insertion; the needle is removed and a trocar and sheath are inserted into the peritoneal cavity; multiple trocars may be inserted at the pubic hairline to allow access for other instruments.
- After removal of the trocar, the laparoscope is inserted through the sheath to examine the pelvis and abdomen.
- To evaluate tubal patency, the physician infuses a dye through the cervix and observes the tubes for spillage.
- After the examination, minor surgical procedures, such as ovarian biopsy, may be performed.

**ACTION STAT!**

 Monitor the patient's vital signs and urine output. Report sudden changes immediately; they may indicate complications.

- Monitor the patient for adverse or allergic reactions. After administration of a general anesthetic, monitor her electrolyte balance, hemoglobin level, and hematocrit. Help her ambulate after recovery.
- Tell the patient that she may resume her usual diet.
- Instruct the patient to restrict activity for 2 to 7 days, as necessary.
- Reassure the patient that some abdominal and shoulder pain is normal and should disappear within 24 to 36 hours.

If pain continues or worsens, notify the practitioner immediately because this may be a sign of bowel perforation. Provide analgesics, as ordered, and monitor her for adverse effects.

### Precautions

- Laparoscopy is contraindicated in the patient with advanced abdominal wall cancer, advanced pulmonary or cardiovascular disease, intestinal obstruction, palpable abdominal mass, large abdominal hernia, chronic tuberculosis, or a history of peritonitis.
- During the procedure, check for proper catheter drainage.

### Complications

- Punctured visceral organ
- Peritonitis

---

## Direct graphic recording

## External fetal monitoring

In external fetal monitoring, a noninvasive test, an electronic transducer and a cardiotachometer amplify and record fetal heart rate (FHR) while a pressure-sensitive transducer (tocodynamometer) records uterine contractions. Fetal monitoring records the baseline FHR (average FHR over two contraction cycles or 10 minutes), periodic fluctuations in the baseline FHR, and beat-to-beat heart rate variability. (See *Understanding fetal monitoring terminology.*) External fetal monitoring is also used during other tests of fetal health, notably the nonstress test and the contraction stress test (CST).

---

### Understanding fetal monitoring terminology

- Baseline fetal heart rate (FHR): Average FHR over two contraction cycles or 10 minutes
- Baseline changes: Fluctuations in FHR unrelated to uterine contractions
- Periodic changes: Fluctuations in FHR related to uterine contractions
- Amplitude: Difference in beats per minute between baseline readings and fluctuation in FHR
- Recovery time: Difference between the end of the contraction and the return to the baseline FHR
- Acceleration: Transient rise in FHR lasting longer than 15 seconds and associated with a uterine contraction
- Deceleration: Transient fall in FHR related to a uterine contraction
- Lag time: Difference between the peak of the contraction and the lowest point of deceleration

---

### Normal results

- FHR ranges from 120 to 160 beats/minute, with a variability of 5 to 25 beats/minute.
- During an antepartum nonstress test, the fetus is considered healthy and should remain so for another week if two fetal movements causing a heart rate acceleration of more than 15 beats/minute from baseline FHR occur in a 20-minute period.
- During nonstress testing, a normal, healthy fetus usually has three rises in FHR within 10 to 15 minutes, but fetuses may sleep up to 45 minutes at a time. If there's no change in FHR in a 10-minute period, consider shaking the patient's abdomen gently, clapping loudly, or having the patient drink ice water or apple juice. If the FHR remains unchanged, a contraction stress test or biophysical profile test should be ordered.

The fetus is assessed by watching fetal movements, muscle tone, fetal breathing, and the amniotic fluid index.

■ During a CST, the fetus is assumed to be healthy and should remain so for another week if three contractions occur during a 10-minute period, with no late decelerations.

### Abnormal results

■ Bradycardia (FHR ≤ 120 beats/minute) may indicate fetal heart block, malposition, or hypoxia. Fetal bradycardia may also be drug induced.

■ Tachycardia (FHR > 160 beats/minute) may result from maternal fever, tachycardia, hyperthyroidism, or use of vagolytic drugs or opioids; early fetal hypoxia; or fetal infection or arrhythmia.

■ Decreased variability (a fluctuation of < 5 beats/minute in the FHR) may be caused by fetal arrhythmia or heart block; fetal hypoxia, central nervous system malformation, or infections; or vagolytic drugs.

■ FHR accelerations may result from early hypoxia. They may precede or follow variable decelerations and may indicate that the fetus is in a breech position.

■ In an antepartum nonstress test, a positive result (fewer than two accelerations of FHR that last longer than 15 seconds each, with a heart rate acceleration of over 15 beats/minute) indicates an increased risk of perinatal morbidity and mortality and usually requires a CST.

■ During a CST, persistent late decelerations during two or more contractions may indicate an increased risk of fetal morbidity or mortality. Hyperstimulation (long or frequent uterine contractions) or suspicious results require biophysical profile assessment. If findings are unsatisfactory, cesarean birth may be indicated.

**DRUG CHALLENGE**

Drugs that affect the sympathetic and parasympathetic nervous systems (possible low FHR)

### Purpose

■ To measure FHR and the frequency of uterine contractions

■ To evaluate antepartum and intrapartum fetal health during stress and nonstress situations

■ To detect fetal distress

■ To determine the necessity for internal fetal monitoring

### Patient preparation

■ Explain that external fetal monitoring assesses fetal health.

■ Assure the patient that external fetal monitoring is painless and won't hurt the fetus or interfere with normal labor.

■ If monitoring is to be performed antepartum, instruct the patient to eat a meal just before the test to increase fetal activity, which decreases the test time.

■ If the patient smokes, advise her to abstain for 2 hours before testing because smoking decreases fetal activity.

■ Explain to the patient that she may have to restrict movement during baseline readings, but that she may change position between the readings.

■ Make sure that the patient or a responsible family member has signed an informed consent form.

### Procedure and posttest care

■ Confirm the patient's identity using two patient identifiers according to facility policy.

■ Place the patient in a semi-Fowler or left lateral position with her abdomen exposed. Cover the ultrasound transducer receiver crystal with conductive gel.

- Palpate the patient's abdomen to identify the fetal chest area, locate the most distinct fetal heart sounds, and then secure the ultrasound transducer over this area with the elastic band, stockinette, or abdominal strap.
- Check the recording equipment to ensure an adequate printout and verify the fetal monitor's alarm boundaries.
- During monitoring, check the elastic band, stockinette, or abdominal strap to ensure that the fit is comfortable yet tight enough to produce a good tracing.
- As labor progresses, reposition the pressure transducer as necessary so that it remains on the fundal portion of the uterus. You may have to reposition the ultrasound transducer as fetal or maternal position changes.

### For antepartum monitoring with nonstress tests

- Tell the patient to hold the pressure transducer in her hand and to push it each time she feels the fetus move.
- Within a 20-minute period, monitor baseline FHR until you record two fetal movements that last longer than 15 seconds each and cause heart rate accelerations of more than 15 beats/minute from the baseline. If you can't obtain two FHR accelerations within 30 minutes, shake the patient's abdomen to stimulate the fetus and repeat the test.

### For antepartum monitoring with a CST

- Induce contractions by oxytocin infusion or nipple stimulation (endogenous oxytocin).
- When giving oxytocin, infuse a dilute solution at a rate of 1 milliunit/minute, increasing the oxytocin rate until the patient experiences three contractions within 10 minutes, each lasting longer than 45 seconds.
- When using nipple stimulation, tell the patient to stimulate one nipple by

hand until contractions begin. If a second contraction doesn't occur in 2 minutes, have her stimulate the nipple again. Stimulate both nipples if contractions don't occur in 15 minutes. Continue the test until three contractions occur in 10 minutes.
- If no decelerations occur during three contractions, the patient may be discharged. Late decelerations during any of the contractions require notification of the practitioner and further tests.

### For intrapartum monitoring

- Secure the pressure transducer with an elastic band, a stockinette, or an abdominal strap over the area of greatest uterine electrical activity during contractions (usually the fundus).
- Adjust the machine to record 0 to 10 mm Hg of pressure between palpable contractions.
- Reposition the ultrasound and pressure transducers as necessary to ensure continuous accurate readings. Review the tracings frequently for baseline abnormalities, periodic changes, variability of changes, and uterine contraction abnormalities.
- Record maternal movement, administration of drugs, and procedures performed directly on the tracing to assist in the evaluation of changes in the tracing.
- Report abnormalities immediately.
- Repeat antepartum monitoring weekly as long as indications, such as pregnancy over 42 weeks' gestation or fetal growth retardation, persist.

## Precautions
- During a CST, watch for fetal distress with oxytocin infusion or nipple stimulation.

# Internal fetal monitoring

Internal fetal monitoring is an invasive procedure that involves attaching an electrode to the fetal scalp to directly monitor fetal heart rate (FHR). A catheter introduced into the uterine cavity measures the frequency and pressure of uterine contractions. Internal monitoring is performed only during labor, after the membranes have ruptured and the cervix has dilated 3 cm, with the fetal head lower than the –2 station and only if external monitoring provides inadequate data.

Internal monitoring provides more accurate information about fetal health than external monitoring and is especially useful in determining whether cesarean delivery is necessary. (See *Understanding internal fetal monitoring*.)

### Reference values

▪ FHR ranges from 120 to 160 beats/minute, with a variability of 5 to 25 beats/minute.

### Abnormal results

▪ Bradycardia (FHR < 120 beats/minute) may indicate fetal heart block, malposition, or hypoxia. It may also result from maternal ingestion of certain drugs, such as propranolol and opioid analgesics. A severe drop in FHR (< 70 beats/minute for more than 60 seconds) with a decrease in variability indicates fetal distress and may result in a compromised neonate.
▪ Tachycardia (FHR > 160 beats/minute) may result from early fetal hypoxia, fetal infection or arrhythmia, prematurity, or maternal fever, tachycardia, hyperthyroidism, or use of vagolytic drugs.
▪ Decreased variability (fluctuation of < 5 beats/minute from baseline) may result from fetal arrhythmia or heart block, hypoxia, central nervous system malformation, or infections or from maternal use of opioids or vagolytic drugs.

▪ Early decelerations (slowing of FHR at the onset of a contraction with recovery to baseline within no more than 15 seconds after the contraction ends) are related to fetal head compression and usually ensure fetal health.
▪ Late decelerations (slowing of FHR after a contraction begins, a lag time of more than 20 seconds, and a recovery time of more than 15 seconds) may be related to uteroplacental insufficiency, fetal hypoxia, or acidosis.
▪ Recurrent and persistently late decelerations with decreased variability usually indicate serious fetal distress, possibly resulting from conduction (spinal, caudal, or epidural) anesthesia or fetal hypoxia.
▪ Variable decelerations (sudden precipitous drops in FHR unrelated to uterine contractions) are commonly related to cord compression.
▪ Poor beat-to-beat variability without periodic patterns may indicate fetal distress, requiring further evaluation such as analysis of fetal blood gas levels.
▪ Decreased intrauterine pressure during labor that isn't progressing normally may require oxytocin stimulation.
▪ Elevated intrauterine pressure readings may indicate abruptio placentae or overstimulation from oxytocin, possibly resulting in fetal distress due to decreased placental perfusion.

#### DRUG CHALLENGE

 Drugs that affect the parasympathetic and sympathetic nervous systems

### Purpose

▪ To monitor FHR, especially beat-to-beat variability (short-term variability)
▪ To measure the frequency and pressure of uterine contractions to assess the progress of labor
▪ To evaluate intrapartum fetal health

## Understanding internal fetal monitoring

In internal fetal monitoring, an electrode is attached to the fetal scalp. The resultant fetal electrocardiograms (FECGs) are transmitted to an amplifier. Subsequently, a cardiotachometer measures the interval between FECGs and plots a continuous fetal heart rate (FHR) graph, which is displayed on a two-channel oscilloscope screen. Intrauterine catheters attached to a transducer in the leg plate measure the frequency and pressure of uterine contractions, which are plotted below the FHR graph.

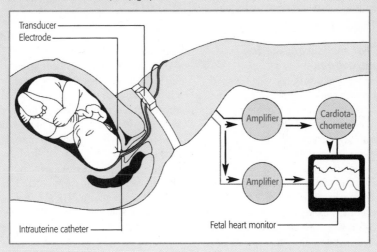

### Patient preparation

■ To supplement or replace external fetal monitoring

### Patient preparation
■ Explain that internal fetal monitoring accurately assesses fetal health and uterine activity and that it doesn't necessarily mean that there's a problem. Describe the procedure and answer all questions.
■ Warn the patient that she may feel mild discomfort when the uterine catheter and scalp electrode are inserted.
■ Make sure the patient or a responsible family member has signed an informed consent form.

### Procedure and posttest care
■ Confirm the patient's identity using two patient identifiers according to facility policy.

### *For measuring FHR*
■ Place the patient in the dorsal lithotomy position and prepare her perineal area for a vaginal examination, explaining each step of the procedure as it's performed by a practitioner or certified nurse-midwife. As the procedure begins, ask the patient to breathe through her mouth and relax her abdominal muscles.
■ After the vaginal examination, the fetal scalp is palpated and an appropriate site is identified. A plastic tube carrying the small electrode is introduced into the cervix, pressed firmly against the fetal scalp, and rotated clockwise to attach the electrode to the scalp. The electrode wire is tugged gently to ensure proper attachment and the tube is withdrawn, leaving the electrode in place.

■ A conduction medium is applied to a leg plate, which is then strapped to the patient's thigh. Electrode wires are attached to the leg plate, and a cable from the leg plate is plugged into the fetal monitor. To check proper placement of the scalp electrode, the monitor is turned on and the electrocardiogram button is pressed; an FHR signal indicates proper electrode attachment. (See *Understanding internal fetal monitoring,* page 450.)

### For measuring uterine contractions

■ Before inserting the uterine catheter, fill it with sterile normal saline solution to prevent air emboli. Explain each step of the procedure to the patient.
■ Ask the patient to breathe deeply through her mouth and to relax her abdominal muscles.
■ After the vagina has been examined and the presenting part of the fetus palpated, the catheter and guide are inserted ⅜" to ¾" (1 to 2 cm) into the cervix, usually between the fetal head and the posterior cervix.
■ The catheter is then gently advanced into the uterus until the black mark on the catheter is flush with the vulva. (The catheter guide should never be passed deeply into the uterus.)
■ The guide is removed and the catheter is connected to a transducer that converts the intrauterine pressure, as measured by the fluid in the catheter, to an electrical signal.

### For both procedures

■ After removing the fetal scalp electrode, apply antiseptic or antibiotic solution to the attachment site.

**Do's & don'ts**

 Watch for signs of fetal scalp abscess or maternal intrauterine infection.

### Precautions

■ Internal fetal monitoring is contraindicated if there's uncertainty about the fetus's presenting part or a technical impediment to attaching the lead.
■ Prevent artifactual pressure readings by flushing the pressure transducer with normal saline solution; to relieve catheter obstruction (by vernix caseosa, for example), inject a small amount of sterile normal saline solution into the catheter while the transducer is isolated from the system.
■ Make sure a low heart rate is actually the FHR, not the maternal heart rate.
■ If FHR patterns indicate distress, fetal oxygenation commonly can be improved by loading maternal fluids to increase placental perfusion, turning the mother on her side (preferably left) to alleviate supine hypotension, and administering oxygen to the mother. If these measures return FHR patterns to normal, labor may continue. If abnormal patterns persist, cesarean birth may be necessary.
■ Make sure the fetal scalp electrode and the uterine catheter are removed before cesarean delivery.

### Complications
■ Fetal scalp abscess
■ Maternal intrauterine infection

# Radiography

## Hysterosalpingography

Hysterosalpingography is a radiologic examination for visualizing the uterine cavity, the fallopian tubes, and the peritubal area. In this procedure, fluoroscopic X-ray films are taken as a contrast medium flows through the uterus and the fallopian tubes.

This test is generally performed as part of an infertility study.

## Normal results
- The uterine cavity is symmetrical.
- The contrast medium courses through fallopian tubes of normal caliber, spills freely into the peritoneal cavity, and doesn't leak from the uterus.

## Abnormal results
- An asymmetrical uterus suggests intrauterine adhesions or masses, such as fibroids or foreign bodies.
- Impaired contrast flow through the fallopian tubes suggests partial or complete blockage, resulting from intraluminal agglutination, extrinsic compression by adhesions, or perifimbrial adhesions.
- Leakage of the contrast medium through the uterine wall suggests fistulas.

## Purpose
- To confirm tubal abnormalities, such as adhesions and occlusion
- To confirm uterine abnormalities, such as the presence of foreign bodies, congenital malformations, and traumatic injuries
- To confirm the presence of fistulas or peritubal adhesions

## Patient preparation
- Explain that the hysterosalpingography confirms uterine and fallopian tube abnormalities.
- Tell the patient who will perform the test and where it will take place. The test should be performed 2 to 5 days after menstruation ends.
- Advise the patient that she may experience moderate cramping from the procedure; however, she may receive a mild sedative, such as diazepam, or a nonprescription prostaglandin inhibitor, if ordered, 30 minutes before the procedure.

## Procedure and posttest care
- Confirm the patient's identity using two patient identifiers according to facility policy.
- With the patient in the lithotomy position, a scout film is taken.
- A speculum is inserted in the vagina, the tenaculum is placed on the cervix, and the cervix is cleaned.
- The cannula is inserted into the cervix and anchored to the tenaculum. After the contrast medium is injected through the cannula, the uterus and the fallopian tubes are viewed fluoroscopically and radiographs are taken. To take oblique views, the X-ray table may be tilted or the patient asked to change position. Films may also be taken later to evaluate spillage of contrast medium into the peritoneal cavity.
- Assure the patient that cramps and vagal reaction (slow pulse rate, nausea, and dizziness) are transient.
- Watch for signs of infection, such as fever, pain, increased pulse rate, malaise, and muscle ache.

## Precautions
- Hysterosalpingography is contraindicated in the patient with menses, undiagnosed vaginal bleeding, or pelvic inflammatory disease.

**ALERT** Watch for an allergic reaction to the contrast medium, such as urticaria, itching, or hypotension.

## Complications
- Uterine perforation
- Infection
- Bleeding
- Adverse reaction to the contrast medium

## Digital mammography

Digital mammography produces pictures of the breast using X-rays. Instead of film, this process uses detectors that change the X-rays into electrical signals, which are then converted to an image. Digital mammography is used for screening and diagnosis. For the patient, the procedure is the same as with ordinary mammography.

Digital mammography may offer the following advantages over conventional mammography:

■ The images can be stored and retrieved electronically, which makes long-distance consultations with other mammography specialists easier.

■ Because the images can be adjusted by the radiologist, subtle differences between tissues may be noted.

■ The number of follow-up procedures that are necessary may be reduced.

■ The need for fewer exposures with digital mammography can reduce the already low levels of radiation.

Digital mammography is effective in the detection of breast cancer and other abnormalities.

## ▌Mammography

Mammography is used as a screening test for breast cancer. It helps to detect breast cysts or tumors, especially those not palpable on physical examination. Biopsy of suspicious areas may be required to confirm malignancy. Mammography may follow screening procedures, such as ultrasonography or thermography. Although mammography can detect 90% to 95% of breast cancers, this test produces many false-positive results.

The American College of Radiologists and the American Cancer Society have established separate guidelines for the use and potential risks of mammography. Both groups agree that despite low radiation levels, the test is contraindicated during pregnancy. Magnetic resonance imaging, which is highly sensitive, is becoming a more popular method of breast imaging; however, it isn't very specific and leads to biopsies of many benign lesions. A digital image approved by the U.S. Food and Drug Administration is similar in use to mammography. (See *Digital mammography*.)

### Normal results

■ Normal duct, glandular tissue, and fat architecture are observed. No abnormal masses or calcifications are seen.

### Abnormal results

■ Well-outlined, regular, and clear spots suggest benign cysts.

■ Irregular, poorly outlined, and opaque areas suggest a malignant tumor.

■ Malignant tumors are generally solitary and unilateral; benign cysts tend to occur bilaterally.

### Purpose

■ To screen for malignant breast tumors

■ To investigate palpable and unpalpable breast masses, breast pain, or nipple discharge

■ To help differentiate between benign breast disease and breast cancer

■ To monitor the patient with breast cancer who has been treated with breast-conserving surgery and radiation

### Patient preparation

■ Assess the patient's understanding of the mammogram, answer her questions, and correct any misconceptions.

■ Tell the patient who will perform the test and where it will take place.

■ Tell the patient not to use underarm deodorant or powder on the day of the examination.

- If the patient has breast implants, tell her to inform the staff when she schedules the mammogram so that a technologist familiar with imaging implants is on duty.
- Inform the patient that although the test takes only about 15 minutes to perform, she may be asked to wait while the films are checked to make sure they're readable. Advise her that there's a high rate of false-positive results.
- Just before the test, give the patient a gown to wear that opens in the front, and ask her to remove all jewelry and clothing above the waist.

### Procedure and posttest care
- The patient stands and is asked to rest one of her breasts on a table above an X-ray cassette.
- The compression plate is placed on the breast and the patient is told to hold her breath. A radiograph is taken of the craniocaudal view. The machine is rotated, the breast is compressed again, and a radiograph of the lateral view is taken.
- The procedure is repeated on the other breast.
- After the films are developed, they're checked to make sure they're readable.

### Complications
- Vasovagal reaction during compression

# Ultrasonography

## Pelvic ultrasonography

In pelvic ultrasonography, high-frequency sound waves are reflected to a transducer to provide images of the interior pelvic area on a monitor. Techniques of sound imaging include A-mode (amplitude modulation, recorded as spikes), B-mode (brightness modulation), gray

scale (a representation of organ texture in shades of gray), and real-time imaging (instantaneous images of the tissues in motion, similar to fluoroscopic examination). Selected views may be photographed for later examination and a permanent record of the test.

### Normal results
- The uterus is normal in size and shape.
- The ovaries' size, shape, and sonographic density are normal.
- The body of the uterus lies on the superior surface of the bladder; the uterine tubes are attached laterally.
- The ovaries are located on the lateral pelvic walls, with the external iliac vessels above the ureter posteroinferiorly and covered by the fimbria of the uterine tubes medially.
- No other masses are visible.
- If the patient is pregnant, the gestational sac and fetus are of normal size in relation to gestational age.

### Abnormal results
- Cystic and solid masses have homogeneous densities, but solid masses (such as fibroids) appear denser.
- Inappropriate fetal size may indicate miscalculated conception or delivery date, fetal anomalies, or a dead fetus.
- Abnormal echo patterns may indicate foreign bodies (such as an intrauterine device), multiple pregnancy, maternal abnormalities (such as placenta previa or abruptio placentae), fetal abnormalities (such as molar pregnancy or abnormalities of the arms and legs, spine, heart, head, kidneys, and abdomen), fetal malpresentation (such as breech or shoulder presentation), and cephalopelvic disproportion.

## Purpose

- To detect foreign bodies and distinguish between cystic and solid masses (tumors)
- To measure organ size
- To evaluate fetal viability, position, gestational age, and growth rate
- To detect multiple pregnancy
- To confirm fetal and maternal abnormalities
- To guide amniocentesis by determining placental location and fetal position

## Patient preparation

- Describe pelvic ultrasonography to the patient and tell her the reason it's being performed.
- Assure the patient that this procedure is safe, noninvasive, and painless.
- Because this test requires a full bladder as a landmark to define pelvic organs, instruct the patient to drink liquids and not to void before the test.
- Tell the patient who will perform the procedure and where it will take place.
- Explain that a water enema may be necessary to produce a better outline of the large intestine.
- Reassure the patient that the test won't harm the fetus, and provide emotional support throughout.

## Procedure and posttest care

- Confirm the patient's identity using two patient identifiers according to facility policy.
- With the patient in a supine position, the pelvic area is coated with mineral oil or water-soluble conductive gel to increase sound wave conduction.
- The transducer is guided over the area, images are observed on the monitor, and good images are photographed.
- Remove the conductive gel from the patient's skin.
- Allow the patient to immediately empty her bladder after the test.

# Vaginal ultrasonography

In vaginal ultrasonography, a probe inserted into the vagina reflects high-frequency sound waves to a transducer, forming an image of the pelvic structures. This study allows better evaluation of pelvic anatomy and earlier diagnosis of pregnancy. It also circumvents the poor visualization encountered with obese patients.

## Normal results

- If the patient isn't pregnant, the uterus and ovaries are normal in size and shape.
- The body of the uterus lies on the superior surface of the bladder; the uterine tubes are attached laterally.
- The ovaries are located on the lateral pelvic walls, with the external iliac vessels above the ureter posteroinferiorly and covered by the fimbria of the uterine tubes medially.
- If the patient is pregnant, the gestational sac and fetus are of normal size for the gestational date.

## Abnormal results

- Vaginal ultrasonography may reveal an empty uterus if the patient was pregnant.
- Free peritoneal fluid may be visible in the pelvic cavity, indicating possible peritonitis.
- Ectopic pregnancies may also be visible in the pelvic cavity.

## Purpose

- To establish pregnancy with fetal heart motion as early as 5 to 6 weeks' gestation
- To determine ectopic pregnancy
- To evaluate abnormal pregnancy
- To diagnose fetal abnormalities and placental location

- To visualize retained products of conception
- To evaluate adnexal pathology, such as tubo-ovarian abscess, hydrosalpinx, and ovarian masses
- To evaluate the uterine lining (in cases of dysfunctional uterine bleeding and postmenopausal bleeding)
- To monitor follicular growth during infertility treatment

## Patient preparation
- Describe the vaginal ultrasonography to the patient and explain the reason for the test.
- Assure the patient that the procedure is safe.

## Procedure and posttest care
- The patient is placed in the lithotomy position. If the sonographer is a male, a female assistant should be present during the examination.
- Water-soluble conductive gel is placed on the transducer tip to allow better sound transmission and a protective sheath is placed over the transducer.
- Place more lubricant on the sheathed transducer tip to allow for its gentle insertion into the vagina by the patient or the sonographer. Allowing the patient to introduce the probe may decrease her anxiety.
- To observe the pelvic structures, rotate the probe 90 degrees to one side and then the other.

# Nervous system

## Noninvasive tests

### Electroencephalography
[EEG]

In EEG, electrodes attached to areas of the patient's scalp record the brain's electrical activity and transmit this information to an electroencephalograph, which records the resulting brain waves on recording paper. The procedure may be performed in a special laboratory or by a portable unit at the bedside. Intracranial electrodes are surgically implanted to record EEG changes for localization of the seizure focus.

#### Normal results
- Alpha waves occur at a frequency of 8 to 11 cycles/second in a regular rhythm; present only in the waking state when the patient's eyes are closed, but he's mentally alert; usually, they disappear with visual activity or mental concentration.
- Beta waves (13 to 30 cycles/second)— generally associated with anxiety, depression, and use of sedatives—are seen most readily in the frontal and central regions of the brain.
- Theta waves (4 to 7 cycles/second) are most common in children and young adults and appear in the frontal and temporal regions.

- Delta waves (0.5 to 3.5 cycles/second) normally occur only in young children and during sleep. (See *Comparing EEG tracings.*)

#### Abnormal results
- In absence seizures, the EEG shows spikes and waves at a frequency of 3 cycles/second.
- In generalized tonic-clonic seizures, it generally shows multiple, high-voltage, spiked waves in both hemispheres.
- In temporal lobe epilepsy, the EEG usually shows spiked waves in the affected temporal region.
- In the patient with focal seizures, it usually shows localized, spiked discharges.
- In the patient with an intracranial lesion, such as a tumor or abscess, the EEG may show slow waves (usually delta waves but possibly unilateral beta waves).
- Vascular lesions, such as cerebral infarcts and intracranial hemorrhages, generally produce focal abnormalities in the injured area.
- Any condition that causes a diminishing level of consciousness alters the EEG pattern in proportion to the degree of consciousness lost. For example, in a patient with a metabolic disorder, an inflammatory process (such as meningitis or encephalitis), or increased intracra-

## Comparing EEG tracings

The following tracings are examples of regular and irregular brain electrical activity as recorded by an EEG.

Normal (top, right temporal; bottom, parietal-occipital)

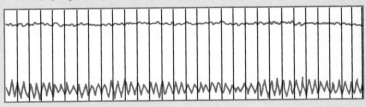

Absence seizures (spikes and waves, 3 per second)

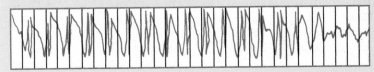

Generalized tonic-clonic seizures (multiple high-voltage spiked waves)

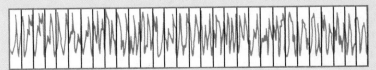

Right temporal lobe epilepsy (focal spiked waves)

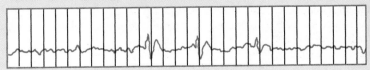

nial pressure, the EEG shows generalized, diffuse, and slow brain waves.

- The most pathologic finding of all is an absent EEG pattern—a "flat" tracing (except for artifacts), which may indicate brain death.

### DRUG CHALLENGE

 Anticonvulsants, barbiturates, tranquilizers, and other sedatives (possible masking of seizure activity); acute drug intoxication resulting in loss of consciousness (flat EEG)

### Purpose

- To determine the presence and type of seizure disorder
- To aid in the diagnosis of intracranial lesions, such as abscesses and tumors
- To evaluate the brain's electrical activity in metabolic disease, cerebral ischemia, head injury, meningitis, en-

cephalitis, mental retardation, psychological disorders, and drugs

■ To evaluate altered states of consciousness or brain death

## Patient preparation

■ Explain that the EEG records the brain's electrical activity.

■ Describe the procedure to the patient and family members and answer all questions.

■ Tell the patient that he must avoid caffeine before the test; other than this, there are no food or fluid restrictions. Tell him that skipping the meal before the test can cause relative hypoglycemia and alter the brain wave pattern.

■ Inform the patient that smoking is prohibited for at least 8 hours before the test.

■ Thoroughly wash and dry the patient's hair to remove hair sprays, creams, and oils.

■ Explain to the patient that during the test, he'll relax in a reclining chair or lie on a bed and that electrodes will be attached to his scalp with a special paste. Assure him that the electrodes won't shock him.

■ If needle electrodes are used, explain to the patient that he'll feel a pricking sensation as they're inserted; however, flat electrodes are more commonly used.

■ Try to allay the patient's fears because nervousness can affect brain wave patterns.

■ Check the patient's medication history for drugs that may interfere with test results. Anticonvulsants, tranquilizers, barbiturates, and other sedatives should be withheld for 24 to 48 hours before the test, as ordered by the practitioner. Infants and very young children occasionally require sedation to prevent crying and restlessness during the test, but sedation itself may alter test results.

■ A patient with a seizure disorder may require a "sleep EEG." In this case, keep the patient awake the night before the test and administer a sedative (such as chloral hydrate) to help him sleep during the test.

■ If the test is performed to confirm brain death, provide the patient's family members with emotional support.

## Procedure and posttest care

■ Position the patient on the bed or in a reclining chair. Reassure him as the electrodes are attached to his scalp.

■ Before the recording procedure begins, instruct the patient to close his eyes, relax, and remain still.

■ During the recording, observe the patient carefully; note blinking, swallowing, talking, or other movements and record these findings on the tracing. These activities may cause artifacts on the tracing and be misinterpreted as an abnormal tracing.

■ The recording may be stopped at intervals to let the patient rest or reposition himself. This is important because restlessness and fatigue can alter brain wave patterns.

■ After an initial baseline recording, the patient may be tested under various stress-producing conditions to elicit patterns not observable while he's at rest. For example, he may be asked to breathe deeply and rapidly for 3 minutes (hyperventilation), which may elicit brain wave patterns-typical of seizure disorders or other abnormalities. This technique is commonly used to detect absence seizures. Also, photic stimulation tests centralized cerebral activity in response to bright light, accentuating abnormal activity in absence or myoclonic seizures. In this procedure, a strobe light placed in front of the patient is flashed 1 to 20 times/second; recordings are made with the patient's eyes opened and closed.

- Review carefully the reinstatement of anticonvulsant medication or other drugs withheld before the test.
- Carefully observe the patient for seizure activity and provide a safe environment.
- Use acetone or witch hazel to help the patient remove electrode paste from his hair.
- If the patient received a sedative before the test, take safety precautions such as raising the bed's side rails.
- If brain death is confirmed, provide the patient's family members with emotional support.
- If clinical events are found to be non-epileptic, a psychological evaluation may be needed.

### Precautions
- Observe the patient carefully for seizure activity.
- If seizure activity occurs, record seizure patterns and be prepared to provide assistance. Have suction equipment readily available.

### Complications
- Adverse effects of sedation, if used
- Possible seizure activity

# Evoked potential studies

Evoked potential studies evaluate the integrity of visual, somatosensory, and auditory nerve pathways by measuring evoked potentials—the brain's electrical response to stimulation of the sensory organs or peripheral nerves. Evoked potentials are recorded as electronic impulses by surface electrodes attached to the scalp and skin over various peripheral sensory nerves. A computer extracts these low-amplitude impulses from background brain wave activity and averages the signals from repeated stimuli.

(See *Visual and somatosensory evoked potentials,* pages 462 and 463.)

Three types of responses are measured:
- Visual evoked potentials, produced by exposing the eye to a rapidly reversing checkerboard pattern, help evaluate demyelinating diseases, traumatic injury, and puzzling visual complaints.
- Somatosensory evoked potentials, produced by electrically stimulating a peripheral sensory nerve, help diagnose peripheral nerve disease and locate brain and spinal cord lesions.
- Auditory brain stem evoked potentials, produced by delivering clicks to the ear, help locate auditory lesions and evaluate brain stem integrity.

Evoked potential studies are also useful for monitoring comatose or anesthetized patients, monitoring spinal cord function during spinal cord surgery, and evaluating neurologic function in an infant whose sensory system normally can't be adequately assessed.

### Normal results
#### Visual evoked potentials
- The most significant wave is P100, a positive wave appearing about 100 msec after the pattern-shift stimulus is applied. Because many physical and technical factors affect P100 latency, normal results vary greatly among laboratories and patients.

#### Somatosensory evoked potentials
- Waveforms obtained vary, depending on locations of the stimulating and recording electrodes.

### Abnormal results
- Information from evoked potential studies is useful but insufficient to confirm a specific diagnosis. Test data must be interpreted in light of clinical information.

# Visual and somatosensory evoked potentials

## Visual (pattern-shift) evoked potentials

In the visual (pattern-shift) evoked potentials test, visual neural impulses are recorded as they travel along the pathway from the eye to the occipital cortex. Wave P100 is the most significant component of the resultant waveform. Normal P100 latency is about 100 msec after the application of a visual stimulus, as shown in the top diagram. Increased P100 latency, shown in the bottom diagram, is an abnormal finding, indicating a lesion along the visual pathway.

Normal tracing

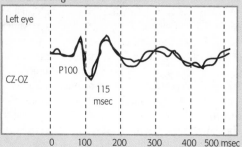

Tracing in multiple sclerosis

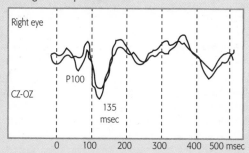

Key: CZ = vertex; OZ = midocciput; FZ = midfrontal; Cc = sensoparietal cortex contralateral to stimulated limb.

## Visual evoked potentials

- Extended P100 latencies confined to one eye indicate a visual pathway lesion anterior to the optic chiasm. A lesion posterior to the optic chiasm usually doesn't produce abnormal P100 latencies.
- Bilateral abnormal P100 latencies have been found in patients with multiple sclerosis, optic neuritis, retinopathies, amblyopia (although abnormal latencies don't correlate well with impaired visual acuity), spinocerebellar degeneration, adrenoleukodystrophy, sarcoidosis, Parkinson's disease, and Huntington's disease.

## Somatosensory evoked potentials

- Abnormal interwave latency indicates a conduction defect between the generators of the two peaks involved. This commonly identifies a precise location of a neurologic lesion.
- Abnormal upper-limb interwave latencies may indicate cervical spondylosis, intracerebral lesions, or sensorimotor neuropathies.
- Abnormalities in the lower limb demonstrate peripheral nerve and root lesions, such as those in Guillain-Barré syndrome, compressive myelopathies,

## Somatosensory evoked potentials

The somatosensory evoked potentials test measures the conduction time of an electrical impulse traveling along a somatosensory pathway to the cortex. Interwave latency is the most significant component of the resultant waveform. On the set of upper- and lower-limb tracings shown at right, the top tracings represent normal interwave latencies; the bottom tracings, typical abnormal latencies found in a patient with multiple sclerosis. Because of the close correlation between waveforms and the anatomy of somatosensory pathways, such tracings allow precise location of lesions that produce conduction defects.

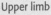

Upper limb

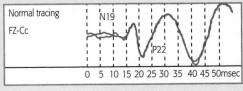

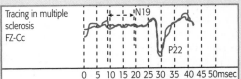

Lower limb

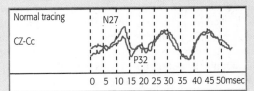

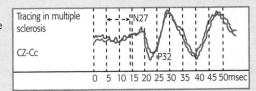

multiple sclerosis, transverse myelitis, and traumatic spinal cord injury.

### Purpose
- To help diagnose nervous system lesions and abnormalities
- To assess the patient's neurologic function

### Patient preparation
- Tell the patient that evoked potential studies measure the electrical activity of his nervous system. Explain who will perform the test and where it will take place.

- Tell the patient that he'll sit in a reclining chair or lie on a bed. If visual evoked potentials will be measured, electrodes will be attached to his scalp; if somatosensory evoked potentials will be measured, electrodes will be placed on his scalp, neck, lower back, wrist, knee, and ankle.
- Assure the patient that the electrodes won't hurt him. Encourage him to relax; tension can affect neurologic function and interfere with test results.
- Have the patient remove all jewelry and other metal objects.

## Procedure and posttest care

- Confirm the patient's identity using two patient identifiers according to facility policy.
- Position the patient in a reclining chair or on a bed and tell him to relax and remain still.

### For visual evoked potentials

- Electrodes are attached to the patient's scalp at occipital, parietal, and vertex sites; a reference electrode is placed on the midfrontal area or ear.
- The patient is positioned 3′ (1 m) from the pattern-shift stimulator.
- One eye is occluded, and the patient is instructed to fix his gaze on a dot in the center of the screen.
- A checkerboard pattern is projected and then rapidly reversed or shifted 100 times, once or twice per second.
- A computer amplifies and averages the brain's response to each stimulus, and the results are plotted as a waveform.
- The procedure is repeated for the other eye.

### For somatosensory evoked potentials

- Electrodes are attached to the patient's skin over somatosensory pathways—typically the wrist, knee, and ankle—to stimulate peripheral nerves. Recording electrodes are placed on the scalp over the sensory cortex of the hemisphere opposite the limb to be stimulated. Additional electrodes may be placed at Erb's point (above the clavicle overlying the brachial plexus), at the second cervical vertebra, and over the lower lumbar vertebrae. Midfrontal or noncephalic electrodes are placed for reference.
- Painless electrical stimulation is delivered to the peripheral nerve through the electrode. The intensity is adjusted to produce a minor muscle response such as a thumb twitch on median nerve stimulation at the wrist.

- Electrical stimuli are delivered 500 or more times at a rate of 5 per second.
- A computer measures and averages the time it takes for the electric current to reach the cortex; the results, expressed in milliseconds (msec), are recorded as waveforms.
- The test is repeated once to verify results, and then the electrodes are repositioned and the entire procedure is repeated for the other side.

# Intracranial computed tomography
## [CT of the brain]

Intracranial computed tomography (CT) provides a series of tomograms, translated by a computer and displayed on a monitor, representing cross-sectional images of various layers of the brain. This technique can reconstruct cross-sectional, horizontal, sagittal, and coronal plane images.

In many cases, intracranial CT scanning eliminates the need for painful and hazardous invasive procedures, such as pneumoencephalography and cerebral angiography. CT scans, which usually use contrast enhancement, are especially valuable in assessing a patient with focal neurologic abnormalities and other clinical features that suggest an intracranial mass. In a patient with a suspected head injury, intracranial CT scans may allow the diagnosis of a subdural hematoma before characteristic symptoms appear.

## Normal results

- Tissue densities appear as white, black, or shades of gray on the computed image obtained by intracranial CT scanning.
- Bone, the densest tissue, appears white; ventricular and subarachnoid cerebrospinal fluid, the least dense, appears black.

- Brain matter appears in shades of gray.
- Structures are evaluated according to their density, size, shape, and position.

## Abnormal results

- Areas of altered density (they may be lighter or darker) or displaced vasculature or other structures may indicate an intracranial tumor, a hematoma, cerebral atrophy, an infarction, edema, or congenital anomalies such as hydrocephalus.
- Intracranial tumors vary significantly in appearance and characteristics. Metastatic tumors generally cause extensive edema in early stages and can usually be defined by contrast enhancement. Primary tumors vary in density and in their capacity to cause edema, displace ventricles, and absorb the contrast medium in contrast enhancement.
- Because the high density of blood contrasts markedly with low-density brain tissue, it's normally easy to detect subdural and epidural hematomas and other acute hemorrhages.
- Cerebral atrophy customarily appears as enlarged ventricles with large sulci.
- Cerebral infarction may appear as low-density areas at the obstruction site or may not be apparent, especially within the first 24 hours or if the infarction is small or doesn't cause edema.
- In the patient with arteriovenous malformation, cerebral vessels may appear with slightly increased density. Contrast enhancement allows a better view of the abnormal area, but magnetic resonance imaging is now the preferred procedure for imaging cerebral vessels.
- Another technology for obtaining brain images is positron emission tomography. (See *Understanding PET and SPECT,* page 466.)

## Purpose

- To diagnose intracranial lesions and abnormalities

- To monitor the effects of surgery, radiation therapy, or chemotherapy on intracranial tumors
- To serve as a guide for cranial surgery

## Patient preparation

- Explain that intracranial CT permits assessment of the brain.
- Unless contrast enhancement is scheduled, inform the patient that there are no food or fluid restrictions. If contrast enhancement is scheduled, instruct him to fast for 4 hours before the test.
- Tell the patient that a series of X-rays will be taken of his brain. Describe who will perform the test and where it will take place. Explain that the test will cause minimal discomfort.
- Tell the patient that he'll be positioned on a moving CT bed with his head immobilized and his face uncovered. The head of the table will then be moved into the scanner, which rotates around his head and makes loud clacking sounds.
- If a contrast medium is used, tell the patient that he may feel flushed and warm and may experience a transient headache, a salty or metallic taste, or nausea and vomiting after the contrast medium is injected.
- Instruct the patient to wear a gown (outpatients may wear comfortable clothing) and to remove all metal objects from the CT scan field.
- If the patient is restless or apprehensive, a sedative may be prescribed.
- Check the patient's history for hypersensitivity to shellfish, iodine, or contrast media, and mark your findings in his chart. Inform the practitioner of any sensitivities because he may order prophylactic medications or may choose not to use contrast enhancement.

# Understanding PET and SPECT

Like computed tomography (CT) scanning and magnetic resonance imaging, positron emission tomography (PET) and single-photon emission computed tomography (SPECT) provide brain images through sophisticated computer reconstruction algorithms. However, PET and SPECT images detail brain function as well as structure and thus differ significantly from the images provided by these other advanced techniques. PET and SPECT combine elements of CT scanning and conventional radionuclide imaging. For example, they measure the emissions of injected radioisotopes and convert them to a tomographic image of the brain. SPECT scanning uses gamma radiation with radionucleotides within the brain, and PET uses radioisotopes of biologically important elements—oxygen, nitrogen, carbon, and fluorine—that emit particles called positrons.

## How it works

During PET and SPECT, pairs of gamma rays are emitted; the scanner detects them and relays the information to a computer for reconstruction as an image. SPECT scanners use radionucleotides labeled with iodine or hexamethyl-propylene amineoxime to detect blood flow. PET scanners omit positrons that can be chemically "tagged" to biological-ly active molecules, such as carbon monoxide, neurotransmitters, hormones, and metabolites (especially glucose), enabling study of their uptake and distribution in brain tissue. For example, blood tagged with 11C-carbon monoxide allows study of hemodynamic patterns in brain tissue; tagged neurotransmitters, hormones, and drugs allow mapping of receptor distribution.

Isotope-tagged glucose (which penetrates the blood-brain barrier rapidly) allows dynamic study of brain function because PET scans can pinpoint the sites of glucose metabolism in the brain under various conditions. Researchers expect SPECT and PET scanning to prove useful in the diagnosis of psychiatric disorders, transient ischemic attacks, amyotrophic lateral sclerosis, Parkinson's disease, Wilson's disease, multiple sclerosis, seizure disorders, cerebrovascular disease, and Alzheimer's disease. The reason is that all of these disorders may alter the location and patterns of cerebral glucose metabolism.

## Cost factors

PET scanning is a costly test because the radioisotopes used have very short half-lives and must be produced at an onsite cyclotron and attached quickly to the desired tracer molecules.

## Procedure and posttest care

■ Confirm the patient's identity using two patient identifiers according to facility policy.

■ Place the patient in a supine position on an X-ray table with his head immobilized by straps, if required, and ask him to lie still.

■ The head of the table is moved into the scanner, which rotates around the patient's head, taking radiographs at 1-degree intervals in an 180-degree arc.

■ When this series of radiographs is completed, contrast enhancement is performed. Usually 50 to 100 ml of contrast medium is given by I.V. injection or I.V. drip over 1 to 2 minutes.

**ALERT**

 Monitor the patient for hypersensitivity reactions, such as urticaria, respiratory difficulty, or rash. Reactions usually develop within 30 minutes.

• After injection of the contrast medium, another series of scans is taken. Information from the scans is stored on magnetic tapes, fed into a computer, and converted into images on an oscilloscope. Photographs of selected views are taken for further study.

• Tell the patient that he may resume his usual diet after the test.

### Precautions

• Intracranial CT scanning with contrast enhancement is contraindicated in the patient who's hypersensitive to iodine or contrast medium.

• Iodine or contrast medium may be harmful or fatal to a fetus, especially during the first trimester.

# Intracranial magnetic resonance imaging

Intracranial magnetic resonance imaging (MRI) produces highly detailed, cross-sectional images of the brain and spine in multiple planes. The primary advantage of MRI is its ability to "see through" bone and to delineate fluid-filled soft tissue. It has proved useful in the diagnosis of cerebral infarction, tumors, abscesses, edema, hemorrhage, nerve fiber demyelination (as in multiple sclerosis), and other disorders that increase the fluid content of affected tissues. MRI can show irregularities of the spinal cord with a resolution and detail previously unobtainable. It can also produce images of organs and vessels in motion.

MRI technology makes use of magnetic fields and radio-frequency waves, which are imperceptible by the patient; no harmful effects have been documented. Research continues on the optimal magnetic fields and radio-frequency waves for each type of tissue. (See *New methods of monitoring cerebral function,* page 468.)

### Normal results

• Brain and spinal cord structures appear distinct and sharply defined.

• Tissue color and shading vary, depending on the radio-frequency energy, magnetic strength, and degree of computer enhancement.

### Abnormal results

• Structural changes resulting from disorders that increase tissue water content, such as cerebral edema, demyelinating disease, and pontine and cerebellar tumors, are detected.

• Areas of demyelination appear as curdlike, gray or gray-white areas around the edges of ventricles.

• Tumors appear as changes in normal anatomy, which computer enhancement may further delineate.

### Purpose

• To help diagnose intracranial and spinal lesions and soft-tissue abnormalities

### Patient preparation

• Explain that intracranial MRI assesses bone and soft tissue. Tell the patient who will perform the test and where it will take place.

• Explain that MRI is painless and involves no exposure to radiation from the scanner. A radioactive contrast dye may be used, depending on the type of tissue being studied.

• Advise the patient that he'll have to remain still for the entire procedure.

• Inform him that the opening for the head and body is quite small and deep. Tell him that he'll hear the scanner clicking, whirring, and thumping as it moves inside its housing.

• Explain to the patient he may receive a sedative if he suffers from claustrophobia or if extensive time is required for scanning. As an alternative, an open

# New methods of monitoring cerebral function

## Optical imaging

Optical imaging uses fiber-optic light and a camera to produce visual images of the brain as it responds to stimulation. This technique produces higher-resolution pictures of the brain than magnetic resonance imaging (MRI) or positron emission tomography scans. Researchers believe it may be valuable during neurosurgery to minimize damage to crucial areas of the brain that control speech, movement, and other

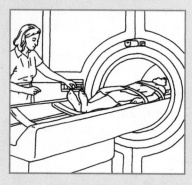

activities. Because the procedure scans only the brain's surface, it's meant to be used in combination with other diagnostic techniques.

## Fast MRI

Fast MRI produces pictures less than a second apart. These images display blood flow through the brain and the changes that occur in blood flow when the patient performs different tasks. Neuroscientists believe that active areas of the brain must consume more oxygen and that areas of the brain that are currently working become laden with oxygen. Fast MRI can distinguish between oxygen-laden and oxygen-depleted blood. Thus, this test may be used to help identify which areas of the normal brain are involved in certain activities and emotions. Possible applications for fast MRI include guiding neurosurgeons during surgery and helping researchers better understand epilepsy, brain tumors, and even psychiatric illnesses.

MRI scanner may be used, which delivers accurate results, but may take longer to complete.

■ Reassure the patient that he'll be able to communicate with the technician at all times.

### Do's & don'ts

 Instruct the patient to remove all metallic objects, including jewelry, hairpins, and watch. Also ask him if he has any surgically implanted joints, pins, clips, valves, pumps, or pacemakers containing metal that could be attracted to the strong MRI magnet. If he does, he won't be able to undergo the test.

■ Make sure that the patient or a responsible family member has signed an informed consent form, if required.

### Procedure and posttest care

■ Confirm the patient's identity using two patient identifiers according to facility policy.
■ The patient is placed in a supine position on a narrow bed, which then slides him to the desired position inside the scanner, where radio-frequency energy is directed at his head or spine.
■ The resulting images are displayed on a monitor and recorded on film or magnetic tape for permanent storage.
■ The radiologist may vary radio-frequency waves and use the computer to manipulate and enhance the images.

- During the procedure, the patient must remain still.
- Tell the patient that he may resume his usual activity after the test.
- If the patient was sedated, ensure that a responsible person drives him home.
- If the test took a long time and the patient was lying flat for an extended period, observe him for orthostatic hypotension.

### Precautions

- Because MRI works through a powerful magnetic field, it can't be performed on the patient with a pacemaker, an intracranial aneurysm clip, or other ferrous metal implants or on a patient with gunshot wounds to the head.
- Because of the strong magnetic field, metallic or computer-based equipment (for example, ventilators and I.V. pumps) can't enter the MRI area. Extension tubing may be added if needed for an I.V. pump.

# Skull radiography

Although skull radiography is of limited value in assessing patients with head injuries, skull X-rays are extremely valuable for studying abnormalities of the skull base and cranial vault, congenital and perinatal anomalies, and systemic diseases that produce bone defects of the skull. For more accurate assessment of head injuries as well as of skull and head abnormalities, nonenhanced computed tomography studies of the head are done.

Skull radiography evaluates the three groups of bones that comprise the skull: the calvaria (vault), the mandible (jaw bone), and the facial bones. The calvaria and the facial bones are closely connected by immovable joints with irregular serrated edges called sutures. The skull bones form an anatomic structure so complex that a complete skull examination requires several radiologic views of each area.

### Normal results

- The size, shape, thickness, and position of the cranial bones as well as the vascular markings, sinuses, and sutures are normal for the patient's age.

### Abnormal results

- Structural abnormalities suggest possible fractures of the vault or base of the skull or congenital anomalies.
- Erosion, enlargement, or decalcification of the sella turcica suggests possible increased intracranial pressure.
- Areas of calcification suggest possible conditions, such as osteomyelitis, or the presence of neoplasm within the brain substance that contain calcium, such as oligodendrogliomas or meningiomas.
- Midline shifting of a calcified pineal gland suggests a possible space-occupying lesion.
- Changes in bone structure suggest possible metabolic disorders, such as acromegaly or Paget's disease.

### Purpose

- To detect fractures in the patient with head trauma
- To aid in the diagnosis of pituitary tumors
- To detect congenital anomalies
- To detect metabolic and endocrinologic disorders

### Patient preparation

- Explain to the patient that his head will be immobilized and that several X-rays of his skull will be taken from various angles.
- Tell the patient that skull radiography helps to determine the presence of anomalies and helps establish a diagnosis.
- Tell the patient who will perform the test and where it will take place.

# Positioning the skull for radiography

### Right lateral and left lateral

The sagittal plane is parallel to the tabletop and the film. A support, such as a folded towel or the patient's clenched fist, is placed under the chin. (Adequate film shows both halves of the mandible directly superimposed.)

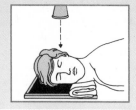

### Anteroposterior Towne's

The patient lies in a supine position with his chin flexed toward the neck; the canthomeatal line is perpendicular to the tabletop and the film. The X-ray beam is angled 30 degrees toward the feet.

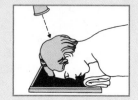

### Posteroanterior Caldwell

The patient lies in a prone position; his chin may be supported by a folded towel or his fist. The sagittal plane and the canthomeatal line are perpendicular to the tabletop and the film. The X-ray beam is angled 15 degrees toward the feet.

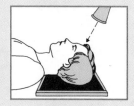

### Axial (base)

The patient lies in a prone position with his chin fully extended; his head rests in such a way that the line of the face is perpendicular and the canthomeatal line is parallel to the tabletop and the film.

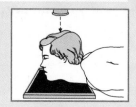

■ Explain to the patient that he doesn't need to restrict food and fluids and that the test will cause no discomfort.

■ Tell the patient to remove glasses, dentures, jewelry, or any metallic objects that would be in the X-ray field.

## Procedure and posttest care

■ Have the patient recline on the X-ray table or sit in a chair.

■ Tell the patient to remain still during the procedure.

■ Use foam pads, sandbags, or a headband to immobilize the patient's head and increase comfort.

### DO'S & DON'TS

Don't hyperextend or flex the head if cervical injuries are unknown or suspected.

■ Five views of the skull are routinely taken: left and right lateral, anteroposterior Towne's, posteroanterior Caldwell, and axial (or base). (See *Positioning the skull for radiography.*)

- Films are developed and checked for quality before the patient leaves the area.

# Spinal computed tomography

Much more versatile than conventional radiography, spinal computed tomography (CT) provides detailed high-resolution images in the cross-sectional, longitudinal, sagittal, and lateral planes. Multiple X-ray beams from a computerized body scanner are directed at the spine from different angles; these pass through the body and strike radiation detectors, producing electrical impulses. A computer then converts these impulses into digital information, which is displayed as a three-dimensional image on a monitor. Storage of the digital information allows electronic recreation and manipulation of the image, creating a permanent record of the images to enable reexamination without repeating the procedure.

CT scans are helpful in defining the lesions causing spinal cord compression. Metastatic disease and discogenic disease with osteophyte formation and calcification are examples of pathologic processes diagnosed by CT scans. Since the advent of magnetic resonance imaging, CT scans are used less frequently to diagnose infection, abscesses, hematomas, and some disk herniations.

## Normal results

- Spinal tissue appears white, black, or gray, depending on its density.
- Vertebrae, the densest tissues, are white.
- Cerebrospinal fluid is black.
- Soft tissues appear in shades of gray.

## Abnormal results

- Spinal lesions and abnormalities are present.
- Tumors appear as masses varying in density. Measuring this density and noting the configuration and location relative to the spinal cord can usually identify the type of tumor. For example, a neurinoma (schwannoma) appears as a spherical mass dorsal to the cord. A darker, wider mass lying more laterally or ventrally to the cord may be a meningioma.
- Degenerative processes and structural changes can be seen in detail.
- Herniated nucleus pulposus shows as an obvious herniation of disk material with unilateral or bilateral nerve root compression; if the herniation is midline, spinal cord compression will be evident.
- Cervical spondylosis shows as cervical cord compression due to bony hypertrophy of the cervical spine; lumbar stenosis, as hypertrophy of the lumbar vertebrae, causing cord compression by decreasing space within the spinal column.
- Facet disorders show as soft-tissue changes, bony overgrowth, and spurring of the vertebrae, which result in nerve root compression.
- Fluid-filled arachnoidal and other paraspinal cysts show as dark masses displacing the spinal cord.
- Vascular malformations, evident after contrast enhancement, show as masses or clusters, usually on the dorsal aspect of the spinal cord.
- Congenital spinal malformations, such as meningocele, myelocele, and spina bifida, show as abnormally large, dark gaps between the white vertebrae.

## Purpose

- To diagnose spinal lesions and abnormalities

- To monitor the effects of spinal surgery or therapy

## Patient preparation

- Explain that spinal CT allows visualization of his spine.
- If contrast medium isn't ordered, tell the patient that he doesn't need to restrict food and fluids. If contrast medium is ordered, instruct him to fast for 4 hours before the test.
- Tell the patient that a series of scans will be taken of his spine. Explain who will perform the procedure and where it will take place.
- Reassure the patient that the procedure is painless but that he may find having to remain still for a prolonged period uncomfortable.
- Explain to the patient that he'll be positioned on an X-ray table inside a CT body scanning unit and he'll be told to lie still because movement during the procedure may cause distorted images. The computer-controlled scanner will revolve around him, taking multiple scans.
- If a contrast medium is used, tell the patient that he may feel flushed and warm and may experience a transient headache, a salty taste, and nausea or vomiting after injection of the contrast medium. Reassure him that these reactions are normal.
- Instruct the patient to wear a radiologic examining gown and to remove all metal objects and jewelry.
- Check the patient's history for hypersensitivity reactions to iodine, shellfish, or contrast media. If such reactions have occurred, note them in the patient's chart and notify the practitioner, who may order prophylactic medications or choose not to use contrast enhancement.

- If the patient appears restless or apprehensive about the procedure, a mild sedative may be prescribed.
- Make sure that the patient or a responsible family member has signed an informed consent form, if required.

## Procedure and posttest care

- Confirm the patient's identity using two patient identifiers according to facility policy.
- Place the patient in a supine position on an X-ray table and tell him to lie as still as possible.
- The table slides into the circular opening of the CT scanner and the scanner revolves around the patient, taking radiographs at preselected intervals.
- After the first set of scans is taken, the patient is removed from the scanner. Contrast medium may be administered.

**ALERT**

 Observe the patient for signs and symptoms of a hypersensitivity reaction, including pruritus, rash, and respiratory difficulty, for 30 minutes after the contrast medium has been injected.

- After contrast medium injection, the patient is moved back into the scanner, and another series of scans is taken. The images obtained from the scan are displayed on a monitor during the procedure and stored on magnetic tape.
- After testing with contrast enhancement, observe the patient for residual effects, such as headache, nausea, and vomiting.
- Inform the patient that he may resume his usual diet, as ordered.

## Precautions

- Body CT scanning with contrast enhancement is contraindicated in the patient who's hypersensitive to iodine, shellfish, or contrast media used in radiographic studies.

- The patient may experience strong feelings of claustrophobia or anxiety when inside the CT body scanner. In such cases, a mild sedative to help reduce anxiety may be ordered.

Do's & don'ts

 For the patient with significant back pain, give prescribed analgesics before the scan.

# Transcranial Doppler studies

Transcranial Doppler studies provide information about the presence, quality, and changing nature of circulation to an area of the brain by measuring the velocity of blood flow through cerebral arteries. Narrowed blood vessels produce high velocities, indicating possible stenosis or vasospasm. High velocities may also indicate an arteriovenous malformation.

### Normal results

- Waveforms and velocities are normal.

### Abnormal results

- Velocities are high, suggesting that blood flow is too turbulent or the vessel is too narrow. (See *Comparing velocity waveforms,* page 474.)

### Purpose

- To measure the velocity of blood flow through certain cerebral vessels
- To detect and monitor the progression of cerebral vasospasm
- To determine whether collateral blood flow exists before surgical ligation or radiologic occlusion of diseased vessels

### Patient preparation

- Explain the purpose of the transcranial Doppler study to the patient (or to his family).
- Tell the patient that the test will be done while he lies on a bed or stretcher or sits in a reclining chair (or it can be performed at the bedside if he's too ill to be moved to the laboratory).
- Describe the procedure. Explain that a small amount of conductive gel will be applied to his skin and that a probe will be used to transmit a signal to the artery being studied. Tell the patient that it usually takes less than 1 hour, depending on the number of vessels to be examined and any interfering factors.
- Tell the patient that he doesn't need to restrict food and fluids.

### Procedure and posttest care

- Confirm the patient's identity using two patient identifiers according to facility policy.
- Have the patient recline in a chair or on a stretcher or bed.
- A small amount of conductive gel is applied to the transcranial window (an area where bone is thin enough to allow the Doppler signal to enter and be detected); the most common approaches are temporal, transorbital, and through the foramen magnum.
- The technician directs the signal toward the artery being studied and records the velocities detected. In a complete study, the middle cerebral arteries, anterior cerebral arteries, posterior cerebral arteries, ophthalmic arteries, carotid siphon, vertebral arteries, and basilar artery are studied.
- The Doppler signal waveforms may be printed out for later analysis and can be transmitted to varying depths (measured in millimeters).
- When the study is completed, wipe away the conductive gel.

## Comparing velocity waveforms

A normal transcranial Doppler signal is usually characterized by mean velocities that fall within the normal reported values. Additional information can be gathered by evaluating the shape of the velocity waveform.

**Effect of significant proximal vessel obstruction**
A delayed systolic upstroke can be seen in a waveform when significant proximal vessel obstruction is present.

Normal

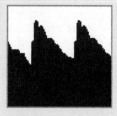

Proximal vessel obstruction

**Effect of increased cerebrovascular rsistance**
Changes in cerebrovascular resistance, as occur with increased intracranial pressure, cause a decrease in diastolic flow.

Normal

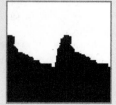

Increased resistance

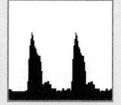

### Precautions
■ Make sure to remove turban head dressings or thick dressings over the test site.

## Invasive tests

### ▌Cerebral angiography

Cerebral angiography involves injecting a contrast medium to allow radiographic examination of the cerebral vasculature. Possible injection sites include the femoral, carotid, and brachial arteries. Because it allows visualization of four vessels (the carotid and the vertebral arteries), the femoral artery is used most commonly.

Usually, this test is performed on patients with suspected abnormality of the cerebral vasculature; abnormalities may be suggested by intracranial computed tomography, lumbar puncture, magnetic resonance imaging, or magnetic resonance angiography.

### Normal results
■ Cerebral vasculature is normal.
■ During the arterial phase of perfusion, the contrast medium fills and opacifies superficial and deep arteries and arterioles.
■ During the venous phase, the contrast medium opacifies superficial and deep veins.

### Abnormal results
■ Changes in the caliber of vessel lumina suggest vascular disease, possibly due to

spasms, plaques, fistulas, arteriovenous malformation (AVM), or arteriosclerosis.
■ Diminished blood flow to vessels may be related to increased intracranial pressure (ICP).
■ Vessel displacement may reflect the presence and size of a tumor, areas of edema, or obstruction of the cerebrospinal fluid pathway.

## Purpose
■ To detect cerebrovascular abnormalities, such as aneurysm or AVM, thrombosis, narrowing, or occlusion
■ To study vascular displacement caused by tumor, hematoma, edema, herniation, vasospasm, increased ICP, or hydrocephalus
■ To locate clips applied to blood vessels during surgery and to evaluate the postoperative status of affected vessels

## Patient preparation
■ Explain that cerebral angiography shows blood circulation in the brain.
■ Describe the test, including who will perform it and where it will take place.
■ Tell the patient to fast for 8 to 10 hours before the test.
■ Make sure that any pretest blood work results are on the chart to determine bleeding tendency or kidney function.
■ Explain to the patient that he'll wear a gown and that he must remove all jewelry, dentures, hairpins, and other metallic objects in the radiographic field.
■ If ordered, give him a sedative and an anticholinergic 30 to 45 minutes before the test.
■ Make sure the patient voids before leaving his room.
■ Tell the patient that he'll be positioned on an X-ray table with his head immobilized and that he should remain still.
■ Explain that he'll receive a local anesthetic (although some patients—especially children—receive a general anesthetic).

■ Explain to the patient that he'll feel a transient burning sensation as the medium is injected; a warm, flushed feeling; a transient headache; a salty or metallic taste in his mouth; or nausea and vomiting after the dye is injected.
■ Make sure that the patient or a responsible family member has signed an informed consent form, if required.

**ALERT**

 Check the patient's history for hypersensitivity to iodine, iodine-containing substances (such as shellfish), or other contrast media. Note any hypersensitivities on his chart and report them as appropriate.

## Procedure and posttest care
■ Confirm the patient's identity using two patient identifiers according to facility policy.
■ Have the patient recline on an X-ray table and instruct him to lie still with his arms at his sides.
■ Clip the hair at the injection site (femoral, carotid, or brachial artery) and clean it with alcohol and povidone-iodine.
■ A local anesthetic is injected. Then the artery is punctured with the appropriate needle and catheterized.
■ In the femoral artery approach, a catheter is threaded to the aortic arch.
■ In the brachial artery approach (least common), a blood pressure cuff is placed distal to the puncture site and inflated before injection to prevent the contrast medium from flowing into the forearm and hand.
■ After X-rays or fluoroscopy verify placement of the needle or catheter, the contrast medium is injected. Observe the patient for an adverse reaction, such as hives, flushing, or laryngeal stridor.
■ An initial series of lateral and anteroposterior X-rays is taken, developed,

and reviewed. Depending on the results, more contrast medium may be injected and another series taken.

- During the test, maintain arterial catheter patency by continuous or periodic flushing. Monitor the patient's vital and neurologic signs.
- When a satisfactory series of X-rays is obtained, the needle (or catheter) is withdrawn. Apply firm pressure to the puncture site for 15 minutes.
- After the test, observe the patient for bleeding, check distal pulses, and apply a pressure bandage.
- Typically, the patient will be on bed rest for 6 to 8 hours. Give prescribed pain medications, and monitor his vital signs and neurologic status for 6 hours. The patient is usually discharged the same day.
- Observe the puncture site for signs of extravasation (redness, swelling) and apply an ice bag to ease the patient's discomfort and minimize swelling. If bleeding occurs, apply firm pressure to the puncture site and inform the practitioner.

### Do's & don'ts

If the femoral approach was used, keep the patient's affected leg straight for 6 hours or longer and routinely check pulses distal to the site (dorsalis pedis, popliteal). Monitor the leg for temperature, color, and sensation. Thrombosis or hematoma can occlude blood flow; extravasation can also impede blood flow by exerting pressure on the artery.

- Monitor the patient for disorientation and weakness or numbness in the extremities (signs of thrombosis or hematoma) and for arterial spasms, which may produce symptoms of transient ischemic attacks (TIAs).
- If the brachial approach was used, immobilize the affected arm for 6 hours or longer and routinely check the radial pulse.
- Place a sign near the patient's bed warning personnel not to take blood pressure readings from the affected arm.
- Observe the patient's arm and hand for changes in color, temperature, or sensation. If they become pale, cool, or numb, report these changes at once.
- After the test, tell the patient he may resume his usual diet. Encourage him to drink fluids to help him pass the contrast medium.

### Precautions
- Cerebral angiography is contraindicated in the patient with hepatic, renal, or thyroid disease.
- This test is also contraindicated in the patient with a hypersensitivity to iodine or contrast media.
- If the patient has been receiving aspirin or other anticoagulants daily, take extra care when compressing the puncture site. Anticoagulants may need to be discontinued for 3 days before testing.

**ACTION STAT!**

Monitor the catheter puncture site frequently and closely for hemorrhage or hematoma formation. If either occurs, notify the practitioner immediately.

### Complications
- Adverse reaction to contrast media
- Bleeding
- Embolism
- Hematoma
- Infection
- Thrombosis, TIA, stroke
- Vasospasm

# Cerebrospinal fluid analysis

Cerebrospinal fluid (CSF), a clear substance that circulates in the subarachnoid space, has many vital functions. It protects the brain and spinal cord from injury and transports products of neurosecretion, cellular biosynthesis, and cellular metabolism through the central nervous system (CNS).

For qualitative analysis, CSF is most commonly obtained by lumbar puncture (usually between the third and fourth lumbar vertebrae) and, rarely, by cisternal or ventricular puncture. A CSF specimen may also be obtained during other neurologic tests such as myelography.

## Normal and abnormal results

- For a summary of normal and abnormal findings in CSF analysis, see *Findings in cerebrospinal fluid analysis,* pages 478 and 479.

## Purpose

- To measure CSF pressure as an aid in detecting an obstruction of CSF circulation
- To aid in the diagnosis of viral or bacterial meningitis, subarachnoid or intracranial hemorrhage, tumors, and brain abscesses
- To aid in the diagnosis of neurosyphilis and chronic CNS infections
- To check for Alzheimer's disease

## Patient preparation

- Describe the procedure to the patient and explain that CSF analysis analyzes the fluid around the spinal cord.
- Inform the patient that he doesn't need to restrict food and fluids.
- Tell the patient who will perform the procedure and where it will take place.
- Advise the patient that a headache is the most common adverse effect of a lumbar puncture, but reassure him that his cooperation during the test helps minimize this effect.
- Make sure that the patient or a responsible family member has signed an informed consent form.
- If the patient is unusually anxious, assess and report his vital signs.

## Procedure and posttest care

- Confirm the patient's identity using two patient identifiers according to facility policy.
- Position the patient on his side at the edge of the bed with his knees drawn up to his abdomen and his chin on his chest. Provide pillows to support the spine on a horizontal plane. This position allows full flexion of the spine and easy access to the lumbar subarachnoid space. Help him maintain this position by placing one arm around his knees and the other arm around his neck.
- If the sitting position is preferred, have the patient sit up and bend his chest and head toward his knees. Help him maintain this position throughout the procedure.
- After the skin is prepared for injection, the area is draped. Warn the patient that he'll probably experience a transient burning sensation when the local anesthetic is injected.
- Tell the patient that when the spinal needle is inserted, he may feel slight local pain as the needle transverses the dura mater.
- Ask the patient to report pain or sensations that differ from or continue after this expected discomfort because such sensations may indicate irritation or puncture of a nerve root, requiring needle repositioning.
- Instruct the patient to remain still and breathe normally; movement and hyperventilation can alter pressure readings or cause injury.

# Findings in cerebrospinal fluid analysis

| Test | Normal | Abnormality |
|---|---|---|
| Pressure | 50 to 180 mm $H_2O$ | Increase |
| | | Decrease |
| Appearance | Clear, colorless | Cloudy |
| | | Xanthochromic or bloody |
| | | Brown, orange, or yellow |
| Protein | 15 to 50 mg/dl (SI, 0.15 to 0.5 q/L) | Marked increase |
| | | Marked decrease |
| Gamma globulin | 3% to 12% of total protein | Increase |
| Glucose | 50 to 80 mg/dl (SI, 2.8 to 4.4 mmol/L) | Increase |
| | | Decrease |
| Cell count | 0 to 5 white blood cells | Increase |
| | No RBCs | RBCs |
| Venereal Disease Research Laboratories test for syphilis and other serologic tests | Nonreactive | Positive |
| Chloride | 118 to 130 mEq/L (SI, 118 to 130 mmol/L) | Decrease |
| Gram stain | No organisms | Gram-positive or gram-negative organisms |

## Implications

Increased intracranial pressure

Spinal subarachnoid obstruction above puncture site

Infection

Subarachnoid, intracerebral, or intraventricular hemorrhage; spinal cord obstruction; traumatic tap (usually noted only in initial specimen)

Elevated protein levels, red blood cell (RBC) breakdown (blood present for at least 3 days)

Tumors, trauma, hemorrhage, diabetes mellitus, polyneuritis, blood in cerebrospinal fluid (CSF)

Rapid CSF production

Demyelinating disease, neurosyphilis, Guillain-Barré syndrome

Systemic hyperglycemia

Systemic hypoglycemia, bacterial or fungal infection, meningitis, mumps, postsubarachnoid hemorrhage

Active disease: meningitis, acute infection, onset of chronic illness, tumor, abscess, infarction, demyelinating disease

Hemorrhage or traumatic lumbar puncture

Neurosyphilis

Infected meninges

Bacterial meningitis

■ The anesthetic is injected, and the spinal needle is inserted in the midline, between the spinous processes of the vertebrae (usually between the third and fourth lumbar vertebra). At this point, initial (or opening) CSF pressure is measured and a specimen is obtained.

■ After the specimen is collected, label the containers in the order in which they were filled and find out if specific instructions are required for the laboratory.

■ Next, a final pressure reading is taken, and the needle is removed.

■ Clean the puncture site with a local antiseptic, such as povidone-iodine solution, and apply a small adhesive bandage.

■ Check whether the patient must lie flat or if the head of his bed may be slightly elevated. In most cases, you'll be instructed to keep the patient lying flat for 8 hours after lumbar puncture. Some practitioners, however, allow a 30-degree elevation at the head of the bed. Remind the patient that although he must not raise his head, he can turn from side to side.

■ Encourage the patient to drink fluids. Provide a flexible straw.

■ Check the puncture site for redness, swelling, and drainage every hour for the first 4 hours, and then every 4 hours for the first 24 hours.

■ If CSF pressure is elevated, assess the patient's neurologic status every 15 minutes for 4 hours. If he's stable, assess him every hour for 2 hours and then every 4 hours or according to the pretest schedule.

## Precautions

■ Infection at the puncture site contraindicates removal of CSF; in a patient with increased intracranial pressure, CSF should be removed with extreme caution because the rapid reduction in pressure that follows withdrawal of fluid can cause cerebellar tonsillar herniation and medullary compression.

■ During the procedure, observe closely for adverse reactions, such as elevated pulse rate, pallor, or clammy skin. Report any significant changes immediately.

■ If the patient is crying, coughing, or straining, the CSF pressure may be increased.

### Alert

 Watch the patient for complications of lumbar puncture, such as reaction to the anesthetic, meningitis, bleeding into the spinal canal, and cerebellar tonsillar herniation and medullary compression. Signs of meningitis include fever, neck rigidity, a positive Kernig's or Brudzinski's sign, and irritability; signs of herniation include decreased level of consciousness, changes in pupil size and equality, altered vital signs (including widened pulse pressure, decreased pulse rate, and irregular respirations), and respiratory failure.

## Digital subtraction angiography
### [DSA]

Digital subtraction angiography (DSA) is a sophisticated radiographic technique that uses video equipment and computer-assisted image enhancement to examine the vascular systems. As in conventional angiography, X-ray images are obtained after injecting a contrast medium. However, unlike conventional angiography, in which images of bone and soft tissue commonly obscure vascular detail, DSA provides a high-contrast view of blood vessels without interfering images or shadows.

This unique view is made possible by digital subtraction, in which fluoroscopic images are taken before and after in-

jection of a contrast medium. A computer converts these images into digital information and then "subtracts" the first image from the second, eliminating most information (mainly bone and soft tissue) common to both images. The result is a better image of the contrast-enhanced vasculature.

### Normal results

■ The contrast medium should fill and opacify all superficial and deep arteries, arterioles, and veins, allowing visualization of normal cerebral vasculature.

### Abnormal results

■ Vascular filling defects may indicate arteriovenous occlusion or stenosis, possibly due to vasospasm, vascular malformation or angiomas, arteriosclerosis, or cerebral embolism or thrombosis.

■ Outpouchings in vessel lumina may reflect cerebral aneurysms; such aneurysms frequently rupture, causing subarachnoid hemorrhage.

■ Vessel displacement or vascular masses may indicate an intracranial tumor.

### Purpose

■ To visualize extracranial and intracranial cerebral blood flow

■ To detect and evaluate cerebrovascular abnormalities

■ To aid postoperative evaluation of cerebrovascular surgery, such as arterial grafts and endarterectomies

### Patient preparation

■ Explain that DSA visualizes cerebral blood vessels.

■ Tell the patient that he'll need to fast for 4 hours before the test, but he doesn't need to restrict fluids.

■ Explain to the patient that he'll receive an injection of a contrast medium, either by needle or through a venous catheter inserted in his arm, and that a series of X-rays will be taken of his head. Tell him who will perform the test, where it will take place, and that it takes 30 to 90 minutes.

■ Inform the patient that he'll be positioned on an X-ray table with his head immobilized and will be asked to lie still. (Some patients—especially children—may be given a sedative to prevent movement during the procedure.)

■ Instruct the patient to remove all jewelry, dentures, and other radiopaque objects from the X-ray field.

■ Tell the patient that he'll probably feel some transient pain from insertion of the needle or catheter and that he may experience a feeling of warmth, a headache, a metallic taste, and nausea or vomiting after the contrast agent is injected.

■ Make sure that the patient or a responsible family member has signed an informed consent form, if required.

## ALERT

 Check the patient's history for hypersensitivity to iodine, iodine-containing substances (such as shellfish), or other contrast media. Note any hypersensitivities on his chart and report them as appropriate.

## Procedure and posttest care

■ Confirm the patient's identity using two patient identifiers according to facility policy.

■ Place the patient in the supine position on an X-ray table and tell him to lie still with his arms at his sides.

■ After an initial series of fluoroscopic pictures (mask images) of the patient's head is taken, the injection site—most commonly the antecubital basilic or cephalic vein—is clipped and cleaned with an antiseptic solution.

■ If catheterization is ordered, a local anesthetic is administered, a venipuncture is performed, and a catheter is in-

serted and advanced to the superior vena cava.

■ After placement is verified by X-ray, I.V. lines from a bag of normal saline solution and from an automatic contrast medium injector are connected. While the saline is administered, the injector delivers the contrast medium at a rate of about 14 ml/second.

■ Monitor the patient's vital signs and neurologic status and observe for signs of a hypersensitivity reaction, such as urticaria, flushing, and respiratory distress.

■ After allowing time for the contrast medium to clear the pulmonary circulation and enter the cerebral vasculature, a second series of fluoroscopic images (contrast images) is taken. The computer digitizes the information received from both series and compares mask and contrast images, subtracting the information (images of bone and soft tissue) common to both. A detailed image of the contrast medium-filled vessels is displayed on a video monitor; the image may be stored on videotape or a compact disc for future reference.

■ Because the contrast medium acts as a diuretic, encourage the patient to increase his fluid intake for 24 hours after this test. Advise him that extra fluid intake will also speed excretion of the contrast medium. Monitor his intake and output, as ordered.

■ Check the venipuncture site for signs of extravasation, such as redness or swelling. If bleeding occurs, apply firm pressure to the puncture site. If a hematoma develops, elevate the arm and apply warm soaks.

■ Observe the patient for a delayed hypersensitivity reaction to the contrast medium. A delayed reaction can occur up to 18 hours after the procedure.

■ Tell the patient that he may resume his usual diet.

## Precautions
- DSA may be contraindicated in the patient with a hypersensitivity to iodine or contrast media; poor cardiac function; renal, hepatic, or thyroid disease; diabetes; or multiple myeloma.

## Complications
- Bleeding
- Infection
- Thrombotic and embolic events

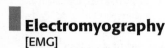
# Electromyography
[EMG]

Electromyography (EMG) records the electrical activity of selected skeletal muscle groups at rest and during voluntary contraction. It involves percutaneous insertion of a needle electrode into a muscle. The electrical discharge of the muscle is then measured by an oscilloscope. Nerve conduction time is often measured simultaneously. (See *Nerve conduction studies.*)

## Normal results
- At rest, a normal muscle exhibits minimal electrical activity.
- During voluntary contraction, electrical activity increases markedly.
- A sustained contraction or one of increasing strength causes a rapid "train" of motor unit potentials that can be heard as a crescendo of sounds over the audio amplifier.

## Abnormal results
- In primary muscle diseases, such as muscular dystrophy, motor unit potentials are short (low amplitude), with frequent, irregular discharges.
- In disorders such as amyotrophic lateral sclerosis (ALS) (as well as in peripheral nerve disorders), motor unit potentials are isolated and irregular, but show increased amplitude and duration.
- In myasthenia gravis, motor unit potentials initially may be normal, but progressively diminish in amplitude with continuing contractions.

**DRUG CHALLENGE**

 Drugs affecting myoneural junctions, such as cholinergics, anticholinergics, and skeletal muscle relaxants

## Purpose
- To aid in differentiating between primary muscle disorders, such as the muscular dystrophies, and secondary disorders

---

### Nerve conduction studies

Nerve conduction studies aid in the diagnosis of peripheral nerve injuries and diseases affecting the peripheral nervous system such as peripheral neuropathies. To measure nerve conduction time, a nerve is stimulated electrically through the skin and underlying tissues. The patient experiences a mild electric shock with each stimulation. At a known distance from the point of stimulation, a recording electrode detects the response from the stimulated nerve.

The time between stimulation of the nerve and the detected response is measured on an oscilloscope. The speed of conduction along the nerve is then calculated by dividing the distance between the point of stimulation and the recording electrode by the time between stimulus and response. In peripheral nerve injuries and diseases, such as peripheral neuropathies, nerve conduction time is abnormal.

- To help assess diseases characterized by central neuronal degeneration such as ALS
- To aid in the diagnosis of neuromuscular disorders such as myasthenia gravis
- To aid in the diagnosis of radiculopathies

### Patient preparation

- Explain that EMG measures the electrical activity of his muscles.
- Tell the patient that there are usually no restrictions on food and fluids (in some cases, cigarettes, coffee, tea, and cola may be restricted for 2 to 3 hours before the test).
- Describe the test, including who will perform it and where it will take place.
- Tell the patient that he may wear a hospital gown or comfortable clothing that permits access to the muscles to be tested.
- Advise the patient that a needle will be inserted into selected muscles and that he may experience discomfort. Reassure him that adverse effects and complications are rare.
- Make sure that the patient or a responsible family member has signed an informed consent form, if required.
- Check the patient's history for medications that may interfere with the results of the test—for example, cholinergics, anticholinergics, and skeletal muscle relaxants. If the patient is receiving such medications, note this on the chart and withhold medications, as ordered.

### Procedure and posttest care

- Confirm the patient's identity using two patient identifiers according to facility policy.
- Position the patient on a stretcher or bed or in a chair, depending on the muscles to be tested. Position his arm or leg so that the muscle to be tested is at rest.

- The skin is cleaned with alcohol, the needle electrodes are quickly inserted, and a metal plate is placed under the patient to serve as a reference electrode. Then the muscle's electrical signal (motor unit potential), recorded during rest and contraction, is amplified 1 million times and displayed on an oscilloscope or computer screen.
- The recorder lead wires are attached to an audio amplifier so that the fluctuation of voltage within the muscle can be heard.
- If the patient experiences residual pain, apply warm compresses and give prescribed analgesics.
- Tell the patient that he may resume his usual medications, as ordered.

### Precautions

- EMG is contraindicated in the patient with a bleeding disorder.

### Complications

- Infection at the insertion site

# Tensilon test

The Tensilon test involves careful observation of the patient after I.V. administration of Tensilon (edrophonium chloride), a rapid, short-acting anticholinesterase that improves muscle strength by increasing muscle response to nerve impulses.

It's especially useful in diagnosing myasthenia gravis, an abnormality of the myoneural junction in which nerve impulses fail to induce normal muscular responses. Patients with myasthenia gravis experience extreme fatigue at the end of the day and after repetitive activity or stress. Results of other procedures, including electromyography, may supplement Tensilon test findings in diagnosing this disease.

## Normal results
- Fasciculations develop.

## Abnormal results
- If the patient has myasthenia gravis, muscle strength should improve promptly after administration of Tensilon.
- A positive response is elicited in motor neuron disease and in some neuropathies and myopathies. The response is usually less dramatic and less consistent than in myasthenia gravis.
- The patient in myasthenic crisis shows brief improvement in muscle strength after Tensilon administration.
- The patient in cholinergic crisis (anticholinesterase overdose) may experience exaggerated muscle weakness.

### DRUG CHALLENGE

 Prednisone (possible delay of Tensilon's effect on muscle strength); quinidine and anticholinergics (inhibit the action of Tensilon); procainamide and muscle relaxants (inhibit normal muscle response)

## Purpose
- To aid in the diagnosis of myasthenia gravis
- To aid in differentiating between myasthenic and cholinergic crises
- To monitor oral anticholinesterase therapy

## Patient preparation
- Explain that the Tensilon test helps determine the cause of muscle weakness.
- Describe the test, including who will perform it, where it will take place, and how long it will last.
- Don't describe the exact response that will be evaluated; foreknowledge can affect the test's objectivity.
- Explain to the patient that a small tube will be inserted into a vein in his arm and that a drug will be administered periodically. He'll be asked to make repetitive muscle movements and his reactions will be observed. To ensure accuracy, the test may be repeated several times.
- Advise the patient that the Tensilon may produce some unpleasant adverse effects, but reassure him that someone will be with him at all times and that any reactions will quickly disappear.
- Check the patient's history for medications that affect muscle function, anticholinesterase therapy, drug hypersensitivities, and respiratory disease. Withhold medications, as ordered. If the patient is receiving anticholinesterase therapy, note this on the requisition request; include the time of the most recent dose.
- Make sure that the patient or a responsible family member has signed an informed consent form.

## Procedure and posttest care
- Confirm the patient's identity using two patient identifiers according to facility policy.
- Begin an I.V. infusion of dextrose 5% in water or normal saline solution.
- When performing the test on an adult patient suspected of having myasthenia gravis, 2 mg of Tensilon are given initially. Before the rest of the dose is administered, the practitioner may want to fatigue the muscles by asking the patient to perform various exercises, such as looking up until ptosis develops, counting to 100 until his voice diminishes, or holding his arms above his shoulders until they drop. When the muscles are fatigued, the remaining 8 mg of Tensilon are administered over 30 seconds.
- Some practitioners may prefer to begin the test with a placebo injection to evaluate the patient's muscle response more accurately. The placebo isn't necessary if cranial muscles are being tested because

cranial strength can't be simulated voluntarily.

■ After Tensilon is administered, the patient is asked to perform repetitive muscle movements, such as opening and closing his eyes and crossing and uncrossing his legs. Closely observe the patient for improved muscle strength. If muscle strength doesn't improve within 3 to 5 minutes, the test may be repeated.

■ To differentiate between a myasthenic and cholinergic crisis, 1 to 2 mg of Tensilon is infused. After the infusion, continually monitor the patient's vital signs. Watch closely for respiratory distress and be prepared to provide respiratory assistance.

■ If muscle strength doesn't improve, more Tensilon is infused cautiously— 1 mg at a time up to a maximum of 5 mg—and the patient is observed for distress.

■ Neostigmine is given immediately if the test demonstrates myasthenic crisis; atropine is given for cholinergic crisis.

■ To evaluate oral anticholinesterase therapy, 2 mg of Tensilon is infused 1 hour after the patient's last dose of the anticholinesterase. The patient is observed carefully for adverse effects and muscle response.

■ After Tensilon administration, the I.V. line is kept open at a rate of 20 ml/hour until all of the patient's responses have been evaluated.

■ When the test is complete, stop the I.V. and check the patient's vital signs.

■ Check the puncture site for hematoma, excessive bleeding, and swelling.

■ Tell the patient that he may resume his usual medications, as ordered.

### Precautions

■ Because of the systemic adverse reactions Tensilon may produce, this test may be contraindicated in the patient with hypotension, bradycardia, apnea, or mechanical obstruction of the intestine or urinary tract.

■ The patient with a respiratory ailment, such as asthma, should receive atropine during the test to minimize adverse reactions to Tensilon.

■ Stay with the patient during the test and observe him closely for adverse reactions.

**ACTION STAT!**

 Keep resuscitation equipment handy in case of respiratory failure.

### Complications

■ Bradycardia, heart block, respiratory arrest

■ Bronchospasms, laryngospasm

■ Paralysis of respiratory muscles

■ Respiratory arrest

■ Respiratory depression

■ Seizures

# Gastrointestinal system

## Esophageal, gastric, and peritoneal content tests

### Acid perfusion test
[Bernstein test]

The acid perfusion test helps to distinguish pain caused by esophagitis (burning epigastric or retrosternal pain that radiates to the back or arms) from pain caused by angina pectoris or other disorders. It requires infusion of saline and acidic solutions into the esophagus through a nasogastric (NG) tube.

#### Normal results
- Absence of pain or burning during infusion of either solution indicates a healthy esophageal mucosa.

#### Abnormal results
- In the patient with esophagitis, the acidic solution causes pain or burning, and the normal saline solution should produce no adverse effects.
- Occasionally, both solutions cause pain in the patient with esophagitis, but they may not cause pain in the patient with asymptomatic esophagitis.

#### Purpose
- To distinguish chest pain caused by esophagitis from chest pain caused by cardiac disorders

#### Patient preparation
- Explain that the acid perfusion test helps determine the cause of heartburn.
- Explain the following restrictions to the patient: no antacids for 24 hours before the test, no food for 12 hours before the test, and no fluids or smoking for 8 hours before the test.
- Describe the test, including who will perform it, where it will take place, and how long it will last.
- Explain to the patient that the test involves passing a tube through his nose into the esophagus and that he may experience some discomfort, a desire to cough, or a gagging sensation during tube passage.
- Tell the patient that liquid is slowly infused through the tube into the esophagus and that he should immediately report pain or burning during the infusion.

- Just before the test, check the patient's pulse rate and blood pressure. Ask him whether he's experiencing any heartburn and, if so, to describe it.
- Make sure that the patient or a responsible family member has signed an informed consent form.

## Procedure and posttest care

- Confirm the patient's identity using two patient identifiers according to facility policy.
- After the patient is seated, insert an NG tube that has been marked 12″ (30.5 cm) from the tip into his stomach. Attach a 20-ml syringe to the tube and aspirate stomach contents. Withdraw the tube into the esophagus (to the 12″ mark).
- Hang labeled containers of normal saline solution and a prescribed acidic solution (0.1 Na HCl) on an I.V. pole behind the patient, and then connect the NG tube to the I.V. tubing.
- Open the line from the normal saline solution and infuse it at a rate of 60 to 120 drops/minute. Continue infusion for 5 to 10 minutes.
- Ask the patient whether he's experiencing any discomfort and record his response.
- Without the patient's knowledge, close the line from the normal saline solution and open the line from the acidic solution. Infuse the acidic solution into the esophagus at the same rate used for the saline solution. Continue infusion for 30 minutes.
- Ask the patient again whether he's experiencing discomfort and record his response.
- If the patient experiences discomfort, without the patient's knowledge, close the line from the acidic solution immediately and open the line from the normal saline solution. Continue to infuse this solution until the discomfort subsides.

- If ordered, repeat infusion of the acidic solution to verify the patient's response. If this isn't required or if the patient experiences no discomfort after infusion of the acidic solution for 30 minutes, stop the solution and withdraw the NG tube.
- If the patient complains of pain or burning, give him an antacid, as ordered. If he complains of a sore throat, provide soothing lozenges or obtain an order for an ice collar.
- Tell the patient that he may resume his usual diet and medications, as ordered.

## Precautions

- The acid perfusion test is contraindicated in the patient with esophageal varices, heart failure, acute myocardial infarction, or other cardiac disorders.
- During intubation, make sure that the tube enters the esophagus and not the trachea. Withdraw the tube immediately if the patient develops cyanosis or paroxysmal coughing.
- Assess the patient's pulse rate and rhythm to detect arrhythmias that may develop.
- Clamp the tube before removing it to prevent fluid aspiration into the lungs.

# Peritoneal fluid analysis

Peritoneal fluid analysis assesses a specimen of peritoneal fluid obtained by paracentesis. This procedure requires inserting a trocar and cannula through the abdominal wall while the patient receives a local anesthetic. If the fluid specimen is removed for therapeutic purposes, the trocar may be connected to a drainage system. However, if only a small amount of fluid is removed for diagnostic purposes, an 18G needle may be used in place of the trocar and cannula. In a four-quadrant tap, fluid is aspirated from each quadrant of the ab-

## Normal findings in peritoneal fluid analysis

Use this chart to determine the normal findings in peritoneal fluid.

| Element | Normal value or finding |
| --- | --- |
| Alkaline phosphatase | Males > age 18: 90 to 239 units/L (SI, 90 to 239 units/L)<br>Females < age 45: 76 to 196 units/L (SI, 76 to 196 units/L)<br>Females > age 45: 87 to 250 units/L (SI, 87 to 250 units/L) |
| Ammonia | < 50 mcg/dl (SI, < 29 µmol/L) |
| Amylase | 138 to 404 units/L (SI, 138 to 404 units/L) |
| Bacteria | None |
| Cytology | No malignant cells present |
| Fungi | None |
| Glucose | 70 to 100 mg/dl (SI, 3.5 to 5 mmol/L) |
| Gross appearance | Sterile, odorless, clear to pale yellow color; scant amount (< 50 ml) |
| Protein | 0.3 to 4.1 g/dl (SI, 3 to 41 g/L) |
| Red blood cells | None |
| White blood cells | < 300/µl (SI, < 300 × 10^9/L) |

domen to verify abdominal trauma and confirm the need for surgery.

### Reference values

- See *Normal findings in peritoneal fluid analysis.*

### Abnormal results

- Milk-colored peritoneal fluid may result from chyle or lymph fluid escaping from a thoracic duct that's damaged or blocked by a malignant tumor, lymphoma, tuberculosis, parasitic infestation, adhesion, or hepatic cirrhosis; a pseudochylous condition may result from the presence of leukocytes or tumor cells.

- Differential diagnosis of true chylous ascites depends on the presence of elevated triglyceride levels (≥ 400 mg/dl [SI, ≥ 4.36 mmol/L]) and microscopic fat globules.
- Cloudy or turbid fluid may indicate peritonitis due to primary bacterial infection, a ruptured bowel (after trauma), pancreatitis, a strangulated or an infarcted intestine, or appendicitis.
- Bloody fluid may result from a benign or malignant tumor, hemorrhagic pancreatitis, or a traumatic tap; however, if the fluid fails to clear on continued aspiration, a traumatic tap isn't the cause.
- Bile-stained green fluid may indicate a ruptured gallbladder, acute pancreatitis,

or a perforated intestine or duodenal ulcer.

■ A red blood cell count over 100/µl (SI, > 100/L) indicates neoplasm or tuberculosis; a count over 100,000/µl (SI, > 100,000/L) indicates intra-abdominal trauma.

■ An elevated white blood cell count with more than 25% neutrophils occurs in 90% of patients with spontaneous bacterial peritonitis and in 50% of those with cirrhosis.

■ A high percentage of lymphocytes suggests tuberculous peritonitis or chylous ascites. Numerous mesothelial cells indicate tuberculous peritonitis.

■ Protein levels rise above 3 g/dl in malignancy (SI, > 3 g/L) and above 4 g/dl (SI, > 4 g/L) in tuberculosis.

■ Peritoneal fluid glucose levels fall in the patient with tuberculous peritonitis or peritoneal carcinomatosis.

■ Amylase levels rise with pancreatic trauma, pancreatic pseudocyst, or acute pancreatitis and may also rise in intestinal necrosis or strangulation.

■ Peritoneal alkaline phosphatase levels rise to more than twice the normal serum levels in the patient with ruptured or strangulated small intestines.

■ Peritoneal ammonia levels also exceed twice the normal serum levels in ruptured or strangulated large and small intestines and in a ruptured ulcer or an appendix.

■ A protein ascitic fluid to serum ratio of 0.5 or greater may suggest a malignancy or tuberculous or pancreatic ascites. The presence of this finding indicates a non-hepatic cause; its absence suggests uncomplicated hepatic disease.

■ An albumin gradient between ascitic fluid and serum greater than 1 g/dl (SI, > 1 g/L) indicates chronic hepatic disease; a lesser value suggests malignancy.

■ Cytologic examination of peritoneal fluid accurately detects malignant cells.

■ Microbiological examination can reveal coliforms, anaerobes, and enterococci, which can enter the peritoneum from a ruptured organ or from infections accompanying appendicitis, pancreatitis, tuberculosis, or ovarian disease.

■ Gram-positive cocci commonly indicate primary peritonitis; gram-negative organisms, secondary peritonitis.

■ The presence of fungi may indicate histoplasmosis, candidiasis, or coccidioidomycosis.

### Purpose

■ To determine the cause of ascites
■ To detect abdominal trauma and peritonitis

### Patient preparation

■ Explain that peritoneal fluid analysis helps determine the cause of ascites or detects abdominal trauma.

■ Inform the patient that he need not restrict food and fluids.

■ Tell the patient that the test requires a peritoneal fluid specimen, that he'll receive a local anesthetic to minimize discomfort, and that the procedure takes about 45 minutes to perform.

■ Provide psychological support to decrease the patient's anxiety and assure him that complications are rare.

■ If the patient has severe ascites, inform him that the procedure will relieve his discomfort and allow him to breathe more easily.

■ Make sure that the patient or a responsible family member has signed an informed consent form.

■ Record the patient's baseline vital signs, weight, and abdominal girth.

■ Tell the patient that a blood sample may be taken for analysis.

■ Tell the patient to void just before the test. This helps to prevent accidental bladder injury during needle insertion.

■ X-rays may be performed before peritoneal analysis to ensure reliability.

## Procedure and posttest care

- Confirm the patient's identity using two patient identifiers according to facility policy.
- Have the patient sit on a bed or in a chair with his feet flat on the floor and his back well-supported. If he can't tolerate being out of bed, place him in high Fowler's position and make him as comfortable as possible.
- Except for the puncture site, keep the patient covered to prevent chilling.
- Provide a plastic sheet or absorbent pad to collect spillage and to protect the patient and bed linens.
- The puncture site is shaved, the skin prepared, and the area draped.
- The local anesthetic is injected.
- The physician inserts the needle or trocar and cannula 1" to 2" (2.5 to 5 cm) below the umbilicus. (However, it may also be inserted through the flank, the iliac fossa, the border of the rectus, or at each quadrant of the abdomen.)
- If a trocar and cannula are used, a small incision is made to facilitate insertion. When the needle pierces the peritoneum, it "gives" with an audible sound. The trocar is removed and a sample of fluid is aspirated with a 50-ml luer-lock syringe.
- If additional fluid is to be drained, assist in attaching one end of an I.V. tube to the cannula and the other end to a collection bag. The fluid is then aspirated (no more than 1,500 ml). If aspirating is difficult, reposition the patient, as ordered.
- After aspiration, the trocar needle is removed and a pressure dressing is applied. Occasionally, the wound may be sutured first.
- Label the specimens in the order they were drawn. If the patient has received antibiotic therapy, note this on the laboratory request.
- Apply a gauze dressing to the puncture site. Make sure it's thick enough to absorb all drainage. Check the dressing frequently (for example, whenever you check vital signs) and reinforce or apply a pressure dressing, if needed.
- Monitor the patient's vital signs until they're stable. If his recovery is poor, check his vital signs every 15 minutes. Weigh him and measure his abdominal girth; compare these with his baseline values.
- Allow the patient to rest and, if possible, withhold treatment or procedures that may cause undue stress such as linen changes.
- Monitor the patient's urine output for at least 24 hours, and watch for hematuria, which may indicate bladder trauma.

### ALERT

 Watch the patient for signs of hemorrhage or shock and for increasing pain or abdominal tenderness. These may indicate a perforated intestine or, depending on the site of the tap, puncture of the inferior epigastric artery, hematoma of the anterior cecal wall, or rupture of the iliac vein or bladder.

- If a large amount of fluid was aspirated, watch the patient for signs of vascular collapse (color change, elevated pulse and respiratory rates, decreased blood pressure and central venous pressure, mental changes, and dizziness). Administer fluids orally if the patient is alert and can accept them.

### ALERT

 Observe the patient with severe hepatic disease for signs of hepatic coma, which may result from sodium and potassium loss accompanying hypovolemia. Watch him for mental changes, drowsiness, and stupor. Such a patient is also prone to uremia, infection, hemorrhage, and protein depletion.

- As ordered, administer I.V. infusions and albumin. Check the laboratory report for electrolyte (especially sodium) and serum protein levels.

### Precautions
- Peritoneal fluid analysis should be performed cautiously in a pregnant patient and in the patient with bleeding tendencies or unstable vital signs.
- Check the patient's vital signs every 15 minutes during the procedure. Watch for deviations from baseline findings. Observe for dizziness, pallor, perspiration, and increased anxiety.

##### ACTION STAT!
 If rapid fluid aspiration induces hypovolemia and shock, reduce the vertical distance between the trocar and the collection bag to slow the drainage rate. If necessary, stop the drainage by turning off the stopcock or clamping the tubing.

- Avoid contamination of the specimens, which alters their bacterial content. Send them to the laboratory immediately after collection.

## *Fecal content tests*

 **Fecal lipids**

Lipids excreted in stool include monoglycerides, diglycerides, triglycerides, phospholipids, glycolipids, soaps (fatty acids and fatty acid salts), sterols, and cholesterol esters. When biliary and pancreatic secretions are adequate, emulsified dietary lipids are almost completely absorbed in the small intestine.

Excessive excretion of fecal lipids (steatorrhea) occurs in several malabsorption syndromes. Qualitative and quantitative tests are used to detect excessive excretion of lipids in patients exhibiting signs of malabsorption, such as weight loss, abdominal distention, and scaly skin.

The qualitative test involves staining a specimen of stool with Sudan III dye and then examining it microscopically for evidence of malabsorption, such as undigested muscle fibers and various fats. The quantitative test involves drying and weighing a 72-hour specimen and then using a solvent to extract the lipids, which are subsequently evaporated and weighed. Only the quantitative test confirms steatorrhea.

### Normal results
- The normal amount of lipids excreted in stool is less than 20% of excreted solids, with excretion of more than 7 g/24 hours.

### Abnormal results
- Digestive and absorptive disorders cause steatorrhea. Digestive disorders may affect the production and release of pancreatic lipase or bile; absorptive disorders may affect the intestine's integrity.
- Scleroderma, radiation enteritis, fistulas, intestinal tuberculosis, small intestine diverticula, and altered intestinal flora may also cause steatorrhea.
- In pancreatic insufficiency, impaired lipid digestion may result from insufficient lipase production.
- Pancreatic resection, cystic fibrosis, chronic pancreatitis, or ductal obstruction by stone or tumor may prevent the normal release or action of lipase.
- In impaired hepatic function, faulty lipid digestion may result from inadequate bile salt production.
- Biliary obstruction, which may accompany gallbladder disease, may prevent

the normal release of bile salts into the duodenum.

- Extensive small-bowel resection or bypass may also interrupt normal enterohepatic bile salt circulation.
- Diseases of the intestinal mucosa affect the normal absorption of lipids.
- Regional ileitis and atrophy due to malnutrition cause gross structural changes in the intestinal wall; celiac disease and tropical sprue produce mucosal abnormalities.
- Whipple's disease and lymphomas cause lymphatic obstruction that may inhibit fat absorption.

**DRUG CHALLENGE**

 Azathioprine, bisacodyl, cholestyramine, kanamycin, neomycin, colchicine, aluminum hydroxide, calcium carbonate, alcohol, potassium chloride, and mineral oil (possible increase or decrease due to inhibited absorption or altered chemical digestion)

### Purpose
- To confirm steatorrhea

### Patient preparation
- Explain that the fecal lipid test evaluates fat digestion.
- Instruct the patient to abstain from alcohol and to maintain a high-fat diet (100 g/day) for 3 days before the test and during the collection period.
- Tell the patient that the test requires a 72-hour stool collection.
- Notify the laboratory and practitioner of medications the patient is taking that may affect test results; they may need to be restricted. If these drugs must be continued, note this on the laboratory request.
- Teach the patient how to collect a timed stool specimen and provide him with the necessary equipment.

- Inform the patient that the laboratory requires 1 to 2 days to complete the analysis.

### Procedure and posttest care
- Confirm the patient's identity using two patient identifiers according to facility policy.
- Collect a 72-hour stool specimen.
- Instruct the patient to resume his usual diet and medications, as ordered.

### Precautions
**DO'S & DON'TS**

 Don't use a waxed collection container because the wax may become incorporated in the stool and interfere with accurate testing.

- Tell the patient to avoid contaminating the stool specimen with toilet tissue or urine.
- Refrigerate the collection container and keep it tightly covered.

## Fecal occult blood

Fecal occult blood is detected by microscopic analysis or by chemical tests for hemoglobin, such as the guaiac test. Normally, stool contains small amounts of blood (2 to 2.5 ml/day); therefore, tests for occult blood detect quantities larger than this. Testing is indicated when clinical symptoms and preliminary blood studies suggest GI bleeding. Additional tests are required to pinpoint the origin of the bleeding. (See *Common sites and causes of GI blood loss.*)

### Normal results
- Less than 2.5 ml of blood should be present in stool, resulting in a green reaction.

### Abnormal results
- A positive test indicates GI bleeding, which may result from many disorders,

# Common sites and causes of GI blood loss

Illustrated here are potential areas that can cause blood loss, resulting in positive fecal occult blood testing. Further clinical assessment and testing is necessary to determine the area involved.

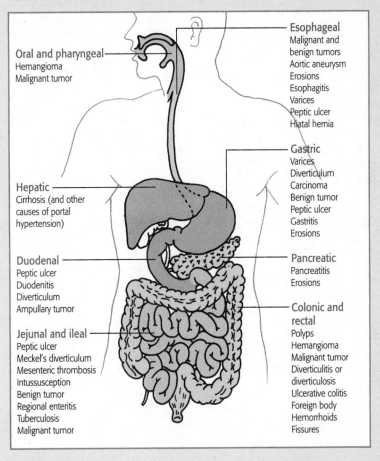

**Oral and pharyngeal**
Hemangioma
Malignant tumor

**Esophageal**
Malignant and
benign tumors
Aortic aneurysm
Erosions
Esophagitis
Varices
Peptic ulcer
Hiatal hernia

**Gastric**
Varices
Diverticulum
Carcinoma
Benign tumor
Peptic ulcer
Gastritis
Erosions

**Hepatic**
Cirrhosis (and other
causes of portal
hypertension)

**Duodenal**
Peptic ulcer
Duodenitis
Diverticulum
Ampullary tumor

**Pancreatic**
Pancreatitis
Erosions

**Jejunal and ileal**
Peptic ulcer
Meckel's diverticulum
Mesenteric thrombosis
Intussusception
Benign tumor
Regional enteritis
Tuberculosis
Malignant tumor

**Colonic and
rectal**
Polyps
Hemangioma
Malignant tumor
Diverticulitis or
diverticulosis
Ulcerative colitis
Foreign body
Hemorrhoids
Fissures

such as varices, a peptic ulcer, carcinoma, ulcerative colitis, dysentery, or hemorrhagic disease.

**DRUG CHALLENGE**

 Iron preparations, bromides, rauwolfia derivatives, indomethacin, colchicine, phenylbutazone, and steroids (possible increase due to association with GI blood

loss); ascorbic acid (false-normal, even with significant bleeding)

## Purpose
- To detect GI bleeding
- To aid in the early diagnosis of colorectal cancer

## Patient preparation

- Explain that the fecal occult blood test helps detect abnormal GI bleeding.
- Instruct the patient to maintain a high-fiber diet and to refrain from eating red meats, turnips, and horseradish for 48 to 72 hours before the test as well as throughout the collection period.
- Tell the patient that the test requires the collection of three stool specimens. Occasionally, only a random specimen is collected.
- Notify the laboratory and practitioner of medications the patient is taking that may affect test results; they may need to be restricted. If these drugs must be continued, note this on the laboratory request.

## Procedure and posttest care

- Confirm the patient's identity using two patient identifiers according to facility policy.
- Collect three stool specimens or a random stool specimen, as ordered. Obtain specimens from two different areas of each stool. Testing may take place in the laboratory or in a utility room on the nursing unit, depending on your facility's policy. Two of the most commonly used screening tests are Hematest and Hemoccult. Hematest uses orthotolidine to detect hemoglobin, and Hemoccult uses guaiac.
- After any of the tests described here are performed, tell the patient that he may resume his usual diet and medications.

### Hematest reagent tablet test

- Use a wooden applicator to smear a bit of the stool specimen on the filter paper supplied with the kit. Alternatively, after performing a digital rectal examination, wipe the finger you used for the examination on a square of the filter paper. Place the filter paper with the stool smear on a glass plate.
- Remove a reagent tablet from the bottle, and immediately replace the cap tightly. Place the tablet in the center of the stool smear on the filter paper. Add one drop of water to the tablet, and allow it to soak in for 5 to 10 seconds. Add a second drop, letting it run from the tablet onto the specimen and filter paper. If necessary, tap the plate gently to dislodge any water from the top of the tablet.
- After 2 minutes, the filter paper will turn blue if the test is positive. Don't read the color that appears on the tablet itself or develops on the filter paper after the 2-minute period. Note the results and discard the filter paper. Remove and discard your gloves and wash your hands thoroughly.

### Hemoccult slide test

- Open the flap on the slide pack and use a wooden applicator to apply a thin smear of the stool specimen to the guaiac-impregnated filter paper exposed in box A. Alternatively, after performing a digital rectal examination, wipe the finger you used for the examination on a square of filter paper. Apply a second smear from another part of the specimen to the filter paper exposed in box B because some parts of the specimen may not contain blood.
- Allow the specimen to dry for 3 to 5 minutes. Open the flap at the rear of the slide package and place 2 drops of Hemoccult developing solution on the paper over each smear. A blue reaction will appear in 30 to 60 seconds if the test is positive. Record the results and discard the slide package. Remove and discard your gloves and wash your hands thoroughly.

### Instant-View fecal occult blood test

- Add a stool sample to the collection tube. Shake it to mix the sample with the extraction buffer, and then dispense 4 drops into the sample well of the cassette. Results will appear on the test region and the control region of the cassette in 5 to 10 minutes, indicating whether the level of hemoglobin is greater than 0.05 mcg/ml of stool. Results will also indicate if the device is performing properly.

### Precautions

- Ingestion of 2 to 5 ml of blood such as from bleeding gums may result in a false-positive test.
- Active bleeding from hemorrhoids may cause possible false-positive results.

# Endoscopy

## Capsule endoscopy
[camera pill]

Capsule endoscopy is an imaging system that consists of a tiny video camera with a light source and transmitter inside a capsule, allowing recording of images along its path. The capsule endoscope measures about 11 × 30 mm and is propelled along the digestive tract by peristalsis. The clear end records images of the stomach walls and, particularly, the small intestine, where many other diagnostic techniques may not reach or otherwise visualize. (See *Detecting disorders in the stomach and small intestine,* page 496.) The images are transmitted to a data recorder on a belt placed around the patient's waist. After swallowing the pill, the patient doesn't need to stay at the hospital and can return to work or other activities of daily living.

### Normal results

- Images reveal normal anatomy of the stomach and small intestine.

### Abnormal results

- Bleeding sites or abnormalities of the stomach and small bowel, such as erosions, Crohn's disease, celiac disease, benign and malignant tumors of the small intestine, vascular disorders, medication-related small-bowel injuries, and pediatric small-bowel disorders may be observed.

### Purpose

- To detect polyps or cancer
- To detect causes of bleeding and anemia
- To determine the cause of recurring symptoms, such as pain or diarrhea
- To obtain motility data, such as gastric or small bowel passage time

### Patient preparation

- Explain that this test helps visualize the stomach and small intestine, helping to detect disorders.
- Tell the patient who will perform the test and where it will take place.
- Inform the patient that he may need to fast for 12 hours before the test but may have fluids for up to 2 hours before the test, unless ordered otherwise.
- Explain to the patient that he'll need to swallow the camera pill and that it will send information to a receiver he'll wear on his belt.
- Tell the patient that the procedure is painless and after swallowing the pill he can go home or go to work.
- Tell the patient he may eat 4 hours after swallowing the pill, unless otherwise ordered.
- Explain that walking helps facilitate movement of the pill.
- Tell the patient that he'll need to return to the facility in 24 hours (or as directed) so the recorder can be removed from his belt.
- Tell the patient that the pill will be excreted normally in his stool in 8 to 72 hours.

## Detecting disorders in the stomach and small intestine

In capsule endoscopy, after the patient swallows the capsule, it travels through the body by the natural movement of the digestive tract. A receiver worn outside the body records the images. The strength of the signal indicates the capsule's location.

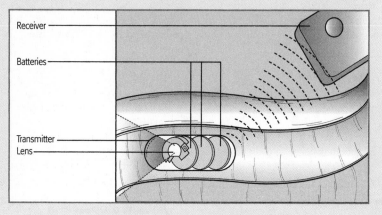

### Procedure and posttest care

- Confirm the patient's identity using two patient identifiers according to facility policy.
- The patient ingests the camera pill, as ordered, and a receiver is attached to his belt.
- The pill records images for up to 6 hours along its path of the stomach, small intestine, and mouth of the large intestine, transmitting the information to the receiver.
- The patient returns to the facility, as ordered, so the images can be transmitted into the computer, where they're displayed on the screen.
- Tell the patient that he may resume his usual diet after the images are obtained.
- The pill is excreted normally in the stool.

### Precautions

- The procedure is contraindicated in the patient with a suspected obstruction, fistula, or stricture and in the patient who can't swallow (an infant, a young child, or someone with a swallowing impairment).
- It's also contraindicated in a patient with cardiac pacemakers or other implanted medical devices.
- The battery is short-lived, so images of the large intestine are unobtainable.
- The pill can't be used to stop bleeding, take tissue samples, remove growths, or repair any problems detected. Other invasive studies may be needed.

## Colonoscopy

Colonoscopy uses a flexible fiber-optic video endoscope to permit visual examination of the lining of the large intestine. It's indicated for patients with a history of constipation or diarrhea, persistent rectal bleeding, and lower abdominal pain when the results of proctosigmoidoscopy and a barium enema test are negative or inconclusive.

## Normal results

- The mucosa of the large intestine beyond the sigmoid colon appears light pink-orange and is marked by semilunar folds and deep tubular pits.
- Blood vessels are visible beneath the intestinal mucosa, which glistens from mucus secretions.

## Abnormal results

- Proctitis, granulomatous or ulcerative colitis, Crohn's disease, and malignant or benign lesions may be seen with visual examination and histologic and cytologic testing.
- Diverticular disease or the site of lower GI bleeding can be detected through colonoscopy alone.

## Purpose

- To detect or evaluate inflammatory and ulcerative bowel disease
- To locate the origin of lower GI bleeding
- To aid in the diagnosis of colonic strictures and benign or malignant lesions
- To evaluate the colon postoperatively for recurrence of polyps and malignant lesions

## Patient preparation

- Check the patient's medical history for allergies, medications, and information pertinent to the current complaint.
- Tell the patient that colonoscopy permits examination of the lining of the large intestine.
- Instruct the patient to maintain a clear liquid diet for 24 to 48 hours before the test and to take nothing by mouth after midnight the night before.
- Describe the procedure and tell the patient who will perform it and where it will take place.
- Explain that the large intestine must be thoroughly cleaned to be clearly visible. Instruct the patient to take a laxative, as ordered, or 1 gallon of GoLYTE-

LY solution in the evening (drinking the chilled solutions at 8 oz [236.6 ml] every 10 minutes until the entire gallon is consumed).
- If fecal results aren't clear, the patient will receive a laxative, suppository, or tap water enema.

### DO'S & DON'TS

 Don't give a soapsuds enema because this irritates the mucosa and stimulates mucus secretions that may hinder the examination.

- Inform the patient that an I.V. line will be started before the procedure and that a sedative will be given just before the procedure. Advise him to arrange for someone to drive him home if he receives sedation.
- Assure the patient that the colonoscope is well lubricated to ease its insertion, that it initially feels cool, and that he may feel an urge to defecate when it's inserted and advanced.
- Explain that air may be introduced through the colonoscope to distend the intestinal wall and to facilitate viewing the lining and advancing the instrument. Tell the patient that flatus normally escapes around the instrument because of air insufflation and that he shouldn't attempt to control it.
- Tell the patient that suction may be used to remove blood or liquid stools that obscure vision, but that this won't cause discomfort.
- Make sure that the patient or a responsible family member has signed an informed consent form.

## Procedure and posttest care

- Confirm the patient's identity using two patient identifiers according to facility policy.
- Place the patient on his left side with his knees flexed and drape him.

# Virtual colonoscopy

Virtual colonoscopy combines computed tomography (CT) scanning and X-ray images with sophisticated image processing computers to generate three-dimensional (3-D) images of the patient's colon. These images are interpreted by a skilled radiologist to recreate and evaluate the colon's inner surface. Although this procedure isn't as accurate as a routine colonoscopy, it's less invasive and is useful in screening the patient with small polyps. The colon must be free from residue and fecal material. Bowel preparation consists of following a clear liquid diet for 24 hours before the procedure; also, the patient performs GoLYTELY bowel preparation the evening before and takes a rectal suppository on the morning of the test.

Before performing the CT scan, a thin red rectal tube is placed, and air is introduced into the colon to distend the bowel. This may produce mild cramping. The CT scan is done with the patient in the supine position and again while prone. The scans are then shipped over a network to a 3-D image processing computer, and a radiologist evaluates the images obtained. If polyps are identified, a colonoscopy may be scheduled to remove them.

■ Obtain the patient's baseline vital signs. Be prepared to monitor vital signs through the procedure. If the patient has known cardiac disease, continuous electrocardiographic monitoring should be instituted. Continuous or periodic pulse oximetry is advisable, particularly in the high-risk patient with possible respiratory depression secondary to sedation.
■ Instruct the patient to breathe deeply and slowly through his mouth as the practitioner palpates the mucosa of the anus and rectum and inserts the lubricated colonoscope through the patient's anus into the sigmoid colon under direct vision.
■ A small amount of air is insufflated to locate the bowel lumen and then the scope is advanced through the rectum.
■ When the instrument reaches the descending sigmoid junction, assist the patient to a supine position to aid the scope advance, if necessary. After passing the splenic flexure, the scope is advanced through the transverse colon, through the hepatic flexure, and into the ascending colon and cecum.
■ Abdominal palpation or fluoroscopy may be used to help guide the colonoscope through the large intestine.
■ Suction may be used to remove blood and secretions that obscure vision.
■ Biopsy forceps or a cytology brush may be passed through the colonoscope to obtain specimens for histologic or cytologic examination; an electrocautery snare may be used to remove polyps.
■ If the practitioner removes a tissue specimen, immediately place it in a specimen bottle containing 10% formalin; immediately place cytology smears in a Coplin jar containing 95% ethyl alcohol. Send specimens to the laboratory immediately. Specimens should be collected in accordance with laboratory and pathology guidelines.
■ Observe the patient closely for signs and symptoms of bowel perforation, including abdominal tenderness, fever, sudden pain, and absent bowel sounds. Report such signs immediately.
■ Check the patient's vital signs and document them according to your facility's policy.
■ After the patient has recovered from sedation, he may resume his usual diet as ordered.

- Provide privacy while the patient rests after the test; tell him that he may pass large amounts of flatus after insufflation.
- If a polyp has been removed, inform the patient that his stool may contain some blood, but excessive bleeding should be reported immediately.

### Precautions
- This procedure is contraindicated in the pregnant woman near term, the patient who has had a recent acute myocardial infarction or abdominal surgery, and one with ischemic bowel disease, acute diverticulitis, peritonitis, fulminant granulomatous colitis, perforated viscus, or fulminant ulcerative colitis. For these cases or for screening purposes, a virtual colonoscopy may be an option to help visualize polyps early before they become concerns. (See *Virtual colonoscopy*.)

ACTION STAT!

 Watch the patient closely for adverse effects of the sedative. Have available emergency resuscitation equipment and an opioid antagonist, such as naloxone, for I.V. use if necessary.

- If a polyp is removed but not retrieved during the examination, give enemas and strain stools to retrieve it if the practitioner requests it.
- Blood from acute colonic hemorrhage hinders visualization.

### Complications
- Perforation of the large intestine
- Excessive bleeding
- Retroperitoneal emphysema

# ▌Endoscopic ultrasonography

Endoscopic ultrasonography (EUS) combines ultrasonography and en-

doscopy to visualize the GI wall and adjacent structures. The incorporation of the ultrasound probe at the distal end of the ultrasonic endoscope allows high-resolution ultrasound imaging.

### Normal results
- A normal anatomy is seen with no evidence of tumor.

### Abnormal results
- Refer to the abnormal results for colonoscopy, page 497; esophagogastroduodenoscopy (EGD), page 500; and proctosigmoidoscopy, page 503.

### Purpose
- To evaluate or stage lesions of the esophagus, stomach, duodenum, pancreas, ampulla, biliary ducts, gallbladder, colon, and rectum
- To evaluate submucosal tumors and large folds
- To localize endocrine tumors

### Patient preparation
- Explain that EUS permits visual examination of tumors and large folds in the GI tract.
- Check the patient's medical history for allergies, medications, and information pertinent to the current complaint.
- Instruct the patient to fast for 6 to 8 hours before the test.
- Describe the procedure to the patient. Tell him who will perform it and where it will take place.
- For an EGD EUS, explain that a flexible instrument will be passed through the mouth and into the esophagus, as in an EGD.
- If a sigmoid EUS is to be performed, tell the patient that the scope is well lubricated to ease its insertion through the anus, that it initially feels cool, and that he may feel an urge to defecate when it's inserted and advanced.

■ For the sigmoid EUS, the patient may have to take a laxative the evening before if ordered.

■ Inform the patient that he may receive an I.V. sedative to help him relax before the endoscope is inserted. If the procedure is being done on an outpatient basis, advise the patient to arrange for someone to drive him home because conscious sedation may affect his reaction time and reflexes, even though he may feel fine.

■ Make sure that the patient or a responsible family member has signed an informed consent form.

### Procedure and posttest care

■ Confirm the patient's identity using two patient identifiers according to facility policy.

■ Obtain the patient's baseline vital signs and monitor him throughout the procedure according to your facility's policy.

■ Follow the procedures for EGD or sigmoidoscopy, depending on which type of EUS will be performed.

### Complications

■ Perforation
■ Bleeding

# ∎ Esophagogastro-duodenoscopy
### [EGD]

Esophagogastroduodenoscopy (EGD) permits visual examination of the lining of the esophagus, stomach, and upper duodenum using a flexible fiber-optic or video endoscope. It's indicated for patients with GI bleeding, hematemesis, melena, substernal or epigastric pain, gastroesophageal reflux disease, dysphagia, anemia, strictures, or peptic ulcer disease; those requiring foreign body retrieval; and postoperative patients with recurrent or new symptoms.

### Normal results

■ The smooth mucosa of the esophagus is normally yellow-pink and marked by a fine vascular network.

■ A pulsation on the anterior wall of the esophagus between 8″ and 10″ (20 and 25.5 cm) from the incisor teeth represents the aortic arch.

■ The orange-red mucosa of the stomach begins the "Z" line, an irregular transition line slightly above the esophagogastric junction.

■ The stomach has rugal folds, and its blood vessels aren't visible beneath the gastric mucosa.

■ The reddish mucosa of the duodenal bulb is marked by a few shallow longitudinal folds.

■ The mucosa of the distal duodenum has prominent circular folds, is lined with villi, and appears velvety.

### Abnormal results

■ Results may indicate acute or chronic ulcers, benign or malignant tumors, and inflammatory disease, including esophagitis, gastritis, and duodenitis.

■ Diverticula, varices, Mallory-Weiss syndrome, esophageal rings, esophageal and pyloric stenoses, and esophageal hiatal hernia may be detected.

■ Gross abnormalities of esophageal motility may be present.

DRUG CHALLENGE

 Anticoagulants (increased risk for bleeding)

### Purpose

■ To diagnose inflammatory disease, malignant and benign tumors, ulcers, Mallory-Weiss syndrome, and structural abnormalities

■ To evaluate the stomach and duodenum postoperatively

- To obtain emergency diagnosis of duodenal ulcer or esophageal injury such as that caused by chemical ingestion

## Patient preparation

- Explain that EGD permits visual examination of the lining of the esophagus, stomach, and upper duodenum.
- Check the patient's medical history for allergies, medications, and information pertinent to the current complaint. Check for hypersensitivity to the medications and anesthetics ordered for the test.
- Instruct the patient to fast for 6 to 12 hours before the test.
- Tell the patient that a flexible instrument with a camera on the end will be passed through his mouth; explain who will perform this procedure, where it will take place, and that it takes about 30 minutes.
- Instruct the patient to remain still while the test is being performed; movement could alter the test results, and the test may have to be repeated.
- If emergency EGD is to be performed, tell the patient that stomach contents may be aspirated through a nasogastric tube.
- Inform the patient that a bitter-tasting local anesthetic will be sprayed into his mouth and throat to calm the gag reflex and that his tongue and throat may feel swollen, making swallowing seem difficult. Advise him to let the saliva drain from the side of his mouth; a suction machine may be used to remove saliva if necessary.
- Explain that a mouth guard will be inserted to protect his teeth and the endoscope; assure him that this won't obstruct his breathing.
- Inform the patient that an I.V. line will be started and a sedative will be given before the endoscope is inserted to help him relax. If the procedure is being done on an outpatient basis, advise the patient to arrange for someone to drive him home because he may feel drowsy from the sedative. Drugs that retard peristalsis of the upper GI tract may be given in some circumstances.
- Tell the patient that he may experience pressure in the stomach as the endoscope is moved about and a feeling of fullness when air or carbon dioxide is insufflated. If he's apprehensive, give meperidine (Demerol) or another analgesic I.M. about 30 minutes before the test as ordered; also give atropine sulfate subcutaneously at this time, as ordered, to decrease gastric secretions, which would interfere with test results.
- Make sure that the patient or a responsible family member has signed an informed consent form.
- Just before the procedure, instruct the patient to remove dentures, eyeglasses, and constricting undergarments.

## Procedure and posttest care

- Confirm the patient's identity using two patient identifiers according to facility policy.
- Obtain the patient's baseline vital signs and leave the blood pressure cuff in place for monitoring throughout the procedure.
- If the patient has known cardiac disease, continuous electrocardiographic monitoring should be instituted. Continuous or periodic pulse oximetry is advisable, particularly in the patient with pulmonary compromise.
- Ask the patient to hold his breath while his mouth and throat are sprayed with a local anesthetic, if requested by the practitioner.
- Place the patient in a left lateral position, bend his head forward, and ask him to open his mouth.
- Remind the patient to let saliva drain from the side of his mouth. Provide an emesis basin to spit out saliva and tis-

sues to wipe saliva from his mouth or use oropharyngeal suction as needed.

■ The practitioner guides the tip of the endoscope to the back of the patient's throat and downward. As the endoscope passes through the posterior pharynx and the cricopharyngeal sphincter, the patient's neck is slowly extended. His chin must be kept at midline. The endoscope is then passed along the esophagus under direct vision.

■ When the endoscope is well into the esophagus (about 12″ [30 cm]), the patient's head is positioned with his chin toward the table so that saliva can drain out of his mouth.

■ After examination of the esophagus and the cardiac sphincter, the endoscope is rotated clockwise and advanced to allow examination of the stomach and duodenum. During the examination, air or water may be introduced through the endoscope to aid visualization, and suction may be applied to remove insufflated air and secretions.

■ A camera may be attached to the endoscope to photograph areas for later study, or a measuring tube may be passed through the endoscope to determine the size of a lesion.

■ Biopsy forceps or a cytology brush may be passed through the scope to obtain specimens for histologic or cytologic study.

■ The endoscope is slowly withdrawn, and suspicious-looking areas of the gastric and esophageal lining are reexamined.

■ Specimens should be collected in accordance with laboratory and pathology guidelines. Place tissue specimens immediately in a specimen bottle containing 10% formalin solution; cell specimens are smeared on glass slides and placed in a Coplin jar containing 95% ethyl alcohol.

**ALERT**

 Observe the patient for signs of perforation. Cervical perforation of the esophagus produces pain on swallowing and with neck movement, thoracic perforation causes substernal or epigastric pain that increases with breathing or movement of the trunk, diaphragmatic perforation produces shoulder pain and dyspnea, and gastric perforation causes abdominal or back pain, cyanosis, fever, and pleural effusion.

■ Observe the patient for evidence of aspiration of gastric contents, which could precipitate aspiration pneumonia.

■ Monitor the patient's vital signs and document them according to your facility's policy.

■ Test the patient's gag reflex by touching the back of the throat with a tongue blade. Withhold food and fluids until the gag reflex returns (usually in 1 hour), and then allow fluids and a light meal.

■ Tell the patient that he may burp some insufflated air and have a sore throat for 3 to 4 days. Throat lozenges and warm saline gargles may ease his discomfort.

■ If the patient experiences soreness at the I.V. site, apply warm soaks.

■ Because of sedation, an outpatient should avoid alcohol for 24 hours and shouldn't drive for 12 hours. Make sure the patient has transportation home.

■ Instruct the patient to notify the practitioner immediately if he experiences persistent difficulty with swallowing, pain, fever, black stools, or bloody vomitus.

■ If tissue or cell specimens are obtained during the procedure, label and send them to the appropriate laboratory immediately.

## Precautions

- EGD is usually contraindicated in the patient with Zenker's diverticulum, a large aortic aneurysm, recent ulcer perforation (known as suspected viscus perforation), or an unstable cardiac or pulmonary condition.
- EGD shouldn't be performed within 2 days after an upper GI series.
- The patient requiring dental prophylaxis may also require antibiotics before this procedure.

### ACTION STAT!

 Observe closely for adverse effects of the sedative: respiratory depression, apnea, hypotension, excessive diaphoresis, bradycardia, and laryngospasm. Have available emergency resuscitation equipment and an opioid antagonist such as naloxone. Be prepared to intervene as necessary.

## Complications

- Adverse reaction to sedation
- Aspiration of gastric contents
- Aspiration pneumonia
- Perforation of the esophagus, stomach, or duodenum

# Proctosigmoidoscopy

Proctosigmoidoscopy uses a proctoscope, sigmoidoscope, and digital examination to evaluate the lining of the distal sigmoid colon, rectum, and anal canal. It's indicated in patients with recent changes in bowel habits, lower abdominal and perineal pain, prolapse on defecation, pruritus, and passage of mucus, blood, or pus in the stool. Specimens may be obtained from suspicious areas of the mucosa by biopsy, lavage or cytology brush, or culture swab.

## Normal results

- Mucosa of the sigmoid colon appears light pink-orange and is marked by semilunar folds and deep tubular pits.
- The rectal mucosa is redder due to its rich vascular network, deepens to purple at the pectinate line (the anatomic division between the rectum and anus), and has three distinct valves.
- The lower two-thirds of the anus (anoderm) is lined with smooth gray-tan skin and joins with the hair-fringed perianal skin.

## Abnormal results

- Visual examination and palpation demonstrate abnormalities of the anal canal and rectum, including internal and external hemorrhoids, hypertrophic anal papilla, anal fissures, anal fistulas, and anorectal abscesses.
- The examination may also reveal ulcerative colitis, ischemic colitis, Crohn's disease, polyposis, bacterial infection, syphilis, polyps, and benign or malignant tumors.
- Biopsy, culture, and other laboratory tests are typically necessary to detect various disorders.

## Purpose

- To aid in the diagnosis of inflammatory, infectious, and ulcerative bowel disease
- To detect hemorrhoids, hypertrophic anal papilla, polyps, fissures, fistulas, and abscesses in the rectum and anal canal
- To diagnose malignant or benign growths

## Patient preparation

- Explain that proctosigmoidoscopy allows visual examination of the lining of the distal sigmoid colon, rectum, and anal canal.
- Tell the patient that the test requires passage of two special instruments

through the anus; tell him who will perform the procedure, and where it will take place.

■ Check the patient's history for allergies, medications, and information pertinent to the current complaint. Find out if he has had a barium test within the past week because barium in the colon hinders accurate examination.

■ Because dietary and bowel preparations for this procedure vary according to the physician's preference, follow the orders carefully. If a special bowel preparation is ordered, explain to the patient that this clears the intestine to ensure a better view.

■ Instruct the patient to maintain a clear liquid diet for 24 to 48 hours before the test, to avoid eating fruits and vegetables before the procedure, and to fast the morning of the procedure, according to the physician's preference.

■ Describe the position the patient will be asked to assume and assure him that he'll be adequately draped.

■ As ordered, give a warm tap water or sodium biphosphate enema 3 to 4 hours before the procedure. The procedure may be started without bowel preparation because enemas can alter intestinal markings and traumatize mucous membranes. For this reason, irritating soapsuds enemas are inappropriate before this test. If the examination is hindered by excessive fecal matter, an enema may be ordered before the examination proceeds.

■ Tell the patient that he may be secured to a tilting table that rotates into horizontal and vertical positions.

■ Tell the patient that the examiner's finger and the instrument are well lubricated to ease insertion, that the instrument initially feels cool, and that he may experience the urge to defecate when the instrument is inserted and advanced.

■ Inform the patient that the instrument may stretch the intestinal wall and cause

transient muscle spasms or colicky lower abdominal pain.

■ Instruct the patient to breathe deeply and slowly through his mouth to relax the abdominal muscles; this reduces the urge to defecate and eases discomfort.

■ Explain that air may be introduced through the endoscope into the intestine to distend its walls. Tell the patient that this causes flatus to escape around the endoscope and that he shouldn't attempt to control it.

■ Inform the patient that a suction machine may remove blood, mucus, or liquid stool that obscures vision but that it won't cause discomfort.

■ Explain that an I.V. line may be started if an I.V. sedative is to be used. If the procedure is being done on an outpatient basis, advise the patient to arrange for someone to drive him home.

■ Make sure that the patient or a responsible family member has signed an informed consent form.

■ If the patient has rectal inflammation, provide a local anesthetic about 15 to 20 minutes before the procedure to minimize discomfort.

## Procedure and posttest care

■ Confirm the patient's identity using two patient identifiers according to facility policy.

■ Obtain the patient's baseline vital signs and monitor him throughout the procedure.

■ Place the patient in a knee-chest or left lateral position with his knees flexed and drape him.

■ If a left lateral position is used, a sandbag may be placed under the patient's left hip so that the buttocks project over the edge of the table. The right buttock is gently raised, and the anus and perianal region are examined under good lighting.

■ Instruct the patient to breathe deeply and slowly through his mouth as the examiner palpates the anal canal, rectum, and rectal mucosa for induration and tenderness; the physician then withdraws his finger and checks for the presence of blood, mucus, or stool.

■ The sigmoidoscope is lubricated, and the patient is told that the instrument is about to be inserted. The right buttock is raised, and the sigmoidoscope is inserted into the anus. As the scope is passed with steady pressure through the anal sphincters, instruct the patient to bear down as though defecating to aid its passage. The sigmoidoscope is advanced through the anal canal into the rectum.

■ At the rectosigmoid junction, a small amount of air may be insufflated to open the bowel lumen. The scope is then gently advanced to its full length into the distal sigmoid colon.

■ As the sigmoidoscope is slowly withdrawn, air is carefully insufflated, and the intestinal mucosa is thoroughly examined.

■ If stool obscures vision, the eyepiece on the scope is removed, a cotton swab is inserted through the scope, and the bowel lumen is swabbed. A suction machine may remove blood, excessive secretions, or liquid stool.

■ To obtain specimens from suspicious areas of the intestinal mucosa, a biopsy forceps, cytology brush, or culture swab is passed through the sigmoidoscope.

■ Polyps may be removed for histologic examination by inserting an electrocautery snare through the sigmoidoscope.

■ Specimens are collected in accordance with laboratory and pathology guidelines and immediately placed in a specimen bottle containing 10% formalin, cytology slides are placed in a Coplin jar containing 95% ethyl alcohol, and culture swabs are placed in a culture tube.

■ After the sigmoidoscope is withdrawn, the proctoscope is lubricated and the patient is told that it's about to be inserted. Assure him that he'll experience less discomfort during passage of the proctoscope.

■ The right buttock is raised, and the proctoscope is inserted through the anus and gently advanced to its full length.

■ The obturator is removed, and the light source is inserted through the proctoscope handle.

■ As the instrument is slowly withdrawn, the rectal and anal mucosa are carefully examined. Specimens may be obtained from suspicious areas of the intestinal mucosa.

■ If a biopsy of the anal canal is required, a local anesthetic may be administered first.

■ Withdraw the proctoscope after the examination is completed.

■ If the patient has been examined in a knee-chest position, instruct him to rest in a supine position for several minutes before standing to prevent orthostatic hypotension.

■ Observe the patient closely for signs of bowel perforation and for vasovagal attack due to emotional stress. Report such signs immediately.

■ Allow the patient nothing by mouth until he's alert.

■ Monitor the patient's vital signs as according to your facility's protocol until he's alert.

■ If air was introduced into the intestine, tell the patient that he may pass large amounts of flatus. Provide privacy while he rests after the test.

■ If a biopsy or polypectomy was performed, inform the patient that blood may appear in his stool.

■ If a tissue specimen or culture swab has been obtained, label it and send it to the appropriate laboratory immediately.

## Precautions

■ If the patient received sedation, he should avoid alcohol for 24 hours and shouldn't drive for 12 hours, so make sure he has transportation home.

### Complications
- Bowel perforation
- Rectal bleeding

# Contrast radiography

## ▌Barium enema
### [lower GI exam]

Barium enema is the radiographic examination of the large intestine after rectal instillation of barium sulfate (single-contrast technique) or barium sulfate and air (double-contrast technique).

The single-contrast technique provides a profile view of the large intestine; the double-contrast technique provides profile and frontal views. The latter technique best detects small intraluminal tumors (especially polyps), the early mucosal changes of inflammatory disease, and subtle intestinal bleeding caused by ulcerated polyps or the shallow ulcerations of inflammatory disease.

### Normal results
- In the single-contrast enema, the intestine is uniformly filled with barium, and colonic haustral markings are clearly apparent. The intestinal walls collapse as the barium is expelled, and the mucosa has a regular, feathery appearance on the postevacuation film.
- In the double-contrast enema, the intestines uniformly distend with air and have a thin layer of barium, providing excellent detail of the mucosal pattern. As the patient is assisted to various positions, the barium collects on the dependent walls of the intestine by the force of gravity.

### Abnormal results
- Adenocarcinoma and, rarely, sarcomas occur higher in the intestine.
- Carcinoma usually appears as a localized filling defect, with a sharp transition between the normal and necrotic mucosa. If it's circumferential, it will have an "apple core" appearance. These characteristics help distinguish carcinoma from the more diffuse lesions of inflammatory disease, but endoscopic biopsy may be necessary to confirm the diagnosis.
- Inflammatory disease, such as diverticulitis, ulcerative colitis, and granulomatous colitis, may be seen.
- Saccular adenomatous polyps, broad-based villous polyps, structural changes in the intestine (such as intussusception, telescoping of the bowel, sigmoid volvulus [a 360-degree turn or greater], and sigmoid torsion [up to a 180-degree turn]); gastroenteritis; irritable colon; vascular injury due to arterial occlusion; and selected cases of acute appendicitis may be present.

### Purpose
- To help diagnose colorectal cancer and inflammatory disease
- To detect polyps, diverticula, and structural changes in the large intestine

### Patient preparation
- Explain that the barium enema test permits examination of the large intestine through X-ray films taken after a barium enema.
- Describe the test, including who will perform it and where it will take place.
- Because residual fecal material in the colon obscures normal anatomy on X-rays, instruct the patient to carefully follow the prescribed bowel preparation, which may include diet, laxatives, or an enema. However, in certain conditions, such as ulcerative colitis and active GI bleeding, their use may be prohibited.

- Stress that accurate test results depend on the patient's cooperation with prescribed dietary restrictions and bowel preparation. A common bowel preparation technique includes restricted intake of dairy products and maintenance of a liquid diet for 24 hours before the test. The patient is encouraged to drink five 8-oz glasses of water or clear liquids 12 to 24 hours before the test. Administer a bowel preparation supplied by the radiography department. (A GoLYTELY preparation isn't recommended because it leaves the bowel too wet for the barium to coat the walls of the bowel.)
- Advise the patient to administer prescribed enemas until the return is clear.
- Tell the patient not to eat breakfast before the procedure; if the test is scheduled for late afternoon (or delayed), he may have clear liquids.
- Tell the patient that he'll be placed on a tilting X-ray table and adequately draped. Assure him that he'll be secured to the table and will be assisted to various positions.
- Tell the patient that he may experience cramping pains or the urge to defecate as the barium or air is introduced into the intestine. Instruct him to breathe deeply and slowly through his mouth to ease discomfort.
- Tell the patient to keep his anal sphincter tightly contracted against the rectal tube; this holds the tube in position and helps prevent leakage of barium. Stress the importance of retaining the barium enema; if the intestinal walls aren't adequately coated with barium, test results may be inaccurate.
- Assure the patient that the barium enema is fairly easy to retain because of its cool temperature.

### Procedure and posttest care
- Confirm the patient's identity using two patient identifiers according to facility policy.
- After the patient is in a supine position on a tilting X-ray table, spot films of the abdomen are taken.
- The patient is assisted to Sims' position, and a well-lubricated rectal tube is inserted through the anus. If the patient has anal sphincter atony or severe mental or physical debilitation, a rectal tube with a retaining balloon may be inserted.
- The barium is administered slowly and the filling process is monitored fluoroscopically. To aid filling, the table may be tilted or the patient assisted to supine, prone, and lateral decubitus positions.
- As barium flow is observed, spot films are taken of significant findings. When the intestine is filled with barium, overhead films of the abdomen are taken. The rectal tube is withdrawn, and the patient is escorted to the toilet or provided with a bedpan and is instructed to expel as much barium as possible.
- After evacuation, an additional overhead film is taken to record the mucosal pattern of the intestine and to evaluate the efficiency of colonic emptying.
- A double-contrast barium enema may directly follow this examination or may be performed separately. If it's performed immediately, a thin film of barium remains in the patient's intestine, coating the mucosa, and air is carefully injected to distend the bowel lumen.
- When the double-contrast technique is performed separately, a colloidal barium suspension is instilled, filling the patient's intestine to either the splenic flexure or the middle of the transverse colon. The suspension is then aspirated and air is forcefully injected into the intestine. If the intestine is filled to the lower descending colon, air is forcefully injected without previous aspiration of the suspension.
- The patient is then assisted to erect, prone, supine, and lateral decubitus po-

sitions in sequence. Barium filling is monitored fluoroscopically, and spot films are taken of significant findings. After the required films are taken, the patient is escorted to the toilet or provided with a bedpan.

■ Make sure further studies haven't been ordered before allowing the patient food and fluids. Encourage extra fluid intake because bowel preparation and the test itself can cause dehydration.

■ Encourage rest because this test and the bowel preparation that precedes it are usually exhausting.

■ Because barium retention after this test can cause intestinal obstruction or fecal impaction, give a mild cathartic or an enema. Tell the patient his stool will be light-colored for 24 to 72 hours. Record and describe any stool passed by the patient in the hospital.

### Precautions

■ This test should be performed cautiously in the patient with obstruction, acute inflammatory conditions (such as ulcerative colitis and diverticulitis), acute vascular insufficiency of the bowel, acute fulminant bloody diarrhea, and suspected pneumatosis cystoides intestinalis.

■ The test is contraindicated in the patient with tachycardia, fulminant ulcerative colitis associated with systemic toxicity and megacolon, toxic megacolon, or suspected perforation.

■ The test is contraindicated in the pregnant patient because of radiation's possible teratogenic effects.

### Complications

■ Barium embolism
■ Barium granulomas
■ Intraperitoneal and extraperitoneal extravasation of barium
■ Perforation of the colon
■ Water intoxication

# ▌Barium swallow
### [esophagography]

Barium swallow is the cineradiographic, radiographic, or fluoroscopic examination of the pharynx and the fluoroscopic examination of the esophagus after ingestion of thick and thin mixtures of barium sulfate. This test, most commonly performed as part of the upper GI series, is indicated in patients with histories of dysphagia and regurgitation. Further testing is usually required for definitive diagnosis. (See *Gastroesophageal reflux scanning.*)

### Normal results

■ The swallowed barium bolus pours over the base of the tongue into the pharynx.

■ A peristaltic wave propels the bolus through the entire length of the esophagus in about 2 seconds.

■ When the peristaltic wave reaches the base of the esophagus, the cardiac sphincter opens, allowing the bolus to enter the stomach. After passage of the bolus, the cardiac sphincter closes. The bolus evenly fills and distends the lumen of the pharynx and esophagus, and the mucosa appears smooth and regular.

### Abnormal results

■ Hiatal hernia, diverticula, and varices may be present. Aspiration into the lungs will also be revealed.

■ Strictures, tumors, polyps, ulcers, and motility disorders (pharyngeal muscular disorders, esophageal spasms, and achalasia) may be detected.

### Purpose

■ To diagnose hiatal hernia, diverticula, and varices
■ To detect strictures, ulcers, tumors, polyps, and motility disorders

# Gastroesophageal reflux scanning

When the results of a barium swallow are inconclusive, gastroesophageal reflux scanning may be conducted to evaluate esophageal function and detect reflux. This test delivers less radiation than a barium swallow and is a much more sensitive indicator of reflux. It also allows reflux to be measured without insertion of an esophageal tube, an important consideration in testing infants, small children, and other patients for whom intubation is contraindicated.

## Procedure

The patient is instructed to fast beginning at midnight the day of the test. As the test begins, he's placed in a supine or upright position and asked to swallow a solution containing a radiopharmaceutical such as technetium 99m ($^{99m}$Tc) sulfur colloid. A gamma counter placed over the patient's chest records its passage through the esophagus into the stomach to determine transit time and evaluate esophageal function.

If reflux is suspected, the patient is repositioned as his stomach distends, and continuous recordings visualize reflux and estimate its quantity. In reflux, radioactivity may be detected in the esophagus.

## Findings and contraindications

Normally, $^{99m}$Tc sulfur colloid descends through the esophagus in about 6 seconds; radioactivity is then detected only in the stomach and small bowel. However, diffuse spasm of the esophagus, achalasia, or other esophageal motility disorders may prolong transit time. In gastroesophageal reflux, radioactivity may be detected in the esophagus. As with other radionuclide studies, this scan is usually contraindicated during pregnancy and lactation. It can be modified for use in the infant or child.

## Patient preparation

- Explain that the barium swallow test evaluates the function of the pharynx and esophagus.
- Instruct the patient to fast after midnight the night before the test. (If the patient is an infant, delay feeding to ensure complete digestion of barium.) He may also be given a restricted diet for 2 to 3 days before the test.
- Describe the test, including who will perform it and where it will take place.
- Describe the milk-shake consistency and chalky taste of the barium preparation the patient is required to ingest. Although it's flavored, he may find it unpleasant to swallow. Tell the patient that he'll first receive a thick mixture, then a thin one, and that he must drink 12 to 14 oz (355 to 420 ml) during the examination.
- Inform the patient that he'll be placed in various positions on a tilting X-ray table and that X-rays will be taken. Reassure him that safety precautions will be maintained.
- Withhold antacids, histamine-2 blockers, and proton pump inhibitors, as ordered, if gastric reflux is suspected.
- Just before the procedure, instruct the patient to put on a gown without snap closures and to remove jewelry, dentures, hair clips, or other radiopaque objects from the X-ray field.

## Procedure and posttest care

- Confirm the patient's identity using two patient identifiers according to facility policy.
- The patient is placed in an upright position behind the fluoroscopic screen and his heart, lungs, and abdomen are examined.

- The patient is then instructed to take one swallow of the thick barium mixture, and the pharyngeal action is recorded using cineradiography. (This action occurs too rapidly for adequate fluoroscopic evaluation.)
- The patient is then told to take several swallows of the thin barium mixture. The passage of the barium is examined fluoroscopically, and spot films of the esophageal region are taken from lateral angles and from right and left postero-anterior angles. Esophageal strictures and obstruction of the esophageal lumen by the lower esophageal ring are best detected when the patient is upright. To accentuate small strictures or demonstrate dysphagia, the patient may be requested to swallow a special "barium marshmallow" (soft white bread that has been soaked in barium) or a barium pill.
- The patient is then secured to the X-ray table and is rotated to the Trendelenburg position to evaluate esophageal peristalsis or demonstrate hiatal hernia and gastric reflux.
- The patient is instructed to take several swallows of barium while the esophagus is examined fluoroscopically, and spot films of significant findings are taken when indicated. After the table is rotated to a horizontal position, the patient is told to take several swallows of barium so that the esophagogastric junction and peristalsis may be evaluated. The passage of the barium is fluoroscopically observed, and spot films of significant findings are taken with the patient in the supine and prone positions.
- During fluoroscopic examination of the esophagus, the cardiac and fundus of the patient's stomach are also carefully studied because neoplasms in these areas may invade the esophagus and cause obstruction.
- Check that additional spot films and repeat fluoroscopic evaluation haven't been ordered before allowing the patient to resume his usual diet.
- Instruct the patient to drink plenty of fluids, unless contraindicated, to help eliminate the barium.
- Administer a cathartic, if prescribed.
- Inform the patient that stools will be chalky and light-colored for 24 to 72 hours. Record a description of all stools passed by the patient in the hospital. Notify the practitioner if the patient fails to expel barium in 2 or 3 days.

### Precautions
- Barium swallow is usually contraindicated in the patient with intestinal obstruction, as well as in the pregnant patient because of radiation's possible teratogenic effects.

### Complications
- Abdominal distention and absent bowel sounds, which may indicate constipation and suggest barium impaction
- Obstruction or fecal impaction from barium retained in the intestine hardening

# ▌Celiac and mesenteric arteriography

Celiac and mesenteric arteriography involves the radiographic examination of the abdominal vasculature after intra-arterial injection of a contrast medium through a catheter. Most commonly, the catheter is passed through the femoral artery into the aorta and then, using fluoroscopy, is positioned in the celiac, superior mesenteric, or inferior mesenteric artery. Injection of a contrast medium into one or more of these arteries provides a map of abdominal vasculature; injection into specific arterial branches, called *superselective angiography,* permits detailed visualization of a particular area. As the contrast medium flows through the abdominal vasculature, serial radiographs outline abdominal vessels in the arterial, capillary, and venous phases of perfusion.

Celiac and mesenteric arteriography is indicated when endoscopy can't locate the source of GI bleeding or when barium studies, ultrasonography, and nuclear medicine or computed tomography scanning prove inconclusive in evaluating neoplasms. It's also used to evaluate cirrhosis and portal hypertension (especially when a portacaval shunt is being considered); to evaluate vascular damage, particularly in the spleen and liver, after abdominal trauma; and to detect vascular abnormalities. Because arteriography can demonstrate the portal vein even when portal venous flow is reversed, it's used more commonly than splenoportography.

### Normal results
- The arteries normally taper in size, becoming gradually smaller with subsequent divisions.
- The contrast medium spreads evenly within the sinusoids.
- The portal vein appears 10 to 20 seconds after the injection as the contrast medium empties from the spleen into the splenic vein or from the intestine into the superior mesenteric vein and further into the portal vein.

### Abnormal results
- GI hemorrhage appears on the angiogram as the extravasation of contrast medium from the damaged vessels.
- Upper GI hemorrhage can result from such conditions as Mallory-Weiss syndrome, a gastric or peptic ulcer, hemorrhagic gastritis, and an eroded hiatal hernia.
- Abdominal neoplasms—carcinoid tumors, adenomas, leiomyomas, angiomas, and adenocarcinomas—can disrupt the normal vasculature in several ways. Neoplasms can invade or encase

nearby arteries and veins, distorting their regular channel-like appearance and, in late stages, displacing them. Vessels within the neoplasm, known as *neovasculature,* appear as abnormal vascular areas.
- Areas of necrosis appear as puddles of contrast medium.
- Contrast medium may also remain in the neoplasm longer during capillary perfusion, producing a tumor blush or stain on the angiogram.
- Arteriovenous shunting may also be present, depending on the size and location of the tumor.
- In cirrhosis, portal venous flow to the liver remains relatively unaffected, and the hepatic artery and its branches appear normal.
- Abdominal trauma commonly causes splenic injury; less commonly, hepatic injury.
- Splenic rupture usually displaces intrasplenic arterial branches, causing the contrast medium to leak from splenic arteries into the splenic pulp.
- Other identifiable vascular abnormalities include aneurysms, thrombi, and emboli.

### Purpose
- To locate the source of GI bleeding
- To help distinguish between benign and malignant neoplasms
- To evaluate cirrhosis and portal hypertension
- To evaluate vascular damage after abdominal trauma
- To detect vascular abnormalities

### Patient preparation
- Explain that celiac and mesenteric arteriography permits examination of the abdominal blood vessels after injection of a contrast medium.
- Tell the patient who will perform the test, where it will take place, and that it

takes 30 minutes to 3 hours, depending on the number of vessels studied.

- Instruct the patient to fast for 8 hours before the test.
- Tell the patient that a laxative may be given the day before the test.
- Tell the patient that he'll receive I.V. conscious sedation and a local anesthetic and that he may feel a brief, stinging sensation as the anesthetic is injected. He may also feel pressure when the femoral artery is palpated, but the local anesthetic will minimize the pain when the needle is introduced into the artery.
- Tell the patient that he may feel a transient burning as the contrast medium is injected.
- Tell the patient that the X-ray equipment makes loud, clacking sounds as the films are taken.
- Instruct the patient to lie still during the test to avoid blurring the films and inform him that restraints may be used to help him remain still.
- Warn the patient that he may feel some temporary stiffness after the test from lying still on the hard X-ray table.
- Make sure that the patient or a responsible family member has signed an informed consent form.
- Check the patient's history for hypersensitivity to iodine, shellfish, or the contrast medium.
- Make sure blood studies (hemoglobin and hematocrit levels; clotting, prothrombin, and partial thromboplastin times; and platelet count) have been completed.
- Just before the procedure, instruct the patient to put on a gown and to remove jewelry and other objects that might obscure anatomic detail on X-ray films.
- Tell the patient to void, and then record his baseline vital signs.
- Administer a sedative, if prescribed.

## Procedure and posttest care

- Confirm the patient's identity using two patient identifiers according to facility policy.
- After the patient is placed in a supine position on the X-ray table, an I.V. infusion is started to maintain hydration and to permit emergency administration of medication. The patient is attached to a heart monitor and pulse oximeter and his blood pressure is monitored according to your facility's policy.
- Spot films of the patient's abdomen are taken, and the peripheral pulses are palpated and marked.
- The puncture site is cleaned with soap and water; the area is clipped, cleaned with povidone-iodine preparation, and surrounded by sterile drapes.
- The local anesthetic is injected and the femoral artery is located by palpation. The needle is gently inserted until a pulsing blood flow is obtained.
- A guide wire is passed through the needle into the aorta, and then the needle is removed, leaving the guide wire in place.
- The catheter is inserted over the guide wire and then withdrawn to inject the contrast medium to check for catheter placement. The guide wire is again inserted into the selected artery for fluoroscopic guidance.
- When the wire is in position, the catheter is advanced over it into the artery. The wire is then removed and placement verified by hand injection of contrast medium.
- The automatic injector is then attached to the catheter. As the contrast medium is injected, a series of films is taken in rapid sequence.
- After injecting into one or more major arteries, superselective angiography may be performed. Using fluoroscopy, the catheter is repositioned in a specific branch of a major artery, contrast medium is injected, and rapid-sequence films

are taken. If necessary, several specific branches may be catheterized.

■ If an occlusion is detected, balloon angioplasty is performed.

■ After filming, the catheter is withdrawn and firm pressure is applied to the puncture site for about 15 minutes.

■ Observe the puncture site for hematoma formation and check peripheral pulses.

■ Inform the patient that he'll be on bed rest for 4 to 6 hours and that he must keep the leg with the puncture site straight. Don't raise the bed further than 30 degrees. He'll be able to logroll and may use the unaffected leg to reposition himself to use the bedpan.

■ Monitor the patient's vital signs until stable and check peripheral pulses. Note the color and temperature of the leg that was used for the test.

■ Check the puncture site for bleeding and hematoma. If bleeding develops, apply pressure to the site. If a hematoma develops, apply warm soaks.

■ Confirm whether the patient can resume his usual diet. If the patient isn't receiving I.V. infusions, encourage intake of fluids to speed excretion of the contrast medium.

### Precautions

■ Celiac and mesenteric arteriography should be performed cautiously in the patient with coagulopathy.

■ The test is contraindicated in the pregnant patient because of radiation's possible teratogenic effects.

### Complications

■ Reactions to the contrast medium

■ Hemorrhage, thrombosis, and emboli

■ Cardiac arrhythmias and infection

# Endoscopic retrograde cholangiopancreatography
[ERCP]

Endoscopic retrograde cholangiopancreatography (ERCP) is the radiographic examination of the pancreatic ducts and hepatobiliary tree after injection of a contrast medium into the duodenal papilla. It's indicated in the patient with confirmed or suspected pancreatic disease or obstructive jaundice of unknown etiology. Complications may include cholangitis and pancreatitis.

### Normal results

■ The duodenal papilla appears as a small red (or sometimes pale) erosion protruding into the lumen.

■ The pancreatic and hepatobiliary ducts usually unite in the ampulla of Vater and empty through the duodenal papilla, separate orifices are sometimes present.

■ The contrast medium uniformly fills the pancreatic duct, hepatobiliary tree, and gallbladder.

### Abnormal results

■ Obstructive jaundice may result from various abnormalities of the hepatobiliary tree and pancreatic duct. Examination of the hepatobiliary tree may reveal stones, strictures, or irregular deviations that suggest biliary cirrhosis, primary sclerosing cholangitis, or carcinoma of the bile ducts.

■ Examination of the pancreatic ducts may also show stones, strictures, and irregular deviations that may indicate pancreatic cysts and pseudocysts, a pancreatic tumor, carcinoma of the head of the pancreas, chronic pancreatitis, pancreatic fibrosis, carcinoma of the duodenal papilla, and papillary stenosis.

## Purpose

- To evaluate obstructive jaundice
- To diagnose cancer of the duodenal papilla, pancreas, and biliary ducts
- To locate calculi and stenosis in the pancreatic ducts and hepatobiliary tree
- To identify leaks from trauma or surgery

## Patient preparation

- Explain that ERCP permits examination of the liver, gallbladder, and pancreas through X-ray films taken after injection of a contrast medium.
- Instruct the patient to fast after midnight before the test.
- Describe the test, including who will perform it and where it will take place.
- Inform the patient that a local anesthetic will be sprayed into his mouth to calm the gag reflex. Warn him that the spray has an unpleasant taste and makes the tongue and throat feel swollen, causing difficulty swallowing.
- Instruct the patient to let saliva drain from the side of his mouth and tell him that suction may be used to remove saliva. Tell him a mouth guard will be inserted to protect his teeth and the endoscope; assure him that it won't obstruct his breathing.
- Tell the patient that he'll receive a sedative before insertion of the endoscope to help him relax, but that he'll remain conscious.
- Tell the patient that he'll also receive an anticholinergic or I.V. glucagon after endoscope insertion. Describe the possible adverse effects of anticholinergics (dry mouth, thirst, tachycardia, urine retention, and blurred vision) or of glucagon (nausea, vomiting, urticaria, and flushing).

- Warn the patient that he may experience transient flushing on injection of the contrast medium. Advise him that he may have a sore throat for 3 or 4 days after the examination.
- Make sure that the patient or a responsible family member has signed an informed consent form.

### ALERT

 Check the patient's history for hypersensitivity to iodine, seafood, or contrast media used for other diagnostic procedures and inform the practitioner of sensitivities.

- Just before the procedure, obtain the patient's baseline vital signs. Instruct him to remove all metallic or other radiopaque objects and constricting undergarments. Then tell him to void to minimize the discomfort of urine retention that may follow the procedure.

## Procedure and posttest care

- Confirm the patient's identity using two patient identifiers according to facility policy.
- An I.V. infusion is started with 150 ml of normal saline solution. The local anesthetic is then given and usually takes effect in about 10 minutes.
- If an anesthetic spray is used, ask the patient to hold his breath while his mouth and throat are sprayed.
- Place the patient in a left lateral position and give him an emesis basin; provide tissues. Because the anesthetic causes the patient to lose some control of his secretions and thus increases the risk of aspiration, encourage him to allow saliva to drain from the side of his mouth.
- Insert a mouth guard.
- While the patient remains in the left lateral position, 5 to 20 mg of I.V. diazepam (Valium) or midazolam (Versed)

is given, as well as an opioid analgesic, if needed.

- When ptosis or dysarthria develops, the patient's head is bent forward and he's asked to open his mouth.

- The physician inserts his left index finger in the patient's mouth and guides the tip of the endoscope along his finger to the back of the patient's throat. The scope is then deflected downward with the left index finger and advanced. As the endoscope passes through the posterior pharynx and cricopharyngeal sphincter, the patient's head is slowly extended to assist the advance of the endoscope. The patient's chin must be kept midline. When the endoscope has passed the cricopharyngeal sphincter, the scope is advanced under direct vision. When it's well into the esophagus, the patient's chin is moved toward the table so saliva can drain from the mouth. The endoscope is advanced through the remainder of the esophagus and into the stomach under direct vision.

- When the pylorus is located, a small amount of air is insufflated, and the tip of the endoscope is angled upward and passed into the duodenal bulb.

- After the endoscope is rotated clockwise to enter the descending duodenum, the patient is assisted to a prone position.

- An anticholinergic or I.V. glucagon is given to induce duodenal atony and to relax the ampullary sphincter.

- A small amount of air is insufflated, and the endoscope is manipulated until the optic lies opposite the duodenal papilla. Then the cannula filled with contrast medium is passed through the biopsy channel of the endoscope, the duodenal papilla, and into the ampulla of Vater.

- The pancreatic duct is visualized first under fluoroscopic guidance with injection of contrast medium.

- The cannula is repositioned at a more cephalad angle, and the hepatobiliary tree is visualized with injection of contrast medium.

- After each injection, rapid-sequence X-ray films are taken.

- Instruct the patient to remain prone while the films are developed and reviewed. If necessary, additional films may be taken.

- When the required radiographs have been obtained, the cannula is removed. Before the endoscope is withdrawn, a tissue specimen may be obtained or fluid aspirated for histologic and cytologic examination, respectively.

- Observe the patient closely for signs of cholangitis and pancreatitis. Hyperbilirubinemia, fever, and chills are the immediate signs of cholangitis; hypotension associated with gram-negative septicemia may develop later. Left upper quadrant pain and tenderness, elevated serum amylase levels, and transient hyperbilirubinemia are the usual signs of pancreatitis. Draw blood samples for amylase and bilirubin determinations, if necessary, but remember that these levels usually rise after ERCP.

- Observe the patient for signs of perforation, such as abdominal pain, bleeding, and fever.

- Tell the patient that he may experience a feeling of fullness, some cramping, and passage of flatus several hours after the test.

- Continue to watch the patient for signs of respiratory depression, apnea, hypotension, excessive diaphoresis, bradycardia, and laryngospasm. Check his vital signs every 15 minutes for 1 hour, every 30 minutes for the next 2 hours, every hour for the next 4 hours, and then every 4 hours for 48 hours.

- Withhold food and fluids until the patient's gag reflex returns. Test the gag reflex by touching the back of his throat with a tongue blade. When the gag reflex returns, allow fluids and a light meal.

- Discontinue or maintain the I.V. infusion, as ordered.
- Check for signs of urine retention. Notify the practitioner if the patient hasn't voided within 8 hours.
- If the patient has a sore throat, provide soothing lozenges and warm saline gargles to ease discomfort.
- If a tissue biopsy or polypectomy occurred, a small amount of blood in the patient's first stool is normal. Report excessive bleeding immediately.
- If this test is performed on an outpatient basis, be sure that transportation is available. The patient who has undergone anesthesia or sedation shouldn't operate an automobile for at least 12 hours postprocedure. Alcohol should be avoided for 24 hours.

### Precautions

- The test is contraindicated in the pregnant patient because of radiation's possible teratogenic effects.
- The test is contraindicated in the patient with infectious disease, pancreatic pseudocysts, stricture or obstruction of the esophagus or duodenum, or acute pancreatitis, cholangitis, or cardiorespiratory disease.

ACTION STAT!

 Monitor the patient's vital signs and airway patency throughout the procedure. Watch him for signs of respiratory depression, apnea, hypotension, excessive diaphoresis, bradycardia, and laryngospasm. Be sure to have available emergency resuscitation equipment and an opioid antagonist such as naloxone.

- If the patient has cardiac disease, continuous electrocardiographic monitoring should be instituted. Continuing periodic pulse oximetry is advisable, particularly in the patient with pulmonary compromise.

### Complications

- Adverse drug reactions
- Ascending cholangitis
- Cardiac arrhythmias
- Pancreatitis
- Perforation of the bowel
- Respiratory depression
- Urine retention

 **Enteroclysis**
[small bowel enema]

Enteroclysis is the fluoroscopic examination of the small bowel using a contrast medium. In this procedure, a small-lumen catheter is inserted through the nose or mouth and passed through the stomach into the distal duodenum or jejunum. Metoclopramide may be given to facilitate peristalsis (which helps pass the catheter into the small bowel). A small balloon at the tip of the catheter may be inflated to prevent reflux of the contrast medium into the stomach. Barium is infused, and then methylcellulose may be infused to obtain a double-contrast study of the small bowel.

The contrast media distend and opacify the bowel loops to allow evaluation and diagnosis. Fluoroscopy and spot films are used to demonstrate and evaluate the small bowel.

### Normal results

- The bowel loops and walls are visible and are free from tumors, ulcers, and constrictions.

### Abnormal results

- Anatomy of the bowel loops can be evaluated by observing Kerckring's folds, lumen diameters, and wall thickness. Abnormalities may indicate Crohn's disease, tumors, partial or complete bowel obstruction, Meckel's diverticula, or congenital disorders.

## Purpose

- To diagnose and evaluate Crohn's disease
- To diagnose Meckel's diverticulum
- To aid in the diagnosis of small-bowel obstruction
- To detect tumors

## Patient preparation

- Explain that enteroclysis evaluates the small bowel.
- Tell the patient that contrast media will be instilled into his bowel and that X-ray films will then be taken to track the flow of the media and allow evaluation of small-bowel function.
- Inform the patient that he'll receive a laxative (such as bisacodyl) the afternoon before the examination, and then he'll receive nothing by mouth until the test. (If the test is being done on an emergency basis, no preparation is required.)
- Inform the patient that he shouldn't take peristalsis-inhibiting drugs (such as meperidine [Demerol] or oxycodone) and aspirin on the day of the test.
- Tell the patient that the examination will take about 45 minutes and that just before the test, he'll be asked to change into a gown, remove his undergarments and jewelry, and empty his bladder.
- Explain that an I.V. line will be inserted for medication administration.
- Tell the patient that he may receive an I.V. sedative, if needed, and that a local anesthetic will be injected inside his nose to make the catheter insertion more comfortable. A GI stimulant (such as metoclopramide) will be administered to aid passage of the tube and to speed the flow of barium by increasing peristalsis.
- Tell him that he'll be asked to turn from side to side and sometimes onto

his abdomen during the procedure. Inform the patient that his cooperation will help the test proceed smoothly.

- Tell the patient that he'll go to a recovery area after the test until he's ready for discharge.
- If the patient is having the procedure as an outpatient, make sure that he has someone to drive him home if he receives I.V. sedation.
- Make sure that the patient or a responsible family member has signed an informed consent form.

## Procedure and posttest care

- Confirm the patient's identity using two patient identifiers according to facility policy.
- Place the patient in the supine position on the X-ray table with his neck slightly extended.
- Administer I.V. medication to help relax the patient and to ease the tube's passage, as ordered.
- The local anesthetic is given nasally; instruct the patient to swallow if he feels it at the back of his throat. The tube is passed through the nose into the nasopharynx, and the patient's chin is brought down to the chest; the tube is advanced into the stomach and duodenum and, if possible, into the jejunum.
- A small balloon is inflated at the catheter tip to prevent reflux of the contrast medium into the patient's stomach.
- The barium contrast is administered by infusion pump. Methylcellulose is then given to help propel the barium into the distal bowel. This double-contrast administration distends the bowel walls and opacifies the bowel loops, allowing clearer evaluation.
- Spot films and overhead films are taken. Barium flow is followed on fluoroscopy.
- The physician examines individual bowel loops as they are opacified and

compresses the abdomen to better evaluate the loops.

- The patient is asked to turn from side to side during the examination.
- After the examination, the balloon is deflated and the catheter is removed.
- Assist the patient to the bathroom to expel the barium through defecation.
- Observe the patient in the recovery area until he's ready for discharge.
- Monitor the patient's vital signs until he's alert.

### Precautions

- The patient may experience discomfort with the passage of the catheter. Provide support, and give the prescribed anesthetic and sedative when needed.

### Complications

- Adverse reaction to sedation, if used
- Constipation

# Percutaneous transhepatic cholangiography

Percutaneous transhepatic cholangiography is the fluoroscopic examination of the biliary ducts after injection of an iodinated contrast medium directly into a biliary radicle. This test is especially useful for evaluating patients with persistent upper abdominal pain after cholecystectomy or severe jaundice.

Although a computed tomography scan or ultrasonography is usually performed first when obstructive jaundice is suspected, percutaneous transhepatic cholangiography may provide the most detailed view of the obstruction; however, this invasive procedure carries a potential risk of complications that include bleeding, septicemia, bile peritonitis, extravasation of the contrast medium into the peritoneal cavity, and subcapsular injection.

### Normal results

- The biliary ducts are of normal diameter and appear as regular channels homogeneously filled with contrast medium.

### Abnormal results

- Obstructive jaundice is associated with dilated ducts; nonobstructive jaundice, with normal-sized ducts. Obstruction may result from cholelithiasis, biliary tract carcinoma, or carcinoma of the pancreas or papilla of Vater that impinges on the common bile duct, causing deviation or stricture.
- When ducts are of normal size and intrahepatic cholestasis is indicated, liver biopsy may be performed to distinguish among hepatitis, cirrhosis, and granulomatous disease.
- A short and irregular stricture with a rat-tail appearance and gross dilation of the proximal ducts may suggest pancreatic or biliary carcinoma.
- Diffuse intrahepatic and extrahepatic stricture may suggest advanced sclerosing cholangitis or infiltrating cholangiocarcinoma.
- Ducts filled with debris, with possible abscesses of various sizes in communication with ducts, may suggest acute supportive cholangitis.

### Purpose

- To determine the cause of upper abdominal pain following cholecystectomy
- To distinguish between obstructive and nonobstructive jaundice
- To determine the location, the extent and, commonly, the cause of mechanical obstruction

### Patient preparation

- Explain that percutaneous transhepatic cholangiography allows examination of the biliary ducts through X-ray films taken after a contrast medium is injected into the liver.

- Instruct the patient to fast for 8 hours before the test.
- Describe the test, including who will perform it and where it will take place.
- Inform the patient that he may receive a laxative the night before and an enema the morning of the test.
- Inform the patient that he'll be placed on a tilting X-ray table that rotates into vertical and horizontal positions during the procedure.
- Assure the patient that he'll be adequately secured to the table and assisted to supine and side-lying positions throughout the procedure.
- Warn him that injection of the local anesthetic may sting the skin and produce transient pain when it punctures the liver capsule.
- Advise the patient that injection of the contrast medium may produce a sensation of pressure and epigastric fullness and may cause transient upper back pain on his right side.
- Tell the patient that he must rest for at least 6 hours after the procedure.
- Make sure that the patient or a responsible family member has signed an informed consent form.

- Advise him of possible adverse effects of contrast medium administration, such as nausea, vomiting, excessive salivation, flushing, urticaria, sweating and, rarely, anaphylaxis; tachycardia and fever may accompany intraductal injection.
- Check the patient's history for normal bleeding, clotting, and prothrombin times and a normal platelet count. If prescribed, give antibiotics 24 hours before the procedure.
- Just before the procedure, give a sedative, if prescribed.

## Procedure and posttest care

- Confirm the patient's identity using two patient identifiers according to facility policy.
- After the patient is placed in a supine position on the X-ray table and is adequately secured, the right upper quadrant of the abdomen is cleaned and draped; the skin, subcutaneous tissue, and liver capsule are infiltrated with a local anesthetic.
- While the patient holds his breath at the end of expiration, the flexible needle is inserted under fluoroscopic guidance through the 10th or 11th intercostal space at the right midclavicular line.
- The needle is aimed toward the xiphoid process and is advanced through the liver parenchyma. It's then slowly withdrawn, injecting the contrast medium to locate a biliary radicle. When fluoroscopy reveals placement in a radicle, the needle is held in position and the remaining contrast medium is injected.
- With the use of a fluoroscope and television monitor, biliary duct opacification is observed, and spot films of significant findings are taken with the patient in supine and lateral recumbent positions. When the required films have been taken, the needle is removed.
- Apply a sterile dressing to the puncture site.
- Check the patient's vital signs until they're stable.
- Enforce bed rest for at least 6 hours after the test, preferably with the patient lying on his right side, to help prevent hemorrhage.
- Check the injection site for bleeding, swelling, and tenderness. Watch for signs of peritonitis: chills, temperature of 102° to 103° F (38.8° to 39.4° C),

and abdominal pain, tenderness, and distention. Notify the practitioner immediately if such complications develop.
▪ Tell the patient that he may resume his usual diet.

### Precautions
▪ The test is contraindicated in the patient with cholangitis, massive ascites, uncorrectable coagulopathy, or hypersensitivity to iodine, as well as in the pregnant patient because of radiation's possible teratogenic effects.

### Complications
▪ Adverse effects of iodinated contrast media
▪ Adverse effects of sedation
▪ Bile leakage
▪ Bleeding
▪ Infection or sepsis
▪ Peritonitis
▪ Pneumothorax
▪ Vasovagal reactions

# Postoperative cholangiography

During cholecystectomy or common bile duct exploration, a T-shaped rubber tube may be inserted into the common bile duct to facilitate drainage. Postoperative cholangiography—radiographic and fluoroscopic examination of the biliary ducts—may be performed 7 to 10 days after surgery.

This procedure requires injection of contrast medium through the T-tube. The contrast medium flows through the biliary ducts and outlines the size and patency of the ducts, revealing any obstruction overlooked during surgery.

### Normal results
▪ Biliary ducts demonstrate homogeneous filling with contrast medium and are normal in diameter.

▪ Contrast flows unimpeded into the duodenum.

### Abnormal results
▪ Negative shadows or filling defects within the biliary ducts associated with dilation may indicate calculi or neoplasms overlooked during surgery.
▪ Abnormal channels of contrast medium departing from the biliary ducts indicate fistulae.

### Purpose
▪ To detect calculi, strictures, neoplasms, and fistulae in the biliary ducts

### Patient preparation
▪ Explain that postoperative cholangiography permits examination of the biliary ducts through X-ray films taken after the injection of a contrast medium.
▪ Describe the test, including who will perform it and where it will take place.
▪ Warn the patient that he may feel a bloating sensation (not pain) in the right upper quadrant as the contrast medium is injected.
▪ Clamp the T-tube the day before the procedure, if necessary. Because bile fills the tube after clamping, this helps prevent air bubbles from entering the ducts.
▪ Withhold the meal just before the test and administer an enema about 1 hour before the procedure.
▪ Make sure that the patient or a responsible family member has signed an informed consent form.

ALERT

 Check the patient's history for hypersensitivity to iodine, seafood, or contrast media used in other diagnostic tests. Notify the practitioner of any previous sensitivities.

▪ Tell the patient that the adverse effects of intraductal administration may in-

clude nausea, vomiting, excessive salivation, flushing, urticaria, sweating and,
rarely, anaphylaxis.

### Procedure and posttest care
▪ Confirm the patient's identity using
two patient identifiers according to facility policy.
▪ After the patient is in a supine position
on the X-ray table, the injection area of
the T-tube is cleaned with sponges
soaked with povidone-iodine solution.
The T-tube is held in a vertical position,
which allows trapped air to surface, and
a needle attached to a long transparent
catheter is carefully inserted into the end
of the T-tube. Care must be taken to
avoid injecting air into the biliary tree
because air bubbles may affect the clarity of the X-ray films.
▪ About 5 ml of contrast medium (usually sodium diatrizoate) is injected under fluoroscopic guidance, and a spot
film is taken in the anteroposterior position. Additional injections are then administered, and spot films and plain
films are taken with the patient in
supine and right lateral decubitus positions.
▪ The T-tube is then clamped and the
patient is assisted to an erect position for
additional films; in this position, air
bubbles may be distinguished from calculi or other pathology.
▪ A final film is taken 15 minutes after
contrast injection to record the emptying of contrast-laden bile into the duodenum. If emptying is delayed, additional films may be taken at 15- or
30-minute intervals until this action is
demonstrated.
▪ If a sterile dressing is applied after
T-tube removal, observe and record any
drainage. Change the dressing, as necessary.
▪ If the T-tube is left in place, attach it to
the drainage system.

▪ Tell the patient that he may resume his
usual diet and activity, as directed.

### Precautions
▪ Postoperative cholangiography is contraindicated in the patient who's hypersensitive to iodine, seafood, or contrast
media used in other tests.

### Complications
▪ Adverse reaction to the contrast media
▪ Infection

# Upper GI and small-bowel series

The upper GI and small-bowel series
is the fluoroscopic examination of the
esophagus, stomach, and small intestine
after ingestion of barium sulfate, a contrast agent. As the barium passes through
the digestive tract, fluoroscopy outlines
peristalsis and the mucosal contours of
the respective organs, and spot films
record significant findings. This test is
indicated in patients who have upper GI
symptoms (difficulty swallowing, regurgitation, burning or gnawing epigastric
pain), signs of small-bowel disease (diarrhea, weight loss), and signs of GI
bleeding (hematemesis, melena).

Although this test can detect various
mucosal abnormalities, subsequent
biopsy is typically necessary to rule out
malignancy or distinguish specific inflammatory diseases. Oral cholecystog-
raphy and routine X-rays should always
precede this test because retained barium clouds anatomic detail on X-ray
films.

### Normal results
▪ After the barium suspension is swallowed, it pours over the base of the
tongue into the pharynx and is propelled by a peristaltic wave through the
entire length of the esophagus in about
2 seconds.

- The bolus evenly fills and distends the lumen of the pharynx and esophagus, and the mucosa appears smooth and regular.
- When the peristaltic wave reaches the base of the esophagus, the cardiac sphincter opens, allowing the bolus to enter the stomach. After passage of the bolus, the cardiac sphincter closes.
- As barium enters the stomach, it outlines the characteristic longitudinal folds called rugae, which are best observed using the double-contrast technique.
- When the stomach is completely filled with barium, its outer contour appears smooth and regular without evidence of flattened, rigid areas suggestive of intrinsic or extrinsic lesions.
- After barium enters the stomach, it quickly empties into the duodenal bulb through relaxation of the pyloric sphincter.
- Although the mucosa of the duodenal bulb is relatively smooth, circular folds become apparent as barium enters the duodenal loop. These folds deepen and become more numerous in the jejunum. The barium temporarily lodges between these folds, producing a speckled pattern on the X-ray film.
- As barium enters the ileum, the circular folds become less prominent and, except for their broadness, resemble those in the duodenum.
- The diameter of the small intestine tapers gradually from the duodenum to the ileum.

## Abnormal results

- X-ray studies of the esophagus may reveal strictures, tumors, hiatal hernia, diverticula, varices, and ulcers (particularly in the distal esophagus).
- Benign strictures usually dilate the esophagus, whereas malignant ones cause erosive changes in the mucosa.

- Tumors produce filling defects in the column of barium, but only malignant ones change the mucosal contour.
- Achalasia (cardiospasm) is strongly suggested when the distal esophagus has a beaklike appearance.
- Gastric reflux appears as a backflow of barium from the stomach into the esophagus.
- Benign tumors, such as adenomatous polyps and leiomyomas, appear as outpouchings of the gastric mucosa and generally don't affect peristalsis.
- Ulcers occur most commonly in the stomach and duodenum (particularly in the duodenal bulb), and these two areas are thus examined together. Benign ulcers usually demonstrate evidence of partial or complete healing and are characterized by radiating folds extending to the edge of the ulcer crater. Malignant ulcers, usually associated with a suspicious mass, generally have radiating folds that extend beyond the ulcer crater to the edge of the mass.
- Pancreatitis or pancreatic carcinoma is indicated by changes in the mucosa of the antrum or duodenal loop or dilation of the duodenal loop.
- X-ray studies of the small intestine may reveal regional enteritis, malabsorption syndrome, and tumors.
- Edematous changes, segmentation of the barium column, and flocculation characterize malabsorption syndrome.
- Filling defects occur with Hodgkin's disease and lymphosarcoma.

## Purpose

- To detect hiatal hernia, diverticula, and varices
- To help diagnose strictures, blockages, ulcers, tumors, regional enteritis, and malabsorption syndrome
- To help detect motility disorders

## Patient preparation

- Explain that the upper GI and small-bowel series uses ingested barium and X-ray films to examine the esophagus, stomach, and small intestine.
- Tell the patient to consume a low-residue diet for 2 to 3 days before the test and then to fast and avoid smoking after midnight the night before the test.
- Describe the test, including who will perform it and where it will take place.
- Inform the patient that he'll be placed on an X-ray table that rotates into vertical, semivertical, and horizontal positions.
- Explain to the patient that he'll be adequately secured and assisted to the supine, prone, and side-lying positions.
- Describe the milk-shake consistency and chalky taste of the barium mixture. Although it's flavored, the patient may find its taste unpleasant, but tell him he must drink 16 to 20 oz (475 to 590 ml) for a complete examination.
- Inform the patient that his abdomen may be compressed to ensure proper coating of the stomach or intestinal walls with barium or to separate overlapping bowel loops.
- As ordered, withhold most oral medications after midnight and anticholinergics and opioids for 24 hours because these drugs affect small intestinal motility. Antacids, histamine-2 receptor antagonists, and proton pump inhibitors are also sometimes withheld for several hours if gastric reflux is suspected.
- Just before the procedure, instruct the patient to put on a gown without snap closures and to remove jewelry, dentures, hair clips, or other objects that might obscure anatomic detail on the X-ray films.

## Procedure and posttest care

- Confirm the patient's identity using two patient identifiers according to facility policy.

- After the patient is secured in a supine position on the X-ray table, the table is tilted until the patient is erect, and the heart, lungs, and abdomen are examined fluoroscopically.
- The patient is instructed to take several swallows of the barium suspension, and its passage through the esophagus is observed. (Occasionally, the patient is given a thick barium suspension, especially when esophageal pathology is strongly suspected.)
- During fluoroscopic examination, spot films of the esophagus are taken from lateral angles and from right and left posteroanterior angles.
- When barium enters the stomach, the patient's abdomen is palpated or compressed to ensure adequate coating of the gastric mucosa.
- To perform a double-contrast examination, the patient is instructed to sip the barium through a perforated straw. As he does so, a small amount of air is also introduced into the stomach; this permits detailed examination of the gastric rugae, and spot films of significant findings are taken. The patient is then instructed to ingest the remaining barium suspension and the filling of the stomach and emptying into the duodenum are observed fluoroscopically.
- Two series of spot films of the stomach and duodenum are taken from posteroanterior, anteroposterior, lateral, and oblique angles, with the patient erect and then in a supine position.
- The passage of barium into the remainder of the small intestine is then observed fluoroscopically, and spot films are taken at 30- to 60-minute intervals until the barium reaches the region of the ileocecal valve. If abnormalities in the small intestine are detected, the area is palpated and compressed to help clarify the defect, and a spot film is taken. The examination ends when the barium enters the cecum.

- Make sure additional X-rays haven't been ordered before allowing the patient food, fluids, and oral medications (if applicable).
- Tell the patient to drink plenty of fluid (unless contraindicated) to help eliminate the barium.
- Give the patient a cathartic or enema. Tell him that his stool will be light-colored for 24 to 72 hours. Record and describe any stool passed by the patient in the hospital. Barium retention in the intestine may cause obstruction or fecal impaction, so notify the practitioner if the patient doesn't pass the barium within 2 to 3 days. Also, barium retention may affect scheduling of other GI tests.
- Instruct the patient to tell the practitioner of abdominal fullness or pain or a delay in return to brown stools.

### Precautions

- The upper GI and small-bowel series may be contraindicated in the patient with obstruction or perforation of the digestive tract. Barium may intensify the obstruction or seep into the abdominal cavity. Sometimes a small-bowel series is performed to find a "transition zone." If a perforation is suspected, Gastrografin (a water-soluble contrast medium) rather than barium may be used.
- The test is contraindicated in the pregnant patient because of radiation's possible teratogenic effects.

### Complications

- Bowel obstruction
- Fecal impaction

# Computed tomography

## Computed tomography of the liver and biliary tract

In computed tomography (CT) of the liver and biliary tract, multiple X-rays pass through the upper abdomen and are measured while detectors record differences in tissue attenuation. A computer reconstructs these data as a two-dimensional image on a monitor. CT scanning accurately distinguishes the biliary tract and the liver if the ducts are large. Use of I.V. contrast media during CT scanning can accentuate different densities.

Although CT scanning and ultrasonography detect biliary tract and liver disease equally well, the latter technique is performed more commonly. CT scanning is more expensive than ultrasonography and requires exposure to moderate amounts of radiation. However, it's the test of choice in patients who are obese and in those with livers positioned high under the rib cage because bone and excessive fat hinder ultrasound transmission.

### Normal results

- The liver has a uniform density that's slightly greater than that of the pancreas, kidneys, and spleen.
- Linear and circular areas of slightly lower density, representing hepatic vascular structures, may interrupt this uniform appearance.
- The portal vein is usually visible; the hepatic artery usually isn't.
- I.V. contrast medium enhances the isodensity of vascular structures and liver parenchyma.

- Intrahepatic biliary radicles aren't visible, but the common hepatic and bile ducts may be visible as low-density structures.
- Because bile has the same density as water, use of an I.V. contrast medium improves demarcation of the biliary tract by enhancing the surrounding parenchyma and vascular structures.
- Like the biliary ducts, the gallbladder is visible as a round or elliptic low-density structure.
- A contracted gallbladder may be impossible to visualize.

## Abnormal results

- Most focal hepatic defects appear less dense than the normal parenchyma, and CT scans can detect small lesions. Use of rapid-sequence scanning with an I.V. contrast medium helps distinguish between the two because the normal parenchyma shows greater enhancement than focal defects.
- Primary and metastatic neoplasms may appear as well-circumscribed or poorly defined areas of slightly lower density than the normal parenchyma. Some lesions have the same density as the liver parenchyma and may be undetectable. Neoplasms that are especially large may distort the liver's contour.
- Hepatic abscesses appear as relatively low-density, homogeneous areas, usually with well-defined borders.
- Hepatic cysts appear as sharply defined round or oval structures and have a density lower than abscesses and neoplasms.
- The density of a hepatic hematoma varies with its age.
- Subcapsular hematomas are usually crescent-shaped and compress the liver away from the capsule.
- Biliary duct dilation indicates obstructive jaundice; an absence of dilation indicates nonobstructive jaundice.

- Dilated intrahepatic bile ducts appear as low-density linear and circular branching structures.
- Dilation of the common hepatic duct, common bile duct, and gallbladder may also be apparent, depending on the site and severity of obstruction. Usually, CT scanning can identify the cause of the obstruction.

## Purpose

- To distinguish between obstructive and nonobstructive jaundice
- To detect intrahepatic tumors and abscesses, subphrenic and subhepatic abscesses, cysts, and hematomas

## Patient preparation

- Explain that CT scanning helps detect biliary tract and liver disease.
- Tell the patient that he'll be given a contrast medium to drink and then he should fast until after the examination. If contrast isn't ordered, fasting isn't necessary.
- Explain who will perform the test and where it will take place.
- Inform the patient that he'll be placed on an adjustable table, which is positioned inside a scanning gantry. Assure him that the test will be painless.
- Tell the patient that he'll be asked to remain still during the test and to hold his breath when instructed. Stress the importance of remaining still during the test because movement can cause artifacts, thereby prolonging the test and limiting its accuracy.
- If I.V. contrast medium is being used, inform the patient that he may experience transient discomfort from the needle puncture and a localized feeling of warmth on injection as well as a salty or metallic taste. Tell him to immediately report nausea, vomiting, dizziness, headache, and hives.

Check the patient's history for hypersensitivity to iodine, seafood, or the contrast media used in other diagnostic tests. Notify the practitioner of any sensitivity to contrast media.

- If a contrast medium has been ordered, give the patient the oral contrast medium supplied by the radiology department.
- Make sure that the patient or a responsible family member has signed an informed consent form.

### Procedure and posttest care

- Confirm the patient's identity using two patient identifiers according to facility policy.
- The patient is placed in a supine position on an X-ray table, and the table is positioned within the opening in the scanning gantry.
- A series of transverse X-ray films is taken and recorded on magnetic tape. This information is reconstructed by a computer and appears as images on a television screen.
- These images are studied, and selected ones are photographed. When the first series of films is completed, the images are reviewed.
- Contrast enhancement may be performed. After the contrast medium is injected, a second series of films is taken, and the patient is carefully observed for an allergic reaction.

### Precautions

- CT scanning of the biliary tract and liver is usually contraindicated during pregnancy.
- Use of an I.V. contrast medium is contraindicated in the patient with hypersensitivity to iodine or with severe renal or hepatic disease.

### Complications

- Adverse effects from contrast medium

# Computed tomography of the pancreas

In computed tomography (CT) of the pancreas, multiple X-rays penetrate the upper abdomen while a detector records the differences in tissue attenuation, which is then displayed as an image on a television screen. A series of cross-sectional views can provide a detailed look at the pancreas. CT scanning accurately distinguishes the pancreas and surrounding organs and vessels if enough fat is present between the structures. Use of an I.V. or oral contrast medium, or both, further accentuate differences in tissue density.

CT scanning is replacing ultrasonography as the test of choice for examining the pancreas. Although ultrasonography costs less and involves less risk for the patient, it's also less accurate. In retroperitoneal disorders, specifically when pancreatitis is suspected, CT scanning goes beyond ultrasonography by showing the general swelling that accompanies acute inflammation of the gland. In chronic cases, CT scanning easily detects calcium deposits commonly missed by simple radiography, particularly in obese patients.

### Normal results

- The pancreatic parenchyma displays a uniform density, especially when an I.V. contrast medium is used.
- The gland normally thickens from tail to head and has a smooth surface.
- A contrast medium administered orally opacifies the adjacent stomach and duodenum and helps outline the pancreas, particularly in the patient with little

peripancreatic fat, such as a child or a thin adult.

## Abnormal results

- Because the tissue density of pancreatic carcinoma resembles that of the normal parenchyma, changes in pancreatic size and shape help demonstrate carcinoma and pseudocysts. Usually, carcinoma first appears as a localized swelling of the head, body, or tail of the pancreas and may spread to obliterate the fat plane, dilate the main pancreatic duct and common bile duct by obstructing them, and produce low-density focal lesions in the liver from metastasis.
- Use of an I.V. contrast medium helps detect metastases by opacifying the pancreatic and hepatic parenchyma.
- Adenocarcinoma and islet cell tumors are the most common carcinomas of the pancreas.
- Cystadenomas and cystadenocarcinomas, usually multilocular, occur most frequently in the body and tail of the pancreas, and appear as low-density focal lesions marked by internal septa. Contrast medium administered by mouth helps distinguish between bowel loops and tumors in the tail of the pancreas.
- Acute pancreatitis, either edematous (interstitial) or necrotizing (hemorrhagic), produces diffuse enlargement of the pancreas.
- In acute edematous pancreatitis, parenchyma density is uniformly decreased.
- In acute necrotizing pancreatitis, the density is nonuniform because of the presence of necrosis and hemorrhage. The areas of tissue necrosis have diminished density.
- In acute pancreatitis, inflammation typically spreads into the peripancreatic fat, causes stranding in the mesenteric fat, and blurs the gland margin. Abscesses, phlegmons, and pseudocysts may oc-

cur as complications of acute pancreatitis.
- In chronic pancreatitis, the pancreas may appear normal, enlarged (localized or generalized), or atrophic, depending on disease severity.

## Purpose

- To detect pancreatic carcinoma or pseudocysts
- To detect or evaluate pancreatitis
- To distinguish between pancreatic disorders and disorders of the retroperitoneum

## Patient preparation

- Explain that CT scanning helps detect disorders of the pancreas.
- Instruct the patient to fast after administration of the oral contrast medium.
- Describe the test, including who will perform it and where it will take place.
- Tell the patient that he'll be placed on an adjustable table that's positioned inside a scanning gantry. Assure him that the procedure is painless.
- Explain to the patient that he'll need to remain still during the test and periodically hold his breath.
- Inform the patient that he may be given an I.V. contrast medium, an oral contrast medium, or both to enhance visualization of the pancreas. Describe possible adverse reactions to the medium, such as nausea, flushing, dizziness, and sweating, and tell him to report these symptoms.

ALERT

 Check the patient's history for recent barium studies and for hypersensitivity to iodine, seafood, or contrast media used in previous tests. Notify the practitioner of any patient sensitivity to contrast media.

- Administer the oral contrast medium.

## Procedure and posttest care

- Confirm the patient's identity using two patient identifiers according to facility policy.
- Help the patient into the supine position on the X-ray table and position the table within the opening in the scanning gantry.
- A series of transverse X-rays is taken and recorded on magnetic tape. The varying tissue absorption is calculated by a computer, and the information is reconstructed as images on a television screen. These images are studied, and selected ones are photographed.
- After the first series of films is completed, the images are reviewed. Then contrast enhancement may be ordered. After the contrast medium is administered, another series of films is taken, and the patient is observed for an allergic reaction, such as itching, hypotension, hypertension, diaphoresis, or dyspnea.
- After the procedure, tell the patient he may resume his usual diet.
- Observe for a delayed allergic reaction to the contrast dye, such as urticaria, headache, and vomiting.

## Precautions

- The test is contraindicated in the pregnant patient because of radiation's possible teratogenic effects.
- If a contrast medium is used, the test is contraindicated in the patient with a history of hypersensitivity to iodine or severe renal or hepatic disease.

## Complications

- Adverse reaction to the contrast media

# Ultrasonography

## ▌Ultrasonography of the gallbladder and biliary system

In ultrasonography of the gallbladder and biliary system, a focused beam of high-frequency sound waves passes into the right upper quadrant of the abdomen, creating echoes that vary with changes in tissue density. These echoes are converted to images on a screen, indicating the size, shape, and position of the gallbladder and biliary system.

## Normal results

- The gallbladder is sonolucent; it appears circular on transverse scans and pear-shaped on longitudinal scans.
- Although the size of the gallbladder varies, its outer walls normally appear sharp and smooth.
- Intrahepatic radicles seldom appear.
- The cystic duct may also be indistinct and has a serpentine appearance.
- The common bile duct has a linear appearance, but is sometimes obscured by overlying bowel gas.

## Abnormal results

- Gallstones within the gallbladder lumen or the biliary system typically appear as mobile, echogenic areas, usually associated with an acoustic shadow. The size of gallstones generally parallels the size of their shadows; gallstones 5 mm or larger usually produce shadows.
- When the gallbladder is shrunken or fully impacted with gallstones, inadequate bile may likewise make gallstone detection difficult, and the gallbladder itself might not be detectable.
- An acoustic shadow in the gallbladder fossa indicates cholelithiasis; the presence of such a shadow in the cystic and

common bile ducts can also indicate cholelithiasis.

- Polyps and carcinoma within the gallbladder lumen are distinguished from gallstones by their fixity. Polyps usually appear as sharply defined, echogenic areas; carcinoma appears as a poorly defined mass, commonly associated with a thickened gallbladder wall.

- Biliary sludge within the gallbladder lumen appears as a fine layer of echoes that slowly gravitates to the dependent portion of the gallbladder as the patient changes position.

- Acute cholecystitis is indicated by an enlarged gallbladder with thickened, double-rimmed walls, usually with gallstones within the lumen.

- In chronic cholecystitis, the walls of the gallbladder appear thickened; the organ itself, however, is generally contracted.

- In obstructive jaundice, ultrasonography readily demonstrates a dilated biliary system and, usually, a dilated gallbladder. Dilated intrahepatic radicles appear tortuous and irregular; a dilated gallbladder usually loses its characteristic pear shape, becoming spherical.

## Purpose
- To confirm a diagnosis of cholelithiasis
- To diagnose acute cholecystitis
- To distinguish between obstructive and nonobstructive jaundice

## Patient preparation
- Explain that ultrasonography allows examination of the gallbladder and the biliary system.
- Instruct the patient to eat a fat-free meal in the evening and then to fast for 8 to 12 hours before the procedure, if possible; this promotes accumulation of bile in the gallbladder and enhances ultrasonic visualization.
- Tell the patient who will perform the procedure and where it will take place.

- Tell the patient that the room may be darkened slightly to aid visualization on the screen.
- Describe the procedure. Tell the patient that a transducer will pass smoothly over his abdomen in direct contact with his skin, but assure him that he'll feel only mild pressure.
- Instruct the patient to remain as still as possible during the procedure and to hold his breath when requested to ensure that the gallbladder is in the same position for each scan.

## Procedure and posttest care
- Confirm the patient's identity using two patient identifiers according to facility policy.
- The patient is placed in a supine position.
- A water-soluble conductive gel is applied to the face of the transducer.
- Transverse and longitudinal oblique scans of the gallbladder are taken at 3/8" (1-cm) intervals, starting at the level of the xiphoid and moving laterally to the right subcostal area. Longitudinal oblique scans are taken at 5-mm intervals parallel to the long axis of the gallbladder marked on the patient's skin, beginning medial to the gallbladder and continuing through to its lateral border.
- During each scan, the patient is asked to inhale deeply and to hold his breath. (If the gallbladder is positioned deeply under the right costal margin, a scan may be taken through the intercostal spaces while the patient holds his breath.)
- The patient is then placed in a left lateral decubitus position and is scanned beneath the right costal margin. (This position and scanning angle may displace and allow detection of stones lodged in the gallbladder neck and cystic duct region.)
- Scanning with the patient erect helps demonstrate mobility or fixity of suspi-

cious echogenic areas. Views may be photographed for later study.
- Remove the conductive gel from the patient's skin.
- Inform the patient that he may resume his usual diet.

## Precautions
- Keep the patient in a fasting state to prevent the excretion of bile in the gallbladder. Even smelling greasy foods, such as popcorn, can cause the gallbladder to empty.

# Ultrasonography of the liver

Ultrasonography of the liver produces images by channeling high-frequency sound waves into the right upper quadrant of the abdomen. Resultant echoes are converted to cross-sectional images on a monitor; different shades of gray depict various tissue densities. Ultrasonography can show intrahepatic structures and organ size, shape, and position.

This procedure is indicated in patients with jaundice of unknown etiology, unexplained hepatomegaly and abnormal biochemical test results, suspected metastatic tumors and elevated serum alkaline phosphatase levels, and recent abdominal trauma.

When used with liver-spleen scanning, ultrasonography can define cold spots (focal defects that fail to pick up the radionuclide) as tumors, abscesses, or cysts; it also provides better views of the periportal and perihepatic spaces than liver-spleen scanning. If ultrasonography fails to provide definitive diagnosis, computed tomography (CT), gallium scanning, or liver biopsy may yield more information.

## Normal results
- The liver normally demonstrates a homogeneous, low-level echo pattern, interrupted only by the different echo patterns of its portal and hepatic veins, the aorta, and the inferior vena cava.
- Hepatic veins appear completely sonolucent; portal veins have margins that are highly echogenic.

## Abnormal results
- Dilated intrahepatic biliary radicles and extrahepatic ducts suggest obstructive jaundice.
- In nonobstructive jaundice, the biliary tree is a normal diameter.
- Cirrhosis demonstrate variable liver size; dilated, tortuous portal branches associated with portal hypertension; and an irregular echo pattern with increased echo amplitude, causing overall increased attenuation.
- In fatty infiltration of the liver, hepatomegaly and a regular echo pattern that, although greater in echo amplitude than that of a normal parenchyma, doesn't alter attenuation are visible.
- Metastasis may appear either hypoechoic or echogenic, poorly defined or well defined. For example, metastatic lymphomas and sarcomas are generally hypoechoic; mucin-secreting adenocarcinoma of the colon is highly echogenic. Liver biopsy is necessary to confirm the tumor type. Serial ultrasonography may be used to monitor the effectiveness of therapy.
- Primary hepatic tumors also present a varied appearance and may mimic metastases, requiring angiography and liver biopsy for definitive diagnosis.
- Abscesses usually appear as sonolucent masses with ill-defined, slightly thickened borders and accentuated posterior wall transmission; scattered internal echoes, caused by necrotic debris, may also be present.

- Cysts usually appear as spherical, sonolucent areas with well-defined borders and accentuated posterior wall transmission.
- Hematomas—either intrahepatic or subcapsular—usually result from trauma. Intrahepatic hematomas appear as poorly defined, relatively sonolucent masses and may have scattered internal echoes due to clotting. Subcapsular hematoma may appear as a focal, sonolucent mass on the periphery of the liver or as a diffuse, sonolucent area surrounding part of the liver.

### Purpose
- To distinguish between obstructive and nonobstructive jaundice
- To screen for hepatocellular disease
- To detect hepatic metastases and hematomas
- To define cold spots as tumors, abscesses, or cysts

### Patient preparation
- Explain that ultrasonography allows examination of the liver.
- Tell the patient who will perform the test and where it will take place.
- Instruct him to fast for 8 to 12 hours before the test to reduce bowel gas, which hinders ultrasound transmission.
- Describe the procedure. Tell the patient a transducer will pass smoothly over his abdomen, channeling sound waves into the liver, but assure him that he'll feel only mild pressure.
- Instruct the patient to remain as still as possible during the procedure and to hold his breath when requested.

### Procedure and posttest care
- Confirm the patient's identity using two patient identifiers according to facility policy.
- The patient is placed in a supine position.

- A water-soluble conductive gel is applied to the face of the transducer.
- Transverse scans are taken at $\frac{3}{8}$" (1-cm) intervals, using a single-sweep technique between the costal margins. Although this technique demonstrates the left lobe of the liver and part of the right lobe, sector scans through the intercostal spaces are used to view the remainder of the right lobe.
- Scans are taken longitudinally from the right border of the liver to the left.
- For better demonstration of the right lateral dome, oblique cephalad-angled scans may be taken beneath the right costal margin.
- Scans are then taken parallel to the hepatic portal, at a 45-degree angle toward the superior right lateral dome, to examine the peripheral anatomy, portal venous system, common bile duct, and biliary tree. Clear images are photographed for later study.
- During each scan, ask the patient to hold his breath briefly in deep inspiration to displace the liver caudally from the costal margin and the ribs to aid visualization.
- Remove the conductive gel from the patient's skin.
- Inform the patient that he may resume his usual diet.

## Ultrasonography of the pancreas

In ultrasonography of the pancreas, cross-sectional images are produced by channeling high-frequency sound waves into the epigastric region and converting the resultant echoes to real-time images, which are displayed on a monitor. The pattern varies with tissue density and indicates the size, shape, and position of the pancreas and surrounding viscera.

## Normal results

- The pancreas normally demonstrates a coarse, uniform echo pattern and usually appears more echogenic than the adjacent liver.

## Abnormal results

- Alterations in the size, contour, and parenchymal texture of the pancreas characterize pancreatic disease.
- An enlarged pancreas with decreased echogenicity and distinct borders suggests pancreatitis.
- A well-defined mass with an essentially echo-free interior indicates pseudocyst.
- An ill-defined mass with scattered internal echoes or a mass in the head of the pancreas (obstructing the common bile duct) and a large noncontracting gallbladder suggest pancreatic cancer.

## Purpose

- To help diagnose pancreatitis, pseudocysts, and pancreatic cancer

## Patient preparation

- Explain that ultrasonography permits examination of the pancreas.
- Instruct the patient to fast for 8 to 12 hours before the procedure to reduce bowel gas.
- Tell the patient who will perform the procedure, where it will take place, and that the room may be darkened slightly to aid visualization on the monitor.
- If the patient is a smoker, ask him to abstain before the test; this eliminates the risk of swallowing air while inhaling, which interferes with test results.
- Describe the procedure. Tell the patient a transducer will pass smoothly over his epigastric region, channeling sound waves into the pancreas, but assure him that he'll only feel mild pressure.
- Tell the patient he'll be asked to inhale deeply during scanning, and instruct

him to remain still during the procedure.

## Procedure and posttest care

- Confirm the patient's identity using two patient identifiers according to facility policy.
- The patient is placed in a supine position.
- A water-soluble conductive gel or mineral oil is applied to the abdomen and, with the patient at full inspiration, transverse scans are taken at 1-cm intervals, starting from the xiphoid and moving caudally; longitudinal scans are taken to view the head, body, and tail of the pancreas in sequence; scanning the right anterior oblique view allows imaging of the head and body of the pancreas; oblique sagittal scans are used to view the portal vein; and scanning from the sagittal view images the vena cava.
- When good ultrasonography views are obtained, they're photographed for later study.
- Remove the conductive gel from the patient's skin.
- Inform the patient that he may resume his usual diet.

## Precautions

- If the patient is dehydrated or obese, the visualization of the pancreas may be altered.

# ▌Ultrasonography of the spleen

In ultrasonography of the spleen, a focused beam of high-frequency sound waves passes into the left upper quadrant of the abdomen, creating echoes that vary with changes in tissue density. These are displayed on a monitor as real-time images that indicate the size, shape, and position of the spleen and surrounding viscera.

Ultrasonography is indicated in patients with an upper left quadrant mass of unknown origin; with splenomegaly, to evaluate changes in splenic size; with left upper quadrant pain and local tenderness; and with recent abdominal trauma.

## Normal results

■ The splenic parenchyma normally demonstrates a homogeneous, low-level echo pattern; its individual vascular channels aren't usually apparent.
■ The superior and lateral splenic borders are clearly defined, each having a convex margin.
■ The undersurface and medial borders, in contrast, show indentations from surrounding organs (stomach, left kidney, and pancreas).
■ The hilar region, where the vascular pedicle enters the spleen, commonly produces an area of highly reflective echoes.
■ The medial surface is generally concave, which helps differentiate between left upper quadrant masses and an enlarged spleen.
■ Even when splenomegaly is present, the spleen generally remains concave medially unless a space-occupying lesion distorts this contour.

## Abnormal results

■ Splenomegaly is generally accompanied by increased echogenicity. Enlarged vascular channels are commonly visible, especially in the hilar region.
■ In splenic rupture, splenomegaly and an irregular, sonolucent area (the presence of free intraperitoneal fluid) are present.
■ In subcapsular hematoma, splenomegaly is seen as well as a double contour, altered splenic position, and a relatively sonolucent area on the spleen's periphery.

■ In subphrenic abscess, ultrasonography shows a sonolucent area beneath the diaphragm.
■ Cysts are spherical, sonolucent areas with well-defined, regular margins with acoustic enhancement behind them.

## Purpose

■ To demonstrate splenomegaly
■ To monitor the progression of primary and secondary splenic disease and to evaluate the effectiveness of therapy
■ To evaluate the spleen after abdominal trauma
■ To help detect splenic cysts and subphrenic abscesses

## Patient preparation

■ Explain that ultrasonography allows examination of the spleen.
■ Tell the patient who will perform the test, where it will take place, and that the room may be darkened slightly to aid visualization on the monitor.
■ Instruct the patient to fast for 8 to 12 hours before the procedure, if possible; this reduces the amount of gas in the bowel, improving sound wave transmission.
■ Describe the procedure. Tell the patient that a transducer will pass smoothly over his abdomen in direct contact with his skin, but assure him that he'll feel only mild pressure.
■ Instruct the patient to remain as still as possible during the procedure and to hold his breath when requested to aid visualization.

## Procedure and posttest care

■ Confirm the patient's identity using two patient identifiers according to facility policy.
■ Because the procedure for ultrasonography varies depending on the size of the spleen and the patient's physique, the patient is usually repositioned sever-

al times; the transducer scanning angle or path is also changed.

■ Generally, the patient is first placed in a supine position, with his chest uncovered.

■ A water-soluble conductive gel is applied to the face of the transducer, and transverse scans of the spleen are taken at ⅜″ to ¾″ (1- to 2-cm) intervals, beginning at the level of the diaphragm and moving posteriorly, while the transducer is angled anteromedially.

■ The patient is then placed in a right lateral decubitus position, and transverse scans are taken through the intercostal spaces using a sectoring motion.

■ A pillow may be placed under the patient's right side to help separate the intercostal spaces, making it easier to position the transducer face between them.

■ Longitudinal scans are taken from the axilla toward the iliac crest.

■ To prevent rib artifacts and to obtain the best view of the splenic parenchyma, oblique scans are taken by passing the transducer face along the intercostal spaces.

■ During each scan, the patient may be asked to hold his breath briefly at various stages of inspiration.

■ Good views are photographed for later study.

■ Remove the conductive gel from the patient's skin.

■ Inform the patient that he may resume his usual diet.

# Cardiovascular system

## Catheterization

### Cardiac catheterization

Cardiac catheterization involves passing a catheter into the right or left side of the heart. Catheterization can determine blood pressure and blood flow in the chambers of the heart, permit blood sample collection, and record films of the heart's ventricles (contrast ventriculography) or arteries (coronary arteriography or angiography).

In catheterization of the left side of the heart, a catheter is inserted into an artery in the antecubital fossa or into the femoral artery through a puncture or cutdown procedure. Guided by fluoroscopy, the catheter is advanced retrograde through the aorta into the coronary artery orifices and left ventricle. Then a contrast medium is injected into the ventricle, permitting radiographic visualization of the ventricle and coronary arteries and filming (cineangiography) of heart activity. Catheterization of the left side of the heart assesses the patency of the coronary arteries, mitral and aortic valve function, and left ventricular function. It helps diagnose left ventricular enlargement, aortic stenosis and insufficiency, aortic root enlargement, mitral insufficiency, aneurysm, and intracardiac shunt.

In catheterization of the right side of the heart, the catheter is inserted into an antecubital vein or the femoral vein and is advanced through the inferior vena cava or right atrium into the right side of the heart and the pulmonary artery. Catheterization of the right side of the heart assesses tricuspid and pulmonic valve function and pulmonary artery pressures.

#### Normal results
■ No abnormalities of heart chamber size or configuration, wall motion or thickness, direction of blood flow, or valve motion are detected.
■ The coronary arteries should have a smooth and regular outline, and vessels should be patent.
■ Cardiac catheterization provides information on pressures in the heart's chambers and vessels.
■ Higher pressures than normal are clinically significant; lower pressures, except in shock, usually aren't significant. (See *Normal pressure curves,* page 536. See also *Normal pressure limits in cardiac chambers and great vessels,* page 537.)

#### Abnormal results
■ Coronary artery disease (CAD), myocardial incompetence, valvular heart disease, and septal defects may be present.
■ Narrowing of the left main coronary artery and occlusion or narrowing high in the left anterior descending artery are

# Normal pressure curves

## Chambers of the right side of the heart

Two pressure complexes are represented for each chamber. Complexes at the far right in this diagram represent simultaneous recordings of pressures from the right atrium, right ventricle, and pulmonary artery.

## Chambers of the left side of the heart

Overall pressure configurations are similar to those of the right side of the heart, but pressures in the left side of the heart, as shown below, are significantly higher because systemic flow resistance is much greater than pulmonary resistance.

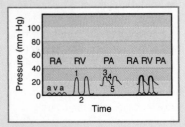

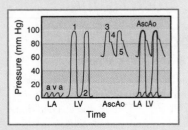

Key:

| | | | | |
|---|---|---|---|---|
| PA | = | Pulmonary artery | LV = Left ventricle | 2 = RV end-diastolic pressure |
| RV | = | Right ventricle | LA = Left atrium | 3 = PA peak systolic pressure |
| RA | = | Right atrium | AscAo = Ascending aorta | 4 = PA dicrotic notch |
| a wave | = | Contraction | 1 = RV peak systolic pressure | 5 = PA diastolic pressure |
| v wave | = | Passive filling | | |

commonly indications for revascularization surgery.

- Impaired wall motion can indicate myocardial incompetence from CAD, aneurysm, cardiomyopathy, or congenital anomalies.
- Valvular heart disease is indicated by a gradient, or difference in pressures, above and below a heart valve.
- Septal defects (atrial and ventricular) can be confirmed by measuring blood oxygen content in both sides of the heart.
- Elevated blood oxygen levels on the right side indicate a left-to-right atrial or ventricular shunt.
- Decreased oxygen levels on the left side indicate a right-to-left shunt.

## Purpose

- To evaluate valvular insufficiency or stenosis, septal defects, congenital anomalies, myocardial function and blood supply, and cardiac wall motion
- To further evaluate the patient after an abnormal stress test
- To evaluate chest pain or angina that isn't controlled with medication or occurs at rest

## Patient preparation

- Explain that cardiac catheterization evaluates the function of the heart and its vessels.
- Instruct the patient to restrict food and fluids for at least 6 hours before the test but to continue his prescribed drug regimen unless directed otherwise.

# Normal pressure limits in cardiac chambers and great vessels

This table details the upper limits of normal pressures within the cardiac chambers and great vessels in recumbent adults. Higher-than-normal pressures are usually clinically significant.

| Chamber or vessel | Pressure (mm Hg) |
|---|---|
| Right atrium | 6 (mean) |
| Right ventricle | 30/6* |
| Pulmonary artery | 30/12* (mean, 18) |
| Left atrium | 12 (mean) |
| Left ventricle | 140/12* |
| Ascending aorta | 140/90* (mean, 105) |
| Pulmonary artery wedge | Almost identical (±1 to 2 mm Hg) to left atrial mean pressure |

* Peak systolic and end-diastolic

■ Describe the test, including who will perform it and where it will be done.

■ Make sure that the patient or a responsible family member has signed an informed consent form.

■ Inform the patient that he may receive a mild sedative, but will remain conscious during the procedure. He'll lie on a padded table as the camera rotates so that his heart can be examined from different angles.

■ Tell the patient that the catheterization team will wear gloves, masks, and gowns to protect him from infection.

■ Inform him that he'll have an I.V. needle inserted in his arm to administer medication. Assure him that the electrocardiography electrodes attached to his chest during the procedure will cause no discomfort.

■ Tell the patient that the catheter will be inserted into an artery or a vein in his arm or leg; if the skin above the vessel is hairy, the hair will be clipped and the skin cleaned with an antiseptic.

■ Explain to the patient that he'll experience a slight stinging sensation when a local anesthetic is injected to numb the incision site for catheter insertion and that he may experience pressure as the catheter moves along the blood vessel. Assure him that these sensations are normal.

■ Inform the patient that injection of a contrast medium through the catheter may produce a hot, flushing sensation or nausea that quickly passes; instruct him to follow directions to cough or breathe deeply.

■ Tell the patient that he'll be given medication if he experiences chest pain during the procedure and that he may also receive nitroglycerin periodically to dilate coronary vessels and aid visualization. Reassure him that complications, such as a myocardial infarction (MI) or thromboembolism, are rare.

**ALERT**

 Check the patient's history for hypersensitivity to shellfish, iodine, or the contrast media used in other diagnostic tests; notify the practitioner of any hypersensitivities.

- Stop anticoagulant therapy, as ordered, to reduce the risk of complications from bleeding.
- Just before the procedure, tell the patient to void and put on a hospital gown.

## Procedure and posttest care

- Confirm the patient's identity using two patient identifiers according to facility policy.
- The patient is placed in the supine position on a tilt-top table and secured by restraints. Elecrocardiogram (ECG) leads are applied for continuous monitoring, and an I.V. line, if not already in place, is started with dextrose 5% in water or normal saline solution at a keep-vein-open rate.
- After a local anesthetic is injected at the catheterization site, a small incision or percutaneous puncture is made into the artery or vein, and the catheter is passed through the needle into the vessel; the catheter is guided to the cardiac chambers or coronary arteries using fluoroscopy.
- When the catheter is in place, the contrast medium is injected through it to visualize the cardiac vessels and structures.
- The patient may be asked to cough or breathe deeply. Coughing helps counteract nausea or light-headedness caused by the contrast medium and can correct arrhythmias produced by its depressant effect on the myocardium; deep breathing can ease catheter placement into the pulmonary artery or the wedge position and moves the diaphragm downward, making the heart easier to visualize.
- During the procedure, the patient may be given nitroglycerin to eliminate catheter-induced spasm or to measure its effect on the coronary arteries.
- Monitor the patient's heart rate and rhythm, respiratory and pulse rates, and blood pressure frequently during the procedure.
- After completion of the procedure, the catheter is removed and pressure should be applied to the incision site for about 30 minutes either manually or with a mechanical compression device. An adhesive bandage or clear occlusive dressing should be applied to protect the site and permit visualization for detection of bleeding or hematoma formation.
- Monitor the patient's vital signs every 15 minutes for 2 hours after the procedure, every 30 minutes for the next 2 hours, and then every hour for 4 hours. If no hematoma or other problems arise, begin checking every 4 hours. If vital signs are unstable, check every 5 minutes and notify the practitioner.
- Observe the insertion site for a hematoma or blood loss. Additional compression may be necessary to control bleeding.
- Check the patient's color, skin temperature, and peripheral pulse below the puncture site. The brachial approach is associated with a higher incidence of vasospasm (characterized by cool fingers and hands and weak pulses on the affected side); this usually resolves within 24 hours.
- Enforce bed rest for 8 hours. If the femoral route was used for catheter insertion, keep the patient's leg extended for 6 to 8 hours; if the antecubital fossa was used, keep the patient's arm extended for at least 3 hours.
- If medications were withheld before the test, check with the practitioner about resuming administration.
- Give prescribed analgesics.
- Unless the patient is scheduled for surgery, encourage intake of fluids high in potassium, such as orange juice, to counteract the diuretic effect of the contrast medium.
- Make sure a posttest ECG is scheduled to check for myocardial damage.

## Precautions

- Coagulopathy, impaired renal function, and debilitation usually contraindicate catheterization of both sides of the heart. Unless a temporary pacemaker is inserted to counteract induced ventricular asystole, left bundle-branch block contraindicates catheterization of the right side of the heart.
- If the patient has valvular heart disease, prophylactic antimicrobial therapy may be indicated to guard against subacute bacterial endocarditis.

## Complications

- Arrhythmias
- Arterial thrombus or embolism and stroke
- Bleeding
- Cardiac tamponade
- Hematoma
- Hypovolemia
- Infective endocarditis
- MI
- Pulmonary edema
- Reaction to contrast media
- Thrombophlebitis

# Electrophysiology studies

Electrophysiology studies (or *bundle of His electrography*) permit measurement of discrete conduction intervals by recording electrical conduction during the slow withdrawal of a bipolar or tripolar electrode catheter from the right ventricle through the bundle of His to the sinoatrial node. The catheter is introduced into the femoral vein, passing through the right atrium and across the septal leaflet of the tricuspid valve.

## Normal results

- Normal conduction intervals in an adult are HV interval (the conduction time from the bundle of His to the Purkinje fibers), 35 to 55 msec; AH interval (atrioventricular nodal conduction time), 45 to 150 msec; and PA interval (intra-atrial conduction time), 20 to 40 msec.

## Abnormal results

- Prolonged HV interval can result from acute or chronic disease.
- AH interval delays can occur from atrial pacing, chronic conduction system disease, carotid sinus pressure, recent MI, and certain drugs.
- PA interval delays can result from acquired, surgically induced, or congenital atrial disease and atrial pacing.

## Purpose

- To diagnose arrhythmias and conduction anomalies
- To determine the need for an implanted pacemaker, an internal cardioverter-defibrillator, and cardioactive drugs and to evaluate their effects on the conduction system and ectopic rhythms
- To locate the site of a bundle-branch block, especially in an asymptomatic patient with conduction disturbances
- To determine the presence and location of accessory conducting structures

## Patient preparation

- Explain to the patient that electrophysiology studies help to evaluate his heart's conduction system.
- Tell the patient not to eat or drink anything for at least 6 hours before the test.
- Describe the test, including who will perform it and where it will be done.
- Explain to the patient that he'll experience a stinging sensation when a local anesthetic is injected to numb the incision site for catheter insertion and that he may experience pressure on catheter insertion.
- Inform the patient that after the hair in the groin area is clipped, a catheter will be inserted into the femoral vein and an I.V. line may be started. Assure him that

the electrocardiography electrodes attached to his chest during the test will cause no discomfort.

- Inform the patient that he'll be conscious during the test, and urge him to report any discomfort or pain.
- Make sure that the patient or a responsible family member has signed an informed consent form.
- Check the patient's history, and inform the practitioner of any ongoing drug therapy.
- Just before the procedure, ask the patient to void and to put on a hospital gown.

### Procedure and posttest care

- Confirm the patient's identity using two patient identifiers according to facility policy.
- Help the patient into the supine position on a padded table.
- Limb electrodes and precordial leads are applied for continuous monitoring. If not already in place, an I.V. line is started and dextrose 5% in water or normal saline solution is administered at a keep-vein-open rate.
- After a local anesthetic is injected at the catheterization site, a small incision or percutaneous puncture is made, and a J-tip electrode is introduced intravenously into the femoral vein (or into the antecubital fossa). The catheter is guided to the cardiac chambers using fluoroscopy. It's advanced until it crosses the tricuspid valve and enters the right ventricle. Then the catheter is slowly withdrawn from the tricuspid area, and recordings of conduction intervals are made from each pole of the catheter, either simultaneously or sequentially.
- Monitor the patient's vital signs frequently during the test, noting especially a drop in blood pressure during an arrhythmia.

- The catheter is removed, and a pressure dressing is applied after completion of the procedure.
- Monitor the patient's vital signs every 15 minutes for 1 hour after the procedure and then every hour for 4 hours until he's stable. If he's unstable, check every 15 minutes and notify the practitioner.
- Observe the patient for shortness of breath, chest pain, pallor, or changes in pulse or blood pressure.
- Enforce bed rest for 4 to 6 hours.
- Check the catheter insertion site for bleeding, as ordered, usually every 30 minutes for 8 hours. If bleeding occurs, notify the practitioner and apply a pressure bandage until the bleeding stops.
- Advise the patient to resume his usual diet.
- Make sure a 12-lead resting electrocardiogram is scheduled to assess for changes.

### Precautions

- Electrophysiology studies are contraindicated in the patient with severe coagulopathy, recent thrombophlebitis, or acute pulmonary embolism.

**ACTION STAT!**

 Have emergency medication and resuscitation equipment available in case the patient develops arrhythmias during the electrophysiology study.

### Complications

- Arrhythmias
- Hemorrhage
- Infection
- Pulmonary emboli and thromboemboli

# Pulmonary artery catheterization

In pulmonary artery (PA) catheterization, also known as *Swan-Ganz catheterization*, a balloon-tipped, flow-directed catheter is threaded through the right atrium to provide intermittent occlusion of the pulmonary artery. PA catheterization permits measurement of pulmonary artery pressure (PAP) and pulmonary artery wedge pressure (PAWP).

The PAWP reading accurately reflects left atrial pressure (LAP) and left ventricular end-diastolic pressure, although the catheter itself never enters the left side of the heart. Obtaining this information is possible because the heart momentarily relaxes during diastole as it fills with blood from the pulmonary veins; at this instant, the pulmonary vasculature, left atrium, and left ventricle act as a single chamber, and all have identical pressures. Thus, changes in PAP and PAWP reflect changes in left ventricular filling pressure, permitting detection of left ventricular impairment.

The procedure is usually performed at bedside in an intensive or coronary care unit. The catheter is inserted through the cephalic vein in the antecubital fossa or the subclavian (sometimes femoral) vein. In addition to measuring atrial and PA pressures, this procedure evaluates pulmonary vascular resistance and tissue oxygenation, as indicated by mixed venous oxygen content. It should be performed cautiously in the patient with left bundle-branch block or an implanted pacemaker.

## Reference values

- Normal pressures are as follows:
  - right atrial pressure (RAP): 1 to 6 mm Hg
  - systolic right ventricular pressure: 20 to 30 mm Hg
  - end-diastolic right ventricular pressure: < 5 mm Hg
  - systolic PAP: 20 to 30 mm Hg
  - diastolic PAP: 10 to 15 mm Hg
  - mean PAP: < 20 mm Hg
  - PAWP: 6 to 12 mm Hg
  - LAP: about 10 mm Hg.

## Abnormal results

- Abnormally high RAP can indicate pulmonary disease, right-sided heart failure, fluid overload, cardiac tamponade, tricuspid stenosis and insufficiency, or pulmonary hypertension.
- Elevated right ventricular pressure can result from pulmonary hypertension, pulmonary valvular stenosis, right-sided heart failure, pericardial effusion, constrictive pericarditis, chronic heart failure, or ventricular septal defects.
- Abnormally high PAP is characteristic in increased pulmonary blood flow, as occurs in a left-to-right shunt secondary to atrial or ventricular septal defect; increased PA resistance, as occurs in pulmonary hypertension or mitral stenosis; chronic obstructive pulmonary disease; pulmonary edema or embolus; and left-sided heart failure from any cause.
- PA systolic pressure is the same as right ventricular systolic pressure.
- PA diastolic pressure is the same as LAP, except in the patient with severe pulmonary disease causing pulmonary hypertension; in such cases, catheterization is still important diagnostically.
- An elevated PAWP can result from left-sided heart failure, mitral stenosis and insufficiency, cardiac tamponade, or cardiac insufficiency
- A depressed PAWP can result from hypovolemia.

## Purpose

- To help assess right and left ventricular function
- To monitor therapy for myocardial infarction, cardiogenic shock, septic

shock, pulmonary edema, fluid-related hypovolemia and hypotension, systolic murmur, unexplained sinus tachycardia, and various cardiac arrhythmias
- To monitor fluid status in the patient with serious burns, renal disease, noncardiogenic pulmonary edema, or acute respiratory distress syndrome
- To monitor the effects of cardiovascular drugs, such as nitroglycerin and nitroprusside
- To establish baseline pressures preoperatively in the patient with existing cardiac disease and then adjust I.V. medications for optimal surgical success
- To differentiate between pulmonary and cardiac pulmonary edema

## Patient preparation
- Explain that PA catheterization evaluates heart function and provides data necessary to determine appropriate therapy or manage fluid status.
- Tell the patient that he doesn't need to restrict food and fluids.
- Describe the test, including who will perform it and where it will be done.
- Tell the patient that he'll be conscious during catheterization and that he may experience discomfort from administration of the local anesthetic.
- Explain that catheter insertion takes about 30 minutes, but that the catheter will remain in place, causing little or no discomfort.
- Instruct the patient to report any discomfort immediately.
- Explain that after insertion, he'll need to have a portable chest X-ray to confirm proper placement of the PA catheter.
- Make sure that the patient or a responsible family member has signed an informed consent form.

## Procedure and posttest care
- Confirm the patient's identity using two patient identifiers according to facility policy.
- Choose an appropriate flexible PA catheter. Catheters used in this test come in 2- to 5-lumen modes and in various lengths. In the 2-lumen catheter, one lumen contains the balloon, 1 mm behind the catheter tip; the other lumen, which opens at the tip, measures pressure in front of the balloon. The 2-lumen catheter measures PAP and PAWP and can be used to sample mixed venous blood and infuse I.V. solutions. The 3-lumen catheter has another proximal lumen that opens 12″ (30.5 cm) behind the tip; when the tip is in the main pulmonary artery, the proximal lumen lies in the right atrium, permitting fluid administration or right atrial pressure (RAP; central venous pressure) monitoring. The 4-lumen type includes a transistorized thermistor for monitoring blood temperature and allows for cardiac output measurement. A 4-lumen catheter with thermodilution and pacer port mode is used in critical care settings to allow for pacing, if necessary. The introducer part of the system may also be used to infuse large amounts of fluids.
- Before catheterization, set up the equipment according to the manufacturer's directions and the facility's protocol.
- If the insertion site is being prepared for a cutdown procedure, prepare the patient's skin and cover it with a sterile drape.
- Assist the patient to the supine position. For antecubital insertion, his arm is abducted with the palm upward on an overbed table for support; for subclavian insertion, the patient is placed in the supine position with his head and shoulders slightly lower than his trunk to make the vein more accessible. If the patient can't tolerate the supine position,

assist him to semi-Fowler's position. During the test, monitor all pressures with the patient in the same position.

■ Check the catheter balloon for defects, using sterile technique, and flush all ports to ensure patency.

■ The catheter introducer is inserted into the vein percutaneously or by cutdown. Then the catheter is inserted through the introducer and directed to the right atrium, and the catheter balloon is partially inflated so that venous flow carries the catheter tip through the right atrium and tricuspid valve into the right ventricle and the pulmonary artery.

■ Observe the monitor for characteristic waveform changes. Obtain a printout of each stage of catheter insertion. (See *PA catheterization: Insertion sites and associated waveforms,* pages 544 and 545.)

■ Instruct the patient to extend the appropriate arm (or leg, if the catheter is inserted into the femoral vein).

### ALERT

During PA catheterization—as the catheter is passed into the chambers of the right side of the heart—watch the monitor for frequent premature ventricular contractions or tachycardia (including ventricular tachycardia), which may result from right ventricular catheter irritation. If irritation occurs, the catheter may be partially withdrawn or medication given to suppress the arrhythmia or right bundle-branch block.

■ To record the PAWP, carefully inflate the catheter balloon with the specified amount of air; the catheter tip will float into the wedge position, as indicated by an altered waveform on the monitor. If a PAWP waveform occurs with less than the recommended inflation volume, don't inflate the balloon further.

■ After the balloon is inflated, record the PAWP. Then allow the balloon to deflate

passively. This allows the catheter to float back into the pulmonary artery. Observe the monitor for a PA waveform.

■ The 1.5-ml syringe that comes in the introducer kit has an indentation along the barrel that won't allow you to inject more than 1.5 cc of air, to prevent over-inflation. The stopcock should be turned so that it's perpendicular to the insertion port to prevent air from the syringe from accidentally inflating the balloon.

### DO'S & DON'TS

Don't overinflate the balloon catheter. Overinflation could distend the pulmonary artery, causing vessel rupture.

■ When the catheter's correct positioning and function are established, it's sutured to the skin. Antimicrobial ointment and an airtight dressing are applied to the insertion site according to facility policy.

■ A chest X-ray is obtained, as ordered, to verify catheter placement.

■ Set alarms on the ECG and pressure monitors.

■ Monitor the patient's vital signs, as ordered or per facility protocol.

■ Document PAP waveforms at the beginning of each shift and monitor them frequently throughout each shift and with changes in treatment. Check PAWP and cardiac output, as ordered (usually every 6 to 8 hours).

■ If the balloon can't be fully deflated after recording the PAWP, don't reinflate it unless the practitioner is present; balloon rupture may cause a life-threatening air embolism. Check all connections for air leaks that may have prevented balloon inflation, particularly if the patient is confused or uncooperative.

■ Take routine aseptic precautions to prevent infection.

■ When the catheter is no longer needed, the dressing is removed and the

# PA catheterization: Insertion sites and associated waveforms

As the pulmonary artery (PA) catheter is directed through the chambers on the right side of the heart to its wedge position, it produces distinctive waveforms on the oscilloscope screen that are important indicators of the catheter's position in the heart.

### Right atrial pressure

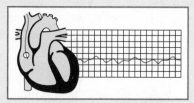

When the catheter tip reaches the right atrium from the superior vena cava, the waveform on the oscilloscope screen or readout strip resembles the one shown above. When this waveform appears, the practitioner inflates the catheter balloon, which floats the tip through the tricuspid valve into the right ventricle.

### Right ventricular pressure

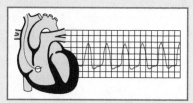

When the catheter tip reaches the right ventricle, the waveform looks like the one shown above.

---

catheter is slowly withdrawn after ensuring that the balloon is deflated. The ECG is monitored for arrhythmias. In some facilities, the practitioner is required to remove the catheter.

- After the catheter is withdrawn, the catheter tip is usually sent to the laboratory for analysis.
- Apply a sterile dressing over the catheter introducer.
- Observe the site for signs of infection, such as redness, swelling, and discharge.
- Watch for complications, such as pulmonary emboli, PA perforation, heart murmurs, thrombi, and arrhythmias.

### Precautions

- Before obtaining a PAWP reading, flush the monitoring system and recalibrate the system according to facility protocol.

- After obtaining a PAWP reading, make sure the balloon is completely deflated.
- Maintain 300 mm Hg of pressure in the pressure bag to permit a fluid flow of 3 to 6 ml/hour. Instruct the patient to extend the appropriate arm (or leg, if the catheter is inserted in the femoral vein).
- If a dampened waveform occurs, the catheter may need to be adjusted. Pulmonary infarct may occur if the catheter is allowed to remain in a wedged position.
- Make sure that the stopcocks are properly positioned and the connections are secure. Loose connections may introduce air into the system or cause blood backup, leakage of deoxygenated blood, or inaccurate pressure readings.
- Make sure that the lumen hubs are properly identified to serve the appropriate catheter ports.

## Pulmonary artery pressure

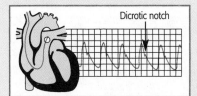

Dicrotic notch

A waveform that resembles the one shown above indicates that the balloon has floated the catheter tip through the pulmonic valve into the pulmonary artery. A dicrotic notch should be visible in the waveform, indicating the closing of the pulmonic valve.

## Pulmonary artery wedge pressure

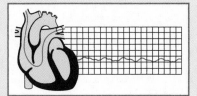

Blood flow in the pulmonary artery then carries the catheter balloon into one of the pulmonary artery's many smaller branches. When the vessel becomes too narrow for the balloon to pass through, the balloon wedges in the vessel, occluding it. The monitor then displays a pulmonary artery wedge pressure waveform such as the one shown above.

---

**ALERT**

 Don't add or remove fluids from the distal PA port; this could cause pulmonary extravasation or damage the artery.

---

- If the catheter hasn't been sutured to the skin, tape it securely to prevent dislodgment.
- If the patient shows signs of sepsis, treat the catheter as the source of infection and send it to the laboratory for culture when removed.

### Complications
- Air emboli
- Infection
- Pulmonary infarction
- Sepsis
- Ventricular arrhythmias

## *Graphic monitoring*

### ■ Electrocardiography

A common test for evaluating cardiac status, electrocardiography graphically records the electric current (electrical potential) generated by the heart. This current radiates from the heart in all directions and, on reaching the skin, is measured by electrodes connected to an amplifier and strip chart recorder. The standard resting (scalar) electrocardiogram (ECG) uses five electrodes to measure the electrical potential from 12 leads: the standard limb leads (I, II, III), the augmented limb leads ($aV_R$, $aV_L$, and $aV_F$), and the precordial, or chest, leads ($V_1$ through $V_6$).

The electrodes are small tabs that peel off a sheet and adhere to the pa-

# Normal ECG waveforms

Because each lead takes a different view of heart activity, it generates its own characteristic tracing. The tracings shown here are representative of each of the 12 leads. Leads $aV_R$, $V_1$, $V_2$, $V_3$, and $V_4$ normally show strong negative deflections. Negative deflections indicate that the current is moving away from the positive electrode; positive deflections, that the current is moving toward the positive electrode.

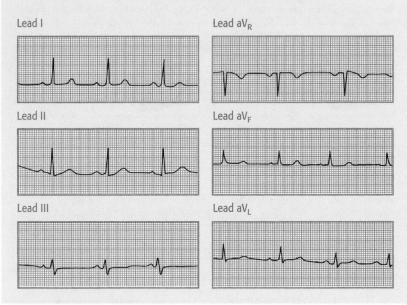

Lead I | Lead $aV_R$

Lead II | Lead $aV_F$

Lead III | Lead $aV_L$

tient's skin. The leads coming from the ECG machine are clearly marked and applied to the electrodes with alligator clamps. The entire tracing is displayed on a screen so that abnormalities (loose leads or artifacts) can be corrected before the tracing is printed or transmitted to a central computer. The electrode tabs can remain on the patient's chest, arms, and legs to provide continuous lead placement for serial ECG studies.

## Normal results

- The normal P wave doesn't exceed 2.5 mm (0.25 mV) in height or last longer than 0.12 second.
- The PR interval, which includes the P wave plus the PR segment, persists for 0.12 to 0.20 second for heart rates above 60 beats/minute.
- The QT interval varies with the heart rate and lasts 0.40 to 0.52 second for heart rates above 60 beats/minute.
- The voltage of the R wave in the $V_1$ through $V_6$ leads doesn't exceed 27 mm.
- The total QRS complex lasts 0.06 to 0.10 second.
- The ST segment is also useful for assessing myocardial ischemia. (See *Normal ECG waveforms*.)
- Negative deflections indicate that the current is moving away from the positive electrode; positive deflections indicate that the current is moving toward the positive electrode.

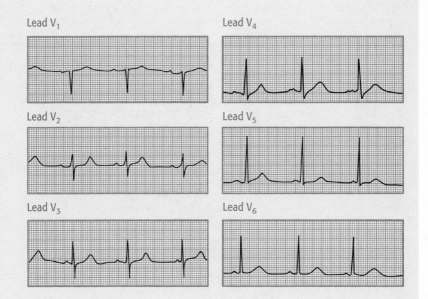

Lead V₁ Lead V₄ Lead V₂ Lead V₅ Lead V₃ Lead V₆

## Abnormal results

- Readings may reveal myocardial infarction (MI), right or left ventricular hypertrophy, arrhythmias, right or left bundle-branch block, ischemia, conduction defects or pericarditis, electrolyte abnormalities (such as hypokalemia), and the effects of cardioactive drugs (such as prolonged QT interval).
- Sometimes an ECG may reveal abnormal waveforms only during angina episodes or during exercise. (See *Abnormal ECG waveforms*, pages 548 and 549.)

## Purpose

- To help identify primary conduction abnormalities, cardiac arrhythmias, cardiac hypertrophy, pericarditis, electrolyte imbalances, myocardial ischemia, and the site and extent of MI
- To monitor recovery from an MI
- To evaluate the effectiveness of cardiac medication (cardiac glycosides, antiarrhythmics, antihypertensives, and vasodilators)
- To assess pacemaker performance
- To determine the effectiveness of thrombolytic therapy and the resolution of ST-segment depression or elevation and T-wave changes

## Patient preparation

- Explain to the patient that an ECG evaluates the heart's electrical activity.
- Tell the patient that he doesn't need to restrict food and fluids.

# Abnormal ECG waveforms

Premature ventricular contractions (PVCs) originate in an ectopic focus of the ventricular wall. They can be unifocal (having the same single focus), as shown in this tracing from lead $V_1$, or multifocal (arising from more than one ectopic focus). In PVCs, the P wave is absent and the QRS complex shows considerable distortion, usually deflecting in the opposite direction from the patient's normal QRS complex. The T wave also deflects in the opposite direction from the QRS complex, and the PVC usually precedes a compensatory pause. Some examples of abnormalities causing PVCs include electrolyte imbalances (especially hypokalemia), myocardial infarction (MI), reperfusion of a new MI or injury, hypoxia, and drug toxicity (cardiac glycosides, beta-adrenergic agents).

### PVC–Lead $V_1$

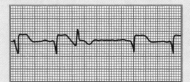

First-degree heart block, the most common conduction disturbance, occurs in healthy hearts as well as diseased hearts and usually is clinically insignificant. It's typically characteristic in elderly patients with chronic degeneration of the cardiac conduction system, and it occasionally occurs in patients receiving cardiac gly-cosides or antiarrhythmic drugs, such as procainamide and quinidine. In children, first-degree heart block may be the earliest sign of acute rheumatic fever. In this lead $V_1$ tracing, the interval between the P wave and the QRS complex (the PR interval) exceeds 0.20 second.

### First-degree heart block–Lead $V_1$

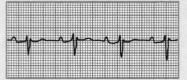

Hypokalemia is a common electrolyte imbalance that's caused by low serum potassium levels and affects the electrical activity of the myocardium. Mild hypokalemia may cause only muscle weakness, fatigue and, possibly, atrial or ventricular irritability; a severe imbalance causes pronounced muscle weakness, paralysis, atrial tachycardia with varying degrees of block, and PVCs that may progress to ventricular tachycardia and fibrillation.

Early signs of hypokalemia, as shown on this lead $V_1$ tracing, include prominent U waves, a prolonged QU interval, and flat or inverted T waves. Usually, T waves don't flatten or invert until potassium depletion becomes severe.

■ Describe the test, including who will perform it, where it will be done, and how long it will last.
■ Tell the patient that electrodes will be attached to his arms, legs, and chest and that the procedure is painless. Explain that during the test, he'll be asked to relax, lie still, and breathe normally.

■ Advise the patient not to talk during the test because the sound of his voice may distort the ECG tracing.
■ Check the patient's medication history for use of cardiac drugs and note the use of such drugs on the test request form.

Hypokalemia—Lead V$_1$

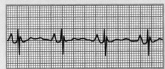

MI produces typical electrocardiogram (ECG) changes in several leads at once, enabling the physician to accurately determine the location and extent of tissue damage. MI causes three changes: an inner zone of tissue necrosis (infarction), a surrounding zone of inflamed tissue, and an outer zone of ischemia. As the infarction progresses, the first ECG change is an elevated ST segment, which indicates formation of an ischemic zone. Then the T wave begins to flatten and finally inverts, and enlarged Q waves appear, indicating developing necrosis—a true infarction. (Abnormal Q waves should be larger than one small square on the chart—0.04 second by 0.1 mV.) The T wave may stay inverted for the rest of the patient's life or it can revert to normal, whereas the deep Q wave remains as a permanent indicator of necrosis. The infarction can be located by studying the characteristic ST-segment, T-wave, and Q-wave changes in various lead combinations. In the three tracings shown here, the ST-segment elevations in leads II, III, and aV$_F$ indicate an infarction in the inferior (diaphragmatic) area of the heart.

## Procedure and posttest care

■ Confirm the patient's identity using two patient identifiers according to facility policy.
■ Place the patient in the supine position. If he can't tolerate lying flat, help him to assume semi-Fowler's position.

■ Have the patient expose his chest, both ankles, and both wrists for electrode placement. If the patient is a woman, provide a chest drape until the chest leads are applied.
■ Turn on the machine and check the paper supply.

### *Multichannel ECG*

■ Place electrodes on the inner aspect of the wrists, the medial aspect of the lower legs, and the chest. If using disposable electrodes, remove the paper backing before positioning.
■ Connect the leadwires after all electrodes are in place.
■ If frequent ECGs will be necessary, use a marking pen to indicate lead positions on the patient's chest to ensure consistent placement.
■ Press the start button and record any required information (for example, the patient's name and room number).
■ The machine produces a printout showing all 12 leads simultaneously. Check to make sure all leads are represented in the tracing. If not, determine which one has come loose, reattach it, and restart the tracing.
■ Make sure the wave doesn't peak beyond the top edge of the recording grid. If it does, adjust the machine to bring the wave inside the boundaries.
■ When the machine finishes the tracing, remove the electrodes and reposition the patient's gown and bed covers.
■ Label each ECG strip with the patient's name and room number (if applicable), date and time of the procedure, and practitioner's name. Note whether the ECG was performed during or on resolution of a chest pain episode.
■ Disconnect the equipment. The electrode patches are usually left in place if the patient is having recurrent chest pain or if serial ECGs are ordered, as with the use of thrombolytics.

- Report any abnormal ECG findings to the practitioner.

### Precautions
- The recording equipment and other nearby electrical equipment should be properly grounded to prevent electrical interference.
- Double-check color codes and lead markings to be sure connectors match.
- Make sure that the electrodes are firmly attached, and reattach them if loose skin contact is suspected. Don't use cables that are broken, frayed, or bare.
- If the patient has a pacemaker in place, an ECG may be performed with or without a magnet. Indicate the presence of a pacemaker and whether a magnet is used. (Many pacemakers function only when the heartbeat falls below a preset rate; a magnet makes the pacemaker fire regularly, which permits evaluation of pacemaker performance.)
- Inaccurate test results may be caused by improper placement of electrodes, patient movement or muscle tremors, strenuous exercise before the test, or medication reactions.
- Mechanical difficulties, such as ECG machine malfunction, faulty adherence of electrode patches (for example, due to diaphoresis), and electromagnetic interference (production of artifact) may occur.

### Complications
- Skin sensitivity to the electrodes

# ■ Exercise electrocardiography
[stress test]

An exercise electrocardiogram (ECG) evaluates the heart's response to physical stress, providing important diagnostic information that can't be obtained from a resting ECG alone.

An ECG and blood pressure readings are taken while the patient walks on a treadmill or pedals a stationary bicycle, and his response to a constant or an increasing workload is observed. Unless complications develop, the test continues until the patient reaches the target heart rate (determined by an established protocol) or experiences chest pain or fatigue. The patient who has recently had a myocardial infarction (MI) or coronary artery surgery may walk the treadmill at a slow pace to determine his activity tolerance before discharge.

### Normal results
- The P and T waves, the QRS complex, and the ST segment change minimally; a slight ST-segment depression occurs in some cases, especially a woman.
- The heart rate rises in direct proportion to the workload and metabolic oxygen demand; blood pressure also rises as workload increases.
- The patient attains the endurance levels predicted by his age and the appropriate exercise protocol. (See *Exercise ECG tracings.*)

### Abnormal results
- A flat or downsloping ST-segment depression of 1 mm or more for at least 0.08 second after the junction of the QRS and ST segments (J point) and a markedly depressed J point, with an upsloping but depressed ST segment of 1.5 mm below the baseline 0.08 second after the J point. T-wave inversion also signifies ischemia.
- Hypotension resulting from exercise, ST-segment depression of 3 mm or more, downsloping ST segments, and ischemic ST segments appearing within the first 3 minutes of exercise and lasting 8 minutes into the posttest recovery period may indicate multivessel or left CAD.

# Exercise ECG tracings

These tracings are from an abnormal exercise electrocardiogram (ECG) obtained during a treadmill test performed on a patient who had just undergone a triple coronary artery bypass graft. The first tracing shows the heart at rest, with a blood pressure reading of 124/80 mm Hg. In the second tracing, the patient worked up to a 10% grade at 1.7 miles per hour before experiencing angina at 2 minutes, 25 seconds. The tracing shows a depressed ST segment; heart rate was 85 beats/minute, and blood pressure was 140/70 mm Hg. The third tracing shows the heart at rest 6 minutes after the test; blood pressure was 140/90 mm Hg.

Resting

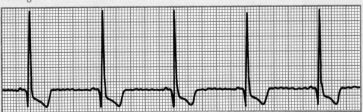

Angina

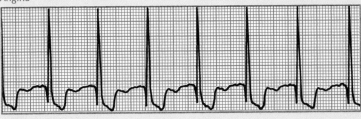

Recovery

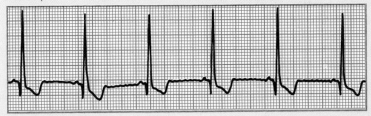

■ ST-segment elevation may indicate dyskinetic left ventricular wall motion or severe transmural ischemia.

Drug challenge

 Cardiac glycoside (possible false-positive); beta-adrenergic

blockers (may make test results difficult to interpret)

## Purpose

■ To help diagnose the cause of chest pain or other possible cardiac pain

- To determine the functional capacity of the heart after surgery or an MI
- To screen for asymptomatic coronary artery disease (CAD), particularly in men older than age 35
- To help set limitations for an exercise program
- To identify arrhythmias that develop during physical exercise
- To evaluate the effectiveness of antiarrhythmic or antianginal therapy
- To evaluate myocardial perfusion
- To determine if coronary artery blockage has recurred after an angioplasty or bypass surgery

### Patient preparation

- Explain to the patient that the exercise ECG records the heart's electrical activity and performance under stress.
- Instruct the patient not to eat, smoke, or drink alcoholic or caffeinated beverages for 3 hours before the test, but to continue his prescribed drug regimen unless directed otherwise. Instruct the patient to inform the practitioner or technician if he has taken an erectile dysfunction drug within the past 24 hours.
- Describe to the patient who will perform the test, where it will be done, and how long it will last.
- Tell the patient that the test will cause fatigue and that he'll be slightly breathless and sweaty, but assure him that the test poses few risks. He may, in fact, stop the test if he experiences fatigue or chest pain.
- Advise the patient to wear comfortable socks and shoes and loose, lightweight shorts or slacks. Men usually don't wear a shirt during the test, and women generally wear a bra and a lightweight short-sleeved blouse or a patient gown with a front closure.
- Explain to the patient that electrodes will be attached to several areas on his chest and, possibly, his back after the

skin areas are cleaned and abraded. Reassure him that he won't feel current from the electrodes; however, they may itch slightly.
- Tell the patient that his blood pressure will be checked periodically throughout the procedure and assure him that his heart rate will be monitored continuously.
- If the patient is scheduled for a multistage treadmill test, explain that the speed and incline of the treadmill will increase at predetermined intervals and that he'll be informed of each adjustment.
- If the patient is scheduled for a bicycle ergometer test, explain that the resistance he experiences in pedaling increases gradually as he tries to maintain a specific speed.
- Encourage the patient to report his feelings during the test. Tell him that his blood pressure and ECG will be monitored for 10 to 15 minutes after the test.
- Check the patient's history for a recent physical examination (within 1 week) and for baseline 12-lead ECG results.
- Make sure that the patient or a responsible family member has signed an informed consent form.

### Procedure and posttest care

- Confirm the patient's identity using two patient identifiers according to facility policy.
- The electrode sites are cleaned with an alcohol swab, and superficial epidermal cell layers and excess skin oils are removed with a gauze pad, fine sandpaper, or a dental burr. After thorough cleaning and abrading, adequately prepared sites will appear slightly red.
- Chest electrodes are placed according to the lead system selected and are secured with adhesive tape, if necessary. The leadwire cable is placed over the patient's shoulder, and the leadwire box is placed on his chest. The cable is secured

by pinning it to the patient's clothing or taping it to his shoulder or back. Then the leadwires are connected to the chest electrodes.

■ The monitor is started, and a stable baseline tracing is obtained and checked for arrhythmias. A blood pressure reading is taken, and the patient is auscultated for the presence of $S_3$ or $S_4$ gallops or crackles.

■ In a treadmill test, the treadmill is turned on to a slow speed, and the patient is shown how to step onto it and how to use the support railings to maintain balance, but not support weight. Then the treadmill is turned off. The patient is instructed to step onto the treadmill, and it's turned on to slow speed until he gets used to walking on it. Exercise intensity is then increased every 3 minutes by slightly increasing the speed of the machine and at the same time increasing the incline by 3%.

■ For a bicycle ergometer test, the patient is instructed to sit on the bicycle while the seat and handlebars are adjusted to comfortable positions. He's instructed not to grip the handlebars tightly, but to use them only for maintaining balance and to pedal until he reaches the desired speed, as shown on the speedometer.

■ In both tests, a monitor is observed continuously for changes in the heart's electrical activity. The rhythm strip is checked at preset intervals for arrhythmias, premature ventricular contractions (PVCs), and ST-segment and T-wave changes. The test level and the time elapsed in the test level are marked on each strip. Blood pressure is monitored at predetermined intervals, usually at the end of each test level, and changes in systolic readings are noted. Some common responses to maximal exercise are dizziness, light-headedness, leg fatigue, dyspnea, diaphoresis, and a

slightly ataxic gait. If symptoms become severe, the test is stopped.

■ Usually, testing stops when the patient reaches the target heart rate. As the treadmill speed slows, he may be instructed to continue walking for several minutes to cool down. Then the treadmill is turned off, the patient is helped to a chair, and his blood pressure and ECG are monitored for 10 to 15 minutes or until the ECG returns to baseline.

■ Auscultate for the presence of an $S_3$ or $S_4$ gallop. An $S_4$ gallop commonly develops after exercise because of increased blood flow volume and turbulence. An $S_3$ gallop is more significant than an $S_4$ gallop, indicating transient left ventricular dysfunction.

■ Tell the patient to resume any activities and medications discontinued before the test, as ordered.

■ Remove the electrodes and clean the electrode sites before the patient leaves.

## Precautions

■ Because an exercise ECG places considerable stress on the heart, it may be contraindicated in the patient with ventricular aneurysm, dissecting aortic aneurysm, uncontrolled arrhythmias, pericarditis, myocarditis, severe anemia, uncontrolled hypertension, unstable angina, or heart failure.

 **ALERT** Stop the test immediately if the ECG shows three consecutive PVCs or a significant increase in ectopy, if the systolic blood pressure falls below resting level, if the heart rate falls to 10 beats/minute below resting level, or if the patient becomes exhausted.

■ Depending on the patient's condition, the test may be stopped if the ECG shows bundle-branch block, ST-segment depression that exceeds 1.5 mm, persistent ST-segment elevation, or frequent or complicated PVCs; if blood pressure fails to rise above the resting level; if systolic pressure exceeds 220 mm Hg; or if the patient experiences angina.

### Complications
- Cardiac arrhythmias and myocardial ischemia or infarction

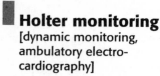

# Holter monitoring
[dynamic monitoring, ambulatory electro-cardiography]

Holter monitoring involves the continuous recording of heart activity over a 24-hour period as the patient follows his normal routine. During this period, the patient wears a small reel-to-reel or cassette tape recorder connected to electrodes placed on his chest and keeps a diary of his activities and any associated symptoms. After the recording period, the tape is analyzed by a computer and a physician to correlate cardiac irregularities, such as arrhythmias and ST-segment changes, with the activities noted in the patient's diary.

### Normal results
- Normal sinus rhythm is recorded with no significant arrhythmias or ST-segment changes.
- Changes in heart rate normally occur during various activities.

### Abnormal results
- Premature ventricular contractions (PVCs), conduction defects, tachyarrhythmias, bradyarrhythmias, and brady-tachy syndrome may be detected.
- Arrhythmias may be associated with dyspnea and CNS symptoms, such as dizziness and syncope.
- ST-T wave changes associated with ischemia may coincide with chest pain or increased patient activity.

### Purpose
- To detect cardiac arrhythmias
- To evaluate chest pain
- To evaluate cardiac status after an acute myocardial infarction or a pacemaker implantation
- To evaluate the effectiveness of antiarrhythmic drug therapy
- To assess and correlate dyspnea, central nervous system (CNS) symptoms (such as syncope and light-headedness), and palpitations with actual cardiac events and the patient's activities

### Patient preparation
- Explain that Holter monitoring helps determine how the heart responds to normal activity or, if appropriate, to cardioactive medication. Tell the patient that electrodes will be attached to his chest, that his chest hair may be clipped, and that he may experience some discomfort during preparation of the electrode sites.
- Explain to the patient that he'll wear a small tape recorder for 24 hours (for 5 to 7 days, if a patient-activated monitor is being used).
- Mention that a shoulder strap or a special belt will be provided to carry the recorder, which weighs about 2 lb (1 kg). Show him how to position the recorder when he lies down.
- Encourage the patient to continue his routine activities during the monitoring period. Stress the importance of logging his usual activities (such as walking, climbing stairs, urinating, sleeping, and having sex), emotional upsets, physical symptoms (dizziness, palpitations, fatigue, chest pain, and syncope), and ingestion of medication; show the patient a sample diary.
- Tell the patient to wear loose-fitting clothing with front-buttoning tops during monitoring.
- Demonstrate the proper use of specific equipment, including how to mark the

tape (if applicable) at the onset of symptoms.

■ If a patient-activated monitor is being used, show the patient how to press the event button to activate the monitor if he experiences an unusual sensation. Instruct him not to tamper with the monitor or disconnect the leadwires or electrodes.

■ Bathing instructions depend on the type of recorder being worn (certain equipment must not get wet).

■ Advise the patient to avoid magnets, metal detectors, high-voltage areas, and electric blankets. Show him how to check the recorder to make sure it's working properly. Instruct him how to troubleshoot problems if the monitor alarm sounds. Explain that if the monitor light flashes, one of the electrodes may be loose and he should depress the center of each one. Tell him to notify you if one comes off.

■ If the patient won't be returning to the health care facility immediately after the monitoring period, show him how to remove and store the equipment. Remind him to bring the diary when he returns.

### Procedure and posttest care

■ Confirm the patient's identity using two patient identifiers according to facility policy.

■ Clean and gently abrade the electrode sites. Peel the backings from the electrodes and apply them to the correct sites, making sure to press the sides and center of each electrode firmly to ensure proper adhesion.

■ Attach the electrode cable securely to the monitor.

■ Position the monitor and case as the patient will wear it, and then attach the leadwires to the electrodes. There shouldn't be too much slack or pull on the wires.

■ Make sure the recorder has a new or fully charged battery, insert the tape, and turn on the recorder.

■ Test the electrode attachment circuit by connecting the recorder to a standard ECG machine. Watch for artifacts while the patient moves normally (stands, sits).

■ Remove all chest electrodes and clean the electrode sites after the test.

### Precautions

■ To eliminate muscle artifact, make sure the lead cable is plugged in firmly. Check to ensure that electrodes aren't placed over large muscle masses such as the pectorals.

### Complications

■ Skin sensitivity to the electrodes

# Impedance plethysmography
### [occlusive impedance phlebography]

Impedance plethysmography is a reliable, widely used, noninvasive test that measures venous flow in the limbs. Electrodes from a plethysmograph are applied to the patient's leg to record changes in electrical resistance (impedance) caused by blood volume variations that may result from respiration or venous occlusion.

### Normal results

■ Temporary venous occlusion normally produces a sharp rise in venous volume; release of the occlusion produces rapid venous outflow.

### Abnormal results

■ When clots in a major deep vein obstruct venous outflow, the pressure in the distal leg (calf) veins rises, and these veins become distended. Such veins are unable to expand further when additional pressure is applied with an occlusive thigh cuff.

- Blockage of major deep veins also decreases the rate at which blood flows from the leg.
- If significant thrombi are present in a major deep vein of the lower leg (popliteal, femoral, or iliac), calf vein filling and venous outflow rates are reduced. In such cases, the practitioner will evaluate the need for further treatment, such as anticoagulant therapy, taking the patient's overall condition into consideration.

## Purpose

- To detect deep vein thrombosis (DVT) in the proximal deep veins of the leg
- To screen the patient at high risk for thrombophlebitis
- To evaluate the patient with suspected pulmonary embolism (because most pulmonary emboli are complications of DVT in the leg)

## Patient preparation

- Explain to the patient that impedance plethysmography helps detect DVT.
- Inform the patient that he doesn't need to restrict food, fluids, and medications.
- Explain that the test requires that both legs be tested and that three to five tracings may be made for each leg.
- Tell the patient who will perform the test and where it will be done.
- Assure the patient that the test is painless and safe.
- Emphasize that accurate testing requires that leg muscles be relaxed and breathing be normal. Reassure the patient that if he experiences pain that interferes with leg relaxation, a mild analgesic will be administered, if ordered.
- Just before the test, instruct the patient to void and to put on a hospital gown.

## Procedure and posttest care

- Confirm the patient's identity using two patient identifiers according to facility policy.
- Place the patient in the supine position, elevating the leg to be tested 30 to 35 degrees. To promote venous drainage, place the calf above the patient's heart level.
- Ask the patient to flex his knee slightly and to rotate his hips by shifting weight to the same side as the leg being tested.
- After the electrodes (connected to the plethysmograph) have been loosely attached to the calf about 3″ to 4″ (7.5 to 10 cm) apart, the pressure cuff (connected to the air pressure system) is wrapped snugly around the thigh about 2″ (5 cm) above the knee.
- The pressure cuff is inflated to 45 to 60 cm $H_2O$, allowing full venous distention without interfering with arterial blood flow. Pressure is maintained for 45 seconds or until the tracing stabilizes. (In a patient with reduced arterial blood flow, pressure is maintained for 2 minutes or longer, after which the pressure cuff is rapidly deflated.)
- The strip chart tracing, which records the increase in venous volume after cuff inflation and the decrease in venous volume 3 seconds after deflation, is checked. Then the test is repeated for the other leg. If necessary, three to five tracings for each leg are obtained to confirm full venous filling and outflow; the tracing showing the greatest rise and fall in venous volume is used as the test result.
- If the result is ambiguous, check the position of the patient's leg as well as cuff and electrode placement.
- Make sure that the conductive gel is removed from the patient's skin after the test.

## Precautions

■ Urge the patient to lie quietly and relax and much as possible.
■ Keep the room temperature as warm as possible to help prevent the patient's extremities from becoming cold.
■ Decreased peripheral arterial blood flow may alter the test results.

# ▌Signal-averaged electrocardiography

Signal averaging is the amplification, averaging, and filtering of an electrocardiogram (ECG) signal that's recorded on the body surface by orthogonal leads. The recording detects high-frequency, low-amplitude cardiac electrical signals in the last part of the QRS complex and in the ST segment. In patients who have survived an acute myocardial infarction (MI) or have coronary artery disease, these distinctive signals, called late potentials, may represent delayed disorganized activity in abnormal areas of the myocardium at the interface of fibrous scar tissue and normal tissue. This activity can lead to life-threatening ventricular arrhythmias.

In this computerized procedure, each electrode lead input is amplified, its voltage is measured or sampled at intervals of 1 msec or less, and each sample is converted into a digital number. The ECG is thereby converted from an analogue voltage waveform into a series of digital numbers that are, in essence, a computer-readable ECG of 100 or more QRS complexes.

### Normal results

■ A QRS complex without low potentials is considered normal.
■ The areas of interest in the signal-averaged ECG are:
 – the duration of the filtered QRS complex (QRST), which indicates how long the completion of the QRS complex is delayed by late potentials
 – the amount of energy in the late potentials, as indicated by the root mean square (RMS) voltage in the terminal 40 msec of the QRS complex (RMS40)
 – the duration of the late potentials, as indicated by the duration of the low-amplitude signals of less than 40 μV in the terminal QRS region.
■ The preceding values can be read either from the signal-averaged ECG itself or from the computer system.

### Abnormal results

■ Late potentials identified after the QRS complex indicates a risk of ventricular arrhythmias.
■ Late potentials are most common and of greater prognostic value in the patient who has had an MI.
■ The patient who doesn't have late potentials is at low risk for serious ventricular arrhythmias and sudden death.
■ Although the predictive accuracy of a positive signal-averaged ECG is relatively low, it's recommended as a screening test for the patient who should undergo electrophysiologic testing.

**DRUG CHALLENGE**

 Antiarrhythmics (may suppress arrhythmias)

### Purpose

■ To detect late potentials and evaluate the risk of life-threatening arrhythmias

### Patient preparation

■ Explain to the patient that signal-averaged ECG is used to evaluate his heart's electrical activity and the potential for developing a life-threatening arrhythmia.
■ Inform the patient that the test will be performed by a technician who has been

specially trained to monitor recording and computerized equipment used to analyze the signal-averaged ECG.

- Describe the test, including who will perform it, where it will be done, and how long it will last.
- Tell the patient that electrodes will be attached to his arms, legs, and chest and that the procedure is painless.
- Explain to the patient that during the test, he'll be asked to lie still and breathe normally. This is important because limb movement or the sound of his voice will distort the recording.
- Inform the patient that he doesn't need to restrict food and fluids.
- Record on the patient's chart any use of antiarrhythmics.

### Procedure and posttest care
- Confirm the patient's identity using two patient identifiers according to facility policy.
- Place the patient in the supine position. If he can't tolerate lying flat, help him into semi-Fowler's position.
- Have the patient expose his chest, both ankles, and both wrists for electrode placement. If the patient is a woman, provide a chest drape until the chest leads are applied.
- The test is performed by a technician who's specially trained to operate the recording and computer equipment used in analyzing the signal-averaged ECG.
- The technician gathers the multiple inputs necessary for signal averaging from standard orthogonal bipolar X, Y, and Z leads over a series of ECG cycles. The average is taken over a large number of beats, typically 100 or more.
- After the test is completed, disconnect the equipment.

### Precautions
- The recording equipment and other nearby electrical equipment should be

properly grounded to prevent electrical interference.
- Tissue-electrode artifacts can be minimized by lightly sanding the skin with fine (no. 220) sandpaper, wiping with alcohol, and using silver-silver chloride electrodes.
- Urge the patient to lie as quiet and motionless as possible to avoid signal distortion.

# Miscellaneous tests

## Cold stimulation test

The cold stimulation test helps detect Raynaud's syndrome by recording temperature changes in the patient's fingers before and after submersion in ice water. Note that digital blood pressure recording or examination of the arteries in the arm and palmar arch should precede this test to rule out arterial occlusive disease.

### Normal results
- Digital temperature returns to baseline levels within 15 minutes.

### Abnormal results
- If digital temperature takes longer than 20 minutes to return to the baseline level, Raynaud's syndrome is indicated.

### Purpose
- To detect Raynaud's syndrome, an arteriospastic disorder characterized by intense vasospasm of the small cutaneous arteries and arterioles of the hands after exposure to cold or stress

### Patient preparation
- Explain that the cold stimulation test detects vascular disorders.

- Tell the patient that he doesn't need to restrict food and fluids.
- Describe the test, including who will perform it, where it will be done, and how long it will last.
- Explain to the patient that he may experience discomfort when his hands are briefly immersed in ice water.
- Have the patient remove his watch and other jewelry and encourage him to relax.

### Procedure and posttest care

- To minimize extraneous environmental stimuli, make sure the test room is neither too warm nor too cold.
- Tape a thermistor to each of the patient's fingers and record the temperature.
- Have the patient submerge his hands in an ice-water bath for 20 seconds.
- When the patient removes his hands from the water, record the temperature of his fingers immediately and every 5 minutes thereafter until it returns to the baseline temperature.

### Precautions

- The cold stimulation test is contraindicated in the patient with gangrenous fingers or open, infected wounds.

# Computed tomography, cardiac scoring

A cardiac scoring computed tomography (CT) scan is a series of tomograms, translated by a computer and displayed on an oscilloscope screen, usually using a contrast medium. This provides layers of cross-sectional images of the heart and reconstructs cross-sectional, horizontal, sagittal, and coronal-plane images.

### Normal results

- A score of 100 or less is normal and indicates that the risk of significant coronary artery disease is minimal, and it is unlikely that the patient has a narrowing of the arteries.

### Abnormal results

- A score between 101 and 400 indicates a significant amount of calcified plaque in the arteries.
- This score indicates an increased risk of myocardial infarction in the future, and further testing is suggested.
- A score greater than 400 signifies extensive calcification and that the patient may have a critical narrowing of the arteries due to plaque. Further assessment is required immediately.

### Purpose

- To diagnose coronary artery calcium content
- To screen for coronary artery calcium content in high-risk patients and patients with chest pain of unknown origin

### Patient preparation

- Make sure the patient has signed an appropriate consent form.
- Note and report allergies.
- Tell the patient that he doesn't need to restrict food or fluid.
- Reassure the patient that he won't receive any contrast media for this test.
- Stress that the patient must remain still during the test because movement can limit accuracy of the test.
- Tell the patient that he may be asked to hold his breath at times during the test.
- Warn the patient that he may experience minimal discomfort because of lying still.
- Caution that the patient will hear clacking sounds as the head of the table

moves into the scanner, which rotates around the patient.

## Procedure and posttest care

■ Confirm the patient's identity using two patient identifiers according to facility policy.
■ The patient is assisted into the supine position on an X-ray table and asked to lie as still as possible.
■ The table slides into the circular opening of the CT scanner, and the scanner revolves around the patient, taking radiographs at preselected intervals.
■ Have him resume his usual diet and medications unless otherwise ordered.

## Precautions

■ The test isn't recommended during pregnancy because of potential risk to the fetus.
■ The presence of coronary stents may alter the quality of the picture.

# Pericardial fluid analysis

Analysis of the fluid inside the pericardial sac of the heart is usually done for the patient with pericardial effusion (an accumulation of excess pericardial fluid), which may result from inflammation (as in pericarditis), rupture, or penetrating trauma.

Obtaining a specimen for analysis requires needle aspiration of pericardial fluid, a procedure called pericardiocentesis. This procedure must be performed cautiously because of the risk of potentially fatal complications, such as myocardial or coronary artery laceration, ventricular fibrillation or vasovagal arrest, pleural infection, or accidental puncture of the lung, liver, or stomach. If possible, echocardiography should determine the effusion site before pericardiocentesis is performed to minimize

the risk of complications. (See *Aspirating pericardial fluid.*)

## Normal results

■ From 10 to 50 ml of sterile fluid is present in the pericardium.
■ Pericardial fluid is clear and straw-colored, without evidence of pathogens, blood, or malignant cells.
■ The fluid contains fewer than 1,000/µl (SI, < 1 × 10⁹/L) white blood cells (WBCs).
■ The glucose concentration approximately equals the levels in whole blood.

## Abnormal results

■ Transudates are protein-poor effusions that usually arise from mechanical factors altering fluid formation or resorption, such as increased hydrostatic pressure, decreased plasma oncotic pressure, or obstruction of the pericardial lymphatic drainage system by a tumor.
■ Exudates result from inflammation and contain large amounts of protein. Exudate effusions may occur in pericarditis, neoplasms, acute myocardial infarction, tuberculosis (TB), rheumatoid disease, and systemic lupus erythematosus.
■ An elevated WBC count or neutrophil fraction may also accompany inflammatory conditions, such as bacterial pericarditis; a high lymphocyte fraction may indicate fungal or tuberculous pericarditis.
■ Turbid or milky effusions may result from lymph or pus accumulation in the pericardial sac or from TB or rheumatoid disease.
■ Bloody pericardial fluid may indicate hemopericardium, hemorrhagic pericarditis, or a traumatic tap.
■ Hemopericardium, the accumulation of blood in the pericardium, may result from myocardial rupture after infarction or aortic rupture secondary to a dissecting aortic aneurysm or thoracic trauma.

# Aspirating pericardial fluid

In pericardiocentesis, a needle and syringe assembly is inserted through the chest wall into the pericardial sac, as illustrated here. Electrocardiographic monitoring with a leadwire attached to the needle and electrodes placed on the limbs (right arm [RA], right leg [RL], left arm [LA], and left leg [LL]) helps to ensure proper needle placement and to avoid damage to the heart.

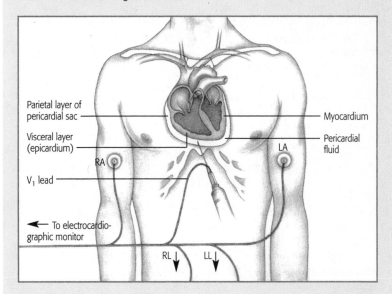

- Hemorrhagic effusions may indicate a malignant tumor, closed chest trauma, Dressler's syndrome, or postcardiotomy syndrome.
- Glucose levels below whole blood levels may reflect increased local metabolism due to malignancy, inflammation, or infection.

### DRUG CHALLENGE

 Antimicrobial therapy (can prevent isolation of the causative organisms)

## Purpose

- To assist in identifying the cause of pericardial effusion and to help determine appropriate therapy

## Patient preparation

- Explain that pericardial fluid analysis detects excessive fluid around the heart, determines its cause, and helps determine appropriate therapy.
- Inform the patient that he doesn't need to restrict food and fluids.
- Tell him who will perform the test and where it will be done.
- Inform the patient that a local anesthetic will be injected before the aspiration needle is inserted.
- Warn him that although fluid aspiration isn't painful, he may experience pressure upon needle insertion into the pericardial sac.
- Advise him that he may be asked to briefly hold his breath to aid needle insertion and placement.

- Tell the patient that an I.V. line will be started at a slow rate in case medications need to be administered.
- Assure him that someone will remain with him during the test and that his pulse and blood pressure will be monitored after the procedure.
- Check the patient's history for current antimicrobial usage and record such usage on the test request form.
- Make sure that the patient or a responsible family member has signed an informed consent form.
- Explain the test to the family if pericardiocentesis is performed to relieve cardiac tamponade and the patient is in shock.

## Procedure and posttest care

- Confirm the patient's identity using two patient identifiers according to facility policy.
- Place the patient in the supine position with the thorax elevated 60 degrees.
- When the patient is comfortable and well supported, instruct him to remain still during the procedure.
- A local anesthetic is given at the insertion site after the skin is prepared with antiseptic solution from the left costal margin to the xiphoid process.
- With the three-way stopcock open, a 50-ml syringe is aseptically attached to one end and the cardiac needle to the other.
- The electrocardiogram (ECG) leadwire is attached to the needle hub with an alligator clip. The ECG is set to lead $V_1$ and turned on (or the patient is connected to a bedside monitor).
- The needle is inserted through the chest wall into the pericardial sac, maintaining gentle aspiration until fluid appears in the syringe.
- The needle is angled 35 to 45 degrees toward the tip of the right scapula between the left costal margin and the xiphoid process. A Kelly clamp is at-

tached at the skin surface after the needle is properly positioned, so it won't advance further.

- While the fluid is being aspirated, label and number the specimen tubes.
- When the needle is withdrawn, apply pressure to the site immediately with sterile gauze pads for 3 to 5 minutes. Then apply a bandage.
- Check blood pressure readings, pulse, respiration, and heart sounds every 15 minutes until stable, every 30 minutes for 2 hours, every hour for 4 hours, and then every 4 hours thereafter. Reassure the patient that such monitoring is routine.

### ALERT

 Be alert for respiratory or cardiac distress. Watch especially for signs of cardiac tamponade: muffled and distant heart sounds, distended neck veins, paradoxical pulse, and shock. Cardiac tamponade may result from rapid reaccumulation of pericardial fluid or puncture of a coronary vessel, causing bleeding into the pericardial sac.

## Precautions

- Carefully observe the ECG tracing during insertion of the cardiac needle; an ST-segment elevation indicates that the needle has reached the epicardial surface and should be retracted slightly; an abnormally shaped QRS complex may indicate perforation of the myocardium. Premature ventricular contractions usually indicate that the needle has touched the ventricular wall.
- Watch for grossly bloody aspirate—a sign of inadvertent puncture of a cardiac chamber.
- If anaerobic organisms are suspected, consult the laboratory concerning the proper collection technique to avoid exposing the aspirate to air. The aspirate

may be placed in an anaerobic collection tube, or the syringe may be filled completely, displacing all air, and the collection tube capped tightly with a sterile rubber tip.

- Have resuscitation equipment on hand.

### Complications
- Inadvertent puncture of a cardiac chamber

---

# *Nuclear medicine*

## ▌Cardiac blood pool imaging

Cardiac blood pool imaging evaluates regional and global ventricular performance after I.V. injection of human serum albumin or red blood cells (RBCs) tagged with the isotope technetium 99m ($^{99m}$Tc) pertechnetate. In first-pass imaging, a scintillation camera records the radioactivity emitted by the isotope in its first pass through the left ventricle. Higher counts of radioactivity occur during diastole because there's more blood in the ventricle; lower counts occur during systole as the blood is ejected. The portion of isotope ejected during each heartbeat can then be calculated to determine the ejection fraction; the presence and size of intracardiac shunts can also be determined.

Gated cardiac blood pool imaging, performed after first-pass imaging or as a separate test, has several forms; however, most forms use signals from an electrocardiogram (ECG) to trigger the scintillation camera. In two-frame gated imaging, the camera records left ventricular end-systole and end-diastole for 500 to 1,000 cardiac cycles; superimposition of these gated images allows as-

sessment of left ventricular contraction to find areas of hypokinesia or akinesia.

In multiple-gated acquisition (MUGA) scanning, the camera records 14 to 64 points of a single cardiac cycle, yielding sequential images that can be studied like motion picture films to evaluate regional wall motion and determine the ejection fraction and other indices of cardiac function. In the stress MUGA test, the same test is performed at rest and after exercise to detect changes in ejection fraction and cardiac output. In the nitroglycerin MUGA test, the scintillation camera records points in the cardiac cycle after sublingual nitroglycerin administration to assess its effect on ventricular function.

Blood pool imaging is more accurate and involves less risk to the patient than left ventriculography in assessing cardiac function.

### Normal results
- The left ventricle contracts symmetrically, and the isotope appears evenly distributed in the scans.
- Normal ejection fraction is 55% to 65%.

### Abnormal results
- Coronary artery disease shows asymmetrical blood distribution to the myocardium, which produces segmental abnormalities of ventricular wall motion.
- Abnormalities may also result from preexisting conditions such as myocarditis.
- Cardiomyopathy shows globally reduced ejection fractions.
- In a left-to-right shunt, the recirculating radioisotope prolongs the downslope of the curve of scintigraphic data.
- Early arrival of activity in the left ventricle or aorta signifies a right-to-left shunt.

## Purpose

- To evaluate left ventricular function
- To detect aneurysms of the left ventricle and other motion abnormalities of the myocardial wall (areas of akinesia or dyskinesia)
- To detect intracardiac shunting

## Patient preparation

- Explain that cardiac blood pooling imaging permits assessment of the heart's left ventricle.
- Describe the test, including who will perform it, where it will be done, and its expected duration.
- Tell the patient that he doesn't need to restrict food and fluids.
- Explain to the patient that he'll receive an I.V. injection of a radioactive tracer and that a detector positioned above his chest will record the circulation of this tracer through the heart.
- Reassure the patient that the tracer poses no radiation hazard and rarely produces adverse effects.
- Inform the patient that he may experience slight discomfort from the needle puncture, but that the imaging itself is painless.
- Instruct the patient to remain silent and motionless during imaging, unless otherwise instructed.
- Make sure that the patient or a responsible family member has signed an informed consent form.

## Procedure and posttest care

- Confirm the patient's identity using two patient identifiers according to facility policy.
- The patient is placed in a supine position beneath the detector of a scintillation camera, and 15 to 20 millicuries of albumin or RBCs tagged with $^{99m}Tc$ pertechnetate are injected intravenously.
- For the next minute, the scintillation camera records the first pass of the isotope through the heart so that the aortic and mitral valves can be located.
- Then, using an ECG, the camera is gated for selected 60-msec intervals, representing end-systole and end-diastole, and 500 to 1,000 cardiac cycles are recorded on X-ray or Polaroid film.
- To observe septal and posterior wall motion, the patient may be assisted to a modified left anterior oblique position or to a right anterior oblique position and given 0.4 mg of nitroglycerin sublingually. The scintillation camera then records additional gated images to evaluate abnormal contraction in the left ventricle.
- The patient may be asked to exercise as the scintillation camera records gated images.
- If the patient is elderly or physically compromised, assist him to a sitting position and make sure he isn't dizzy. Then help him get off the examination table.

## Precautions

- Cardiac blood pool imaging is contraindicated during pregnancy.

# Cardiac magnetic resonance imaging

A great asset in the diagnosis of cardiac disorders, cardiac magnetic resonance imaging (MRI) can "see through" bone and to delineate fluid-filled soft tissue in great detail as well as produce images of organs and vessels in motion.

In this noninvasive procedure, the patient is placed in a magnetic field, into which a radiofrequency beam is introduced. Resulting energy changes are measured and used by the MRI computer to generate images on a monitor. Cross-sectional images of the anatomy are viewed in multiple planes and recorded for the permanent record.

## Normal results

- No anatomic or structural dysfunctions are present in cardiovascular tissue.

## Abnormal results

- Cardiomyopathy and pericardial disease may be seen.
- Atrial or ventricular septal defects or other congenital defects may be detected.
- Paracardiac or intracardiac masses may be revealed.
- Cardiac MRI can also evaluate the extent of pericardial or vascular disease.

## Purpose

- To identify anatomic sequelae related to myocardial infarction, such as formation of ventricular aneurysm, ventricular wall thinning, and mural thrombus
- To detect and evaluate cardiomyopathy
- To detect and evaluate pericardial disease
- To identify paracardiac or intracardiac masses
- To detect congenital heart disease, such as atrial or ventricular septal defects, and the degree of malposition of the great vessel
- To identify vascular disease, such as thoracic aneurysm and thoracic dissection
- To assess the structure of the pulmonary vasculature

## Patient preparation

- Explain that cardiac MRI assesses the heart's function and structure.
- Tell the patient who will perform the test and where it will be done.
- Inform the patient that he'll be positioned on a narrow bed, which slides into a large cylinder that houses the MRI magnets. Tell him that the scanner will make clicking, whirring, and thumping noises as it moves inside its housing and that he may receive earplugs.
- Explain to the patient who's claustrophobic or anxious about the test's duration that he'll receive a mild sedative to reduce his anxiety, or he may need to be scanned in an open MRI scanner, which may take longer but is less confining.
- Explain the need to lie flat and still.
- Reassure the patient that he'll be able to communicate with the technician at all times and that the procedure will be stopped if he feels claustrophobic.
- Immediately before the test, have the patient remove all metal objects. Double-check to make sure that he doesn't have a pacemaker or any surgically implanted joints, pins, clips, valves, or pumps containing metal that could be attracted to the strong MRI magnet. If he does, he won't be able to undergo the test.
- Give the prescribed sedative.

## Procedure and posttest care

- Confirm the patient's identity using two patient identifiers according to facility policy.
- At the scanner room door, check the patient one last time for metal objects.
- The patient is placed supine on a narrow, padded, nonmetallic bed that slides to the desired position inside the scanner. Radiofrequency waves are directed at his chest. The resulting images are displayed on a monitor and recorded on film or magnetic tape for permanent storage.
- The radiologist may vary the waves and use the computer to manipulate and enhance the images.
- Remind the patient to remain still throughout the procedure.
- Assess how the patient responds to the enclosed environment. Provide reassurance, if necessary.

If the patient is sedated, monitor his hemodynamic, cardiac, respiratory, and mental status until the effects of the sedative have worn off.

## Precautions

- The claustrophobic patient may experience anxiety. Monitor the cardiac patient for signs of ischemia (chest pressure, shortness of breath, or changes in hemodynamic status).
- The patient must be able to remain still during the procedure.
- MRI can't be performed on the patient with a pacemaker or an intracranial aneurysm clip.
- If the patient is unstable, make sure an I.V. line with no metal components is in place and that all equipment is compatible with MRI imaging. If necessary, monitor the patient's oxygen saturation, cardiac rhythm, and respiratory status during the test.
- An anesthesiologist may be needed to monitor a heavily sedated patient.
- A nurse or radiology technician should maintain verbal contact with the conscious patient.

## Complications

- Adverse reaction to sedation
- Claustrophobia, possibly leading to a panic attack

# Cardiac positron emission tomography

Cardiac positron emission tomography (PET) scanning combines elements of computed tomography scanning and conventional radionuclide imaging. Like radionuclide imaging, cardiac PET scans measure emissions of injected radioisotopes and convert these values to tomographic images. PET uses radioisotopes of biologically important elements—oxygen, nitrogen, carbon, and fluorine—which emit particles called *positrons*. During positron emissions, gamma rays are detected by the PET scanner and reconstructed to form an image. One distinct advantage of PET scans is that positron emitters can be chemically "tagged" to biologically active molecules, such as carbon monoxide, neurotransmitters, hormones, and metabolites (particularly glucose), enabling study of their uptake and distribution in tissue.

## Normal results

- No areas of ischemic tissue are present.
- If the patient receives two tracers, the flow and distribution should match, indicating normal tissue.

## Abnormal results

- Reduced blood flow with increased glucose use indicates ischemia.
- Reduced blood flow with decreased glucose use indicates necrotic, scarred tissue.

## Purpose

- To detect coronary artery disease
- To evaluate myocardial metabolism and contractility
- To distinguish viable from infarcted cardiac tissue, especially during the early stages of myocardial infarction (MI)

## Patient preparation

- If cardiac PET is ordered to assess myocardial contractility, explain to the patient that the test distinguishes viable tissue from tissue injured by MI and also may help the practitioner assess mitochondrial impairment associated with ischemia or evaluate coronary artery obstruction.
- Describe the test to the patient, including who will perform it and where it will

be done. Take the time to describe the equipment.

■ Tell the patient that the test is painless, unless an I.V. infusion is planned, in which case he may experience slight discomfort from the tourniquet and needle puncture. If the radioisotope will be inhaled, explain to the patient that this procedure is painless.

■ If fasting is ordered, describe food and fluid restrictions to the patient.

■ Instruct the patient to refrain from smoking or drinking alcohol for at least 24 hours before the test.

■ Explain to the patient that he'll be given a radioactive substance by injection, inhalation, or I.V. infusion, and that a highly specialized camera will detect the radioactive decay of this substance and send these data to a computer, which converts the data to an image.

■ Tell the patient that he'll undergo an attenuation scan for about 30 minutes. Then he'll receive the appropriate positron emitter and undergo PET scanning. The entire procedure may take up to 3 hours.

**ALERT**

 Because the radioisotope may be harmful to a fetus, the female patient of child-bearing age should be screened carefully before undergoing cardiac PET.

## Procedure and posttest care

■ Confirm the patient's identity using two patient identifiers according to facility policy.

■ The patient is placed in a supine position with his arms above his head.

■ An attenuation scan is performed lasting about 30 minutes.

■ The appropriate positron emitter is given and scanning is completed.

■ Another positron emitter may be given if comparative studies are needed.

■ Instruct the patient to move slowly after the procedure to avoid postural hypotension.

■ Encourage increased oral fluid intake to flush the radioisotope from the bladder.

### Precautions

■ Stress to the patient the importance of remaining still during the study.

### Complications

■ Orthostatic hypotension

# Radiopharmaceutical myocardial perfusion imaging
[chemical stress imaging]

Radiopharmaceutical myocardial perfusion imaging is an alternative method of assessing coronary vessel function in the patient who can't tolerate exercise electrocardiography.

In this test, I.V. infusion of a selected drug—for example, adenosine, dobutamine, or dipyridamole—is used to simulate the effects of exercise by increasing blood flow in the coronary arteries. Next, a radiopharmaceutical agent is injected intravenously to allow imaging that assists in evaluating the cardiac vessel's response to the drug-induced stress. Resting and stress images are obtained to evaluate coronary perfusion.

### Normal findings

■ Imaging should reveal characteristic distribution of the radiopharmaceutical throughout the left ventricle and show no visible defects.

### Abnormal findings

■ Cold spots are usually caused by coronary artery disease (CAD) but may result from myocardial fibrosis, attenuation due to soft tissue (for example, breasts and diaphragm), or coronary spasm.

■ The absence of cold spots in the presence of CAD may result from insignificant artifact obstruction, single-vessel disease, or collateral circulation.

## Purpose

■ To assess the presence and degree of CAD and myocardial perfusion abnormalities
■ To detect viable ischemic myocardium
■ To evaluate therapeutic procedures, such as bypass surgery or coronary angioplasty
■ To evaluate myocardial perfusion

## Patient preparation

■ Describe to the patient what the radiopharmaceutical myocardial perfusion imaging test is, including who will perform it and where it will take place.
■ Tell him that he'll need to arrive 1 hour before the test and that an I.V. line will be started before the test.
■ If the patient will receive adenosine or dipyridamole, instruct him to avoid taking all theophylline medications for 24 to 36 hours and all caffeinated drinks for 12 hours before the test.
■ If the patient will receive dobutamine, instruct him to withhold beta-adrenergic blockers for 48 hours before the test. Also tell him not to eat for 3 to 4 hours before the test, although he may have water. Instruct him to take his other medications, as prescribed, with sips of water.
■ Tell the patient to continue taking antihypertensive medications. If his systolic blood pressure is higher than 200 mm Hg, the dobutamine stress test can't be done until his blood pressure is under control.
■ Confirm that the female patient of childbearing age isn't pregnant before performing radiopharmaceutical myocardial perfusion imaging.
■ Screen the patient for bronchospastic lung disease or asthma. Adenosine and dipyridamole are contraindicated in these cases; use dobutamine instead. Weigh the patient to determine the appropriate dosage.
■ Tell the patient that a cardiologist, a nurse, an electrocardiography technician, and a nuclear medicine technologist will be present for the medication infusion.
■ Inform the patient that he may experience flushing, shortness of breath, dizziness, headache, chest pain, and increased heart rate during the infusion, but that these will end as soon as the infusion ends and that emergency equipment will be available, if needed.
■ Make sure that the patient or a responsible family member has signed an informed consent form.

## Procedure and posttest care

■ Confirm the patient's identity using two patient identifiers according to facility policy.
■ Place the patient on a bed or an examination table in the electrocardiography or medical imaging department and start an I.V. line.
■ Apply 12 electrocardiogram (ECG) leadwires to appropriate sites and obtain baseline ECG and blood pressure readings.
■ The selected chemical stress medication is infused, and blood pressure, pulse, and cardiac rhythm are monitored continuously.
■ Tell the patient to report the symptoms he's feeling.
■ At the appropriate time, the selected radiopharmaceutical is injected.

- Depending on which radiopharmaceutical is used, the patient either undergoes imaging immediately or is instructed to return for imaging 45 minutes to 2 hours later. Resting imaging may be done before stress imaging or 3 to 4 hours afterward, depending on the radiopharmaceutical used.
- Tell the patient when he needs to return and whether he should continue to fast.
- If the patient must return for further scanning, tell him to rest; he may also need to restrict foods and fluids in the interim.
- Remove the I.V. line after the images are completed.
- When all scans are completed, tell the patient that he may resume his usual diet.

### Precautions
- This test is usually contraindicated in a pregnant patient.
- The use of adenosine or dipyridamole is contraindicated in the patient with bronchospastic lung disease or asthma.

A CTION STAT!

 Keep resuscitation equipment available in case the patient experiences arrhythmias, angina, ST-segment depression, or bronchospasm.

- Aminophylline, the reversal agent for adenosine and dipyridamole, can be administered to reverse severe adverse reactions.
- Contraindications include a myocardial infarction within 10 days of testing, acute myocarditis and pericarditis, unstable angina, arrhythmias, hypertension or hypotension, aortic or mitral stenosis, hyperthyroidism, and severe infection.
- Beta-adrenergic blockers, calcium channel blockers, and angiotensin-converting enzyme inhibitors should be withheld up to 36 hours before testing, as ordered. Nitrates should be withheld 6 hours before testing.

### Complications
- Myocardial ischemia or infarction
- Serious arrhythmias

# Technetium pyrophosphate scanning
### [hot spot myocardial imaging or infarct avid imaging]

Technetium pyrophosphate scanning is used to detect a recent myocardial infarction (MI) and to determine its extent. This test uses an I.V. tracer isotope (technetium 99m [$^{99m}$Tc] pyrophosphate). This isotope accumulates in damaged myocardial tissue (possibly by combining with calcium in the damaged myocardial cells), where it forms a "hot spot" on a scan made with a scintillation camera. Such hot spots first appear within 12 hours of infarction, are most apparent after 48 to 72 hours, and usually disappear after 1 week. Hot spots that persist longer than 1 week usually suggest ongoing myocardial damage.

### Normal findings
- No isotope is found in the myocardium.

### Abnormal findings
- The isotope is taken up by the sternum and ribs, and their activity is compared with the heart's; 2+, 3+, and 4+ activity (equal to or greater than bone) indicates a positive myocardial scan.
- Areas of isotope accumulation, or hot spots, appear in damaged myocardium.

### Purpose
- To confirm a recent MI

- To help define the size and location of an MI
- To assess the prognosis after an acute MI

### Patient preparation

- Explain to the patient that $^{99m}$Tc scanning helps assess if the heart muscle is injured.
- Inform the patient that he need not restrict food and fluids. Tell him who will perform the test and where it will take place.
- Inform the patient that he'll receive an I.V. tracer isotope 2 or 3 hours before the procedure and that multiple images of his heart will be made.
- Reassure the patient that the injection causes only slight discomfort, that the scan itself is painless, and that the test involves less exposure to radiation than a chest X-ray.
- Instruct the patient to remain quiet and motionless while he's being scanned.
- Make sure that the patient or a responsible family member has signed an informed consent form.

### Procedure and posttest care

- Confirm the patient's identity using two patient identifiers according to facility policy.
- Usually, 20 millicuries of $^{99m}$Tc pyrophosphate are injected intravenously into the antecubital vein.
- After 2 or 3 hours, the patient is placed in a supine position and electrocardiography electrodes are attached for continuous monitoring during the test.
- Generally, scans are taken with the patient in several positions, including anterior, left anterior oblique, right anterior oblique, and left lateral. Each scan takes 10 minutes.

### Precautions

- Monitor the patient for adverse reactions to the injected contrast medium.

# ▌Thallium imaging
### [cold spot myocardial imaging, thallium scintigraphy]

Thallium imaging evaluates myocardial blood flow after I.V. injection of the radioisotope thallium-201 or Cardiolite. The main difference between these tracers is that Cardiolite has a better energy spectrum for imaging. Cardiolite requires living myocardial cells for uptake and allows for imaging the myocardial blood flow before and after reperfusion. This allows for better estimation of myocardial salvage. Because thallium, the physiologic analogue of potassium, concentrates in healthy myocardial tissue but not in necrotic or ischemic tissue, areas of the heart with a normal blood supply and intact cells rapidly take it up. Areas with poor blood flow and ischemic cells fail to take up the isotope and appear as "cold spots" on a scan.

This test is performed with the patient in a resting state or after stress. Resting imaging can detect acute myocardial infarction (MI) within the first few hours of symptoms but doesn't distinguish an old from a new infarct. Stress imaging, performed after the patient exercises on a treadmill until he experiences angina or rate-limiting fatigue, can assess known or suspected coronary artery disease (CAD) and can evaluate the effectiveness of antianginal therapy or balloon angioplasty and the patency of grafts after coronary artery bypass surgery. Possible complications of stress testing include arrhythmias, angina pectoris, and MI.

## Normal results

- The isotope distributes normally throughout the left ventricle, and no defects (cold spots) are detected.
- The results may be normal if the patient has narrowed coronary arteries but adequate collateral circulation.

## Abnormal results

- Persistent defects indicate a MI.
- Transient defects (those that disappear after 3 to 6 hours of rest) indicate ischemia from CAD.

## Purpose

- To assess myocardial scarring and perfusion
- To demonstrate the location and extent of acute or chronic MI, including transmural and postoperative infarction (resting imaging)
- To diagnose CAD (stress imaging)
- To evaluate the patency of grafts after coronary artery bypass surgery
- To evaluate the effectiveness of antianginal therapy or balloon angioplasty (stress imaging)

## Patient preparation

- Explain that thallium imaging helps determine if any areas of the heart muscle aren't receiving an adequate blood supply.
- If the patient is undergoing stress imaging, instruct him to restrict alcohol, tobacco, and nonprescribed medications for 24 hours before the test and to have nothing by mouth for 3 hours before the test.
- Describe the test, including who will perform it and where it will be done. Explain that additional scans may be required.
- Tell the patient that he'll receive an I.V. radioactive tracer and that multiple images of his heart will be scanned.
- Explain to the patient that it's important to lie still when images are taken.

- Warn the patient that he may experience discomfort from skin abrasion during preparation for electrode placement. Assure him that the test involves minimal radiation exposure.
- Make sure that the patient or a responsible family member has signed an informed consent form.
- Tell the patient undergoing stress imaging to wear walking shoes during the treadmill exercise and to report fatigue, pain, or shortness of breath immediately.

## Procedure and posttest care

- Confirm the patient's identity using two patient identifiers according to facility policy.

### Resting imaging

- Optimally, within the first few hours of symptoms of a MI, the patient receives an injection of I.V. thallium or Cardiolite and scanning begins after 10 minutes.
- If further scanning is required, have the patient rest and restrict food and beverages other than water.

### Stress imaging

- The patient, wired with electrodes, walks on a treadmill at a regulated pace that's gradually increased, while the electrocardiogram (ECG), blood pressure, and heart rate are monitored.
- When the patient reaches peak stress, the examiner injects 1.5 to 3 millicuries of thallium into the antecubital vein and then flushes it with 10 to 15 ml of normal saline solution or an infusion of Cardiolite.
- The patient exercises an additional 45 to 60 seconds to permit circulation and uptake of the isotope, and then lies on his back under the scintillation camera.
- If the patient is asymptomatic, the precordial leads are removed. Scanning begins after 10 minutes with the patient in the anterior, left anterior oblique, and left lateral positions.

- Additional scans may be taken after the patient rests and occasionally after 24 hours. Taking a scan after the patient rests is helpful in differentiating between an ischemic area and an infarcted or scarred area of the myocardium.

### Precautions

- Contraindications include impaired neuromuscular function, pregnancy, locomotor disturbances, acute MI or myocarditis, aortic stenosis, acute infection, unstable metabolic conditions (such as diabetes), digoxin toxicity, and recent pulmonary infarction.
- Emergency medical equipment should be readily available, if needed.

ACTION STAT!

 Stop stress imaging at once if the patient develops chest pain, dyspnea, fatigue, syncope, hypotension, ischemic ECG changes, significant arrhythmias, or critical signs (pale, clammy skin, confusion, or staggering).

### Complications

- Cardiac arrhythmias or arrest
- Hypotension or hypertension
- Myocardial ischemia or infarction
- Respiratory distress

# Radiography

 ## Cardiac radiography
[cardiac X-ray]

Among the most frequently used tests for evaluating cardiac disease and its effects on the pulmonary vasculature, cardiac radiography provides images of the thorax, mediastinum, heart, and lungs. In a routine evaluation, posteroanterior and left lateral views are taken. The posteroanterior view is preferable to the an-

teroposterior view because it places the heart slightly closer to the plane of the film, providing a sharper, less-distorted image. Cardiac radiography may be performed on a bedridden patient using portable equipment, but such equipment can provide only anteroposterior views.

### Normal results

- In the posteroanterior view, the thoracic cage appears at least twice as wide as the heart.
- In the anteroposterior view, relative heart size and position may look different, and the cardiac silhouette and vascular markings may increase.
- If cardiac radiography is performed to evaluate the position of cardiac catheters and pacemakers, the films should confirm accurate placement.

### Abnormal results

- Cardiac X-ray films must be evaluated based on the patient's history, physical examination, electrocardiography results, and results of previous radiographic tests for cardiac abnormalities.
- Left or right ventricular or left atrial enlargement, or even a multi-chamber enlargement may be revealed.
- In left ventricular enlargement, the posteroanterior view shows the border of the left side of the heart to be rounded and convex, with lateral extension of the lower left border; the lateral view shows posterior bulging of the left ventricle.
- In right ventricular enlargement, the posteroanterior view shows secondary prominence of the pulmonary artery segment at the border of the left side of the heart; the lateral view shows anterior bulging in the region of the right ventricular outflow tract.
- In left atrial enlargement, the posteroanterior view shows double density of the enlarged left atrium, straightening

of the border of the left side of the heart, elevation of the left mainstem bronchus and, rarely, lateral extension of the border of the right side of the heart superior to the right ventricle; the lateral view shows a posterior bulge at the level of the left atrium.

■ In the posteroanterior view, dilation of pulmonary venous shadows in the superior lateral aspect of the hilus and vascular shadows horizontally and inferiorly along the margin of the right side of the heart may be the first signs of pulmonary vascular congestion.

■ Chronic pulmonary venous hypertension produces an antler pattern, caused by dilated superior pulmonary veins and normal or constricted inferior pulmonary veins.

■ Acute alveolar edema may produce a butterfly appearance, with increased densities in central lung fields; interstitial pulmonary edema, a cloudy or cotton-puff appearance.

## Purpose

■ To help detect cardiac disease and abnormalities that change the size, shape, or appearance of the heart and lungs

■ To ensure correct positioning of pulmonary artery and cardiac catheters and of pacemaker wires

## Patient preparation

■ Explain that cardiac radiography reveals the size and shape of the heart. Tell the patient who will perform the test and where it will be done. Reassure him that the test uses little radiation and is harmless.

■ Instruct the patient to remove jewelry, other metallic objects, and clothing above his waist and to put on a gown that has ties instead of metal snaps.

## Procedure and posttest care

■ Confirm the patient's identity using two patient identifiers according to facility policy.

### Posteroanterior view

■ The patient stands erect about 6′ (2 m) from the X-ray machine with his back to the machine and his chin resting on top of the film cassette holder.

■ The holder is adjusted to slightly hyperextend the patient's neck. The patient places his hands on his hips, with his shoulders touching the holder, and centers his chest against it.

■ The patient is asked to take a deep breath and hold it during the X-ray film exposure.

### Left lateral view

■ The patient is positioned with his arms extended over his head and his left torso flush against the cassette and centered.

■ The patient is asked to take a deep breath and hold it during the X-ray film exposure.

### Anteroposterior view of a bedridden patient

■ The head of the bed is elevated as much as possible.

■ The patient is assisted to an upright position to reduce visceral pressure on the diaphragm and other thoracic structures.

■ The film cassette is centered under the patient's back. Although the distance between the patient and the X-ray machine may vary a little, the path between the two should be clear.

■ The patient is instructed to take a deep breath and hold it during the X-ray film exposure.

## Precautions

■ Cardiac radiography is usually contraindicated during the first trimester of pregnancy. If it's performed during pregnancy, a lead shield or apron should cover the patient's abdomen and pelvic area during the X-ray exposure.

■ When testing an ambulatory patient, make sure the radiographic order stipulates a posteroanterior view and not an anteroposterior view. Include on the order any pertinent findings from previous cardiac radiographs as well as the indication for this test.

■ When testing a bedridden patient, make sure anyone else in the room is protected from X-rays by a lead shield, a room divider, or sufficient distance.

■ A thoracic deformity such as scoliosis may cause misleading results.

# Lower limb venography
## [ascending contrast phlebography]

Lower limb venography is the radiographic examination of a vein. Commonly used to assess the condition of the deep leg veins after injection of a contrast medium, it's the definitive test for deep vein thrombosis (DVT), an acute condition marked by inflammation and thrombus formation in the deep veins of the legs. Venography shouldn't be used for routine screening because it exposes the patient to relatively high doses of radiation and can cause complications, such as phlebitis, local tissue damage and, occasionally, DVT itself.

Venography is also expensive and not easily repeated. A combination of three noninvasive tests—Doppler ultrasonography, impedance plethysmography, and $^{125}I$ fibrinogen scan—is an acceptable though less accurate alternative to venography. Radionuclide tests, such as the $^{125}I$ fibrinogen scan, are used to screen for DVT or to attempt to detect the disorder in a patient who's too ill for

venography or is hypersensitive to the contrast medium.

## Normal results
■ Opacification of the superficial and deep vasculature with no filling defects is observed.

## Abnormal results
■ Consistent filling defects on repeat views, abrupt termination of a column of contrast material, unfilled major deep veins, or diversion of flow (for example, through collateral veins) is diagnostic of DVT.

## Purpose
■ To confirm a diagnosis of DVT
■ To distinguish clot formation from venous obstruction (for example, a large tumor of the pelvis impinging on the venous system)
■ To evaluate congenital venous abnormalities
■ To assess deep vein valvular competence (especially helpful in identifying underlying causes of leg edema)
■ To evaluate lower extremities edema of unknown origin
■ To locate a suitable vein for arterial bypass grafting

## Patient preparation
■ Explain that lower limb venography helps detect abnormal conditions in the veins of the legs.
■ Instruct the patient to restrict food and to drink only clear liquids for 4 hours before the test.
■ Describe the test, including who will perform it and where it will be done.
■ Tell the patient that pretest blood work for coagulation and kidney function may be needed.
■ Warn the patient that he may feel a burning sensation in his leg on injection of the contrast medium and some discomfort during the procedure.

# Patient positioning for lower limb venography

In lower limb venography, the patient lies on an X-ray table that's inclined 40 to 60 degrees, while keeping his weight off the leg being tested. Fluoroscopy monitors the progress of the contrast medium, and spot films are taken as the contrast circulates through the venous system of the leg.

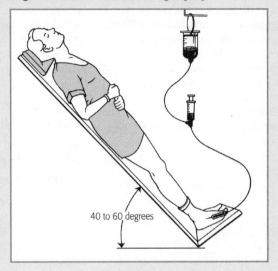

40 to 60 degrees

■ Make sure that the patient or a responsible family member has signed an informed consent form.

**A**LERT

 Check the patient's history for hypersensitivity to iodine or iodine-containing foods or to contrast media. Mark any sensitivities on the chart and notify the practitioner.

■ Reassure the patient that contrast media complications are rare, but tell him to report nausea, severe burning or itching, constriction in the throat or chest, or dyspnea immediately. Restrict anticoagulant therapy, if ordered.

■ Just before the test, instruct the patient to void, to remove all clothing below the waist, and to put on a gown.

■ If ordered, give a prescribed sedative to an anxious or uncooperative patient.

## Procedure and posttest care

■ Confirm the patient's identity using two patient identifiers according to facility policy.

■ The patient is positioned on a tilting radiographic table so that the leg being tested doesn't bear any weight. (See *Patient positioning for lower limb venography*.) He's instructed to relax this leg and keep it still; a tourniquet may be tied around the ankle to expedite venous filling.

■ A superficial vein in the dorsum of the patient's foot is injected with normal saline solution.

■ When needle placement is correct, 100 to 150 ml of the contrast medium is slowly injected over 90 seconds to 3 minutes and the presence of extravasation is checked.

■ If a suitable superficial vein can't be found (due to edema), a surgical cutdown of the vein may be performed.

■ Using a fluoroscope, the distribution of the contrast medium is monitored, and spot films are taken from the anteroposterior and oblique projections and over the thigh and femoroiliac regions. Then, overhead films are taken of the calf, knee, thigh, and femoral area.

▪ After filming, the patient is repositioned horizontally, the leg is quickly elevated, and normal saline solution is infused to flush the contrast medium from the veins.

▪ The fluoroscope is checked to confirm complete emptying. Then the needle is removed.

▪ Apply an adhesive bandage to the injection site.

▪ Monitor the patient's vital signs until he's stable; check his pulse rate and quality on the dorsalis pedis, popliteal, and femoral arteries.

▪ Administer prescribed analgesics, as ordered, to counteract the irritating effects of the contrast medium.

▪ If the venogram indicates DVT, initiate the prescribed therapy (heparin infusion, bed rest, leg elevation or support, or blood chemistry tests).

▪ Tell the patient that he may resume his usual diet and medications, as ordered.

▪ Observe the patient for signs and symptoms of a latent reaction to the dye. Encourage fluids to flush the dye from the kidneys.

### Precautions

**ALERT**

 Most allergic reactions to the contrast medium occur within 30 minutes of injection. Carefully observe the patient for signs of anaphylaxis (flushing, urticaria, laryngeal stridor).

▪ Lower limb venography is contraindicated in the patient with previous thrombosis, severe edema or obesity, or cellulitis (may limit visualization of the deep venous system).

### Complications

▪ Adverse reactions to contrast media or drugs
▪ Renal insufficiency or failure
▪ Thrombophlebitis
▪ Tissue necrosis or ulceration with extravasation of the contrast media

# Ultrasonography

## Doppler ultrasonography

Doppler ultrasonography is a type of ultrasound test used to evaluate blood flow in the major veins and arteries of the arms and legs and in the extracranial cerebrovascular system. An alternative to arteriography and venography, it's safer, less costly, and faster than invasive tests.

In Doppler ultrasonography, a hand-held transducer directs high-frequency sound waves to the artery or vein being tested. The sound waves strike moving red blood cells and are then reflected back to the transducer, allowing direct listening and graphic recording of blood flow.

Measurement of systolic pressure during this test is used to detect the presence, location, and extent of peripheral arterial occlusive disease. Changes in sound wave frequency during respiration are observed to detect venous occlusive disease. Compression maneuvers detect occlusion of the veins and occlusion or stenosis of carotid arteries.

Pulse volume recorder testing may be performed with Doppler ultrasonography to record changes in blood volume or flow in an extremity or organ.

### Normal results

▪ Arterial waveforms of the arms and legs are triphasic, with a prominent systolic component and one or more diastolic sounds.

- The ankle-arm pressure index—the ratio between ankle systolic pressure and brachial systolic pressure—is normally equal to or greater than 1. (The ankle-arm pressure index is also known as the *arterial ischemia index*, the *ankle-brachial index*, or the *pedal-brachial index*.)
- Proximal thigh pressure is normally 20 to 30 mm Hg higher than arm pressure, but pressure measurements at adjacent sites are similar.
- In the arms, pressure readings should remain unchanged despite postural changes.
- Venous blood flow velocity is normally phasic with respiration and is of a lower pitch than arterial flow.
- Distal compression or release of proximal limb compression increases blood flow velocity.
- In the legs, abdominal compression eliminates respiratory variations, but release increases blood flow; Valsalva's maneuver also interrupts venous flow velocity.
- In cerebrovascular testing, a strong velocity signal is present. In the common carotid artery, blood flow velocity increases during diastole due to low peripheral vascular resistance of the brain.
- The direction of periorbital arterial flow is normally anterograde out of the orbit.

### Abnormal results

- Arterial stenosis or occlusion diminishes the blood flow velocity signal, with no diastolic sound and a less prominent systolic component distal to the lesion.
- If complete occlusion is present and collateral circulation hasn't taken over, the velocity signal may be absent.
- A pressure gradient exceeding 20 mm Hg at adjacent sites of measurement in the leg may indicate occlusive disease.

- An abnormal gradient between the proximal thigh and the above- or below-knee cuffs indicates superficial femoral or popliteal artery occlusive disease; an abnormal gradient between the below-knee and ankle cuffs indicates tibiofibular disease.
- Abnormal gradients of arm and forearm pressure readings may indicate brachial artery occlusion.
- If venous blood flow velocity is unchanged by respirations, doesn't increase in response to compression or Valsalva's maneuver, or is absent, venous thrombosis is indicated.
- In chronic venous insufficiency and varicose veins, the flow velocity signal may be reversed. Confirmation of results may require venography.
- Inability to identify Doppler signals during cerebrovascular examination implies total arterial occlusion.
- Reversed periorbital arterial flow indicates significant arterial occlusive disease of the extracranial internal carotid artery.

### Purpose

- To help diagnose venous insufficiency and superficial and deep vein thrombosis (popliteal, femoral, iliac)
- To help diagnose peripheral artery disease and arterial occlusion
- To monitor the patient who has had arterial reconstruction and bypass grafts
- To detect abnormalities of carotid artery blood flow associated with conditions such as aortic stenosis
- To evaluate possible arterial trauma

### Patient preparation

- Explain that Doppler ultrasonography evaluates blood flow in the arms and legs or neck.
- Tell the patient who will perform the test and where it will be done.
- Reassure the patient that the test doesn't involve risk or discomfort.

- Tell the patient that he'll be asked to move his arms to different positions and to perform breathing exercises as measurements are taken. A small ultrasonic probe resembling a microphone is placed at various sites along veins or arteries, and blood pressure is checked at several sites.
- Check with the vascular laboratory about special equipment or instructions.

## Procedure and posttest care

- Confirm the patient's identity using two patient identifiers according to facility policy.
- Water-soluble conductive gel is applied to the tip of the transducer.

### Peripheral arterial evaluation

- Peripheral arterial evaluation is always performed bilaterally. The usual test sites in each leg are the common femoral, superficial femoral, popliteal, posterior tibial, and dorsalis pedis arteries; in each arm, the test sites are usually the subclavian, brachial, radial, ulnar and, occasionally, the palmar arch and digital arteries.
- The patient is instructed to remove all clothing above or below the waist, depending on the test site, and he's placed in a supine position on the examining table or bed, with his arms at his sides.
- Brachial blood pressure is measured, and the transducer is placed at various points along the test arteries.
- The signals are monitored and the waveforms recorded for later analysis.
- Segmental limb blood pressure is obtained to localize arterial occlusive disease.
- During lower extremity tests, a blood pressure cuff is wrapped around the calf, pressure readings are obtained, and waveforms are recorded from the dorsalis pedis and posterior tibial arteries. Then the cuff is wrapped around the thigh, and waveforms are recorded at the popliteal artery.
- In upper extremity tests, examination is performed on one arm, with the patient first placed in a supine position and then sitting; and then on the other arm. A blood pressure cuff is wrapped around the forearm, pressure readings are taken, and waveforms are recorded over the radial and ulnar arteries. Then, the cuff is wrapped around the upper arm, pressure readings are taken, and waveforms are recorded with the transducer over the brachial artery.
- Blood pressure readings and waveform recordings are repeated with the arm in extreme hyperextension and hyperabduction to check for possible compression factors that may interfere with arterial blood flow. The upper extremity examination is performed on one arm, with the patient first in a supine position and then sitting; it's then repeated on the other arm.

### Peripheral venous evaluation

- Usual test sites for peripheral venous evaluation include the popliteal, superficial femoral, and common femoral veins in the leg and the posterior tibial vein at the ankle; the brachial, axillary, and subclavian veins in the arm; jugular veins; and, occasionally, the inferior and superior vena cava.
- The patient is instructed to remove all clothing above or below the waist, depending on the test site.
- He's placed in a supine position and instructed to breathe normally.
- The transducer is placed over the appropriate vein, waveforms and compressibility are recorded, and respiratory modulations are noted.
- Proximal limb compression maneuvers are performed and augmentation is noted after release of compression, to evaluate venous valve competency.

# How to detect thrombi with a Doppler probe

The Doppler probe is typically used to detect venous thrombi by first positioning the transducer and then occluding the blood vessel by compression (as shown in the illustration of the normal leg below). Water-soluble conductive gel is applied to the tip of the transducer to provide coupling between the skin and transducer.

When pressure is released, allowing blood flow to resume, the transducer picks up the sudden augmentation of the flow sound and permits graphic recording of blood flow. If a thrombus is present, a compression maneuver fails to produce the augmented flow sound because the blood flow (as shown below in the femoral vein) is significantly impaired.

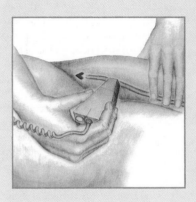
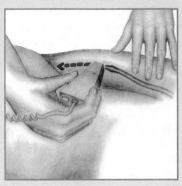

- Changes in respiration are monitored.
- During lower-extremity tests, the patient is asked to perform Valsalva's maneuver, and venous blood flow is recorded.
- The procedure is repeated for the other arm or leg.

### *Extracranial cerebrovascular evaluation*
- Usual test sites for extracranial cerebrovascular evaluation include the supraorbital, common carotid, external carotid, internal carotid, and vertebral arteries.
- The patient is placed in a supine position on the examining table or bed, with a pillow beneath his head for support.
- Brachial blood pressure is then recorded using the Doppler probe.

- The transducer is positioned over the test artery, and blood flow velocity is monitored and recorded.
- The influence of compression maneuvers on blood flow velocity is measured, and the procedure is repeated on the opposite side. (See *How to detect thrombi with a Doppler probe.*)

### *All procedures*
- Remove the conductive gel from the patient's skin.

### Precautions
- Don't place the Doppler probe over an open or draining lesion.

### Complications
- Bradyarrhythmia (if probe placed near carotid sinus)

# Echocardiography
[echo]

Echocardiography is a noninvasive test that shows the size, shape, and motion of cardiac structures. It's useful for evaluating patients with chest pain, enlarged cardiac silhouettes on X-ray films, electrocardiographic changes unrelated to coronary artery disease (CAD), and abnormal heart sounds on auscultation.

In this test, a transducer directs ultra-high-frequency sound waves toward cardiac structures, which reflect these waves. The echoes are converted to images that are displayed on a monitor and recorded on a strip chart or videotape. Results are correlated with clinical history, physical examination, and findings from additional tests.

The techniques most commonly used in echocardiography are M-mode (motion-mode), for recording the motion and dimensions of intracardiac structures, and two-dimensional (cross-sectional), for recording lateral motion and providing the correct spatial relationship between cardiac structures.

## Normal results

- Anterior and posterior mitral valve leaflets normally separate in early diastole, with the anterior leaflet moving toward the chest wall and the posterior leaflet moving away from it. The leaflets attain maximum excursion rapidly, and then move toward each other during ventricular diastole; after atrial contraction, they come together and remain so during ventricular systole. On an M-mode echocardiogram, the leaflets appear as two fine lines within the echo-free, blood-filled left ventricular cavity.
- The aortic valve cusps lie between the parallel walls of the aortic root, which move anteriorly during systole and posteriorly during diastole. During ventricular systole, these cusps separate and

appear as a boxlike configuration on an M-mode echocardiogram. They remain open throughout systole and normally demonstrate a characteristic fine fluttering motion. During diastole, the cusps come together and appear as a single or double line within the aortic root on an M-mode echocardiogram.

- The motion of the tricuspid valve resembles that of the mitral valve.
- During diastole, the pulmonic valve gradually moves posteriorly; during atrial systole, it's displaced posteriorly; during ventricular systole, it quickly moves posteriorly; during right ventricular ejection, the cusp moves anteriorly, attaining its most anterior position during diastole.
- The left ventricular cavity normally appears as an echo-free space between the interventricular septum and the posterior left ventricular wall. Echoes produced by the chordae tendineae and the mitral leaflet appear within this cavity.
- The right ventricular cavity normally appears as an echo-free space between the anterior chest wall and the interventricular septum.

## Abnormal results

- In mitral stenosis, the valve narrows abnormally due to the leaflets' thickening and disordered motion. Instead of moving in opposite directions during diastole, both mitral valve leaflets move anteriorly.
- In mitral valve prolapse, one or both leaflets balloon into the left atrium during systole.
- When blood regurgitates through the aortic valve during diastole, it strikes this leaflet, causing the flutter seen in M-mode echocardiography.
- In stenosis, due to conditions such as rheumatic fever or bacterial endocarditis, the aortic valve thickens and thus generates more echoes.

■ In rheumatic fever, the valve may thicken slightly and allow normal motion during systole, or it may thicken severely and curtail motion.

■ In bacterial endocarditis, valve motion is disrupted, and shaggy or fuzzy echoes usually appear on or near the valve.

■ A large chamber size may indicate cardiomyopathy, valvular disorders, or heart failure; a small chamber, restrictive pericarditis.

■ Hypertrophic obstructive cardiomyopathy can also be identified by the echocardiogram, with systolic anterior motion of the mitral valve and asymmetric septal hypertrophy.

■ Left atrial tumors are usually on a pedicle and can thus shift in and out of the mitral opening. During diastole, the tumor appears as a mass of echoes against the anterior mitral valve leaflet. During ventricular systole, these echoes shift back into the body of the atrium.

■ In CAD, ischemia or infarction may cause absent or paradoxical motion in ventricular walls that normally move together and thicken during systole. These affected areas may also fail to thicken or may become thinner, particularly if scar tissue is present.

■ When fluid accumulates between the epicardium and the pericardium, it causes an abnormal echo-free space to appear. In large effusions, pressure exerted by excess fluid can restrict pericardial motion.

## Purpose

■ To diagnose and evaluate valvular abnormalities

■ To measure the size of the heart's chambers

■ To evaluate chambers and valves in congenital heart disorders

■ To aid in the diagnosis of hypertrophic and related cardiomyopathies

■ To detect atrial tumors

■ To evaluate cardiac function or wall motion after myocardial infarction

■ To detect pericardial effusion

■ To detect mural thrombi

## Patient preparation

■ Explain that echocardiography is used to evaluate the size, shape, and motion of various cardiac structures.

■ Inform the patient that he doesn't need to restrict food and fluids.

■ Tell the patient who will perform the test, where it will be done, and that it's safe, painless, and noninvasive.

■ Explain that the room may be darkened slightly to aid visualization on the monitor screen and that other procedures (electrocardiography and phonocardiography) may be performed simultaneously to time events in the cardiac cycle.

■ Describe the procedure to the patient and instruct him to remain still during the test because movement may distort results.

■ Tell the patient that conductive gel will be applied to his chest and a quarter-sized transducer will be placed directly over it. Warn him that he may feel minor discomfort because pressure is exerted to keep the transducer in contact with the skin.

■ Explain to the patient that the transducer is angled to observe different parts of the heart and that he may be repositioned on his left side during the procedure.

■ Inform the patient that he may be asked to inhale a gas with a slightly sweet odor (amyl nitrite) while changes in heart function are recorded; describe the possible adverse effects (dizziness, flushing, and tachycardia), but assure him that such symptoms quickly subside.

## Procedure and posttest care

- Confirm the patient's identity using two patient identifiers according to facility policy.
- The patient is placed in a supine position.
- Conductive gel is applied to the third or fourth intercostal space to the left of the sternum, and the transducer is placed directly over it.
- The transducer is systematically angled to direct ultrasonic waves at specific parts of the patient's heart.
- During the test, the oscilloscope screen, which displays the returning echoes, is observed.
- Significant findings are recorded on a strip chart recorder (M-mode echocardiography) or on a videotape recorder (two-dimensional echocardiography).
- For a different view of the heart, the transducer is placed beneath the xiphoid process or directly above the sternum.
- For a left lateral view, the patient may be positioned on his left side.
- To record heart function under various conditions, the patient is asked to inhale and exhale slowly, to hold his breath, or to inhale amyl nitrite.
- Doppler echocardiography may be used in this examination to assess speed and direction of blood flow. The sound of blood flow may be heard as the continuous-wave and pulsed-wave Doppler sampling of cardiac valves is performed. This technique is used primarily to assess heart sounds and murmurs as they relate to cardiac hemodynamics.
- When the test is completed, remove the conductive gel from the patient's skin.

# Transesophageal echocardiography
## [TEE]

Transesophageal echocardiography combines ultrasound with endoscopy to give a better view of the heart's structures. In this procedure, a small transducer is attached to the end of a gastroscope and inserted into the esophagus, allowing images to be taken from the posterior aspect of the heart. This causes less tissue penetration and interference from chest wall structures and produces high-quality images of the thoracic aorta, except for the superior ascending aorta, which is shadowed by the trachea.

This test is appropriate for inpatients and outpatients, for patients under general anesthesia, and for critically ill, intubated patients.

## Normal results

- No cardiac problems are detected.

## Abnormal results

- Thoracic and aortic disorders, endocarditis, congenital heart disease, intracardiac thrombi, or tumors. Findings may include aortic dissection or aneurysm, mitral valve disease, or congenital defects such as patent ductus arteriosus.

## Purpose

- To visualize and evaluate:
  – thoracic and aortic disorders, such as dissection and aneurysm
  – valvular disease, especially in the mitral valve and in prosthetic devices
  – endocarditis
  – congenital heart disease
  – intracardiac thrombi
  – cardiac tumors
  – valvular repairs

## Patient preparation

- Explain that transesophageal echocardiography allows visual examination of heart function and structures.
- Tell the patient who will perform the test, when it's scheduled, and that he'll need to fast for 6 hours before the test.
- Review the patient's medical history for possible contraindications to the test,

such as esophageal obstruction or varices, GI bleeding, previous mediastinal radiation therapy, or severe cervical arthritis.

■ Ask the patient about allergies and note them on the chart.

■ Before the test, have the patient remove dentures or oral prostheses and note any loose teeth.

■ Explain to the patient that his throat will be sprayed with a topical anesthetic and that he may gag when the tube is inserted.

■ Tell the patient that an I.V. line will be inserted to administer sedation before the procedure and that he may feel slight discomfort from the tourniquet and needle puncture. Reassure him that he'll be made as comfortable as possible and that his blood pressure and heart rate will be monitored continuously.

■ Make sure that the patient or a responsible family member has signed an informed consent form.

### Procedure and posttest care

■ Confirm the patient's identity using two patient identifiers according to facility policy.

■ Connect the patient to a cardiac monitor, the automated blood pressure cuff, and pulse oximetry probe so that all parameters can be assessed during the procedure.

■ Help the patient lie down on his left side and administer the prescribed sedative.

■ The back of the patient's throat is sprayed with a topical anesthetic.

■ A bite block is placed in his mouth, and he's instructed to close his lips around it.

■ A gastroscope is introduced and advanced 12″ to 14″ (30 to 35 cm) to the level of the right atrium. To visualize the left ventricle, the scope is advanced 16″ to 18″ (40 to 45 cm).

■ Ultrasound images are recorded and then reviewed after the procedure.

■ Monitor the patient's vital signs and oxygen levels for any changes.

■ Keep the patient in a supine position until the sedative wears off.

■ Encourage the patient to cough after the procedure while lying on his side or sitting upright.

**Do's & don'ts**

Don't give food or water until the gag response returns.

■ If the procedure is done on an outpatient basis, make sure someone is available to drive the patient home.

■ Treat sore throat symptomatically.

### Precautions

■ Keep resuscitation equipment readily available.

■ Have suction equipment nearby to avoid aspiration if vomiting occurs.

■ Vasovagal responses may occur with gagging, so observe the cardiac monitor closely.

■ Use pulse oximetry to detect hypoxia.

■ If bleeding occurs, stop the procedure immediately.

### Complications

■ Adverse reaction to the sedation
■ Bleeding
■ Cardiac arrhythmias
■ Laryngospasm

## Ultrasonography of the abdominal aorta

In ultrasonography of the abdominal aorta, a transducer directs high-frequency sound waves into the abdomen over a wide area from the xiphoid process to the umbilical region. The echoing sound waves are displayed on a monitor to indicate internal organs, the vertebral column, and the size and course of the abdominal aorta and other major vessels.

## Normal results

- The abdominal aorta tapers from about 1″ to ⅝″ (2.5 to 1.5 cm) in diameter along its length from the diaphragm to the bifurcation.
- It descends through the retroperitoneal space, anterior to the vertebral column and slightly left of the midline.
- Four of its major branches are usually well visualized: the celiac trunk, the renal arteries, the superior mesenteric artery, and the common iliac arteries.

## Abnormal results

- The luminal diameter of the abdominal aorta greater than 1½″ (3.8 cm) suggests aneurysm; greater than 2¾″ (7 cm), aneurysm with high risk of rupture.

## Purpose

- To detect and measure a suspected abdominal aortic aneurysm (findings may be supported and refined by angiography or computed tomography angiography)
- To detect and measure the expansion of a known abdominal aortic aneurysm

## Patient preparation

- Explain that ultrasonography allows examination of the abdominal aorta.
- Instruct the patient to fast for 12 hours before the test to minimize bowel gas and motility.
- Tell the patient who will perform the test, where it will be done, that the lights may be lowered, and that he'll feel only slight pressure.
- Describe the procedure. Tell the patient that mineral oil or a gel, which may feel cool, will be applied to his abdomen.
- Explain that a transducer will pass over his skin, from the costal margins to

the umbilicus or slightly below, directing safe, painless, and inaudible sound waves into the abdominal vessels and organs.
- Reassure the patient with a known aneurysm that the sound waves won't cause rupture.
- Instruct the patient to remain still during scanning and to hold his breath when requested.
- If ordered, give simethicone to reduce bowel gas.

## Procedure and posttest care

- Confirm the patient's identity using two patient identifiers according to facility policy.
- The patient is placed in a supine position, and conductive gel or mineral oil is applied to his abdomen.
- Longitudinal scans are made at ⅛″ to ¾″ (0.5- to 2-cm) intervals left and right of the midline until the entire abdominal aorta is outlined; transverse scans are made at ⅜″ to ¾″ (1- to 2-cm) intervals from the xiphoid to the bifurcation at the common iliac arteries.
- The patient may be placed in the right and left lateral positions.
- Appropriate views are photographed or videotaped.
- Remove the conductive gel from the patient's skin.
- Instruct the patient that he may resume his usual diet and medications, as ordered.

**ACTION STAT!**

Aneurysms may expand and dissect rapidly, so check the patient's vital signs frequently. Remember that the sudden onset of constant abdominal or back pain accompanies rapid expansion of the aneurysm; sudden, excruciating pain with weakness, sweating, tachycardia, and hypotension signals rupture.

# Urinary system

## Structural tests

### ▌Antegrade pyelography

Antegrade pyelography allows examination of the upper collecting system when ureteral obstruction rules out retrograde ureteropyelography or when cystoscopy is contraindicated. It depends on percutaneous needle puncture for injection of contrast medium into the renal pelvis or calyces.

Renal pressure can be measured during this procedure. Also, urine can be collected for cultures and cytologic studies and for evaluation of renal functional reserve before surgery.

After completing radiographic studies, a nephrostomy tube can be inserted to provide temporary drainage or access for other therapeutic or diagnostic procedures.

#### Normal results
- The upper collecting system should fill uniformly and appear normal in size and course. Normal structures should be outlined clearly.

#### Abnormal results
- Enlargements of the upper collecting system and parts of the ureteropelvic junction indicate obstruction.
- In hydronephrosis, the ureteropelvic junction shows marked distention.
- Intrarenal pressure greater than 20 cm $H_2O$ indicates obstruction.

#### Purpose
- To evaluate obstruction of the upper collecting system by stricture, calculus, clot, or tumor
- To evaluate hydronephrosis revealed during excretory urography or ultrasonography and to enable placement of a percutaneous nephrostomy tube
- To evaluate the function of the upper collecting system after ureteral surgery or urinary diversion
- To assess renal functional reserve before surgery

#### Patient preparation
- Explain that antegrade pyelography allows radiographic examination of the kidney.
- Tell the patient that he may be required to fast for 6 to 8 hours before the test.
- Tell him that he may receive antimicrobial drugs before and after the procedure.
- Tell the patient who will perform the test and where it will take place.
- Explain to the patient that a needle will be inserted into the kidney after he's given a sedative and local anesthetic. Explain that urine may be collected from

the kidney for testing and that, if necessary, a tube will be left in the kidney for drainage.

■ Tell the patient that he may feel mild discomfort during injection of the local anesthetic and contrast medium and that he may also feel transient burning and flushing from the contrast medium.

■ Warn him that the X-ray machine makes loud clacking noises as films are taken.

### ALERT

 Check the patient's history for hypersensitivity to iodine-based contrast media or iodine-containing foods such as shellfish. Mark sensitivities on the chart and inform the practitioner because the patient may require prophylactic antiallergenics (diphenhydramine or corticosteroids).

■ Check his history and recent coagulation studies for indications of bleeding disorders.

■ Make sure that the patient or a responsible family member has signed an informed consent form.

■ Administer a sedative just before the procedure, if needed, and check that pretest blood work, such as kidney function, has been performed, if ordered.

## Procedure and posttest care

■ Confirm the patient's identity using two patient identifiers according to facility policy.

■ The patient is placed in a prone position on the X-ray table. The skin over the kidney is cleaned with antiseptic solution, and a local anesthetic is injected.

■ Previous urographic films or ultrasound recordings are studied for anatomic landmarks. (It's important to determine if the kidney to be studied is in the normal position. If not, the angle of

the needle entry must be adjusted during percutaneous puncture.)

■ Under guidance of fluoroscopy or ultrasonography, the percutaneous needle is inserted below the 12th rib at the level of the transverse process of the second lumbar vertebra. Aspiration of urine confirms that the needle has reached the dilated collecting system, which is usually 2¾" to 3⅛" (7 to 8 cm) below the skin surface in adults.

■ Flexible tubing is connected to the needle to prevent displacement during the procedure. If intrarenal pressure is to be measured, the manometer is connected to the tubing as soon as it's in place. Urine specimens are then taken, if needed.

■ An amount of urine equal to the amount of contrast medium to be injected is withdrawn to prevent overdistention of the collecting system.

■ The contrast medium is injected under fluoroscopic guidance. Posteroanterior, oblique, and anteroposterior radiographs are taken. Ureteral peristalsis is observed on the fluoroscope screen to evaluate obstruction.

■ A percutaneous nephrostomy tube is inserted if drainage is needed because of increased renal pressure, dilation, or intrarenal reflux. If drainage isn't needed, the catheter is withdrawn and a sterile dressing is applied.

■ Check the patient's vital signs every 15 minutes for the first hour, every 30 minutes for the second hour, and then every 2 hours for the next 24 hours.

■ Check dressings for bleeding, hematoma, or urine leakage at the puncture site at each vital signs check. For bleeding, apply pressure. For a hematoma, apply warm soaks. Report urine leakage or the patient's failure to void within 8 hours.

■ Monitor the patient's fluid intake and urine output for 24 hours. Observe each

specimen for hematuria. Report hematuria if it persists after the third voiding.
- Watch for and report signs of sepsis or extravasation of contrast medium (chills, fever, rapid pulse or respirations, and hypotension).

 Also watch for and report signs that adjacent organs have been punctured, such as pain in the abdomen or flank, or pneumothorax (sudden onset of pleuritic chest pain, dyspnea, tachypnea, decreased breath sounds on the affected side, and tachycardia).

- If a nephrostomy tube is inserted, make sure it's patent and draining well. Irrigate with 5 to 7 ml of sterile saline solution, as ordered, to maintain patency.
- Give prescribed antibiotics and analgesics for several days after the procedure.
- If hydronephrosis is present, monitor intake and output, edema, hypertension, flank pain, acid-base status, and glucose level.

### Precautions
- Antegrade pyelography is contraindicated in the patient with bleeding disorders.
- This procedure is contraindicated in the pregnant patient unless the benefits outweigh the risks to the fetus.

### Complications
- Adverse reaction to the contrast medium
- Hematoma or infection

 # Cystourethroscopy

Cystourethroscopy, a test that combines two endoscopic techniques, allows visual examination of the bladder and urethra. One of the instruments used in this test is the cystoscope, which has a fiber-optic light source, a magnification system, a right-angled telescopic lens, and an angled beak for smooth passage into the bladder. The other instrument, the urethroscope (or panendoscope), is similar but has a straight-ahead lens and is used for examination of the bladder neck and urethra. The lenses of the cystoscope and urethroscope use a common sheath inserted into the urethra to obtain the desired view.

Other invasive procedures, such as biopsies, lesion resection, calculi removal, dilatation of a constricted urethra, and catheterization of the ureteral orifices for retrograde pyelography, may also be performed through this sheath.

Kidney-ureter-bladder radiography and excretory urography usually precede this test.

### Normal results
- The urethra, bladder, and ureteral orifices appear normal in size, shape, and position.
- The mucosa lining of the lower urinary tract should appear smooth and shiny, with no evidence of erythema, cysts, or other abnormalities.
- No obstructions, tumors, or calculi are present.

### Abnormal results
- Urethral stricture, calculi, tumors, diverticula, ulcers, polyps, and enlarged prostate gland may be detected.
- The test may detect bladder wall trabeculation and various congenital anomalies, such as ureteroceles, duplicate ureteral orifices, or urethral valves in children.

### Purpose
- To diagnose and evaluate urinary tract disorders by direct visualization of urinary structures

## Patient preparation

- Explain that cystourethroscopy permits examination of the bladder and urethra.
- Unless a general anesthetic has been ordered, inform the patient that he doesn't need to restrict food and fluids. If a general anesthetic will be given, instruct the patient to fast for 8 hours before the test.
- Tell the patient who will perform the test, where it will take place, and that it takes about 20 to 30 minutes.
- Inform the patient that he may experience some discomfort after the procedure, including a slight burning when he urinates.
- Make sure that the patient or a responsible family member has signed an informed consent form.
- Before the procedure, give a sedative, if ordered, and instruct the patient to urinate.

## Procedure and posttest care

- Confirm the patient's identity using two patient identifiers according to facility policy.
- After a general or regional anesthetic (as required) has been administered, the patient is placed in the lithotomy position on a cystoscopic table. The genitalia are cleaned with an antiseptic solution, and the patient is draped. (Local anesthetic is instilled at this point.)
- The instrument is moved toward the bladder to visually examine the urethra. A urethroscope is inserted into the well-lubricated sheath (instead of an obturator), and both are passed gently through the urethra into the bladder. The urethroscope is then removed, and a cystoscope is inserted through the sheath into the bladder.
- After the bladder is filled with irrigating solution, the scope is rotated to inspect the entire surface of the bladder

wall and ureteral orifices with the right-angled telescopic lens.
- The cystoscope is then removed, the urethroscope reinserted, and the urethroscope and sheath are slowly withdrawn, permitting examination of the bladder neck and the various portions of the urethra, including the internal and external sphincters. (See *Using a cystourethroscope.*)
- During cystourethroscopy, a urine specimen is routinely taken from the bladder for culture and sensitivity testing, and residual urine is measured.
- If a tumor is suspected, a urine specimen is sent to the laboratory for cytologic examination; if a tumor is found, biopsy may be performed. If a urethral stricture is present, urethral dilatation may be necessary before cystourethroscopy.
- If the patient has received only a local anesthetic, he may complain of a burning sensation when the instrument is passed through the urethra. He may also feel an urgent need to urinate as the bladder fills with irrigating solution. Reassure the patient that these sensations are common and generally transient.
- Monitor the patient's vital signs for 15 minutes for the first hour after the test, and then every hour until they stabilize.
- If local anesthesia was used, keep the patient supine for several minutes, and then help him to sit or stand. Watch for orthostatic hypotension.
- Instruct the patient to drink lots of fluids (or increase I.V. fluids, if ordered) and to take the prescribed analgesic. Reassure him that burning and frequency will soon subside.
- Give antibiotics, as ordered, to prevent bacterial sepsis due to urethral tissue trauma.
- Report flank or abdominal pain, chills, fever, an elevated white blood cell

## Using a cystourethroscope

This cross-sectional illustration shows how a urologic examination is performed with a cystourethroscope, a device that allows direct visualization of the tissues of the lower urinary tract. The sheath of the cystourethroscope permits passage of a cystoscope and urethroscope for illuminating the urethra, bladder, and ureters. This instrument also provides a channel for minor surgical procedures, such as biopsies, excision of small lesions, and calculi removal.

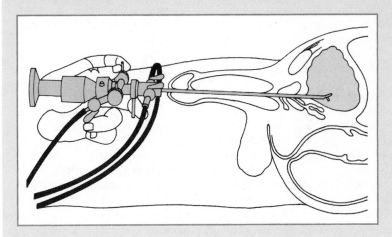

count, or low urine output to the practitioner immediately.

■ Record the patient's intake and output for 24 hours, and observe him for distention. If he doesn't void within 8 hours after the test or if bright red blood continues to appear after three voidings, notify the practitioner.

■ Instruct the patient to abstain from alcohol for 48 hours.

■ Apply heat to the lower abdomen to relieve pain and muscle spasm (if ordered). A warm sitz bath may be ordered.

### Precautions

■ Cystourethroscopy is contraindicated in the patient with acute forms of urethritis, prostatitis, or cystitis because instrumentation can lead to sepsis.

■ The test is also contraindicated in the patient with bleeding disorders because instrumentation can lead to increased bleeding.

### Complications

■ Bleeding
■ Infection
■ Sepsis

## Kidney-ureter-bladder radiography
### [KUB]

Usually the first step in diagnostic testing of the urinary system, kidney-ureter-bladder (KUB) radiography surveys the abdomen to determine the position of the kidneys, ureters, and bladder and to detect gross abnormalities.

This test doesn't require intact renal function and may aid differential diagnosis of urologic and GI diseases, which commonly produce similar signs and symptoms.

## Normal results

- The shadows of the kidneys appear bilaterally, the right slightly lower than the left, and are about the same size, with the superior poles tilted slightly toward the vertebral column, paralleling the shadows (or stripes) produced by the psoas muscles.
- The bladder's shadow can be seen but not as clearly as the kidneys' shadows.

## Abnormal results

- Bilateral renal enlargement may result from polycystic disease, multiple myeloma, lymphoma, amyloidosis, diabetes, hydronephrosis, or compensatory hypertrophy.
- A tumor, a cyst, or hydronephrosis may cause unilateral enlargement.
- Abnormally small kidneys may suggest end-stage glomerulonephritis or bilateral atrophic pyelonephritis.
- An apparent decrease in the size of one kidney suggests possible congenital hypoplasia, atrophic pyelonephritis, or ischemia.
- Renal displacement may be due to a retroperitoneal tumor such as an adrenal tumor.
- Obliteration or bulging of a portion of the psoas muscle stripe may result from a tumor, an abscess, or a hematoma.
- Congenital anomalies, such as abnormal location or absence of a kidney, may be detected.
- Horseshoe kidney may be suggested by renal axes that parallel the vertebral column, especially if the inferior poles of the kidneys can't be clearly distinguished.
- A lobulated edge or border may suggest polycystic kidney disease or patchy atrophic pyelonephritis.

- Opaque bodies may reflect calculi or vascular calcification due to aneurysm or atheroma; opacification may also suggest cystic tumors, fecaliths, foreign bodies, or abnormal fluid collection.
- Calcifications may appear anywhere in the urinary system, but positive identification requires further testing. The lone exception is staghorn calculus, which forms a perfect cast of the renal pelvis and calyces.

## Purpose

- To evaluate the size, structure, and position of the kidneys
- To screen for abnormalities, such as calcifications, in the region of the kidneys, ureters, and bladder

## Patient preparation

- Explain that KUB radiography helps detect urinary system abnormalities.
- Inform the patient that he doesn't need to restrict food and fluids. Tell him who will perform the test, where it will take place, and that it takes only a few minutes.

## Procedure and posttest care

- Confirm the patient's identity using two patient identifiers according to facility policy.
- The patient is placed in a supine position in correct body alignment on an X-ray table. His arms are extended overhead, and the iliac crests are checked for symmetrical positioning.
- If the patient can't extend his arms or stand, he may lie on his left side with his right arm up.
- A single X-ray is taken.

## Precautions

- A male patient should have gonadal shielding to prevent irradiation of the testes. A female patient's ovaries can't be shielded because they're too close to the kidneys, ureters, and bladder.

# Magnetic resonance imaging of the urinary tract

Magnetic resonance imaging (MRI) is becoming more commonly used for diagnosing urinary tract disorders. It's unclear at present whether MRI is better than computed tomography or ultrasound for imaging the urinary system. In most cases, MRI is used when these alternative tests fail to produce a clear image. MRI uses radio-frequency waves and magnetic fields to visualize specific structures (kidney or prostate), which are then converted to computer-generated images.

## Normal results

- Visualization of the soft tissue structures of the kidneys appears normal.
- Visualization of the blood vessels appears normal.

## Abnormal results

- Tumors, strictures, stenosis, thrombosis, malformations, abscess, inflammation, edema, fluid collection, bleeding, hemorrhage, and organ atrophy may be revealed.

## Purpose

- To evaluate genitourinary tumors and abdominal or pelvic masses
- To detect prostate stones and cysts
- To detect cancer invasion into seminal vesicles and pelvic lymph nodes

## Patient preparation

- Explain that MRI of the urinary tract helps evaluate abnormalities in the urinary system.
- Advise the patient to avoid alcohol, caffeine-containing beverages, and smoking for at least 2 hours and food for at least 1 hour before the test.

- Tell the patient who will perform the test, where it will take place, and that it takes about 30 to 90 minutes.
- Explain that he can continue taking medications, except for iron, which interferes with the imaging.
- Tell him that he'll need to remove all clothing, jewelry, and metallic objects and wear a special hospital gown without snaps or closures.
- Inform the patient that he won't feel pain but may feel claustrophobic while lying supine in the tubular MRI chamber. If so, the practitioner may order an anxiolytic.
- Tell the patient that he'll hear loud clacking noises throughout the test. However, he'll probably receive a headset with a choice of music to decrease the noise level.

**A<small>LERT</small>**

If contrast media will be used, obtain a history of allergies or hypersensitivity to these agents. Mark sensitivities on the chart and notify the practitioner.

- Ask if the patient has any implanted metal devices or prostheses, such as vascular clips, shrapnel, pacemakers, joint implants, filters, and intrauterine devices. If so, the patient may not be able to have the test.
- Make sure that the patient or a responsible family member has signed an informed consent form.
- Just before the procedure, have the patient urinate.

## Procedure and posttest care

- Confirm the patient's identity using two patient identifiers according to facility policy.
- The patient is placed in the supine position on a narrow, flat table, and the table is then moved into the enclosed cylindrical scanner.

- Varying radio-frequency waves are directed at the area being scanned.
- The patient is told to lie very still in the scanner while the images are being produced.
- Although his face remains uncovered to allow him to see out, the patient is advised to keep his eyes closed to promote relaxation and prevent a closed-in feeling.
- If nausea occurs because of claustrophobia, the patient is encouraged to take deep breaths.
- If sedatives were given, monitor the patient's vital signs until he's awake and responsive.
- Advise the patient that he may resume his usual diet, fluids, and medications, as ordered.

### Precautions

- This test is contraindicated in the patient with metal implants, rods, or screws or prosthetic devices.
- This test is contraindicated in the pregnant patient unless its benefits greatly outweigh the possible risks to the fetus.

### Complications

- Anxiety
- Adverse reaction to the contrast medium

# Nephrotomography

In nephrotomography, special films are exposed before and after opacification of the renal arterial network and parenchyma with contrast medium. The resulting tomographic slices clearly delineate various linear layers of the kidneys, while blurring structures in front of and behind these selected planes.

Nephrotomography can be performed as a separate procedure or as an adjunct to excretory urography. Nephrotomography is particularly helpful in vi-

sualizing space-occupying lesions suggested by excretory urography or retrograde ureteropyelography. Additional films are exposed to define the wall thickness of the mass and its interior.

### Normal findings

- The size, shape, and position of the kidneys appear within normal range, with no space-occupying lesions or other abnormalities.

### Abnormal findings

- Simple cysts and solid tumors, renal sinus–related lesions, ectopic renal lobes, adrenal tumors, areas of nonperfusion, and renal lacerations following trauma may be detected. (See *Simple cyst or solid tumor: Differential diagnosis in nephrotomography.*)

### Purpose

- To differentiate between a simple renal cyst and a solid neoplasm
- To assess renal lacerations as well as posttraumatic nonperfused areas of the kidneys
- To localize adrenal tumors when laboratory tests indicate their presence

### Patient preparation

- Explain to the patient that nephrotomography provides images of sections or layers of the kidney tissues and blood vessels.
- Instruct the patient to fast for 8 hours before the test. Tell him who will perform the test and where it will take place.
- Tell the patient that he'll be positioned on an X-ray table and that he may hear loud, clacking sounds as the films are exposed. Tell him that he may experience transient adverse effects from the contrast medium injection—usually a burning or stinging sensation at the injection site, flushing, and a metallic taste.

## Simple cyst or solid tumor: Differential diagnosis in nephrotomography

| Feature | Cyst | Tumor |
| --- | --- | --- |
| Consistency | Homogeneous | Irregular |
| Contact with healthy renal tissue | Sharply distinct | Poorly resolved |
| Density | Radiolucent | Variable radiolucent patches (or same as normal renal parenchyma) |
| Shape | Spheric | Variable |
| Wall of lesion | Thin and well defined | Thick and irregular |

■ Make sure that the patient or a responsible family member has signed an informed consent form.

 Check the patient's history for hypersensitivity to iodine or iodine-containing foods or to contrast media used in other diagnostic tests. If he has a history of sensitivity, provide antiallergenic prophylaxis (such as diphenhydramine) or use a non–iodine-containing contrast medium, as necessary.

■ An elderly, diabetic, or dehydrated patient is at increased risk for contrast-induced renal failure. Check serum creatinine levels and inform the practitioner if they're elevated. I.V. fluids may be ordered before the test to ensure hydration and decrease nephrotoxic potential.

### Procedure and posttest care
■ Confirm the patient's identity using two patient identifiers according to facility policy.
■ The test may be performed using either the infusion method or bolus method. Complications resulting from either technique are minor and infrequent.
■ A plain film of the kidneys is exposed to provide general information about their position, size, and shape, and preliminary anteroposterior tomograms are made to determine tomographic levels. Posterior oblique tomograms are made to rule out the presence of radiopaque renal calculi, which would be masked by the contrast medium.

### Infusion method
■ After test tomograms are reviewed, five vertical slices of renal parenchyma ⅜″ (1 cm) apart are selected for filming.
■ Contrast medium is then administered through the antecubital vein—the first half in 4 to 5 minutes (rapid phase) and the second half in the following 8 to 10 minutes (slow phase). Serial tomograms are made as soon as the slow phase begins.

### Bolus method
■ After test tomograms are reviewed, circulation time from arm to tongue is determined by injecting a bolus of a

bitter-tasting agent (dehydrocholic acid or sodium dehydrocholate) into the antecubital vein. Arm-to-tongue circulation time is close to arm-to-kidney circulation time.

- With the needle still in place, a loading dose of a conventional urographic contrast medium is injected to perform excretory urography.
- Five minutes after this injection, a loading dose of a contrast medium is quickly injected to ensure a high concentration of the contrast medium in the kidneys. A multi-film tomographic cassette, exposed at the predetermined arm-to-kidney circulation time, visualizes the main renal vessels and possible vessels within tumors.
- A series of individual tomograms measuring 1 cm are then made in rapid succession through the opacified kidneys.
- If the exposures are poor, this method requires a second infusion of contrast medium because normal kidneys quickly clear the substance.

### Both methods

- If a hematoma develops at the injection site, apply warm soaks.
- Monitor the patient's vital signs and urine output for 24 hours after the test.
- Ensure adequate hydration (unless contraindicated) and monitor serum creatinine levels because of the risk of contrast-induced renal failure.

Alert

 Observe for signs of a posttest allergic reaction (flushing, nausea, urticaria, and sneezing). Have epinephrine (1:1,000) and an antihistamine readily available to counter allergic reactions.

### Precautions

- Nephrotomography should be performed with extreme caution in the patient with hypersensitivity to iodine-based compounds, cardiovascular disease, or multiple myeloma and in an elderly or a dehydrated patient with impaired renal function, as evidenced by elevated serum creatinine.

### Complications

- Adverse reaction to the contrast medium
- Impaired renal function

# Renal computed tomography

Renal computed tomography (CT) scan provides a useful image of the kidneys made from a series of tomograms or cross-sectional slices, which are then translated by a computer and displayed on a monitor. The image density reflects the amount of radiation absorbed by renal tissue and permits identification of masses and other lesions. An I.V. contrast medium may be injected to accentuate the renal parenchyma's density and help differentiate renal masses. This highly accurate test is usually performed to investigate diseases found by other diagnostic procedures such as excretory urography.

### Normal results

- The renal parenchyma is slightly denser than the liver but is much less dense than bone, which appears white on a CT scan.
- The density of the collecting system is generally low (black), unless a contrast medium is used to enhance it to a higher (whiter) density.
- The position of the kidneys is evaluated according to the surrounding structures; their size and shape are determined by counting cuts between the

superior and inferior poles and following the contour of the kidneys' outline.

## Abnormal results

- Renal masses appear as areas of different density than normal parenchyma, possibly altering the kidneys' shape or projecting beyond their margins.
- Renal cysts, for example, appear as smooth, sharply defined masses with thin walls and a lower density than normal parenchyma.
- Tumors, such as renal cell carcinoma, however, are usually not as well delineated; they tend to have thick walls and nonuniform density.
- With contrast enhancement, solid tumors show a higher density than renal cysts, but lower density than normal parenchyma.
- Tumors with hemorrhage, calcification, or necrosis show higher densities.
- Vascular tumors are more clearly defined with contrast enhancement.
- Adrenal tumors are confined masses, usually detached from the kidneys and from other retroperitoneal organs.
- Abnormal accumulations of fluid around the kidneys may indicate hematomas, lymphoceles, and abscesses.
- After nephrectomy, CT can detect abnormal masses, such as recurrent tumors, in a renal fossa, which should be empty.

## Purpose

- To detect and evaluate renal abnormalities, such as a tumor, an obstruction, calculi, polycystic kidney disease, congenital anomalies, and abnormal fluid accumulation around the kidneys
- To evaluate the retroperitoneum

## Patient preparation

- Explain that renal CT permits examination of the kidneys.

- If contrast enhancement isn't scheduled, inform the patient that he doesn't need to restrict food and fluids. If contrast enhancement is scheduled, instruct him to fast for 4 hours before the test.
- Tell the patient who will perform the test and where it will take place.
- Inform him that he'll be positioned on an X-ray table and that a scanner will take films of his kidneys.
- Warn the patient that the scanner may make loud clacking noises as it rotates around his body.
- Tell the patient that he may experience transient adverse effects, such as flushing, a metallic taste, and headache, after contrast medium injection.
- Make sure that the patient or a responsible family member has signed an informed consent form.

**ALERT**

Check the patient's history for hypersensitivity to iodine-based contrast media or iodine-containing foods such as shellfish. Mark sensitivities on the chart and inform the practitioner because the patient may require prophylactic antiallergenics (diphenhydramine or corticosteroids).

- Just before the procedure, instruct the patient to put on a gown and to remove any metallic objects that could interfere with the scan.
- Administer prescribed sedatives.

## Procedure and posttest care

- Confirm the patient's identity using two patient identifiers according to facility policy.
- The patient is placed in a supine position on the X-ray table and secured with straps.
- The table is moved into the scanner.
- Instruct the patient to lie still.

- The scanner then rotates around the patient, taking multiple images at different angles within each cross-sectional slice.
- When one series of tomograms is complete, I.V. contrast enhancement may be performed. Another series of tomograms is then taken.
- After the I.V. contrast medium is given, monitor the patient for allergic reactions, such as respiratory difficulty, urticaria, or skin eruptions.
- Information from the scan is stored on a disk or magnetic tape, fed into a computer, and then converted into an image for display on a monitor. Radiographs and photographs are taken of selected views.
- After the test, tell the patient that he may resume his usual diet.
- If calculi are present, strain urine, hydrate the patient, and discuss nutritional adaptations as indicated.
- Support the patient and his family if surgery is indicated for a neoplasm.
- Monitor the patient's vital signs if a sedative was given.

## Complications
- Hypersensitivity to the contrast medium

# Renal ultrasonography

In renal ultrasonography, high-frequency sound waves are transmitted from a transducer to the kidneys and perirenal structures. The resulting echoes are displayed on a monitor as anatomic images.

Renal ultrasonography can be used to detect abnormalities or clarify those detected by other tests. It's especially useful in cases in which excretory urography is ruled out. Unlike excretory urography, this test isn't dependent on renal function and therefore may be useful in the patient with renal failure. Ultrasonography of the ureter, bladder, and gonads also may be used to evaluate urologic disorders.

## Normal results
- The kidneys are located between the superior iliac crests and the diaphragm.
- The renal capsule should be outlined sharply; the cortex should produce more echoes than the medulla.
- In the center of each kidney, the renal collecting systems appear as irregular areas of higher density than surrounding tissue.
- If the bladder is also being evaluated, its size, shape, position, and urine content can be determined.

## Abnormal results
- Cysts are usually fluid-filled, circular structures that don't reflect sound waves.
- Tumors produce multiple echoes and appear as irregular shapes.
- Abscesses found within or around the kidneys usually echo sound waves poorly; their boundaries are slightly more irregular than those of cysts. A perirenal abscess may displace the kidney anteriorly.
- Hydronephrosis may show a large, echo-free, central mass that compresses the renal cortex. Calyceal echoes are usually circularly diffused and the pelvis significantly enlarged.
- After kidney transplantation, compensatory hypertrophy of the transplanted kidney is normal, but an acute increase in size indicates rejection.
- Increased urine volume or residual urine after voiding may indicate bladder outlet obstruction.

## Purpose
- To determine the size, shape, and position of the kidneys, their internal structures, and perirenal tissues

- To evaluate and localize urinary obstruction and abnormal fluid accumulation
- To assess and diagnose complications after kidney transplantation
- To detect renal or perirenal masses
- To differentiate between renal cysts and solid masses
- To verify placement of a nephrostomy tube

### Patient preparation

- Explain to the patient that renal ultrasonography is used to detect kidney abnormalities.
- Inform the patient that he doesn't need to restrict food and fluids.
- Tell the patient who will perform the test, where it will take place, and that it's safe and painless.

### Procedure and posttest care

- Confirm the patient's identity using two patient identifiers according to facility policy.
- The patient is placed in the prone position, the area to be scanned is exposed, and conductive gel is applied.
- The longitudinal axis of the kidneys is located by using measurements from excretory urography or by performing transverse scans through the upper and lower renal poles.
- These points are marked on the skin and connected with straight lines. Sectional images ⅜″ to ¾″ (1 to 2 cm) apart can then be obtained by moving the transducer longitudinally, transversely, or at any other angle required.
- During the test, the patient may be asked to breathe deeply to visualize upper portions of the kidney.
- After the test, remove the conductive gel from the patient's skin.
- If bladder abnormalities are found, prepare the patient for further testing.
- If rejection of a transplanted kidney is suspected or diagnosed, monitor the patient's intake and output, blood pressure, blood urea nitrogen and creatinine levels, and vital signs. Also, watch for signs of adrenal dysfunction (hypotension, decreased urine output, and electrolyte imbalances) if a tumor is detected on the gland.
- If ultrasonography is used as a guide for nephrostomy tube placement or abscess drainage, monitor the amount and characteristics of drainage and tube patency.

# Retrograde cystography

Retrograde cystography involves the instillation of contrast medium into the bladder, followed by radiographic examination. This procedure is used to diagnose bladder rupture without urethral involvement because it can determine the location and extent of the rupture. Other indications for retrograde cystography include neurogenic bladder; recurrent urinary tract infections (UTIs), especially in children; suspected vesicoureteral reflux; and vesical fistulas, diverticula, and tumors. This test is also performed when cystoscopic examination is impractical, as in male infants, or when excretory urography hasn't adequately visualized the bladder. Voiding cystourethrography is commonly performed concomitantly.

### Normal results

- The bladder has normal contours, capacity, integrity, and urethrovesical angle, with no evidence of a tumor, diverticula, or a rupture.
- Vesicoureteral reflux is absent.
- The bladder isn't displaced or externally compressed; the bladder wall is smooth, not thick.

## Abnormal results

- Vesical trabeculae or diverticula, space-occupying lesions (tumors), calculi or gravel, blood clots, high- or low-pressure vesicoureteral reflux, and a hypotonic or hypertonic bladder may be detected.

## Purpose

- To evaluate the structure and integrity of the bladder

## Patient preparation

- Explain that retrograde cystography permits radiographic examination of the bladder.
- Inform the patient that he doesn't need to restrict food and fluids.
- Tell him who will perform the test and where it will take place.
- Inform the patient that he may experience some discomfort when the catheter is inserted and when the contrast medium is instilled through the catheter.
- Tell him that he may hear loud clacking noises as the X-ray films are exposed.
- Make sure that the patient or a responsible family member has signed an informed consent form.

**A**LERT

Check the patient's history for hypersensitivity to iodine-based contrast media or iodine-containing foods such as shellfish. Mark sensitivities on the chart and inform the practitioner because the patient may require prophylactic antiallergenics (diphenhydramine or corticosteroids).

## Procedure and posttest care

- Confirm the patient's identity using two patient identifiers according to facility policy.
- The patient is placed in a supine position on the X-ray table and a preliminary kidney-ureter-bladder radiograph is taken.
- The radiograph is developed immediately and scrutinized for renal shadows, calcifications, contours of the bone and psoas muscles, and gas patterns in the lumen of the GI tract.
- The bladder is catheterized and 200 to 300 ml of sterile contrast medium (50 to 100 ml for an infant) is instilled by gravity or gentle syringe injection. The catheter is then clamped.
- With the patient in a supine position, an anteroposterior film is taken. The patient is then tilted to one side, then the other, and two posterior oblique (and sometimes lateral) views are taken.
- If the patient's condition permits, he's placed in the jackknife position and a posteroanterior film is taken. A space-occupying vesical lesion may require additional exposures. Rarely, to enhance visualization, 100 to 300 ml of air may be insufflated into the bladder by syringe after removal of the contrast medium (double-contrast technique).
- The catheter is then unclamped, the bladder fluid is allowed to drain, and a radiograph is obtained to detect urethral diverticula, reflux into the ureters, fistulous tracts into the vagina, or intraperitoneal or extraperitoneal extravasation of the contrast medium.
- Monitor the patient's vital signs every 15 minutes for the first hour, every 30 minutes during the second hour, and then every 2 hours for up to 24 hours.
- Record the time of the patient's voidings and the color and volume of the urine. Observe for hematuria that persists after the third voiding and notify the practitioner.
- Watch for signs of urinary sepsis from UTIs (chills, fever, elevated pulse and respiration rates, and hypotension) or similar signs related to extravasation of contrast medium into the general circulation.

- Prepare the patient for surgery and urinary diversion, if indicated. Strain urine if calculi are detected.
- Watch for retention or distention if neurogenic bladder is diagnosed and give medication, as ordered (baclofen for spasms; bethanechol chloride for hypotonic bladder).
- Discuss the use of a percutaneous stimulator if one is being contemplated. Teach self-catheterization, if indicated for neurogenic bladder.

### Precautions

- Retrograde cystography is contraindicated during exacerbation of an acute UTI or when an obstruction prevents passage of a urinary catheter.
- This test shouldn't be performed in the patient with urethral evulsion or transection, unless catheter passage and flow of contrast medium are monitored fluoroscopically.

### Complications

- Hematuria
- Urinary sepsis

# Retrograde ureteropyelography

Retrograde ureteropyelography allows radiographic examination of the renal collecting system after injection of a contrast medium through a ureteral catheter during cystoscopy. The contrast medium is usually iodine-based and although some of it may be absorbed through the mucous membranes, this test is preferred for the patient with hypersensitivity to iodine (in whom I.V. administration of an iodine-based contrast medium, as in excretory urography, is contraindicated). This test is also indicated when visualization of the renal collecting system by excretory urography is inadequate due to inferior films or marked renal insufficiency because

retrograde ureteropyelography isn't influenced by impaired renal function.

### Normal findings

- Opacification of the pelves and calyces should occur immediately.
- Normal structures should be outlined clearly and should appear symmetrical in bilateral testing.
- Ureters should fill uniformly and appear normal in size and course.
- Inspiratory and expiratory exposures, when superimposed, normally create two outlines of the renal pelvis ³/₄" (2 cm) apart.

### Abnormal findings

- Incomplete or delayed drainage reflects an obstruction, most commonly at the ureteropelvic junction.
- Enlargement of the components of the collecting system or delayed emptying of contrast medium may indicate obstruction due to a tumor, a blood clot, a stricture, or calculi.
- Perinephric inflammation or suppuration commonly causes fixation of the kidney on the same side, resulting in a single sharp radiographic outline of the collecting system when inspiratory and expiratory exposures are superimposed.
- Upward, downward, or lateral renal displacement can result from a renal abscess or tumor or from a perinephric abscess.
- Neoplasms can cause displacement of either pole or of the entire kidney.

### Purpose

- To assess the structure and integrity of the renal collecting system (calyces, renal pelvis, and ureter) (see *Sites and types of obstruction indicated by ureteropyelography,* page 600)

## Sites and types of obstruction indicated by ureteropyelography

Ureteropyelography may detect a stricture, neoplasm, blood clot, or calculus that obstructs urine flow in the calyces, pelvis, or ureter. Small calculi may remain in the calyces and pelvis or pass down the ureter. A staghorn calculus (a cast of the calyceal and pelvic collecting system) may form from a calculus that stays in the kidney.

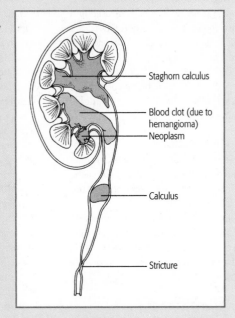

Staghorn calculus

Blood clot (due to hemangioma)

Neoplasm

Calculus

Stricture

### Patient preparation

■ Explain to the patient that retrograde ureteropyelography permits visualization of the urinary collecting system.
■ If a general anesthetic is to be used, instruct the patient to fast for 8 hours before the test. Generally, he should be well hydrated to ensure adequate urine flow.
■ Tell the patient who will perform the test and where it will take place.
■ Inform the patient that he'll be positioned on an examination table, with his legs in stirrups, and that the position may be tiring.
■ If the patient will be awake throughout the procedure, tell him that he may feel pressure as the instrument is passed and a pressure sensation in the kidney area when the contrast medium is intro-

duced. Also, he may feel an urgency to void.
■ Make sure that the patient or a responsible family member has signed an informed consent form.
■ Administer prescribed premedication just before the procedure.

### Procedure and posttest care

■ Confirm the patient's identity using two patient identifiers according to facility policy.
■ Place the patient in the lithotomy position. Care must be taken to avoid pressure points or impairment to circulation while his legs are in the stirrups.
■ After the patient is anesthetized, the urologist first performs a cystoscopic examination.

- After visual inspection of the bladder, one or both ureters are catheterized with opaque catheters, depending on the condition or abnormality suspected. Radiographic monitoring allows correct positioning of the catheter tip in the renal pelvis.
- The renal pelvis is emptied by gravity drainage or aspiration. About 5 ml of contrast medium is then slowly injected through the catheter using the syringe with the special adapter.
- When adequate filling and opacification have occurred, anteroposterior radiographic films are taken and immediately developed. Lateral and oblique films can be taken, as needed, after the injection of more contrast medium.
- After the radiographs of the renal pelvis are examined, a few more milliliters of contrast medium are injected to outline the ureters as the catheter is slowly withdrawn.
- Delayed films (10 to 15 minutes after complete catheter removal) are then taken to check for contrast medium retention, indicating urinary stasis.
- If ureteral obstruction is present, the ureteral catheter may be kept in place and, together with an indwelling urinary catheter, connected to a gravity drainage system until posttest urinary flow is corrected or returns to normal.
- Check the patient's vital signs every 15 minutes for the first hour, every 30 minutes for 1 hour, every hour for the next 4 hours, and then every 4 hours for 24 hours.
- Monitor the patient's fluid intake and urine output for 24 hours. Observe each specimen for hematuria. Gross hematuria or hematuria after the third voiding is abnormal and should be reported. If the patient doesn't void for 8 hours after the procedure or if the patient immediately feels distress and his bladder is distended, urethral catheterization may be necessary.

- Be especially attentive to catheter output if ureteral catheters have been left in place because inadequate output may reflect catheter obstruction, requiring irrigation. Protect ureteral catheters from dislodgment. Note output amounts for each catheter (indwelling, urinary, urethral) separately; this helps determine the location of an obstruction that's causing reduced output.
- Administer prescribed analgesics, tub baths, and increased fluid intake for dysuria, which commonly occurs after retrograde ureteropyelography.

**ALERT**

 Watch for and report severe pain in the area of the kidneys as well as any signs of sepsis (such as chills, fever, and hypotension).

## Precautions

- Retrograde ureteropyelography must be done carefully in the patient with urinary stasis caused by ureteral obstruction to prevent further injury to the ureter.
- This test is contraindicated in the pregnant patient unless the benefits of the procedure outweigh the risks to the fetus.
- The test is contraindicated also in patients with an active UTI.
- If irrigation is ordered, never use more than 10 ml of sterile saline solution.

## Complications
- Hematuria

# Retrograde urethrography

Used almost exclusively in men, retrograde urethrography requires instillation or injection of a contrast medium into the urethra and permits visualization of its membranous, bulbar, and penile portions.

Although visualization of the anterior portion of the urethra is excellent with this test alone, the posterior portion is more effectively outlined by retrograde urethrography in tandem with voiding cystourethrography.

## Normal results

- The membranous, bulbar, and penile portions of the urethra—and occasionally the prostatic portion—appear normal in size, shape, and course.

## Abnormal results

- Radiographs obtained during retrograde urethrography may show urethral diverticula, fistulas, strictures, false passages, calculi, and lacerations; congenital anomalies, such as urethral valves and perineal hypospadias; and, rarely, tumors (in less than 1% of cases).

## Purpose

- To diagnose urethral strictures, diverticula, and congenital anomalies
- To assess urethral lacerations or other trauma
- To assist with follow-up examination after surgical repair of the urethra

## Patient preparation

- Explain that retrograde urethrography diagnoses urethral structural problems.
- Inform the patient that he doesn't need to restrict food and fluids.
- Describe the test, including who will perform it and where it will take place.
- Inform the patient that he may experience some discomfort when the catheter is inserted and when the contrast medium is instilled through the catheter.
- Tell him that he may hear loud clacking noises as the X-ray films are exposed.

- Make sure that the patient or a responsible family member has signed an informed consent form.

**ALERT**

 Check the patient's history for hypersensitivity to iodine-based contrast media or iodine-containing foods such as shellfish. Mark sensitivities on the chart and inform the practitioner because the patient may require prophylactic antiallergenics (diphenhydramine or corticosteroids).

- Give prescribed sedatives just before the procedure, and instruct the patient to void before leaving the unit.

## Procedure and posttest care

- Confirm the patient's identity using two patient identifiers according to facility policy.

### *For men*

- The patient is placed in a recumbent position on the examining table. Anteroposterior exposures of the bladder and urethra are made, and the resulting films studied for radiopaque densities, foreign bodies, or calculi.
- The glans and meatus are cleaned with an antiseptic solution. The catheter is filled with the contrast medium before insertion to eliminate air bubbles.
- Although no lubricant should be used, the tip of the catheter may be dipped in sterile water to ease insertion.
- The catheter is inserted until the balloon portion is inside the meatus; the balloon is then inflated with 1 to 2 ml of water, which prevents the catheter from slipping during the procedure.
- The patient then assumes the right posterior oblique position, with his right thigh drawn up to a 90-degree angle and the penis placed along its axis. The left thigh is extended.

- The contrast medium is injected through the catheter. After three-quarters of the contrast medium has been injected, the first X-ray film is exposed while the remainder of the contrast medium is being injected. Left lateral oblique views may also be taken.
- Fluoroscopic control may be helpful, especially for evaluating urethral injury.

### For women and children
- In women, this test may be used when urethral diverticula are suspected. A double-balloon catheter is used, which occludes the bladder neck from above and the external meatus from below.
- In children, the procedure is the same as for adults except that a smaller catheter is used.

### For all patients
ALERT

 Watch for chills and fever related to extravasation of contrast medium into the general circulation for 12 to 24 hours after retrograde urethrography.

### Precautions
- Retrograde urethrography should be performed cautiously in the patient with a urinary tract infection.

### Complications
- Infection
- Extravasation of the contrast medium

# Structure and function tests

 ## Excretory urography
### [I.V. pyelography, IVP]
The cornerstone of a urologic workup, excretory urography requires I.V. administration of a contrast medium and allows visualization of the renal parenchyma, calyces, and pelvis as well as the ureters, bladder and, in some cases, the urethra.

In some facilities, a nonenhanced computed tomography scan of the urinary tract is commonly performed instead of this test if urinary tract stones are suspected.

### Normal results
- The kidneys, ureters, and bladder show no gross evidence of soft- or hard-tissue lesions.
- Prompt visualization of the contrast medium in the kidneys demonstrates bilateral renal parenchyma and pelvicaliceal systems of normal conformity.
- The ureters and bladder should be outlined, and the postvoiding radiograph should show no mucosal abnormalities and minimal residual urine.

### Abnormal results
- Renal or ureteral calculi; abnormal size, shape, or structure of kidneys, ureters, or bladder; a supernumerary or an absent kidney; polycystic kidney disease associated with renal hypertrophy; a redundant pelvis or ureter; a space-occupying lesion; pyelonephrosis; renal tuberculosis; hydronephrosis; and renovascular hypertension may be detected.

### Purpose
- To evaluate the structure and excretory function of the kidneys, ureters, and bladder

- To support a suspected differential diagnosis of renovascular hypertension

## Patient preparation

- Explain to the patient that excretory urography helps to evaluate the structure and function of the urinary tract.
- Make sure that the patient is well hydrated; then instruct him to fast for 8 hours before the test.
- Tell him who will perform the test and where it will take place.
- Obtain blood urea nitrogen (BUN) and creatinine levels, as ordered.
- Inform the patient that he may experience a transient burning sensation and metallic taste when the contrast medium is injected. Tell him to report other sensations he may experience.
- Warn the patient that the X-ray machine may make loud clacking noises during the test.
- Make sure that the patient or a responsible family member has signed an informed consent form.

ALERT

Check the patient's history for hypersensitivity to iodine, iodine-containing foods, or contrast media containing iodine. Mark sensitivities on the chart and notify the practitioner.

- Administer a laxative, if necessary, the night before the test, to minimize poor resolution of X-ray films due to stool and gas in the GI tract.

## Procedure and posttest care

- Confirm the patient's identity using two patient identifiers according to facility policy.
- The patient is placed in a supine position on the X-ray table.
- A kidney-ureter-bladder radiograph is exposed, developed, and studied for gross abnormalities of the urinary system. Contrast medium is injected (dosage varies according to age), and the patient is observed for signs of hypersensitivity (flushing, nausea, vomiting, hives, or dyspnea).
- The first radiograph, visualizing the renal parenchyma, is obtained about 1 minute after the injection, possibly supplemented by tomography if small space-occupying masses, such as cysts or tumors, are suspected.
- Films are then exposed at regular intervals—usually 5, 10, and 15 or 20 minutes after the injection.
- Ureteral compression is performed after the 5-minute film is exposed. This can be accomplished through inflation of two small rubber bladders placed on the abdomen on both sides of the midline, secured by a fastener wrapped around the patient's torso. The inflated bladders occlude the ureters without causing the patient discomfort and facilitate retention of the contrast medium by the upper urinary tract.
- After the 10-minute film is exposed, ureteral compression is released. As the contrast flows into the lower urinary tract, another film is taken of the lower halves of both ureters and then, finally, one is taken of the bladder.
- At the end of the procedure, the patient voids, and another film is made immediately to visualize residual bladder content or mucosal abnormalities of the bladder or urethra.
- If a hematoma develops at the injection site, apply warm soaks.
- Observe the patient for delayed reactions to the contrast medium.
- Continue I.V. fluids or provide oral fluid to increase hydration. Administer medications, as ordered.

## Precautions

- Premedication with corticosteroids may be indicated for the patient with severe asthma or a history of sensitivity to the contrast medium.

- This test may be contraindicated in the patient with abnormal renal function (as evidenced by increased creatinine and BUN levels) and in a child or an elderly patient with actual or potential dehydration.

- Ureteral compression is contraindicated by ureteral calculi, aortic aneurysm, pregnancy, or recent abdominal trauma or surgical procedure.

### Complications

- Adverse reaction to the contrast medium
- Dehydration
- Impaired renal function

# Radionuclide renal imaging

Radionuclide renal imaging, which involves I.V. injection of a radionuclide followed by scintigraphy, provides a wealth of information for evaluating the kidneys. Observing the uptake concentration and transit of the radionuclide during this test allows assessment of renal blood flow, renal structure, and nephron and collecting system function. Depending on the patient's clinical presentation, this procedure may include dynamic scans to assess renal perfusion and function or static scans to assess structure.

### Normal results

- Renal perfusion should be evident immediately following uptake of the $^{99m}$Tc in the abdominal aorta.
- Within 1 to 2 minutes, a normal pattern of renal circulation should appear.
- The radionuclide should delineate the kidneys simultaneously, symmetrically, and with equal intensity.
- Kidneys are normal in size, shape, and position.

- Maximum counts of the radionuclide in the kidneys occur within 5 minutes after injection (and within 1 minute of each other) and should fall to about one-third or less of the maximum counts in the same kidney within 25 minutes.

- Within this time, kidney function can be compared as the concentration of radionuclide shifts from the cortex to the pelvis and, finally, to the bladder.

- Renal function is best evaluated by comparing these images with the renogram curves.

- Total function is considered normal when the effective renal plasma flow is 420 ml/minute or greater and the percentage of the dose excreted in the urine at 30 to 35 minutes is greater than 66%.

### Abnormal results

- Impeded renal circulation, such as that caused by trauma and renal artery stenosis or renal infarction, may be observed.

- Abnormal perfusion may indicate obstruction of the vascular grafts.

- The function study can detect abnormalities of the collecting system and urine extravasation.

- Markedly decreased tubular function causes reduced radionuclide activity in the collecting system; outflow obstruction causes decreased radionuclide activity in the tubules, with increased activity in the collecting system.

- Static images can demonstrate lesions, congenital abnormalities, and traumatic injury. They may also detect space-occupying lesions within or surrounding the kidney, such as tumors, infarcts, and inflammatory masses (abscesses, for example). Static images can also identify congenital disorders, such as horseshoe kidney and polycystic kidney disease.

- A lower-than-normal total concentration of the radionuclide, as opposed to focal defects, suggests a diffuse renal disorder, such as acute tubular necrosis, severe infection, or ischemia.

■ In a patient who has had a kidney transplant, decreased radionuclide uptake generally indicates organ rejection.

■ Failure of visualization may indicate congenital ectopia or aplasia.

**DRUG CHALLENGE**

Antihypertensives (possible masking of abnormalities)

## Purpose

■ To detect and assess functional and structural renal abnormalities (such as lesions and renovascular hypertension) and acute or chronic disease (such as pyelonephritis or glomerulonephritis)

■ To assess renal transplantation or renal injury due to trauma to the urinary tract or obstruction

## Patient preparation

■ Explain to the patient that radionuclide renal imaging permits the evaluation of the structure, blood flow, and function of the kidneys.

■ Tell the patient who will perform the test and where it will take place.

■ Inform the patient that he'll receive an injection of a radionuclide and that he may experience transient flushing and nausea.

■ Emphasize to the patient that only a small amount of radionuclide is administered and that it's usually excreted within 24 hours.

■ Tell the patient several series of films will be taken of his bladder. (If static scans are ordered, there will be a delay of several hours before the images are taken.)

■ Make sure that the patient or a responsible family member has signed an informed consent form.

■ Make sure that the patient isn't scheduled for other radionuclide scans on the same day as this test.

■ If the patient receives antihypertensive medication, ask the practitioner if it should be withheld before the test.

■ A pregnant patient or a young child may receive supersaturated solution of potassium iodide 1 to 3 hours before the test to block thyroid uptake of iodine.

## Procedure and posttest care

■ Confirm the patient's identity using two patient identifiers according to facility policy.

■ The patient is commonly placed in a prone position so that posterior views may be obtained. If the test is being performed to evaluate transplantation, the patient is positioned supine for anterior views.

■ Instruct the patient not to change his position.

■ A perfusion study (radionuclide angiography) is performed first to evaluate renal blood flow. The $^{99m}$Tc is administered intravenously, and rapid-sequence photographs (one per second) are taken for 1 minute.

■ Next, a function study is performed to measure the transit time of the radionuclide through the kidneys' functional units. After Hippuran is administered I.V., images are obtained at a rate of one per minute for 20 minutes. Alternatively, this entire procedure can be recorded on computer-compatible magnetic tape, and concurrent renogram curves can be plotted.

■ Finally, static images are obtained 4 or more hours later, after the radionuclide has drained through the pelvicaliceal system.

■ Instruct the patient to flush the toilet immediately after each voiding for 24 hours as a radiation precaution.

■ If the patient is incontinent, change bed linens promptly and wear gloves to

maintain standard precautions and prevent unnecessary skin contact.
- Monitor the injection site for signs of hematoma, infection, and discomfort. Apply warm compresses for comfort.
- Monitor the patient's intake and output and electrolyte, acid-base, blood urea nitrogen, and creatinine levels, as indicated.

### Precautions

- This test is contraindicated in a pregnant woman unless the benefits to the mother outweigh the risk to the fetus.

## Renal angiography

Renal angiography requires arterial injection of a contrast medium and permits radiographic examination of the renal vasculature and parenchyma. As the contrast pervades the renal vasculature, rapid-sequence radiographs show the vessels during three phases of filling: arterial, nephrographic, and venous.

This procedure usually follows standard bolus aortography, which shows individual variations in number, size, and condition of the main renal arteries, aberrant vessels, and the relationship of the renal arteries to the aorta.

### Normal results

- Renal arteriographs show normal arborization of the vascular tree and normal architecture of the renal parenchyma.

### Abnormal results

- Renal tumors usually show hypervascularity; renal cysts typically appear as clearly delineated, radiolucent masses.
- Renal artery stenosis caused by arteriosclerosis produces a noticeable constriction in the blood vessels, usually within the proximal portion of its length; this is a crucial finding in confirming renovascular hypertension.

- Renal artery dysplasia usually affects the middle and distal portions of the vessel. Alternating aneurysms and stenotic regions give this rare disorder a characteristic beads-on-a-string appearance.
- In renal infarction, blood vessels may appear to be absent or cut off, with the normal tissue replaced by scar tissue.
- The test may detect renal artery aneurysms (saccular or fusiform) and renal arteriovenous fistula with abnormal widening of and direct passage between the renal artery and renal vein.
- Destruction, distortion, and fibrosis of renal tissue with areas of reduced and tortuous vascularity may be noted in severe or chronic pyelonephritis, and an increase in capsular vessels with abnormal intrarenal circulation may indicate renal abscesses or inflammatory masses.
- In renal trauma, it may detect an intrarenal hematoma, a parenchymal laceration, shattered kidneys, and areas of infarction.
- It may also be useful in distinguishing pseudotumors from tumors or cysts, in evaluating the volume of residual functioning renal tissue in hydronephrosis, and in evaluating donors and recipients before and after renal transplantation.

### Purpose

- To demonstrate the configuration of total renal vasculature before surgical procedures
- To determine the cause of renovascular hypertension, such as from stenosis, thrombotic occlusions, emboli, and aneurysms
- To evaluate chronic renal disease or renal failure
- To investigate renal masses and renal trauma
- To detect complications following kidney transplantation, such as a nonfunctioning shunt or rejection of the donor organ

- To differentiate highly vascular tumors from avascular cysts

## Patient preparation

- Explain to the patient that renal angiography permits visualization of the kidneys, blood vessels, and functional units and aids in diagnosing renal disease or masses.
- Instruct the patient to fast for 8 hours before the test and to drink extra fluids the day before the test and the day after the test to maintain adequate hydration (or to start an I.V. line, if needed). Oral medication may be continued; a special order is needed for the patient with diabetes.
- Tell the patient he may receive a laxative or an enema the evening before the test.
- Tell the patient who will perform the test and where it will take place.
- Describe the procedure to the patient, and inform him that he may experience transient discomfort (flushing, burning sensation, and nausea) during injection of the contrast medium.
- Make sure that the patient or a responsible family member has signed an informed consent form.

### ALERT

Check the patient's history for hypersensitivity to iodine-based contrast media or iodine-containing foods such as shellfish. Mark sensitivities on the chart and inform the practitioner because the patient may require prophylactic antiallergenics (diphenhydramine or corticosteroids).

- Administer prescribed medications (usually a sedative and an opioid analgesic) before the test.
- Instruct the patient to put on a gown and to remove all metallic objects that may interfere with test results.

- Record the patient's baseline vital signs. Ensure that recent laboratory test results (blood urea nitrogen and serum creatinine levels and bleeding studies) are documented on the patient's chart. Verification of adequate renal function and adequate clotting ability is vital.
- Evaluate peripheral pulse sites, and mark them for easy access in postprocedure assessment.
- Ask the patient to void before leaving the unit.

## Procedure and posttest care

- Confirm the patient's identity using two patient identifiers according to facility policy.
- The patient is placed in a supine position, and a peripheral I.V. infusion is started. The skin over the arterial puncture site is cleaned with antiseptic solution, and a local anesthetic is injected.
- The femoral artery is punctured and, under fluoroscopic visualization, cannulated. (If a femoral pulse is absent or the artery is convoluted or plaque-ridden, percutaneous transaxillary, transbrachial, or translumbar catheterization may be performed instead.)
- After passing the flexible guide wire through the artery, the cannula is withdrawn, leaving several inches of wire in the lumen.
- A polyethylene catheter is passed over the wire and advanced, under fluoroscopic guidance, up the femoroiliac vessels to the aorta. The guide wire is removed, and the catheter is flushed with heparin flush solution.
- The contrast medium is injected, and screening aortograms are taken before proceeding.
- On completion of the aortographic study, a renal catheter is exchanged for the vascular catheter.
- To determine the position of the renal arteries and ensure that the tip of the catheter is in the lumen, a test bolus

(3 to 5 ml) of contrast medium is injected immediately.

■ If the patient has no adverse reaction to the contrast medium, 20 to 25 ml of the substance is injected just below the origin of the renal arteries.

■ A series of rapid-sequence X-ray films of the filling of the renal vascular tree is exposed.

■ If additional selective studies are required, the catheter remains in place while the films are examined. If the films are satisfactory, the catheter is removed.

■ Apply a sterile pad firmly to the puncture site for 15 minutes.

■ Before the patient is returned to his room, observe the puncture site for a hematoma.

■ Keep the patient flat in bed and instruct him to keep the punctured leg straight for at least 6 hours or as otherwise ordered.

■ Check the patient's vital signs every 15 minutes for 1 hour, every 30 minutes for 2 hours, and then every hour until they stabilize.

■ Monitor popliteal and dorsalis pedis pulses for adequate perfusion at least every hour for 4 hours. Note the color and temperature of the involved extremity and compare with the uninvolved extremity. Watch for signs of pain or paresthesia in the involved limb.

■ Watch for bleeding or hematomas at the injection site. Keep the pressure dressing in place, and check for bleeding when you check the patient's vital signs. If bleeding occurs, promptly notify the practitioner, and apply direct pressure or a sandbag to the site.

■ Apply cold compresses to the puncture site to reduce edema and lessen pain.

**ALERT**

Provide extra fluids (2,000 to 3,000 ml) in the 24-hour period after the test to prevent nephrotoxicity from the contrast medium. Also monitor the patient for anaphylaxis from the contrast medium. (Signs include cardiorespiratory distress, renal failure, and shock.)

■ Monitor the patient for atrial arrhythmias and evaluate aspartate aminotransferase and lactate dehydrogenase activity if renal stenosis is observed.

### Precautions
■ Renal angiography is contraindicated during pregnancy and in the patient with bleeding tendencies, allergy to contrast media, or renal failure caused by end-stage renal disease.

### Complications
■ Adverse reaction to the contrast medium
■ Hematoma

# Renal venography

Renal venography is a relatively simple procedure allowing radiographic examination of the main renal veins and their tributaries. In this test, contrast medium is injected by percutaneous catheter passed through the femoral vein and inferior vena cava into the renal vein. Indications for renal venography include renal vein thrombosis, a tumor, and venous anomalies.

### Normal results
■ After injection of the contrast medium, opacification of the renal vein and tributaries should occur immediately.
■ Normal renin content of venous blood in an adult in a supine position is 1.5 to 1.6 ng/ml/hour.

## Abnormal results

- Renal vein occlusion near the inferior vena cava or the kidney indicates renal vein thrombosis.
- A clot can usually be identified because it's within the lumen and less sharply outlined than a filling defect.
- A filling defect of the renal vein may indicate obstruction or compression by an extrinsic tumor or retroperitoneal fibrosis. A renal tumor that invades the renal vein or inferior vena cava usually produces a filling defect with a sharply defined border.
- Venous anomalies are indicated by opacification of abnormally positioned or clustered vessels.
- Absence of a renal vein differentiates renal agenesis from a small kidney.
- Elevated renin content in renal venous blood usually indicates essential renovascular hypertension when assay results correspond for both kidneys. Elevated renin levels in one kidney indicate a unilateral lesion and usually require further evaluation by arteriography.

 Salt, antihypertensive drugs, diuretics, estrogen, and hormonal contraceptives

## Purpose

- To detect renal vein thrombosis
- To evaluate renal vein compression due to extrinsic tumors or retroperitoneal fibrosis
- To assess renal tumors and detect invasion of the renal vein or inferior vena cava
- To detect venous anomalies and defects
- To differentiate renal agenesis from a small kidney
- To collect renal venous blood samples for evaluation of renovascular hypertension

## Patient preparation

- Explain to the patient that renal venography permits radiographic study of the renal veins.
- If prescribed, instruct the patient to fast for 4 hours before the test.
- Tell the patient who will perform the test and where it will take place.
- Inform the patient that a catheter will be inserted into a vein in the groin area after he's given a sedative and a local anesthetic.
- Tell the patient that he may feel mild discomfort during injection of the local anesthetic and contrast medium and that he may also feel transient burning and flushing from the contrast medium.
- Warn the patient that the X-ray equipment may make loud, clacking noises as the films are taken.

**A**LERT

 Check the patient's history for hypersensitivity to iodine-based contrast media or iodine-containing foods such as shellfish. Mark sensitivities on the chart and inform the practitioner because the patient may require prophylactic antiallergenics (diphenhydramine or corticosteroids).

- Check the patient's history and any coagulation studies for indications of bleeding disorders.
- If renin assays will be done, check the patient's diet and medications and consult with the health care team. As ordered, restrict the patient's salt intake and discontinue antihypertensive drugs, diuretics, estrogen, and hormonal contraceptives.
- Make sure that the patient or a responsible family member has signed an informed consent form.
- Administer a sedative, if necessary, just before the procedure.

- Record the patient's baseline vital signs. Make sure pretest blood urea nitrogen and urine creatinine levels are adequate because the kidneys clear contrast media.

## Procedure and posttest care

- Confirm the patient's identity using two patient identifiers according to facility policy.
- The patient is placed in a supine position on the X-ray table, with his abdomen centered over the film. The skin over the right femoral vein near the groin is cleaned with antiseptic solution and draped. (The left femoral vein or jugular veins may be used.)
- A local anesthetic is injected and the femoral vein is cannulated.
- Under fluoroscopic guidance, a guide wire is threaded a short distance through the cannula, which is then removed. A catheter is passed over the wire into the inferior vena cava.
- When catheterization of the femoral vein is contraindicated, the right antecubital vein is punctured, and the catheter is inserted and advanced through the right atrium of the heart into the inferior vena cava.
- A test bolus of contrast medium is injected to determine whether the vena cava is patent. If so, the catheter is advanced into the right renal vein and contrast medium (usually 20 to 40 ml) is injected.
- When studies of the right renal vasculature are completed, the catheter is withdrawn into the vena cava, rotated, and guided into the left renal vein.
- If visualization of the renal venous tributaries is indicated, epinephrine can be injected into the ipsilateral renal artery by catheter before contrast medium is injected into the renal vein. Epinephrine temporarily blocks arterial flow and allows filling of distal intrarenal veins. Obstructing the artery briefly with a balloon catheter produces the same effect.

- After anteroposterior films are made, the patient lies in a prone position for posteroanterior films.
- For renin assays, blood samples are withdrawn under fluoroscopy within 15 minutes after venography. After catheter removal, apply pressure to the site for 15 minutes and put on a dressing.
- Check the patient's vital signs and distal pulses every 15 minutes for the first hour, every 30 minutes for the second hour, and then every 2 hours for 24 hours.
- Keep the patient on bed rest for 2 hours.
- Observe the puncture site for bleeding or a hematoma when checking the patient's vital signs; if bleeding occurs, apply pressure. Report bleeding as soon as possible.

**ALERT**

Report signs and symptoms of vein perforation, embolism, and extravasation of contrast medium. These include chills, fever, rapid pulse and respiration, hypotension, dyspnea, and chest, abdominal, or flank pain. Also report complaints of paresthesia or pain in the catheterized limb—symptoms of nerve irritation or vascular compromise.

- Administer prescribed sedatives and antimicrobials.
- Prepare for further arteriography or surgery, as ordered.
- Instruct the patient that he may resume his usual diet and medications as ordered.
- Instruct the patient to increase fluid intake (unless contraindicated) to help clear contrast media.

## Precautions

- Renal venography is contraindicated in severe thrombosis of the inferior vena cava.
- Watch the patient for signs of hypersensitivity to the contrast medium.

## Complications

- Hypersensitivity to the contrast medium
- Paresthesia, vein perforation, and embolism

# Urodynamic tests

# Cystometry

Cystometry assesses the bladder's neuromuscular function by measuring the efficiency of the detrusor muscle reflex, intravesical pressure and capacity, and the bladder's reaction to thermal stimulation. Because results from cystometry can be ambiguous, they're typically supported by results of other tests, such as cystourethrography, excretory urography, and voiding cystourethrography.

## Normal and abnormal results

- For characteristic findings, see *Normal and abnormal cystometry findings.*

**DRUG CHALLENGE**

 Concurrent use of drugs such as antihistamines (possible interference with bladder function)

## Purpose

- To evaluate detrusor muscle function and tonicity
- To help determine the cause of bladder dysfunction

## Patient preparation

- Explain to the patient that cystometry evaluates bladder function.
- Tell the patient that he doesn't need to restrict food and fluids.
- Describe the procedure, including who will perform it, where it will take place, and how long it will last.
- Tell the patient that he'll feel a strong urge to void during the test and that he may feel embarrassed or uncomfortable. Provide reassurance.
- Make sure that the patient or a responsible family member has signed an informed consent form.
- Check the patient's medication history for drugs that may affect test results such as antihistamines.
- Tell the patient to urinate just before the procedure.

## Procedure and posttest care

- Confirm the patient's identity using two patient identifiers according to facility policy.
- Place the patient in a supine position on the examination table.
- A catheter is passed into the bladder to measure the residual urine level. Any difficulty with insertion of the catheter may reflect meatal or urethral obstruction.
- To test the patient's response to thermal sensation, 30 ml of room-temperature physiologic saline solution or sterile water is instilled into the bladder. Then an equal volume of warm (110° to 115° F [43.3° to 46.1° C]) fluid is instilled into the bladder. The patient is asked to report his sensations, such as the need to void, nausea, flushing, discomfort, and a feeling of warmth.
- After the fluid is drained from the patient's bladder, the catheter is connected to the cystometer, and normal saline solution, sterile water, or gas (usually carbon dioxide) is slowly introduced into the bladder. The flow of gas is ad-

# Normal and abnormal cystometry findings

Because cystometry assesses micturition and vesical function, it can aid diagnosis of neurogenic bladder dysfunction. The five main types of neurogenic bladder, as presented in the following chart, result from lesions of the central or peripheral nervous system. Uninhibited neurogenic bladder results from a lesion to the upper motor neuron and causes frequent, usually uncontrollable micturition in the presence of even a small amount of urine. A complete upper motor neuron lesion characterizes reflex neurogenic bladder and causes total loss of conscious sensation and vesical control.

| Feature or response | Normal bladder function | Uninhibited neurogenic bladder (mildly spastic, incomplete upper motor neuron lesion) | Reflex neurogenic bladder (completely spastic, complete upper motor neuron lesion) |
|---|---|---|---|
| Micturition | | | |
| Start | + | +/0 | 0 |
| Stop | + | 0 | 0 |
| Residual urine | 0 | 0 | + |
| Vesical sensation | + | + | 0 |
| First urge to void | 150 to 200 ml | E (< 150 ml) | 0 |
| Bladder capacity | 400 to 500 ml | ↓ | ↓ |
| Bladder contractions | 0 | + | + |
| Intravesical pressure | L | ↑ | ↑ |
| Bulbocavernosus reflex | + | + | ↑ |
| Saddle sensation | + | + | 0 |
| Bethanechol test (exaggerated response) | 0 | + | 0 |
| Ice water test | + | + | + |
| Anal reflex | + | + | + |
| Heat sensation and pain | + | + | 0 |

KEY:
+  = Present/Positive     ↓  = Decreased     D  = Delayed
0  = Absent/Negative     V  = Variable      L  = Low
↑  = Increased           E  = Early

*(continued)*

## Normal and abnormal cystometry findings *(continued)*

In autonomous neurogenic bladder, a lower motor neuron lesion produces a flaccid bladder that fills without contracting. The patient can't perceive bladder fullness or initiate and maintain urination without applying external pressure. Lower motor neuron lesions can cause sensory or motor paralysis of the bladder. In sensory paralysis, the patient experiences chronic urine retention because he can't perceive bladder fullness. In motor paralysis, the patient has full sensation but can't initiate or control urination.

| Feature or response | Autonomous neurogenic bladder (flaccid, incomplete lower motor neuron lesion) | Sensory paralytic bladder (lower motor neuron lesion) | Motor paralytic bladder (lower motor neuron lesion) |
|---|---|---|---|
| Micturition | | | |
|   Start | 0 | + | 0 |
|   Stop | 0 | + | 0 |
| Residual urine | + | + | ++ |
| Vesical sensation | 0 | 0 | + |
| First urge to void | 0 | D | + |
| Bladder capacity | ↑ | ↑ (< 1 L) | V |
| Bladder contractions | 0 | 0 | 0 |
| Intravesical pressure | ↓ | ↓ | L |
| Bulbocavernosus reflex | 0 | +/↓/0 | + |
| Saddle sensation | 0 | V | + |
| Bethanechol test (exaggerated response) | + | + | 0 |
| Ice water test | 0 | 0 | 0 |
| Anal reflex | 0 | V | V |
| Heat sensation and pain | 0 | 0 | + |

KEY:
+ = Present/Positive     ↓ = Decreased     D = Delayed
0 = Absent/Negative     V = Variable     L = Low
↑ = Increased     E = Early

justed automatically to the desired reading (100 ml/minute) by a four-channel cystometer.

- The patient is asked to indicate when he first feels an urge to void and then when he feels he must urinate. The related pressure and volume are automatically plotted on the graph.
- When the bladder reaches its full capacity, the patient is asked to urinate so that the maximal intravesical voiding pressure can be recorded. The patient's bladder is then drained and, if no additional tests are required, the catheter is removed; otherwise, the catheter is left in place to measure urethral pressure profile or to provide supplemental findings.
- If abnormal bladder function is caused by muscle incompetence or disrupted innervation, an anticholinergic (atropine) or cholinergic (bethanechol) medication may be injected and the study repeated in 20 to 30 minutes.
- Encourage the patient to drink lots of fluids, unless contraindicated, to relieve burning on urination, a common adverse effect of the procedure.
- Short-term antibiotics are commonly given to prevent infection.
- Administer a sitz bath or warm tub bath if the patient experiences discomfort after the test.
- Measure fluid intake and urine output for 24 hours. Watch for hematuria that persists after the third voiding and for signs and symptoms of sepsis (such as fever or chills).

### Precautions

- Cystometry is contraindicated in the patient with an acute urinary tract infection because uninhibited contractions may cause erroneous readings and the test may lead to pyelonephritis and septic shock.

- Tell the patient not to strain at voiding; it can cause ambiguous cystometric readings.

### Complications
- Infection or bleeding

# External sphincter electromyography

External sphincter electromyography (EMG) measures electrical activity of the external urinary sphincter using needle electrodes inserted in perineal or periurethral tissues, electrodes in an anal plug, or skin electrodes. Skin electrodes are the most common method used.

Incontinence is the primary indication for external sphincter EMG. Usually, the test is done with cystometry and voiding urethrography as part of a full urodynamic study.

### Normal results

- Increased muscle activity when the patient tightens the external urinary sphincter and decreased muscle activity when he relaxes it are normal results.
- If EMG and cystometrography are performed simultaneously, a comparison of results shows that muscle activity of the normal sphincter increases as the bladder fills. During voiding and bladder contraction, muscle activity decreases as the sphincter relaxes.

### Abnormal results

- Failure of the sphincter to relax or increased muscle activity during voiding demonstrates detrusor–external sphincter dyssynergia.

DRUG CHALLENGE

 Effect of anticholinergic or cholinergic drugs on detrusor and sphincter activity

## Purpose
- To assess neuromuscular function of the external urinary sphincter
- To assess the functional balance between bladder and sphincter muscle activity

## Patient preparation
- Explain to the patient that external sphincter EMG will determine how well his bladder and sphincter muscles work together.
- Describe the test, including who will perform it, where it will take place, and how long it will last.
- If skin electrodes are used, describe their placement and explain the preparatory procedure, which may include clipping the hair in a small area.
- If needle electrodes are used, describe their placement to the patient and explain that the discomfort is equivalent to an I.M. injection. Assure him that he'll feel discomfort only during insertion. Explain that wires connect the needles to the recorder, but pose no danger of electric shock. If the patient is a woman, tell her that she may notice slight bleeding at the first voiding.
- If an anal plug is used, tell the patient that only the tip of the plug will be inserted into the rectum and that he may feel fullness, but no discomfort.
- Check the patient's history for use of cholinergic or anticholinergic drugs and note such use.
- Make sure that the patient or a responsible family member has signed an informed consent form.

## Procedure and posttest care
- Confirm the patient's identity using two patient identifiers according to facility policy.
- Place the patient in the lithotomy position for electrode placement. After placement, he may lie in the supine position. Record the patient's position, the type of electrode and measuring equipment used, and other tests done at the same time.
- Electrode paste is applied to the ground plate, which is taped to the thigh and grounded. The electrodes are positioned and connected to electrode adapters.
- When using skin electrodes, clean the skin with antiseptic solution and then dry the area. If necessary, shave a small area to optimize electrode contact. Apply electrode paste and tape the electrodes in place. For a woman, electrodes are placed in the periurethral area; for a man, in the perineal area beneath the scrotum.
- To position needle electrodes on a male patient, a gloved finger is inserted in the rectum. The needles and wires are inserted through the perineal skin toward the apex of the prostate. Needle positions are 3 o'clock and 9 o'clock. The needles are withdrawn, and the wires are held in place and then taped to the thigh.
- To position needle electrodes on a female patient, the labia are spread and the needles and wires are inserted periurethrally at the 2 o'clock and 10 o'clock positions. The needles are withdrawn, and the wires are taped to the thigh.
- When using anal plug electrodes, the plug is lubricated, and the patient is asked to breathe slowly and deeply and to relax the anal sphincter to accommodate the plug by bearing down.
- After electrode placement, the adapters are inserted in the preamplifier, and recording starts. The patient is asked to alternately relax and tighten the sphincter.
- When sufficient data have been recorded, the patient is asked to bear down and exhale while the anal plug and needle electrodes are removed. Re-

move skin electrodes gently to avoid pulling hair and tender skin.

- Clean and dry the area before the patient dresses.
- In some urodynamic laboratories, cystometrography is done with EMG for a thorough evaluation of detrusor and sphincter coordination.
- For women, watch for and report hematuria after the first voiding if needle electrodes were used.
- Watch for and report symptoms of mild urethral irritation, such as dysuria, hematuria, and urinary frequency.
- Advise the patient to take a warm sitz bath and encourage him to drink 2 to 3 qt (2 to 3 L) of fluids daily, unless contraindicated.

### Precautions

- Insert the needles quickly to minimize discomfort.
- The ground plate should be properly applied and anchored; wires should be taped securely to prevent artifacts.

### Complications

- Bleeding or infection

# Uroflowmetry

Uroflowmetry, a simple, noninvasive test, uses a uroflometer to detect and evaluate dysfunctional voiding patterns. The uroflometer, contained in a funnel into which the patient voids, measures flow rate (volume of urine voided per second), continuous flow (time of measurable flow), and intermittent flow (total voiding time, including any interruptions).

Types of uroflometers include rotary disc, electromagnetic, spectrophotometric, and gravimetric systems. The gravimetric system, which weighs urine as it's voided and plots the weight against time, is the simplest to use.

### Normal results

- Flow rate varies according to the patient's age and sex and the volume of urine voided. (See *Minimum volume flow rates,* page 618.)

### Abnormal results

- Increased flow rate indicates reduced urethral resistance, possibly associated with external sphincter dysfunction. (See *Characteristic uroflow curves,* page 618.)
- A high peak on the curve plotted over the voiding time indicates decreased outflow resistance, possibly due to stress incontinence.
- Decreased flow rate indicates outflow obstruction or hypotonia of the detrusor muscle.
- More than one distinct peak in a normal curve indicates abdominal straining, possibly due to pushing against an obstruction to empty the bladder.

**DRUG CHALLENGE**

 Drugs that affect bladder and sphincter tone, such as urinary spasmolytics and anticholinergics

### Purpose

- To evaluate lower urinary tract function
- To demonstrate bladder outlet obstruction

### Patient preparation

- Explain to the patient that uroflowmetry evaluates his pattern of urination. Advise him not to urinate for several hours before the test and to increase fluid intake so that he'll have a full bladder and a strong urge to void.
- Describe the test, including who will perform it and where it will take place.

## Minimum volume flow rates

This chart lists the minimum volume flow rates needed to obtain adequate recordings.

| Age | Minimum volume (ml/sec) | Male (ml/sec) | Female (ml/sec) |
|-----|-------------------------|---------------|-----------------|
| 4 to 7 | 100 | 10 | 10 |
| 8 to 13 | 100 | 12 | 15 |
| 14 to 45 | 200 | 21 | 18 |
| 46 to 65 | 200 | 12 | 15 |
| 66 to 80 | 200 | 9 | 10 |

## Characteristic uroflow curves

The graphs below illustrate common uroflow curves that may be seen with conditions such as hesitancy, incontinence, abdominal straining, and detrusor muscle weakness and obstruction.

Normal curve

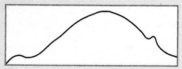

Normal peak with hesitancy may result from the patient's embarrassment or advanced age.

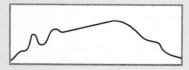

High peak flow over short voiding time may indicate incontinence.

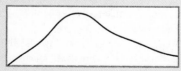

Many peaks over normal voiding time indicate abdominal straining and detrusor muscle weakness.

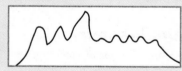

Low peak with long voiding time and urethral dribbling indicates obstruction.

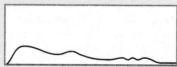

- Instruct the patient to remain still while voiding during the test to help ensure accurate results. Assure him that he'll have complete privacy during the test.
- As ordered, discontinue drugs that may affect bladder and sphincter tone, such as urinary spasmolytics and anticholinergics.

### Procedure and posttest care

- Confirm the patient's identity using two patient identifiers according to facility policy.
- Check cable connections before the test.
- Remind the patient not to strain while voiding.
- Ask the male patient to void while standing and the female patient to void while sitting.
- The patient pushes the start button on the commode chair, counts for 5 seconds (1 one-thousand, 2 one-thousand, and so on), and voids. When finished, he counts for 5 seconds and pushes the button again. The volume of urine voided is then recorded and plotted as a curve over the time of voiding. The patient's position and the route of fluid intake (oral or I.V.) are noted.
- Instruct the patient to resume medications stopped for the test.
- Monitor the patient for urine retention or bladder distention. Also monitor his intake and output. If neurogenic bladder is diagnosed, teach self-catheterization, if indicated; provide bladder training as needed.

### Precautions

- The transducer must be level, and the beaker must be centered beneath the funnel.
- The beaker must be large enough to hold all urine; overflow can invalidate results and damage the transducer.

# Voiding cystourethrography

In voiding cystourethrography, a contrast medium is instilled by gentle syringe pressure or gravity into the bladder through a urethral catheter. Fluoroscopic films or overhead radiographs demonstrate bladder filling and then show excretion of the contrast medium as the patient voids.

### Normal results

- Delineation of the bladder and urethra shows normal structure and function, with no regurgitation of contrast medium into the ureters.

### Abnormal results

- Urethral stricture, vesical or urethral diverticula, ureterocele, cystocele, prostate enlargement, vesicoureteral reflux, or neurogenic bladder may be detected.

### Purpose

- To detect abnormalities of the bladder and urethra, such as vesicoureteral reflux, neurogenic bladder, prostatic hyperplasia, urethral strictures, or diverticula

### Patient preparation

- Explain to the patient that voiding cystourethrography permits assessment of the bladder and the urethra.
- Inform the patient that he doesn't need to restrict food and fluids.
- Tell the patient who will perform the test and where it will take place.
- Inform the patient that a catheter will be inserted into his bladder and that a contrast medium will be instilled through the catheter.
- Tell the patient that he may experience a feeling of fullness and an urge to void when the contrast medium is instilled. Explain that X-rays will be taken of his

bladder and urethra and that he'll be asked to assume various positions.
■ Make sure that the patient or a responsible family member has signed an informed consent form.

 Check the patient's history for hypersensitivity to iodine-based contrast media or iodine-containing foods such as shellfish. Mark sensitivities on the chart and inform the practitioner because the patient may require prophylactic antiallergenics (diphenhydramine or corticosteroids).

■ Administer a sedative, if prescribed, just before the procedure.

## Procedure and posttest care
■ Confirm the patient's identity using two patient identifiers according to facility policy.
■ The patient is placed in a supine position, and an indwelling urinary catheter is inserted into the bladder.
■ The contrast medium is instilled through the catheter until the bladder is full.
■ The catheter is clamped, and X-ray films are exposed with the patient in supine, oblique, and lateral positions.
■ The catheter is removed, and the patient assumes the right oblique position (right leg flexed to 90 degrees, left leg extended, penis parallel to right leg) and begins to void.
■ Four high-speed exposures of the bladder and urethra, coned down to reduce radiation exposure, are usually made on one film during voiding.
■ If the right oblique view doesn't delineate both ureters, the patient is asked to stop urinating and to begin again in the left oblique position.
■ The most reliable voiding cystourethrograms are obtained with the patient recumbent. The patient who can't

void recumbent may do so standing (not sitting).
■ Expression cystourethrography may have to be performed, under a general anesthetic, for a young child who can't void on command.
■ Observe and record the time, color, and volume of the patient's voidings. Report hematuria if present after the third voiding.
■ Encourage the patient to drink large quantities of fluids to reduce burning on urination and to flush out residual contrast medium.

 Monitor the patient for chills and fever related to extravasation of contrast material or urinary sepsis.

■ If stricture is present, prepare for surgery, as indicated.
■ Monitor the patient for symptoms of urinary tract infection.

## Precautions
■ Voiding cystourethrography is contraindicated in the patient with an acute or exacerbated urethral or bladder infection or an acute urethral injury.
■ Hypersensitivity to the contrast medium may also contraindicate this test.

## Complications
■ Bleeding or infection
■ Adverse reaction to the contrast medium

# Whitaker test
### [pressure study, flow study]

The Whitaker test correlates radiographic findings with measurements of pressure and flow in the kidneys and ureters and facilitates assessment of the upper urinary tract's efficiency in emptying.

In this procedure, radiographs are taken after urethral catheterization, I.V. administration of a contrast medium, percutaneous cannulation of the kidney, and renal perfusion of the contrast medium. Intrarenal and bladder pressures are then measured.

### Normal results

- Normal outlines of the renal pelvis and calyces are observed.
- The ureter should fill uniformly and appear normal in size and course.
- The normal value for intrarenal pressure is 15 cm $H_2O$.
- The normal value for bladder pressure may range from 5 to 10 cm $H_2O$.

### Abnormal results

- Enlargement of the renal pelvis, calyces, or ureteropelvic junction may indicate obstruction.
- Subtraction of bladder pressure from intrarenal pressure results in a differential that aids diagnosis. A differential of 12 to 15 cm $H_2O$ indicates obstruction. A differential of less than 10 cm $H_2O$ indicates a bladder abnormality, such as hypertonia or neurogenic bladder.

### Purpose

- To identify and evaluate renal obstruction

### Patient preparation

- Explain to the patient that the Whitaker test helps to evaluate kidney function.
- Instruct the patient to avoid food and fluids for at least 4 hours before the test.
- Tell the patient who will perform the test, where it will take place, and that it will take about 1 hour.
- Describe the procedure to the patient. Inform him that he'll be given a mild sedative before the test, that he may feel some discomfort during insertion of the urethral catheter and injection of the local anesthetic, and that he may also feel transient burning and flushing after injection of the contrast medium.

- Warn the patient that the X-ray machine makes loud clacking noises as films are exposed.
- Check that pretest blood work (such as kidney function) was done, if ordered.
- Make sure that the patient or a responsible family member has signed an informed consent form.

**ALERT**

Check the patient's history and recent coagulation studies for bleeding disorders. Also check for hypersensitivity to iodine-based contrast media or iodine-containing foods such as shellfish. Mark sensitivities on the chart and inform the practitioner because the patient may require prophylactic antiallergenics (diphenhydramine or corticosteroids).

- Give prophylactic antimicrobials, as prescribed, to prevent infection from instrumentation.
- Instruct the patient to void, and give prescribed sedatives just before the procedure.

### Procedure and posttest care

- Confirm the patient's identity using two patient identifiers according to facility policy.
- Place the patient in a supine position on the X-ray table. The table must be horizontal and must remain at the same height throughout the test.
- To prepare for measurement of bladder pressure, a urethral catheter is placed in the bladder. The patient's bladder may be emptied, depending on his suspected condition. (If an obstruction is suspected, the patient will be asked to void before the test. If a condition, such as a bladder hypertonia, is the suspected

cause of insufficient emptying, he shouldn't void.)

- A plain film of the urinary tract is taken to obtain anatomic landmarks.
- The catheter is then connected to a three-way stopcock on a manometer line linked to the transducer and recorder. The line is then filled with sterile water.
- Contrast medium is injected intravenously.
- The patient is placed prone and made comfortable with pillows. When urography demonstrates contrast medium in the kidney, the skin is cleaned with antiseptic solution and draped.
- Pressure recording equipment is calibrated. The renal perfusion tubing is filled with sterile water or normal saline solution and held at the level of the kidney.
- Local anesthetic is injected, and an incision is made through the flank for cannulation of the kidney.
- The patient is asked to hold his breath while the needle is inserted into the renal pelvis. Aspiration of urine confirms that the needle is in position.
- The cannula is then connected by a four-way stopcock to the perfusion tubing and the manometer line.
- Perfusion of the contrast medium is begun, serial X-rays are taken, and intrarenal pressure is measured. Bladder pressure is then measured.
- Perfusion continues at a steady rate of 10 ml/minute until bladder pressure is constant. When pressure holds steady for a few minutes and adequate films have been taken, perfusion is discontinued. Residual fluid is aspirated from the kidney, the cannula is removed, and the wound is dressed.
- Keep the patient in a supine position for 12 hours after the test.
- Check the patient's vital signs every 15 minutes for the first hour, every 30 minutes for the next hour, and then every 2 hours for 24 hours.

- Check the puncture site for bleeding, hematoma, or urine leakage each time vital signs are checked. If bleeding occurs, apply pressure. If a hematoma develops, apply warm soaks. Report urine leakage.
- Monitor fluid intake and urine output for 24 hours. Report hematuria that persists after the third voiding.

### Alert

 Watch the patient for signs of sepsis (chills, fever, tachycardia, tachypnea, or hypotension) or similar signs of contrast medium extravasation.

- Inform the patient that colicky pains are transient.
- Give prescribed analgesics.
- Give antimicrobials for several days after the test, as ordered, to prevent infection.
- If an obstruction is present, prepare the patient for surgery.

### Precautions

- Contraindications include bleeding disorders and severe infection.

### Complications

- Bleeding, hematoma, or urine leakage

# Miscellaneous tests

# Miscellaneous tests

## Miscellaneous tests

### Dexamethasone suppression

The dexamethasone suppression test requires administration of dexamethasone, an oral steroid. Dexamethasone suppresses levels of circulating adrenal steroid hormones in normal people but fails to suppress them in patients with Cushing's syndrome and some forms of clinical depression.

#### Normal results
- A cortisol level of 5 g/dl (140 nmol/L) or greater indicates failure of dexamethasone suppression.

#### Abnormal results
- Failure of suppression occurs in the patient with Cushing's syndrome, severe stress, and depression that's likely to respond to treatment with antidepressants.

##### DRUG CHALLENGE

 Certain drugs, particularly barbiturates or phenytoin, within 3 weeks of the test (possible false-positive); corticosteroids, hormonal contraceptives, lithium, methadone, aspirin, diuretics, morphine, or MAO inhibitors

#### Purpose
- To diagnose Cushing's syndrome
- To help diagnose clinical depression

#### Patient preparation
- Explain the purpose of the dexamethasone suppression test.
- Inform the patient that the test requires two blood samples drawn after administration of dexamethasone. Explain who will perform the venipunctures and when they'll be done.
- Explain to the patient that he may experience discomfort from the tourniquet and needle punctures.
- Restrict food and fluids for 10 to 12 hours before the test.

#### Procedure and posttest care
- Confirm the patient's identity using two patient identifiers according to facility policy.
- On the first day, give the patient 1 mg of dexamethasone at 11 p.m. On the next day, collect blood samples at 4 p.m. and 11 p.m. More frequent sampling may increase the likelihood of measuring a nonsuppressed cortisol peak.

- If a hematoma develops at the venipuncture site, apply warm soaks.

## Precautions

- Many medications, including corticosteroids, oral contraceptives, lithium, methadone, aspirin, diuretics, morphine, and monoamine oxidase (MAO) inhibitors, can affect the accuracy of test results. If possible, don't give any of these medications for 24 to 48 hours before the test, as ordered.
- Diabetes mellitus, pregnancy, and severe stress, such as trauma, severe weight loss, dehydration, and acute alcohol withdrawal can cause a false-positive.

# D-xylose absorption

The D-xylose absorption test evaluates the patient with symptoms of malabsorption, such as weight loss and generalized malnutrition, weakness, and diarrhea. D-xylose is a pentose sugar that's absorbed in the small intestine without the aid of pancreatic enzymes, passes through the liver without being metabolized, and is excreted in the urine. Because of its absorption in the small intestine without digestion, measurement of D-xylose in the urine and blood indicates the absorptive capacity of the small intestine.

## Reference values

- In children, blood D-xylose level is > 30 mg/dl in 1 hour; urine D-xylose level is 16% to 33% of ingested D-xylose excreted in 5 hours.
- In adults, blood D-xylose level is 25 to 40 mg/dl in 2 hours; urine D-xylose level is 3.5 g excreted in 5 hours (in those age 65 or older, the level is > 5 g in 24 hours).

## Abnormal results

- Low blood and urine D-xylose levels most commonly result from malabsorption disorders that affect the proximal small intestine, such as sprue and celiac disease.
- Low D-xylose levels may also result from regional enteritis involving the jejunum, Whipple's disease, multiple jejunal diverticula, myxedema, diabetic neuropathic diarrhea, rheumatoid arthritis, alcoholism, severe heart failure, and ascites.

**DRUG CHALLENGE**

 Aspirin (decreased D-xylose excretion by the kidneys); indomethacin (decreased intestinal D-xylose absorption)

## Purpose

- To aid in the differential diagnosis of malabsorption
- To determine the cause of malabsorption syndrome

## Patient preparation

- Explain that the D-xylose absorption test helps evaluate digestive function by analyzing blood samples and urine specimens after ingestion of a sugar solution.
- Tell the patient that he must fast overnight before the test and that he'll have to fast and remain in bed during the test.
- Tell him that the test requires several blood samples. Explain who will perform the venipunctures and when they'll be done.
- Explain to the patient that he may experience discomfort from the tourniquet and needle punctures.
- Inform the patient that all his urine will be collected for 5 or 24 hours, as ordered.

- Withhold medications that alter test results, such as aspirin and indomethacin, as ordered. Record any medications the patient is taking on the laboratory request.

### Procedure and posttest care

- Confirm the patient's identity using two patient identifiers according to facility policy.
- Perform a venipuncture to obtain a fasting blood sample and collect the sample in a 10-ml tube without additives. Collect a first-voided morning urine specimen. Label these specimens and send them to the laboratory immediately to serve as a baseline.
- Give the patient 25 g of D-xylose dissolved in 8 oz (240 ml) of water, followed by an additional 8 oz of water. If the patient is a child, administer 0.5 g of D-xylose per pound of body weight, up to 25 g. Record the time of D-xylose ingestion.
- For an adult, draw a blood sample 2 hours after D-xylose ingestion; for a child, 1 hour after ingestion. Collect the sample in a 10-ml tube without additives. Occasionally, a 5-hour sample may be drawn to support the findings of the 1- or 2-hour sample.
- Collect and pool all urine during the 5 or 24 hours after D-xylose ingestion.
- If a hematoma develops at the venipuncture site, apply warm soaks.
- Observe the patient for abdominal discomfort or mild diarrhea caused by D-xylose ingestion.
- Instruct the patient that he may resume his usual diet and medications, as ordered.

### Precautions

- Be sure to collect all urine and refrigerate the specimen during the collection period.
- Because patients age 65 and older and those with borderline or elevated creati-

nine levels tend to have low 5-hour urine levels but normal 24-hour levels, the practitioner will have to establish the length of the collection period. At the end of the collection period, send the urine specimen to the laboratory immediately.

- Maintain bed rest and withhold food and fluids (other than D-xylose) throughout the test period.

# Radiology and nuclear medicine

## Gallium scanning

A gallium scan is a total body scan used to assess certain neoplasms and inflammatory lesions that attract gallium. It's usually performed 24 to 48 hours after the I.V. injection of radioactive gallium ($^{67}$Ga) citrate; occasionally, it's performed 72 hours after the injection or, in acute inflammatory disease, 4 to 6 hours after the injection.

Because gallium has an affinity for benign and malignant neoplasms and inflammatory lesions, exact diagnosis requires additional confirming tests, such as ultrasonography and computed tomography scanning. Also, be aware that many neoplasms and a few inflammatory lesions may fail to demonstrate abnormal gallium activity.

### Normal results

- Gallium activity is shown in the liver, spleen, bones, and large bowel. Activity in the bowel results from mucosal uptake of gallium and fecal excretion of gallium.

### Abnormal results

- Abnormally high gallium accumulation is characteristic in inflammatory bowel diseases, such as ulcerative colitis and regional ileitis (Crohn's disease), and in carcinoma of the colon.

- In Hodgkin's disease and malignant lymphoma, gallium scanning can demonstrate abnormal activity in one or more lymph nodes or in extranodal locations.
- Gallium localizes in hepatomas but not in pseudotumors; in abscesses but not in pleural effusions; and in tumors but not in cysts or hematomas.

### Purpose

- To detect primary or metastatic neoplasms and inflammatory lesions when the site of the disease hasn't been clearly defined
- To evaluate malignant lymphoma and identify recurrent tumors after chemotherapy or radiation therapy
- To clarify focal defects in the liver when liver-spleen scanning and ultrasonography prove inconclusive
- To evaluate bronchogenic carcinoma

### Patient preparation

- Explain that gallium scanning helps detect abnormal or inflammatory tissue.
- Tell the patient that he doesn't need to restrict food and fluids.
- Explain to the patient that the test requires a total body scan (usually performed 24 to 48 hours after the I.V. injection of $^{67}$Ga citrate).
- Tell the patient who will perform the test and where it will take place.
- Warn the patient that he may experience transient discomfort from the needle puncture during injection of the $^{67}$Ga citrate. Reassure him, however, that the dosage is only slightly radioactive and isn't harmful.
- If a gamma scintillation camera is to be used, assure the patient that although the uptake probe and detector head may touch his skin, he'll experience no discomfort.

- If a rectilinear scanner will be used, mention to the patient that it makes a soft, irregular clicking noise as it registers the radiation emissions.
- Make sure that the patient or a responsible family member has signed an informed consent form.
- Administer a laxative, an enema, or both, as ordered.

### Procedure and posttest care

- Confirm the patient's identity using two patient identifiers according to facility policy.
- The patient may be positioned erect or recumbent or in an appropriate combination of these positions, depending on his physical condition.
- Scans or scintigrams of the patient are taken 24 to 48 hours after $^{67}$Ga citrate injection, from anterior and posterior views and, occasionally, lateral views.
- If the initial gallium scan suggests bowel disease and additional scans are necessary, give the patient a cleansing enema before continuing the test.

### Precautions

- This test should precede barium studies because barium retention may hinder visualization of gallium activity in the bowel.
- Gallium scanning is usually contraindicated in a child and during pregnancy or lactation; however, it may be performed if the potential diagnostic benefit outweighs the risks of exposure to radiation.

### Complications

- Infection at the venipuncture site

# Lymphangiography

Lymphangiography (or lymphography) is the radiographic examination of the lymphatic system after the injection of an oil-based contrast medium into a lymphatic vessel in each foot or, less commonly, in each hand. This test is no longer used widely.

Injection into the foot allows visualization of the lymphatics of the leg, inguinal and iliac regions, and the retroperitoneum up to the thoracic duct.

Injection into the hand allows visualization of the axillary and supraclavicular nodes. This procedure may also be used to study the cervical region (retroauricular area), but this is less useful and less common.

X-ray films are taken immediately after injection to demonstrate the filling of the lymphatic system and then again 24 hours later to visualize the lymph nodes. Because the contrast medium remains in the nodes for up to 2 years, subsequent X-ray films can assess progression of disease and monitor effectiveness of treatment.

## Normal findings
- Homogeneous and complete filling with contrast medium is seen on the initial films.
- On the 24-hour films, the lymph nodes are fully opacified and well circumscribed; the lymphatic channels are emptied a few hours after injection of the contrast medium.

## Abnormal findings
- Enlarged, foamy-looking nodes indicate Hodgkin's disease or malignant lymphoma.
- Filling defects or lack of opacification indicates metastatic involvement of the lymph nodes.
- Shortened lymphatic vessels and a deficient number of vessels indicate primary lymphedema.
- Abruptly terminating lymphatic vessels, caused by retroperitoneal tumors impinging on the vessels, inflammation,

filariasis, and trauma resulting from surgery or radiation, indicate secondary lymphedema.

## Purpose
- To detect and stage lymphomas and to identify metastatic involvement of the lymph nodes (computed tomography [CT] used more commonly for staging)
- To distinguish primary from secondary lymphedema
- To suggest surgical treatment or evaluate the effectiveness of chemotherapy and radiation therapy in controlling malignancy
- To investigate enlarged lymph nodes detected by CT or ultrasonography

## Patient preparation
- Explain to the patient that lymphangiography permits examination of the lymphatic system through X-ray films taken after the injection of a contrast medium.
- Inform the patient that he need not restrict food and fluids.
- Tell the patient who will perform the procedure and where it will take place.
- Mention to the patient that additional X-ray films are also taken the following day, but that these take less than 30 minutes.
- Inform the patient that blue contrast medium will be injected into each foot to outline the lymphatic vessels, that the injection causes transient discomfort, and that the contrast medium discolors urine and stool for 48 hours and may give his skin and vision a bluish tinge for 48 hours.
- Tell the patient that a local anesthetic will be injected before a small incision is made in each foot.
- Inform the patient that the contrast medium is then injected for the next 1¼ hours using a catheter inserted into a lymphatic vessel.

- Advise the patient that he must remain as still as possible during injection of the contrast medium and that he may experience some discomfort in the popliteal or inguinal areas at the beginning of the injection.
- If this test is performed on an outpatient basis, advise the patient to have a friend or relative accompany him.
- Warn the patient that the incision site may be sore for several days after lymphangiography.
- Make sure that the patient or a responsible family member has signed an informed consent form.

## ALERT

 Check the patient's history to determine if he's hypersensitive to iodine, seafood, or the contrast media used in other diagnostic tests such as excretory urography. Alert the practitioner to any sensitivities.

- Just before the procedure, instruct the patient to void and check his vital signs for a baseline. If prescribed, administer a sedative and an oral antihistamine (if hypersensitivity to the contrast medium is suspected).

### Procedure and posttest care

- Confirm the patient's identity using two patient identifiers according to facility policy.
- A preliminary X-ray of the chest is taken with the patient in an erect or a supine position.
- The skin over the dorsum of each foot is cleaned with antiseptics.
- Blue contrast dye is injected intradermally into the area between the toes, usually the first and fourth toe webs.
- The contrast medium infiltrates the lymphatic system, and within 15 to 30 minutes, the lymphatic vessels appear as small blue lines on the upper surface of the instep of each foot.
- A local anesthetic is then injected into the dorsum of each foot and a transverse incision is made to expose the lymphatic vessel.
- Each vessel is cannulated with a 30G needle attached to polyethylene tubing and a syringe filled with ethiodized oil.
- After the needles are positioned, the patient is instructed to remain still throughout the injection period to avoid dislodging the needles.
- The syringe is then placed within an infusion pump that injects the contrast medium at a constant rate of 0.1 to 0.2 ml/minute for about 1½ hours to avoid injury to delicate lymphatic vessels.
- Fluoroscopy may be used to monitor filling of the lymphatic system.
- The needles are removed, the incisions are sutured, and sterile dressings are applied.
- X-ray films of the legs, pelvis, abdomen, and chest are taken.
- The patient is then taken to his room, but must return 24 hours later for additional films.
- Check the patient's vital signs every 4 hours for 48 hours.

## ALERT

 Watch for pulmonary complications, such as shortness of breath, pleuritic pain, hypotension, low-grade fever, and cyanosis caused by embolization of the contrast medium.

- Enforce bed rest for 24 hours, with the patient's feet elevated to help reduce swelling.
- Apply ice packs to the incision sites to help reduce swelling and give prescribed analgesics.

- Check the incision sites for infection and leave the dressings in place for 2 days, making sure the wounds remain dry. Tell the patient that the sutures will be removed in 7 to 10 days.
- Prepare the patient for follow-up X-rays, as needed.

### Precautions

- Lymphangiography is contraindicated in the patient with hypersensitivity to iodine, pulmonary insufficiencies, cardiac diseases, or severe renal or hepatic disease.

### Complications

- Bleeding or infection

# Red blood cell survival time

Normally, red blood cells (RBCs) are destroyed only when they reach senility. However, in hemolytic diseases, RBCs of all ages are randomly destroyed, resulting in anemia. The RBC survival time test measures the survival time of circulating RBCs and detects sites of abnormal RBC sequestration and destruction.

Survival time is measured by labeling a random sample of RBCs with radioactive chromium-51 sodium chromate ($^{51}Cr$). This labeled group of RBCs is then injected back into the patient. Serial blood samples measure the percentage of labeled cells per unit volume over 3 to 4 weeks until 50% of the cells disappear. (The disappearance rate corresponds to destruction of a random cell population.)

A normal RBC survives about 120 days (half-life of 60 days); the $^{51}Cr$-labeled RBCs have a shorter half-life (25 to 30 days) because about 1% of senescent RBCs are removed from the circulation each day and about 1% of $^{51}Cr$ is spontaneously eluted from the labeled RBCs each day.

During the test period, a gamma camera scans the body for sites of abnormally high radioactivity, which indicates sites of excessive RBC sequestration and destruction. Other tests performed with the RBC survival time test may include spot-checks of the stool to detect GI blood loss, hematocrit, blood volume studies, and radionuclide iron uptake and clearance tests to aid in the differential diagnosis of anemia.

### Normal findings

- The normal half-life for RBCs labeled with $^{51}Cr$ is 25 to 30 days.
- Normal gamma camera scans reveal slight radioactivity in the spleen, liver, and sometimes the bone marrow.

### Abnormal findings

- Decreased RBC survival time indicates a hemolytic disease, such as chronic lymphocytic leukemia, congenital nonspherocytic hemolytic anemia, hemoglobin C disease, hereditary spherocytosis, idiopathic acquired hemolytic anemia, paroxysmal nocturnal hemoglobinuria, elliptocytosis, pernicious anemia, sickle cell anemia, sickle cell hemoglobin C disease, or hemolytic-uremic syndrome.

### Purpose

- To help evaluate unexplained anemia, particularly hemolytic anemia
- To identify sites of abnormal RBC sequestration and destruction

### Patient preparation

- Explain to the patient that the RBC survival time test helps identify the cause of his anemia.
- Advise the patient that he need not restrict food and fluids.
- Explain to the patient that the test involves labeling a blood sample with a radioactive substance and requires regular blood samples at 3-day intervals for 3 to

4 weeks. Tell him who will perform the test and where it will take place.

▪ Tell the patient that he may experience discomfort from the needle punctures and the tourniquet. Reassure him that collecting each sample takes less than 3 minutes and that the small amount of radioactive substance used is harmless.

▪ If stool collection is required to test for GI bleeding, teach the patient the proper collection technique.

▪ Make sure that the patient or a responsible family member has signed an informed consent form.

### Procedure and posttest care

▪ Confirm the patient's identity using two patient identifiers according to facility policy.

▪ A 30-ml blood sample is drawn and mixed with 100 microcuries of $^{51}Cr$ for an adult (less for a child).

▪ After an incubation period, the mixture is injected intravenously into the patient. A blood sample is drawn 30 minutes after injection to determine blood and RBC volumes.

▪ A 6-ml sample is collected in a heparinized tube after 24 hours; follow-up samples are collected at 3-day intervals for 3 to 4 weeks. (Intervals between samples may vary, depending on the laboratory.)

▪ To avoid error from physical decay of the $^{51}Cr$, each sample is measured with a scintillation well counter on the day it's drawn.

▪ Radioactivity per milliliter of RBCs is calculated, and the values are plotted to determine mean RBC survival time. Simultaneous gamma camera scans of the precordium, sacrum, liver, and spleen detect radioactivity at sites of excess RBC sequestration. A hematocrit test is done on a small portion of each blood sample to check for blood loss.

▪ At the end of the study, a sample is drawn to compare ending blood and RBC volumes with beginning volumes.

▪ If a hematoma develops at the venipuncture site, apply warm soaks.

### Precautions

▪ This test is contraindicated during pregnancy because it exposes the fetus to radiation.

▪ Because excess blood loss can invalidate test results, this test is usually contraindicated for a patient with active bleeding or poor clotting function. However, if the test is necessary for a patient with poor clotting function, observe the venipuncture sites carefully for signs of hemorrhage.

DO'S & DON'TS

 The patient shouldn't receive blood transfusions during the test period and shouldn't have blood samples drawn for other tests.

# Skin tests

## Delayed hypersensitivity skin tests

Skin testing for delayed-type hypersensitivity (DTH) is an important method for evaluating T-cell mediated immune response in a patient. (However, positive reactions don't indicate protection against the antigen.) This response requires previous exposure to the antigen and an intact immune system. After initial exposure to the antigen, the body produces antibodies and sensitized T cells. When re-exposed to the antigen (recall antigen), the antibodies react immediately, causing a hypersensitivity reaction; however, the T cells respond over the next few days, causing a delayed hypersensitivity reaction. The immediate response is typically erythema, while the delayed response is induration (hardening). The lack of response to a recall antigen is termed anergy and, in the absence of underlying disease or immunosuppressive therapy, may indicate T-cell immunodeficiency disease.

The most commonly used recall antigen is *Mycobacterium tuberculosis* (purified protein derivative [PPD] Mantoux test). Other antigens used in the clinical setting include Candida, Trichophyton, and mumps. Some antigens previously used for DTH testing, such as fungi and streptococci, are no longer available or recommended for clinical use.

DTH-like reactions may occur with topical contact to Rhus species plants (poison ivy, oak, and sumac), nickel, dinitrochlorobenzene (DNCB), dinitrofluorobenzene (DNFB), and picryl chloride. Contact sensitivity to Rhus and nickel is determined clinically, and skin testing isn't considered necessary. There's a risk of local tissue necrosis when using chemical antigens, specifically DNCB and DNFB, so their use is discouraged; in vitro assessment of cell-mediated immunity is preferred in those circumstances.

DTH testing can be used to assess the status of an individual's immune system in severe infection, cancer, pretransplantation, and malnutrition. Antigens used for this testing must be antigens the patient has been previously exposed to. For example, *C. albicans,* tetanus, or mumps can be used.

DTH testing is performed by injecting a small amount of antigenic material intradermally or applying it topically and measuring the reaction after 48 to 72 hours. Skin testing has limited value in infants because of their immature immune system and lack of previous sensitization. In addition, patch testing may

be used. This involves applying antigenic material topically to the skin, helping to confirm allergic contact sensitization and isolate the causative agent.

## Normal results

- In the recall antigen test, a positive response (5 mm or more of induration at the test site) appears 48 hours after injection.

## Abnormal results

- In the recall antigen test, a positive response to less than two of the test antigens, a persistent unresponsiveness to intradermal injection of higher-strength antigens, or a generalized diminished reaction (causing less than 10 mm combined induration) indicates diminished delayed hypersensitivity.
- Diminished delayed hypersensitivity can result from Hodgkin's disease (common); sarcoidosis; liver disease; congenital immunodeficiency disease, such as ataxia-telangiectasia, DiGeorge syndrome, and Wiskott-Aldrich syndrome; uremia; acute leukemia; viral diseases, such as influenza, infectious mononucleosis, measles, mumps, and rubella; fungal diseases, such as coccidioidomycosis and cryptococcosis; bacterial diseases, such as leprosy and tuberculosis (TB); and terminal cancer. Diminished delayed hypersensitivity can also result from immunosuppressive or steroid therapy or viral vaccination.

### DRUG CHALLENGE

 Hormonal contraceptives (may cause false-negative results by inhibiting lymphocyte mitosis)

## Purpose

- To assess for exposure to or activation of certain diseases, most commonly TB

- To assess the status of a patient's immune system during illness (cancer, transplantation)
- To evaluate sensitivity to environmental antigens in the patient with persistent symptoms (for example, asthma, seasonal rhinitis, recurrent or persistent urticaria)

### Patient preparation

- Explain to the patient that a small amount of antigenic material will be injected superficially or applied to the skin.
- Inform the patient that testing takes only a few minutes for each antigen. Reactions will be evaluated 48 to 72 hours later. Occasionally, the test must be repeated in 2 to 3 weeks when a negative result is displayed initially. The first test "reminds" the body that it was previously exposed to the antigen and a response is noted on retesting. This is commonly done for TB testing and is called the *two-step test.*
- Be sure to ask the patient about sensitivity to the test antigens, whether he has had previous skin testing, and what the outcomes of that testing were. When performing TB testing, ask about previous TB disease or exposure and bacille Calmette-Guérin vaccination.

### Procedure and posttest care

- Confirm the patient's identity using two patient identifiers according to facility policy.
- Inject each antigen being tested intradermally, using a separate tuberculin syringe, on the patient's forearm. (See *Administering test antigens.*)
- Circle each injection site with a pen, and label each according to the antigen given.
- Instruct the patient to avoid washing off the circles until the test is completed.
- Inject the control allergy diluent on the other forearm.

## Administering test antigens

This illustration shows the arm of a patient undergoing a recall antigen test, which determines whether he has previously been exposed to certain antigens. A sample panel of four test antigens has been injected into his forearm, and the test site has been marked and labeled for each antigen.

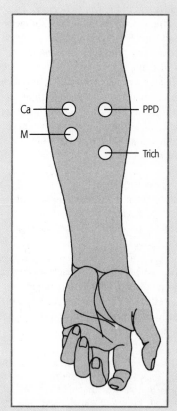

Key:
Ca = *Candida*
M = Mumps
PPD = Purified protein derivative
Trich = *Trichophyton*

- Inspect the injection sites for reactivity after 48 to 72 hours. Record induration and erythema in millimeters. A negative test at the first concentration of antigen should be confirmed using a higher concentration.
- Watch the patient closely for severe local reactions that may occur at the test site, such as pain, blistering, swelling, induration, itching, and ulceration. Scarring or hyperpigmentation also may result. Also observe for swelling and tenderness in the lymph nodes at the elbow or axillary region. Check for tachycardia and fever, although these rarely occur. Symptoms typically appear in 15 to 30 minutes.
- Tell the patient experiencing hypersensitivity that steroids will control the reaction, but that skin lesions may persist for 10 to 14 days. Instruct him to avoid scratching or otherwise disturbing the affected area.

### Precautions

- If the forearms are not free from disease (for example, if the patient has atopic dermatitis), use other sites such as the back.
- The U.S. Food and Drug Administration hasn't approved all vaccines for use in skin testing, though nonapproved substances are commonly used. Currently approved antigens include PPD to *M. tuberculosis* and mumps.

ALERT

 Observe the patient carefully for signs of anaphylactic shock—urticaria, respiratory distress, and hypotension. If such signs develop, give epinephrine, as ordered, and notify the practitioner immediately.

# Selected references

Bishop, M.L., et al. *Clinical Chemistry,* 5th ed. Philadelphia: Lippincott Williams & Wilkins, 2005.

Clark, P.M. Ductal Lavage: A New Look Inside the Breast. *www.cancernews.com/data/Article/223.asp* [Accessed 2006.]

DeGroot, L., and Jameson, J.L., eds. *Endocrinology,* 5th ed. Philadelphia: W.B. Saunders Co., 2006.

Esquerda, A., et al. "Tumor Necrosis Factor-Alpha in Pleural Fluid: A Marker of Complicated Parapneumonic Effusions," *Chest* 127(5):1868, May 2005.

Fischbach, F.T. *A Manual of Laboratory and Diagnostic Tests,* 7th ed. Philadelphia: Lippincott Williams & Wilkins, 2004.

Flisiak, R. "High Concentration of Antimitochondrial Antibodies Predicts Progressive Primary Biliary Cirrhosis," *World Journal of Gastroenterology* 11(36):5706-709, September 2005.

Forbes, B., et al. *Bailey and Scott's Diagnostic Microbiology,* 12th ed. St. Louis: Mosby–Year Book, Inc., 2007.

Fujita, N., MD, et al. "Endoscopic Approach to Early Diagnosis of Pancreatic Cancer," *Pancrease* 28(3):279-81, April 2004.

Gilkeson, R.C., and Ciancibello, L. "Virtual Bronchoscopy: Technical Features and Clinical Applications," *Applied Radiology* 32(4), May 2003. *www.medscape.com/viewarticle/452491*

Ilkhanipour, K., et al. "Combining Clinical Risk with D-dimer Testing to Rule Out Deep Vein Thrombosis," *Journal of Emergency Medicine* 27(3):233-39, October 2004.

Kasper, D., et al., eds. *Harrison's Principles of Internal Medicine,* 16th ed. New York: McGraw-Hill Book Co., 2005.

Kwong, R.Y., et al. "Detecting Acute Coronary Syndrome in the Emergency Department with Cardiac Magnetic Resonance Imaging," *Circulation* 107(4):531-37, February 2003.

Lim, D., et al. "Elevated Cardiac Troponin Levels in Critically Ill Patients: Prevalence, Incidence, and Outcomes," *American Journal of Critical Care* 15(3):280-88, May 2006.

*Lippincott Manual of Nursing Practice Series: Diagnostic Tests.* Philadelphia: Lippincott Williams & Wilkins, 2007.

Lynch, T., and Prahash, A. "B-type Natriuretic Peptide: A Diagnostic, Prognostic, and Therapeutic Tool in Heart Failure," *American Journal of Critical Care* 13(1):46-53, January 2004.

Munro, S.C., et al. "Diagnosis of and Screening for Cytomegalovirus Infection in Pregnant Women," *Journal of Clinical Microbiology* 43(9):4713-18, September 2005.

Nettina, S. *Lippincott Manual of Nursing Practice,* 8th ed. Philadelphia: Lippincott Williams & Wilkins, 2006.

Pagana, K.D., and Pagana, T.J. *Mosby's Diagnostic and Laboratory Test Reference,* 7th ed. St. Louis: Mosby–Year Book Inc., 2005.

*Professional Guide to Diagnostic Tests.* Philadelphia: Lippincott Williams & Wilkins, 2005.

Prue-Owens, K.K., LTC. "Use of Peripheral Venous Access Devices for Obtaining Blood Samples for Measurement of Activated Partial Thromboplastin Times," *Critical Care Nurse* 26(1):30-38, February 2006.

Ryan, K.J., and Ray, C.G. *Sherris Medical Microbiology: An Introduction to Infectious Diseases,* 4th ed. Columbus, Ohio: McGraw-Hill Book Co., 2004.

Smith, G.C., et al. "Pregnancy-associated plasm protein A and alpha-fetoprotein and prediction of adverse perinatal outcome," *Obstetrics and Gynecology* 107(1): 161-66, January 2006.

Stonesifer, E. "Common Laboratory and Diagnostic Testing in Patients with Gastrointestinal Disease," *AACN Clinical Issues* 15(4):582-94, October-December 2004.

Turgeon, M. *Clinical Hematology Theory and Procedures,* 4th ed. Philadelphia: Lippincott Williams & Wilkins, 2005.

Ye, W., et al. "*Helicobacter pylori* Infection and Gastric Atrophy: Risk of Adenocarcinoma and Squamous-cell Carcinoma of the Esophagus and Adenocarcinoma of the Gastric Cardia," *Journal of the National Cancer Institute* 96(5):388-96, March 2004.

# Index

i refers to an illustration; t refers to a table.

i refers to an illustration; t refers to a table.

---

i refers to an illustration; t refers to a table.

i refers to an illustration; t refers to a table.

Fluid overload, red blood cell count in, 6
Fluid retention, total hemoglobin in, 18
Fluorescein angiography, 349-351
Fluorescent treponemal antibody absorption, 228-229
Folacin. *See* Folic acid.
Folate. *See* Folic acid.
Folate deficiency, total homocysteine in, 85
Folic acid, 167-168
Folic acid deficiency, white blood cell differential in, 23t
Follicle-stimulating hormone, 100-102
Food or drug sensitivity, white blood cell differential in, 23t
Fractionated erythrocyte porphyrins, 157-158
Fractures
  bone scan in, 415
  calcium in, 53
  paranasal sinus radiography in, 406t
  phosphate in, 57
  skull radiography in, 469
Free cortisol, urine, 254-255
Free thyroxine and free triiodothyronine, 113-114
Fungal serology, 223-225

# G

Galactosemia, phenylalanine screening in, 155
Galactose-1-phosphate uridyltransferase, 82-84
Gallbladder disorders
  alanine aminotransferase in, 69
  alkaline phosphatase in, 70-71
  endoscopic retrograde cholangiopancreatography in, 513
  gallbladder and biliary system ultrasonography in, 528-529
  percutaneous transhepatic cholangiography in, 518
  protein in, 150i
Gallbladder and biliary system ultrasonography, 528-530
Gallium scanning, 626-627
Gamma-glutamyl transferase, 74-75
Gamma-glutamyl transpeptidase. *See* Gamma-glutamyl transferase.
Gangrene, white blood cell count in, 20

Gastrectomy with dumping syndrome
  fasting plasma glucose in, 159
  2-hour postprandial plasma glucose in, 164
Gastric hormones. *See* Pancreatic and gastric hormones.
Gastrin, 128-129
Gastroesophageal reflux scanning, 509
Gastrointestinal bleeding
  colonoscopy in, 497
  fecal occult blood in, 492-493
  sites and causes of, 493i
Gastrointestinal disorders. *See also specific disorder.*
  barium enema in, 506
  barium swallow in, 508
  capsule endoscopy in, 495
  celiac and mesenteric arteriography in, 511
  colonoscopy in, 497
  electrocardiography in, 500
  endoscopic retrograde cholangiopancreatography in, 513-514
  enteroclysis in, 516-517
  fecal lipids in, 491-492
  pancreatic ultrasonography in, 532
  peritoneal fluid analysis in, 488-489
  postoperative cholangiography in, 520
  proctosigmoidoscopy in, 503
  protein in, 150i
  splenic ultrasonography in, 533
  upper gastrointestinal and small-bowel series in, 522
Gastrointestinal system tests, 486-534
Gaucher's disease
  acid phosphatase in, 79
  angiotensin-converting enzyme in, 80
Gene-based test for human immunodeficiency virus, 216
General cellular tests, 182-185
General humoral tests, 185-192
German measles. *See* Rubella antibodies.
Gigantism
  creatinine in, 154
  growth hormone suppression in, 102
  human growth hormone in, 103
Glomerulonephritis
  complement assays in, 185
  creatinine in, 269
  creatinine clearance in, 268
  fibrinogen in, 33
  glucose oxidase in, 278
  immune complex assays in, 188

i refers to an illustration; t refers to a table.

i refers to an illustration; t refers to a table.

---

i refers to an illustration; t refers to a table.

i refers to an illustration; t refers to a table.

---

i refers to an illustration; t refers to a table.

Myocardial infarction
  alanine aminotransferase in, 69-70
  aspartate aminotransferase in, 73
  cholinesterase in, 82
  complement assays in, 186
  C-reactive protein in, 64
  creatine kinase in, 66
  electrocardiography in, 547
  fasting plasma glucose in, 159
  fibrin split products in, 34
  gamma-glutamyl transferase in, 74-75
  lactate in, 166
  lactate dehydrogenase isoenzymes in, 87t
  myoglobin in, 68
  pericardial fluid analysis in, 560
  potassium in, 59
  thallium imaging in, 571
  white blood cell count in, 20, 23t
  zinc in, 173
Myocarditis, lactate dehydrogenase iso-
    enzymes in, 87t
Myoglobin, 67-68
Myxedema
  antithyroid antibodies in, 199
  D-xylose absorption in, 625
  fasting plasma glucose in, 159
  17-hydroxycorticosteroids in, 257
  17-ketosteroids in, 259
  thyroid imaging in, 339t
  2-hour postprandial plasma glucose
    in, 164

## N

Nasopharyngeal culture, 324-326
  obtaining specimen for, 326i
Nearsightedness, 344, 345i
Neonatal thyroid-stimulating hormone,
    107-108
Nephrotic syndrome
  aldosterone in, 120
  alpha$_1$-antitrypsin in, 72
  fasting plasma glucose in, 159
  immunoglobulins in, 190t
  lysozyme in, 251
  phospholipids in, 140
  thyroxine-binding globulin in, 117
  total cholesterol in, 141
  triglycerides in, 142
  2-hour postprandial plasma glucose
    in, 164
  urinalysis in, 244

Nephrotomography, 592-594
  differential diagnosis in, 593t
Nerve conduction studies, 482
Nervous system tests, 458-485
Neural tube defects, alpha-fetoprotein in, 231
Neutrophil function tests, 183
Nitroblue tetrazolium test, 183
Nucleic acid test, 216
5?-nucleotidase, 76-77

## O

Obstetric complications. See also specific
    complication.
  amniotic fluid analysis in, 424-425
  amylase in, 77
  fibrinogen in, 33
  fibrin split products in, 34
  magnesium in, 56
  pelvic ultrasonography in, 455
  pregnanediol in, 262
  protein in, 150i
  urinalysis in, 240
Occlusive impedance phlebography. See
    Impedance plethysmography.
Ocular ultrasonography, 357-358
One-stage factor assay
  extrinsic coagulation system, 36-37
  intrinsic coagulation system, 37-38
Ophthalmoscopy, 351-352
Oral glucose tolerance, 161-162
Oral lactose tolerance, 162-163
OraQuick rapid human immunodeficiency
    virus-1 antibody test, 216
Orbital computed tomography, 359-360
Orbital radiography, 360-361
Organophosphate insecticide poisoning,
    cholinesterase in, 81-82
Organ transplant rejection
  fibrin split products in, 34
  lysozyme in, 251
  renin activity in, 92
  urinalysis in, 243
Osmotic fragility, 4-5
Osteomalacia
  alkaline phosphatase in, 71
  calcium in, 53
  calcium and phosphates in, 284t
Otoscopy, 367-369
Ovarian biopsy, 297t
Ovarian cysts, progesterone in, 135

i refers to an illustration; t refers to a table.

i refers to an illustration; t refers to a table.

---

i refers to an illustration; t refers to a table.

i refers to an illustration; t refers to a table.

---

i refers to an illustration; t refers to a table.